Medication Safety in Look-Alike Sound-Alike (LASA) Drugs

Teeraporn Sadira Supapaan
https://orcid.org/0000-0002-6887-8181
Ubon Ratchathani University, Thailand

IGI Global
Scientific Publishing
Publishing Tomorrow's Research Today

Vice President of Editorial	Melissa Wagner
Director of Acquisitions	Mikaela Felty
Director of Book Development	Jocelynn Hessler
Production Manager	Mike Brehm
Cover Design	Jose Rosado

Published in the United States of America by
IGI Global Scientific Publishing
701 East Chocolate Avenue
Hershey, PA, 17033, USA
Tel: 717-533-8845 | Fax: 717-533-7115
Website: https://www.igi-global.com E-mail: cust@igi-global.com

Library of Congress Cataloging-in-Publication Data

LCCN: 2025042365 (CIP Data Pending)
ISBN13: 979-8-3373-5478-1
Isbn13Softcover: 979-8-3373-5479-8
EISBN13: 979-8-3373-5480-4
British Cataloguing in Publication Data
A Cataloguing in Publication record for this book is available from the British Library.

Table of Contents

Preface

Medicines prevent illness, alleviate symptoms, manage chronic conditions, assist with complicated procedures, and save lives. However, each step of the medication-use process also opens up chances of error. Look-alike, sound-alike medication errors, also known as LASA medication errors, are some of the most frequent and avoidable. These mistakes happen when a certain medicine is mixed up with another due to similarities of name, pronunciation, packaging, labeling, dosage forms, colors, shapes, strength, concentrations, or the appearance of the medicine in general. Misunderstanding can occur in the prescribing, transcribing, dispensing, preparing, storing, administering, monitoring, or self-administration of medication by a patient. LASA errors thus do not occur in only a single profession, healthcare setting, or single point on the medication-use pathway.

LASA medication errors have been recognized for a long time. However, they continue to pose significant patient safety issues worldwide. They continue to present significant patient safety issues worldwide. They remain among the most significant patient safety issues worldwide. They are usually estimated to contribute 6–15% of reported medication errors and can lead to temporary delays in treatment, minor adverse effects, hospitalization, irreversible harm, and even death. The harm can occur in two ways simultaneously: the patient can receive an unintended medication, and the needed medication to treat the actual illness is either withheld or delayed. This risk is particularly severe when there is confusion with high-alert medications, pharmaceuticals with narrow therapeutic indices, injectable drugs, chemotherapy, insulin, opioids, neuromuscular blockers, concentrated electrolytes, vaccines, or drugs used in frail populations.

In some cases, LASA errors have been defined as deficits in individual attention. This definition is not a complete explanation. The wrong medicine can be chosen, prepared, dispensed, or even administered by a healthcare professional, who may, in turn, be the cause of the circumstances under which the mistake could occur; however, often, the system creates such circumstances. There is a possibility of having similar names in the market without proper differentiation. Packages can have almost the same color, font, image, or container designs. Multiple strengths may be placed next to one another. Electronic systems can show similar spellings next to each other or cut off names in a manner that eliminates differentiating information. Repackaging can destroy original identifiers. Interruptions, exhaustion, time constraints, staffing constraints, insufficient lighting, communication breakdown, and excessive workloads can then transform an already similar situation into a real error. Systems thinking rather than individual blame must be the foundation of the prevention of LASA harm.

Digital transformation has not completely eradicated LASA errors; instead, they have evolved. The search functions can identify a few similar names with a few letters typed. Confusing medicines might be placed adjacent to each other in drop-down menus. Dispensing machines can be automated and store items in adjacent spaces. Electronic medication lists can skip the visual information that would otherwise assist users in differentiating between one product and another. Over-warnings can be a source of alert fatigue, making even the well-intended safety messages less valuable. At the same time, digital tools offer important ways to prevent problems by using computer programs to check names, support clinical decisions, verify barcodes, show product images, use artificial intelligence, recognize text, identify pills, and connect medication databases. The key question is not only the presence of the use of technology but also its design, testing, and implementation based on medication-safety principles and human-factor engineering.

The Medication Without Harm program by the World Health Organization aims to reduce avoidable and severe harmful events related to medication. The direct impact of this priority on LASA medication errors is that they are predictable, systematic, and often preventable. They must be prevented by a concerted effort on the part of regulatory agencies, pharmaceutical firms, health facilities, health care workers, information-technology creators, educators, researchers, patients, and caregivers. No one intervention will suffice. Unsafe packaging cannot be made up of tall man letters. In case of missing, faulty, or circumvented barcodes, patients are not safeguarded by barcode verification. Systems that show electronic alerts cannot prevent errors caused by systems producing too many warnings that clinicians ignore. Confusion generated by the fundamentally unsafe names of products or almost similar containers cannot Education alone cannot fully resolve the confusion caused by the fundamentally unsafe names of products or nearly identical containers. by education in full. Prevention should be multi-layered and carried out throughout the entire lifetime of medicine.

This book was formulated in an effort to fill a research gap in the literature of medication safety. Current sources tend to focus on various individual components of LASA errors, including misidentified drug names, individual incidence reports, packaging, or preventive measures chosen. This book is aimed at relating these dimensions and demonstrating how evidence can be converted into prevention action plans. It is based on the main assumption that LASA errors are not isolated occurrences. They are a consequence of familiar product similarity, vulnerability of the system, human cognition, and environmental conditions, and such combinations can be detected and controlled.

The book is based on the international evidence and original research and practical experience in Thailand. The national survey that underlies some of this work reported over 2,510 reported pairs of LASA drugs in dosage forms and levels of healthcare. This fact proves that LASA risk is not confined to a few well-known international cases. Naming confusion can be among generic names, trade names, varying strengths of the same drug, the products of the same manufacturer, or the drugs of different therapeutic action but similar appearance. The Thai setting also exemplifies issues that are common to most healthcare systems, such as repackaging, incomplete labeling, lack of use of standardized identifiers, use of multilingual drug names, disjointed medicine records, and distribution of unnamed or poorly labeled products. Though the examples have a basis in Thailand, the principles and preventive frameworks can be applied on an international scale.

The target audience is multidisciplinary. Practical guidance on how clinical pharmacists, hospital pharmacists, community pharmacists, physicians, nurses, pharmacy technicians, and other healthcare professionals can identify and manage LASA risks during the medication-use process will be beneficial. The frameworks and examples can be used by medication-safety officers, risk managers, quality-improvement personnel, hospital administrators, and accreditation teams to evaluate institutional vulnerabilities and focus on interventions. The discussions about drug naming, packaging, labeling, product differentiation, and postmarket surveillance can be used by regulators and pharmaceutical manufacturers to enhance the safety of products before and after being introduced to the market.

Pharmacy, medical, nursing, and public-health educators are also targeted in the book to have an organized resource to teach medication safety. The chapters can be used by undergraduate and postgraduate students to relate theory to clinical practice. Conceptual frameworks, examples of surveillance strategies, and areas that need to be developed further will be available to the researchers. The electronic prescribing, barcode verification, artificial intelligence, and drug-identification systems can be discussed to benefit health-information-technology professionals. Patients and caregivers can also learn why identifying medicines with care is important, why it is important to label them clearly and have current medication lists, and why asking about the name, purpose, strength, and appearance of a medicine is encouraged as a type of safe care.

The book is divided into 12 chapters. The initial six chapters lay the conceptual, preventive, technological, design, nomenclature, and specialized clinical underpinnings of LASA medication safety. The following six chapters discuss the implications of LASA errors and unique risks of dietary supplements, oral liquids, vaccines, and injectable medicines. The chapters have been combined to create the progression between the knowledge of the problem and the prevention design and the widely applicable principles and specific high-risk product types and the tools that can be implemented.

CHAPTER OVERVIEW

Chapter 1, Introduction to the Look-Alike, Sound-Alike Medication Errors. It introduces the concept of LASA medication errors and how the similarity of names, labels, packaging, and appearance can result in prescribing, dispensing, and administration mistakes. The chapter places LASA errors in the context of the wider area of medication safety and highlights that its impact is frequently underestimated. It further elaborates why the risks of LASA remain common in digital health technologies and organized medication-management systems, even as improvements are made to enhance safety. The chapter presents the necessity of regulatory, technological, organizational, and professional reaction to the issue by connecting the problem with the Medication Without Harm initiative of the World Health Organization. It is significant as it offers a common multidisciplinary framework by which clinicians, policymakers, educators, and researchers can comprehend LASA-related harm and how this necessitates coordinated prevention.

Chapter 2, Integrated Strategies to Prevent Look-Alike Sound-Alike (LASA) Medication Errors, shifts from definition to prevention. It offers a multifaceted approach that integrates regulatory protection, technological protection, professional practice, and patient involvement. Regulators and manufacturers can minimize risk prior to the arrival of medicines in the market by using name-screening algorithms, differentiated packaging, proper labeling, and other product-design controls. Electronic prescribing alerts, barcode checks, coordinated checkups, and standardized procedures are extra layers of protection within the healthcare organizations. In addition to institutional environments, self-use errors can be avoided by using clear labels, mobile applications, health-literacy interventions, and patient education. The significance of the chapter is that it shows that LASA prevention should be ongoing up to the product development, clinical application, and follow-up of patients where the responsibility belongs to the regulators, manufacturers, healthcare professionals, and patients.

Chapter 3, Challenges in Drug Identification and LASA Errors, discusses a fundamental safety issue: How can original information concerning a medicine be identified correctly when it is missing, incompletely known, or unintelligible?

The chapter discusses the issues of identification in the clinical and community contexts, including similarity by appearance, labeling constraints, and a lack of uniform identifiers. These problems are especially noticeable in cases of repacking medicines, their separation from their original containers, or their supply without proper labeling. The case of Yaa Chud in Thailand demonstrates the additional dangers that arise when multiple drugs are prescribed without sufficient information. Yaa Chud's case in Thailand illustrates the heightened risks associated with prescribing multiple drugs without sufficient information. alongside scanty information. The chapter examines the imprint codes, packaging features, traditional identification resources, and artificial-intelligence-based tools, with a concurrent acknowledgment of their weaknesses in the real world. It is significant in that it demonstrates that dependable identification is a requirement in preventing LASA errors and that technological solutions should be combined with professional verification and extended system support.

Chapter 4, Addressing LASA Medication Errors with Better Drug Packaging and Labeling, introduces the idea of packaging and labeling as proactive safety-promoting systems rather than a container or advertising tool. It looks at typography, color coding, Tallman lettering, barcode validation, trade dress, and other design components with respect to human-factor engineering. Cases of ophthalmic, pediatric, anesthetic, and injectable products demonstrate the impact of visual design in facilitating quick differentiation or causing cognitive overload. Regulatory frameworks and international standards and recommendations of various organizations, including the FDA, WHO, MHRA, ISO, and ADA, are also considered in the chapter. It is important because it shifts individual healthcare professionals' vigilance from product differentiation to product design. Once the packaging and labeling are designed to expose critical differences, they become preventive barriers that facilitate safer selection, preparation, dispensing, and administration.

Chapter 5, Look-Alike, Sound-Alike Medication Errors Caused by Drug Names, orthographic and phonetic similarities are discussed. The names of the drugs should be able to operate in crowded national and global markets, but similar names in spelling or pronunciation might be mixed in oral communication, translation of handwriting, computerized choice, or recalling the names by memory. The chapter summarizes the causes and clinical outcomes of name confusion and addresses severe cases of morphine and hydromorphone and vinblastine and vincristine. It contrasts regulations in the United States, Canada, the United Kingdom, Thailand, and the World Health Organization and shows how standardized naming conventions and systematic name screening can mitigate risk. The chapter also considers hospital measures like tall man lettering, electronic alerts, and clinician education. The significance of the chapter is that risks associated with names are best addressed in a proactive way before they become common in the market, and they are always monitored and mitigated in the clinical practice.

Chapter 6, Look-Alike, Sound-Alike (LASA) Risks in Oncology Pharmacies, implements the overall LASA model is implemented in one of the most complicated and dangerous medication settings. Oncology care is typified by high rates of therapeutic innovation, diversified formularies, narrow therapeutic index, high toxicity, complicated protocols, and stages of prescribing, verifying, preparing, and administering drugs or therapies. The misunderstanding of similar medicines in this case can have especially severe outcomes. The chapter demonstrates that LASA risk does not exist in one generation of cancer treatment or one type of medicine; it is present as the drug-naming conventions, treatment practices, and clinical workflows change. Its significance is that oncology medication safety must be constantly re-evaluated with specialized professional knowledge, tightly checked by verification, and systems that can be adjusted to new therapies without repeating the patterns of misunderstanding in the past.

Chapter 7, Clinical Consequences of Look-Alike, Sound-Alike Medication Errors, discusses the clinical outcomes of LASA vulnerabilities affecting patients. It discusses a spectrum of outcomes based on real-world cases and patient-safety reports, which include treatment failure, mild adverse effects, hospitalization, irreversible harm, and death. The chapter notes that injury can result from both using the wrong medicine and not getting the needed treatment for the underlying condition. Medications with a narrow therapeutic index and high-alert medicines are particularly critical since even minor selection or dosing errors can quickly escalate to severe outcomes. The NCC MERP Index will enable an organized method of understanding the magnitude of medication errors and assist in risk-based reactions. The chapter also acknowledges the psychological and organizational implications of clinical injury other than direct clinical injury. It is significant because it increases the visibility of the LASA errors' burden and shows the necessity of considering the near misses and the less critical incidents as the warning signs of the system's vulnerability instead of ignoring them.

Chapter 8, Look-Alike, Sound-Alike in Dietary Supplements, the LASA medication safety principles are applied to non-traditional pharmaceutical products. Dietary supplements and herbal products are commonly consumed, frequently used in combination with prescription drugs, and are possibly chosen as direct consumer products. They can be introduced in the market rather than medicines that undergo premarket screening to determine similarity in names, indications, packaging, or graphic design. Marketing-driven similarities can cause consumers to select the wrong product, misinterpret its designation, or substitute a supplement for evidence-based therapy. Marketing can lead to consumers choosing the incorrect product, misinterpreting its designation, or replacing a supplement with evidence-based therapy. The chapter explores regulatory loopholes, real-life examples of similarity in the packaging of herbal products in hospitals, and the functions of pharmacists and patient education. Notably, medication-safety systems should consider the overall marketplace where patients are exposed to medicines, supplements, traditional products, and health claims, rather than focusing LASA surveillance on prescription drugs.

Chapter 9, Oral Liquid Medications and LASA Errors, is devoted to the preparations, which are vital in the case of pediatric patients, the elderly, and individuals with swallowing problems. The presence of oral liquids poses unique risks as bottles, labels, colors, flavors, and concentrations might be similar, and proper use also relies on dosing and administration by the caregivers. The chapter combines foreign evidence with Thai epidemiological reports and data demonstrating that oral-liquid LASA pairs constitute 3.39 percent of all LASA pairs in the national database and that packaging similarity is the most common mechanism of action. Vulnerabilities in prescribing, dispensing, measurement, and administration are analyzed using examples of generic-name oral liquids. This chapter is significant since oral liquids might seem less dangerous than injectable or oncology products, but an error in product choice that can be overshadowed by the concentration differences, vulnerability of children, and the need to take doses with the help of a caregiver can cause severe harm.

Chapter 10, Monograph of Look-Alike, Sound-Alike (LASA) Drugs Reported in Thailand (Oral Liquid Preparation), transforms the results of surveillance into a format of a structured risk-management tool. The chapter, with oral-liquid illustrations, presents a standard, component-based LASA drug monograph based on evidence provided in a national survey of Thailand. The framework integrates data on drug identification, similarity mechanisms, NCC MERP severity, and resources on safety and practical prevention. It is valuable not just in relation to the individual products mentioned since the approach can be tailored by hospitals to their respective formularies, incident reports, and high-risk medicine lists. What is significant about the chapter is that it serves as a tool of implementation: it illustrates how a list of reported LASA pairs can be converted to agreed-upon guidance to be used in prioritization, storage, labeling, information-system warning, professional communication, patient counseling, and continued review.

Chapter 11, Introduction to Look-Alike, Sound-Alike Medication Errors in Vaccines, discusses the LASA risk of vaccination systems in the Introduction to Look-Alike, Sound-Alike Medication Errors in Vaccines. Mistakes in vaccination can also occur because of the similarity of names, labels, packing, formulations, or storage facilities and can result in the wrong choice, preparation, or administration of vaccines. This chapter is based on surveillance databases, epidemiological studies, and published research, especially in the areas of pediatric, neonatal, and high-throughput vaccination. The aftermath is not limited to a single clinical incident: a mistake can lead to insufficient immunological coverage, severe adverse effects, repeated vaccinations, and a lack of trust in immunization campaigns. It is thus the concerted effort by manufacturers, healthcare organizations, clinicians, and patients who is needed to prevent these issues. The significance of this chapter is that it shows that vaccine safety is not only determined by the quality of products and the cold chain but also dependable differentiation during storage, preparation, and administration.

Chapter 12, Look-Alike, Sound-Alike Medication Errors in Injectable Drugs, discusses one of the most at-risk groups regarding medication safety. Injectable drugs are able to induce quick systemic responses and may commonly have limited recovery margins once utilized. The neuromuscular blockers, insulin, vasopressors, opioids, and concentrated electrolytes are examples that demonstrate which classes are associated with confusion that may result in serious damage to patients. The chapter examines typical drug combinations, contributing factors, regulatory interventions, systemic preventive interventions, and human-factor-based interventions. It is significant because it demonstrates that safe injectable use cannot be achieved without coordinated controls in manufacturing, procurement, storage, dispensing, preparation, and administration and especially in high-acuity settings where there is the most time pressure and where the effects of error are the most severe.

The twelve chapters reveal that LASA medication errors are not single incidents but system-wide issues that occur due to the drug nomenclature, product design, technology, communication, storage, and human cognition. A drug could be produced properly and be pharmacologically active, but it could be unsatisfactorily safe because its name, packaging, label, or concentration could be confused with another medicine. The quality of medication should thus encompass not only the purity, potency, and stability but also the ability to easily identify and distinguish medicines in their life cycle.

This book is a contribution to the field because it incorporates regulatory, clinical, technological, educational, and patient-centered views. It relates international evidence on medication safety to the experience in Thailand and other healthcare systems with comparable issues. The book expands the knowledge of LASA risk by covering drug identification, artificial intelligence, packaging and labeling, drug nomenclature, oncology, dietary supplements, oral liquids, vaccines, and injectable medicines. The monograph framework that is standardized also illustrates how findings of surveillance can be converted into practical institutional recommendations.

The detection of a perplexing drug similarity is just the first step. Healthcare organizations should decide on actions, participants, risk priorities, and preventive measures. These involve the scrutiny of the incidents and near misses, evaluation of new formulary products, enhancement of storage and labels, setting up of electronic alerts, training of health care professionals, and patient counseling as well as reevaluation of the risks in case of product or system changes. The proactive method aims to identify similarities prior to any damage being caused by conducting name screening, visual screening, usability testing, artificial-intelligence-based identification, and a structured review of new medicines. Near misses are thus beneficial learning and preventive opportunities.

Other partners in medication safety are patients and caregivers. They are expected to be educated about the names, uses, strong points, and appearance of their medicines; have updated medication lists; store medicines in clearly labeled containers; use the correct measuring devices; and raise questions when a product has a different appearance. Their involvement does not substitute professional, organizational, manufacturer, or regulatory responsibility but is an extra protection against errors.

This book highlights that all LASA-related errors result in avoidable damage. The damage could have been avoided. Prevention does not mean we can avoid all risks or that every incident is due to negligence. Instead, it is learning through repetitive patterns and developing systems where the right medicine is easier to locate, prescribe, order, prepare, dispense, administer, and monitor. The roles of regulators, manufacturers, healthcare organizations, professionals, technology developers, educators, patients, and caregivers are important and complementary.

The final objective of this book is to make research returns into safer medication practices and awareness into long-term action. Hopefully, evidence, cases, structures, and recommendations provided in these chapters can assist the reader to identify the weak points and introduce preventive measures that are relevant in their respective environments. Simply because a medicine resembles another medicine, it should not do harm.

My belief in this book is that when a LASA medication error is committed in one hospital, the same (or a similar) mistake can be made in another hospital where there are similar conditions. Nevertheless, the institution where medication events occur can still retain valuable insights. Other healthcare organizations might thus remain unaware of the same vulnerability until a similar incident occurs again. The respectful sharing of these lessons can turn a single case into a more general preventive opportunity.

This is why I have tried to find evidence of real cases and experiences of medication safety in Thailand and integrate these findings with international evidence and recommendations. I hope that by reading this book, pharmacists, other healthcare professionals, educators, students, and healthcare organizations, as well as policymakers, will be able to note LASA risks to ensure that patients are not harmed. I also hope it will inspire institutions to share with each other and to enhance medication systems with a collective, positive, and non-accusing commitment to patient safety.

Acknowledgement

In the name of God, the Most Gracious, the Most Merciful.

The author would like to express her deepest gratitude to her professor, Professor Claire Anderson, whose leadership, dedication, and contributions to pharmacy education, workforce development, and professional practice have been a continuing source of inspiration. The author is sincerely grateful for her example, which encouraged and inspired the development of this book.

The author also wishes to express profound respect and sincere appreciation to Professor Michael R. Cohen for his lifelong dedication to medication safety. His pioneering work has greatly advanced the understanding that medication errors should not be viewed solely as individual failures, but also as consequences of weaknesses within healthcare systems. His scholarship, leadership, and commitment to preventing medication-related harm have deeply influenced the author's work and provided important inspiration for this book.

The author is sincerely grateful to Assoc. Prof. Dr. Payom Wongpoowarak, Assoc. Prof. Wibul Wongpoowarak, Assoc. Prof. Dr. Thida Ningsanond, and Assoc. Prof. Dr. Bancha Yingngam for their valuable guidance, thoughtful suggestions, kindness, and continued support throughout the development of this book. Appreciation is also extended to the Faculty of Pharmaceutical Sciences, Ubon Ratchathani University, Ubon Ratchathani, Thailand, for providing an academic environment that supports research and innovation.

The author would like to thank her advisors and mentors—Assoc. Prof. Sakchai Ausayakhun, Assoc. Prof. Siriwan Suttajit, Prof. Dr. Jiradej Manosroi, Prof. Dr. Aranya Manosroi, Prof. Bungorn Sripanidkulchai, Assoc. Prof. Chutinun Prasitpuripreecha, Assoc. Prof. Warisada Sila-On, Assoc. Prof. Bee Yean Low, Assoc.Prof. Summana Moolasarn, and Assoc. Prof. Aporanee Chaiyakum—for their kindness and invaluable support throughout her academic journey.

The author would also like to acknowledge Dr. Jintana Napaporn, Assoc. Prof. Dr. Chonladda Pitchayajittipong, Asst. Prof. Peerawat Jinatongthai, Asst. Prof. Dr. Nonglek Kunawaradisai, Dr. Saksit Sripa, Dr. Narongchai Chaksupa, Dr. Suttasinee Suwannakul, Ms. Phantiwa Namboon, and Mr. Natthawut Banrueangthong for their valuable support and contributions.

Sincere appreciation is extended to all students, colleagues, and alumni who have participated in and supported research on look-alike, sound-alike medications in Thailand. Their dedication, collaboration, and academic efforts have greatly enriched this field and contributed meaningfully to the body of knowledge presented in this book.

The author is also grateful to all pharmacists who generously shared their knowledge, practical experience, and insights regarding look-alike, sound-alike (LASA) medications. Their contributions have been invaluable to the development of this work and to the advancement of LASA-related research in Thailand. Special thanks are extended to Mr. Peerapat Singkan, Mr. Jakkrit Busapan, Dr. Wannaporn Wattanawong, Ms. Ananya Songmuang, and Mr. Thanatcha Songmuang for their expertise and support.

Finally, the author offers heartfelt thanks to her family for their love, patience, encouragement, and unwavering support, and to everyone who has contributed, directly or indirectly, to this work and to the shared goal of improving medication safety. This book would not have been possible without their kindness, generosity, and support.

Chapter 1
Introduction to Look-Alike, Sound-Alike Medication Errors

ABSTRACT

Medicine safety is vital to the provision of high-quality healthcare and yet, look-alike, sound-alike (LASA) medication errors continue to pose an enormous and often underestimated challenge within the clinical environment. Same names, same labels and same packaging may be dangerous leading to errors in prescription, dispensing and administration. LASA errors continue to experience an outsized proportion of medication mishaps over the globe, such as digital health technologies and structured medication management systems. The WHO campaign of medication without harm is supported by regulatory, technological, and system-level strategies. The chapter aims to present the multidisciplinary framework of LASA-related harm that can be used to prevent and reduce it in clinical practice informed by healthcare professionals, policymakers, and researchers.

INTRODUCTION

Medications are foundational to modern healthcare, enabling the prevention, treatment, and management of a wide range of clinical conditions (Sakai & Morimoto, 2022). With the continuous expansion of global pharmacopeia, the diversity of available formulations and brands has grown exponentially. This diversity, however, presents a significant safety challenge: medication errors related to look-alike, sound-alike (LASA) drugs (Cohen, 2006; Cohen & Smetzer, 2007; Tariq et al., 2021). These errors occur when medications with similar names, labels, or packages are

DOI: 10.4018/979-8-3373-5478-1.ch001

confused at various stages of the medication use process, including prescribing, transcribing, dispensing, and administering (Ostini et al., 2012).

Although LASA drugs constitute a small percentage of all prescriptions, they account for a disproportionately high volume of medication error reports. According to international reviews, six to fifteen percent of all medication errors reported are attributed to LASA confusion, although these medications make up less than 0.01 percent of the pharmaceutical market by volume (Lambert et al., 2019; The Institute for Safe Medication Practices (ISMP), 2023a, 2024). These are not mere accidents: confusion between similar drugs or labels has caused serious adverse drug events, such as overdose, treatment failure, and even death, particularly in high-risk medications, including insulin, chemotherapy agents, and anesthetics (Cohen, Domizio, et al., 2007; Cohen & Smetzer, 2017; The Institute for Safe Medication Practices (ISMP), 2011, 2015).

The seriousness of this problem was acknowledged by the World Health Organization (WHO), which in 2017 introduced its global challenge, medication without harm, to decrease severe preventable medication-related harm by half (World Health Organization, 2017). The WHO (2023) has identified LASA errors as critical intervention targets in their technical report and has provided a comprehensive list of recommendations (World Health Organization, 2023). These are the introduction of national LASA medication lists, the introduction of tall man lettering to highlight specific components of drug names, and the introduction of clear high-contrast labeling and packaging conventions.

Health systems are also advised to integrate electronic prescriptions, barcode medication administration (BCMA), and clinical decision support software into a harmonized safety framework (World Health Organization, 2023). The persistence of LASA errors across regions and care settings implies that structural and cognitive influences still occur even when safeguards are soundly designed. The contributing factors are name similarity, visual packaging similarity, cluttered electronic order entry systems and time pressure during clinical decision-making. When digital interfaces sort drug names alphabetically or default to abbreviated terms, prescribers and pharmacists are more likely to choose the wrong product. Most of these lessons can be learned through pharmaceutical error reporting and assessment. Large LASA error case compilations have demonstrated trends across countries and care settings, indicating the need to collaborate and standardize international cooperation to achieve long-term improvement. Labeling formats and naming conventions are different and are jurisdiction specific, but the potential dangers of sound or appearance similarity do not differ. WHO guidance, peer-reviewed literature, and real-world case studies inform this interdisciplinary study of LASA medication errors. The structural origins of LASA risk, regulator-based and clinical system redesign-based LASA prevention strategies, and emergent medication safety technology are explored. The framework provided in the chapter can enable healthcare professionals, policy makers, and researchers to learn how to achieve this level of LASA medication error reduction.

Objectives of the Chapter

The aims of this chapter are as follows:

(1) To briefly describe LASA concerns and the history of medication errors.
(2) To define LASA errors and explain the terminology of the chapter.
(3) To categorize LASA mistakes by name, by packaging, and by appearance confusion and state their reasons.
(4) To summarize the clinical error prevalence data for LASA
(5) To review the WHO and ISMP-directed international response policies and strategies to limit LASA mistakes.
(6) To examine global and regional LASA drug error regulatory landscapes and reporting patterns.
(7) To assess regulatory and technological LASA error prevention strategies and propose integrated improvements.

Organization of the Chapter

Chapter 1 starts with a brief chronicle of the history of medication errors, including milestone moments that transformed patient safety thinking. It then characterizes LASA errors and ascribes the reason they pose unique risks at every stage of medication use. The narrative next describes the three main LASA error types: name confusion, packaging confusion, and appearance confusion. This background justifies the examination of drug pairs and groups that are particularly likely to mix and is shown with the World Health Organization actions that have led to the global safety of LASA. The existing prevalence statistics provide grounds for comparing international guidelines and joint efforts with the problems and successes of regions. In this context, prevention strategies that span policy measures, human factor principles, and technologies such as electronic prescribing, barcode verification, and emerging machine learning tools are reviewed. Examples of visual illustrations and cases help explain in detail how these interventions can be applied to the real world. The chapter ends with a conclusion on generative insights and possible future directions of integrated safety efforts, policy-making, and cross-sector cooperation to minimize LASA-related harm.

A BRIEF HISTORY OF MEDICATION ERRORS

The World Health Organization (WHO) estimates that in the United States, medication errors result in at least one fatality daily and injure approximately 1.3 million individuals annually (Rodziewicz et al., 2023). Although not all of these mistakes can be avoided worldwide, they are among the main sources of unnecessary harm to one in ten patients in wealthier countries and to 2.6 million deaths annually in poorer countries. Despite advancements in healthcare, overcoming these costly mistakes is still a vulnerability of the system since it is expected to contribute only to the total cost of up to two trillion U.S. dollars to society (World Health Organization, 2021). Medical errors remain a significant public health issue and a leading cause of death (Tariq et al., 2021).

The National Coordinating Council for Medication Error and Prevention (NCC MERP) defines a medication error as any preventable event that may cause or lead to inappropriate medication use or patient harm while healthcare professionals, patients, or consumers control the medication. Prescription, order communication, product labeling, packaging, nomenclature, compounding, dispensing, distribution, administration, education, monitoring, and use are relevant to such events (National Coordinating Council for Medication Error Reporting and Prevention (NCC MERP), 2022).

From prescribing to patient delivery, medication provision is complicated and prone to errors. Medication errors are caused by prescribing errors, dose miscalculations, poor drug distribution, drug- and device-related issues, incorrect drug administration, poor communication, and a lack of patient education. The number of patient deaths due to drug errors increased from 198,000 in 1995 to 218,000 in 2000. Over $177 billion is lost because of these errors (The Academy of Managed Care Pharmacy (AMCP), 2019).

Owing to improper use of prescription and medication ordering systems, preventable errors occur. Illegible handwritten prescriptions, insufficient coprescribed medication information, lab values, and allergic sensitivities can cause errors. Prescription errors can result from choosing the wrong drug or dose or a complicated regimen. Sound-alike names can cause errors when read aloud, whereas similar-looking names can cause errors when handwritten (Tariq et al., 2021; Wheeler et al., 2018).

Dispensing errors can be commission (e.g., dispensing the wrong drug or dose) or omission (e.g., failing to counsel the patient or screen for interactions). These errors can be potential, detected, and corrected before the patient is reached or when the patient is reached or when they can reach the patient and cause harm (Ibrahim et al., 2020; Tariq et al., 2021).

Errors in drug administration can be made by healthcare providers or patients themselves. Communication issues are a significant factor, with patients often unaware of the potential for errors and not fully understanding the information provided to them. Frequently, drug names, appearances, dosages, administration schedules, side effects, interactions, and whether a new drug replaces or supplements other therapy are miscommunicated. Over-the-counter medications may be misread, or healthcare providers may not know they are being used (Samaranayake et al., 2014; Tariq et al., 2021).

DEFINING LASA ERRORS

Healthcare providers make LASA errors when they mix medications with similar names or appearances. These errors can cause harmless or life-threatening consequences, depending on the medications and healthcare scenario. The names of LASA drugs may be similar because of spelling or phonetics. These errors can result from confusing brand names and generic names, two brand names, or two generic names. LASA errors can also result from drug shape, color, packaging, and labeling similarities. The selection of a medication by a shelf or electronic list can be erroneous during the prescribing, dispensing or administration process (Bryan et al., 2015; Bryan et al., 2021b; Cohen, 2007; Cohen, Domizio, et al., 2007; Wongboonnak P, 2018). ISMP Medication Safety Alert enumerates numerous look-alike and sound-alike names of medications in error. The scenarios below involving the names of two similar sounding medications illustrate the issue and the means to prevent them (Cohen, Domizio, et al., 2007).

Bryan et al. reported that LASA drug medication errors can occur at any point in the treatment pathway and can lead to overdosing, underdosing, or inappropriate dosing, putting patient safety at risk. Interventions to reduce LASA errors include typographic changes such as tall-man lettering, barcoding, computerized physician order entry, and indication alerts. These strategies aim to reduce the risk of confusion and improve patient safety by making similar drug names more distinguishable (Bryan et al., 2021a). In conclusion, LASA medication errors constitute a significant healthcare problem because of the confusion of drug names and appearance. Interventions and technological solutions are needed to minimize such errors and enhance medication safety.

TYPE OF LASA ERRORS

LASA medication errors are caused by three fundamental factors: confusion of names, similarity of packaging, and similarity of appearance. These risks overlap and may be visualized as iceberg layers (Figure 1). The tiny tip above the surface is a reflection of wrong-drug events, which clinicians note and report, and the large mass under the surface illustrates the hidden dangers in everyday practice, such as the same cap color on the same vials, new names beginning with the same syllable, or cartons with a thin accent stripe (The Institute for Safe Medication Practices (ISMP), 2015; The Institute for Safe Medication Practices Canada (ISMP Canada), 2016; The Pennsylvania Patient Safety Advisory, 2004).

The latest evidence from Thailand highlights the frequency of the overlap of these three factors. A recent national survey of 128 hospitals revealed 2,510 LASA drug pairs; 2/3 of these pairs were tablets or capsules, and 66.7% of the similarities reported were due to drug-name similarity (Supapaan et al., 2024). A 200-bed general hospital follow-up case study revealed 46 confirmed pairs of LASA; 64.6% of the cases were associated with similar names, 24.6% with look-alike packaging, and 10.8% with a near-identical appearance (Supapaan TS, Songmuang A, et al., 2024). The pharmacists interviewed in that study emphasized that heavy workloads made it easy to rely on memory rather than barcode scans or tall man lettering, allowing multiple risks to combine.

Knowing which root cause is in play can guide the choice of preventive measures. Name-driven errors respond to tall man lettering, read-back procedures, and split electronic pick lists. Packaging similarity calls for barcode verification, segregated storage bins, and bold shelf signage. The appearance overlap benefits from color zoning, auxiliary stickers, and an independent double check at the bedside. Matching defenses to the underlying mechanism helps institutions move toward the World Health Organization goal of reducing serious, avoidable medication harm by 50% before 2030 (World Health Organization, 2022, 2023).

Figure 1. Iceberg model of LASA errors

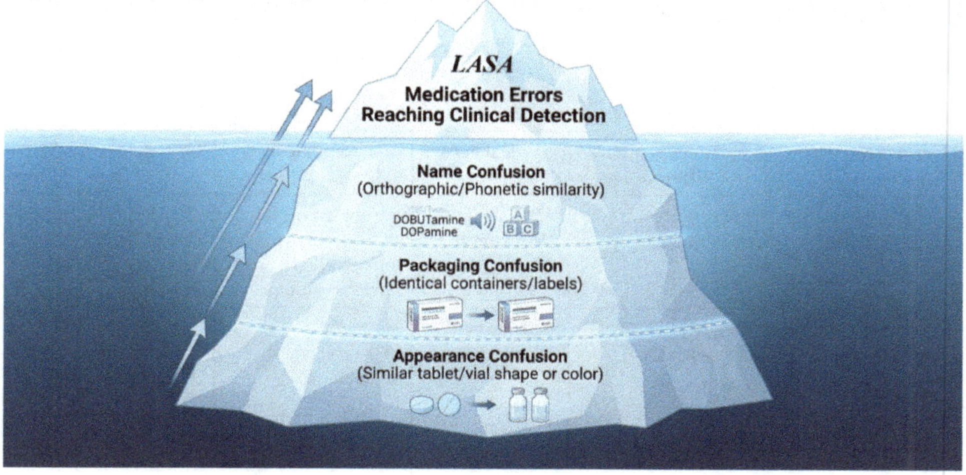

The visible "tip" represents medication errors that reach clinical detection, whereas the submerged tiers illustrate three root-cause domains—name confusion (orthographic or phonetic similarity), packaging confusion (nearly identical containers or labels), and appearance confusion (similar tablets/vial shape or color)—that can independently or jointly trigger incorrect drug selection.

Name Confusion

When two drug names look alike (*orthographic* similarity) or sound alike (*phonetic* similarity), hurried clinicians may misselect, misrecord, or mishear an order, especially when drop-down lists, voice orders, or illegible handwriting are in play. Reviews of voluntary reports to the Institute for Safe Medication Practices (ISMP) indicate that approximately every four wrong-medication events involve a patient being given a different drug than the one that they were supposed to be given (Institute for Safe Medication Practices (ISMP), 2015).

Pennsylvania's statewide reporting program painted a similar picture. In an inaugural annual review, the Pennsylvania Patient Safety Reporting System (PA-PSRS) reported that 11% of all medication-error submissions were wrong-drug events, and 34% of those events stemmed from name confusion; insulin products accounted for 9% of the mix-ups and opiate narcotics for 21%, with a single pair of *morphine/hydromorphone* responsible for one-third of the opiate errors and several fatalities (The Pennsylvania Patient Safety Advisory, 2004). **Table 1** lists common LASA drug pairs, including Humalog/Humulin R, Taxol/Taxotere, and Foradil/Toradol, frequently reported in Pennsylvania safety reports. **Table 2** shows additional pairs highlighted in the ISMP alerts.

Table 1. Representative look-alike (orthographic) drug–name pairs

LASA drug pair	Therapeutic difference	Typical error point	Reported/ potential harm	References
Hydralazine vs HydrOXYzine	Antihypertensive vs. antihistamine	ADC shelf, eMAR drop-down	Severe hypotension or, conversely, uncontrolled allergy/asthma	The Pennsylvania Patient Safety Advisory (2006)
Humalog® (insulin lispro) vs Humulin R® (regular human insulin)	Rapid- vs. short-acting insulin	Bedside pen selection	Hypo- or hyperglycemia; ketoacidosis	The Pennsylvania Patient Safety Advisory (2005)
Morphine vs Hydromorphone	≥5-fold potency gap	Ward dispensing & verbal orders	Fatal respiratory depression	Cohen, Smetzer, et al. (2007); Lowe et al. (2017); The Pennsylvania Patient Safety Advisory (2007)
TAXOL® (paclitaxel) vs TAXOTERE® (docetaxel)	Different chemotherapeutic agent & solvent	Oncology compounding	Underdosing (tumor progression) or severe toxicity	The Pennsylvania Patient Safety Advisory (2004)
Avandia® (rosiglitazone) vs Coumadin® (warfarin)	Antidiabetic vs. anticoagulant	CPOE pick-lists	Poor glycemic control or bleeding	The Pennsylvania Patient Safety Advisory (2004)
vinBLAStine vs vincristine	Vinca-alkaloid doses differ ×10	Chemo preparation	Fatal neuro-toxicity or undertreatment	The Institute for Safe Medication Practices (ISMP) (2015)

Abbreviations

LASA = look-alike sound-alike; ADC = automated dispensing cabinet; eMAR = electronic medication administration record; CPOE = computerized provider order entry.

Table 2. Representative sound-alike (phonetic) drug–name pairs

LASA drug pair	Therapeutic difference	Typical error point	Reported/ potential harm	References
Foradil® (formoterol) vs Toradol® (ketorolac)	Bronchodilator vs. NSAID	Verbal/handwritten orders	Untreated bronchospasm or NSAID renal/ GI ADR	The Pennsylvania Patient Safety Advisory (2004)
Plavix®(clopidogrel) vs Paxil® (paroxetine)	Antiplatelet vs. SSRI	Admission history & e-Rx	Stent thrombosis or serotonin syndrome	The Pennsylvania Patient Safety Advisory (2004)
Zyrtec® (cetirizine) vs Zantac® (ranitidine)	Antihistamine vs. H_2-blocker	Pediatric syrup dispensing	Persistent reflux or untreated allergy	Levine and Cohen (2007); The Institute for Safe Medication Practices (ISMP) (2019)
Morphine vs Meperidine	µ- vs. κ-opioid; dose gap	OR verbal orders	Seizure or respiratory depression	The Pennsylvania Patient Safety Advisory (2004)
OxyContin® (oxycodone) vs MS Contin® (morphine sulfate)	Different opioid & release profiles; OxyContin® (a sustained-release oxycodone preparation)- MS Contin® (morphine sulfate controlled-release)	Ward stock & CPOE	Over- or undersedation; unmanaged pain	Carter D and Sooknanan D (2024); Smith and Lesar (2011); The Pennsylvania Patient Safety Advisory (2004).
Hydromorphone vs Morphine	5- to 7-fold potency gap	Verbal/handwritten orders on surgical wards	Fatal respiratory depression	Lowe et al. (2017)
Inamrinone (formerly *amrinone*) vs Amiodarone	Inotrope vs. anti-arrhythmic	ICU dispensing (name now revised)	Hypotension or arrhythmia due to wrong agent	Cohen, Smetzer, et al. (2007); Pollak et al. (1998)

Abbreviations
ADR = adverse drug reaction; CPOE = computerized provider order entry; CR = controlled-release formulation; e-Rx = electronic prescription; GI = gastrointestinal; H_2 blocker = histamine-2 receptor antagonist; ICU = intensive care unit; NSAID = nonsteroidal anti-inflammatory drug; OR = operating room; SSRI = selective serotonin-reuptake inhibitor; µ-opioid/κ-opioid = mu-/kappa-opioid receptor agonist subclasses.

Packaging Confusion

Packing-related selection errors occur when medications are packaged or labeled such that clinicians unintentionally select the wrong product. The similarity often begins with the primary container, the component in direct contact with the medicine, such as a vial, ampoule, blister pack, or syringe barrel, and then extends to the secondary packaging (U.S. Department of Health and Human Services Food and Drug Administration, 1999, 2022). Secondary packaging may include outer cartons, foil pouches, or wallet cards, also called blister cards or unit dose cards, which are flat cardboard or plastic carriers that hold one or more small blister cavities (U.S. Department of Health and Human Services Food and Drug Administration, 1999). When colors, typefaces, and layout elements match across different products, this visual overlap can mislead healthcare providers and significantly increase the risk of selection errors (U.S. Department of Health and Human Services Food and Drug Administration, 2022; World Health Organization, 2023).

Example

- **Nitroprusside vs dexamethasone vials**

Nitroprusside vials were mixed with look-alike vials of dexamethasone (Cohen, Smetzer, et al., 2007).

- **Digoxin prefilled syringes vs other Carpuject® syringes**

Prefilled syringes of digoxin have been confused with other medications in prefilled syringes, especially if they are from the same manufacturer (e.g., Carpuject® syringes) (Cohen, Smetzer, et al., 2007).

- **Contrast media vials**

Mixups have occurred between look-alike vials of contrast media, especially if the products are from the same manufacturer. (for example, Hypaque [diatrizoate meglumine, used for cerebral angiography] has been confused with nonisonic Omnipaque 300 [iohexol, used for myelography] from the same manufacturer) (Cohen, Smetzer, et al., 2007).

- **Large-volume parenteral**

Bags of 5% sodium chloride injection have been confused with those of 5% dextrose and sodium chloride injection (Cohen, Smetzer, et al., 2007). The bags of 3% sodium chloride injection may be confused with those of 0.3% sodium chloride injection (Cohen, Smetzer, et al., 2007).

Primary Packaging

Primary containers are the components that come into direct contact with a medicine. Common examples include blister packs, vials, and ampoules. As shown in **Figure 2**, 300 mg and 450 mg of rifampicin capsules are packaged in blister packs of identical size and brown color. The foil strips of 25 mg and 10 mg amitriptyline tablets from the same manufacturer are shown in **Figure 3**. The foils appear similar, making the two strengths difficult to distinguish.

Figure 2. Rifampicin (300 mg) and blister packs (450 mg) were used

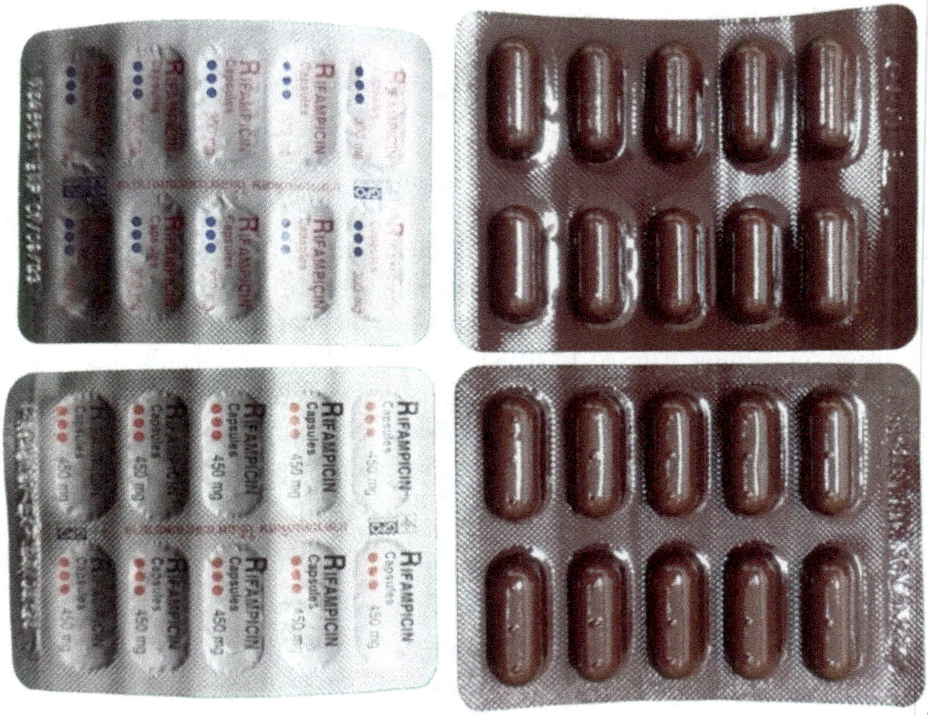

Both strengths exhibit the same brown color and blister size.

Figure 3. Amitriptyline (25 mg and 10 mg tablets)

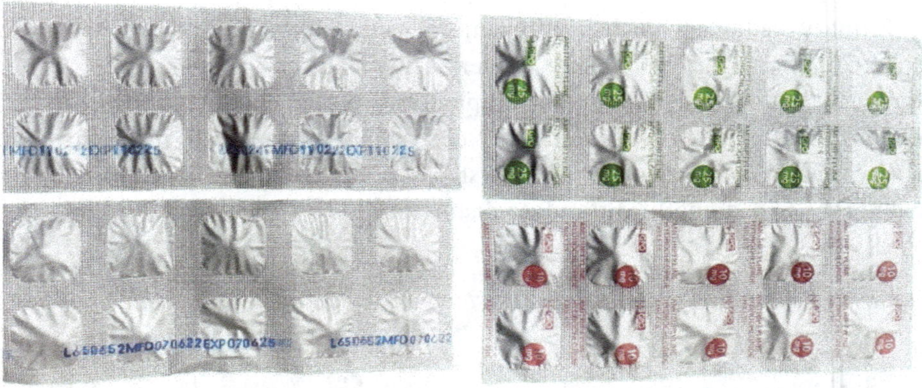

Both strengths are produced by the same manufacturer and exhibit an identical appearance.

A medication error report from the intensive care unit revealed an incident involving 100 mg/mL hydrocortisone and 100 mg/mL levetiracetam injections (**Figure 4**). Hydrocortisone, packaged in a clear glass vial with an orange cap and blue label, was ordered, but an almost identical vial of levetiracetam was dispensed. The corresponding color of the cap, the label, and the shape of the vials also created confusion. According to the NCC MERP taxonomy, the event fell under category B, which means that the error reached the patient but was not harmful. The pharmacy managers advised the involved staff members and reminded all the personnel to be extra cautious with LASA medications, particularly in regard to urgent (STAT) orders (Department of Pharmacy Srinagarind Hospital, 2022a).

Figure 4. Examples of look-alike vials that led to a medication error. In the ICU, a Category B type was mistaken when levetiracetam was filled instead of 100 mg of hydrocortisone because of the similarity of cap colors and the shape of the vials

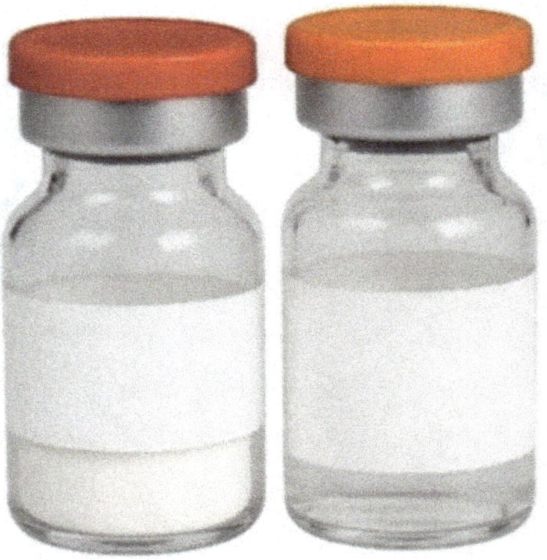

An inpatient department ward received a medication error report about a 600 mg injection of ceftaroline fosamil and a 2 g/0.5 g injection of ceftazidime/avibactam. Errors occurred when a 2 g/0.5 g dose of ceftazidime/avibactam was ordered, but a 600 mg dose of ceftaroline fosamil was dispensed because of the visual resemblance of their vials (Department of Pharmacy Srinagarind Hospital, 2022b), as demonstrated in the example in **Figure 5.** These two products were packaged in glass vials of similar sizes, shapes, and labeling styles, with light-colored labels, a blue accentual text, and a similar color of the caps, which was a source of confusion. This dispensing error is a Category B error (an error that occurred but did not reach the patient) (Devine et al., 2005).

Figure 5. Examples of look-alike vials associated with a medication error. An error involved a Category B error when ceftaroline fosamil was discharged instead of the recommended ceftazidime because of its similarity in terms of its vial look, label design, and blue caps

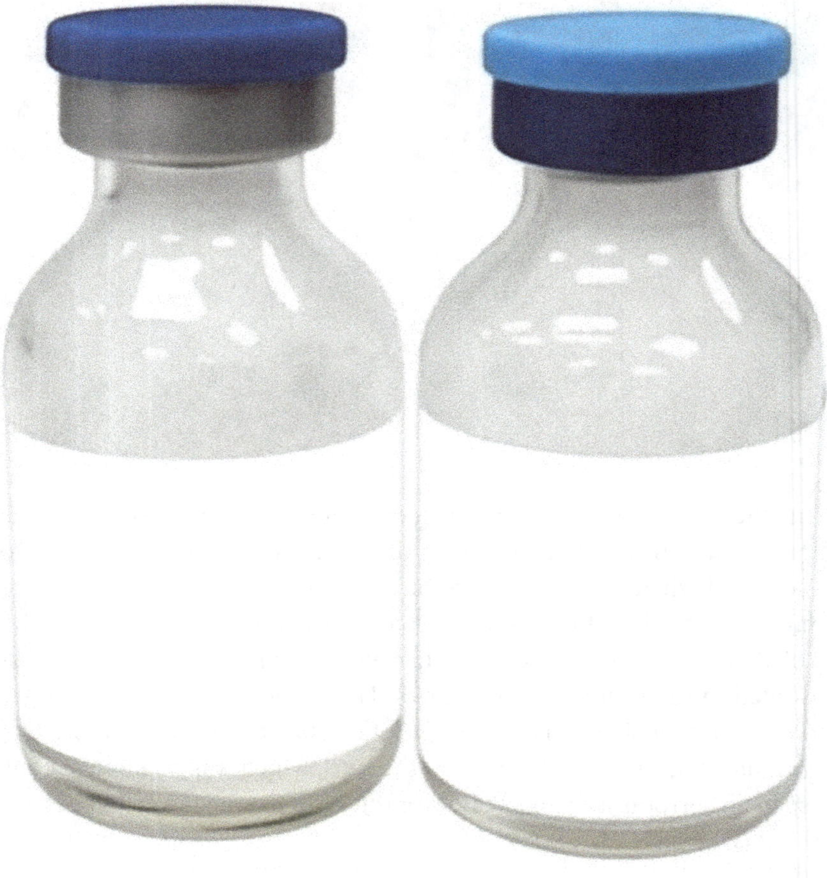

Secondary Packaging

Outer cartons, which are used as secondary packaging, can also be confusing. Illustrations include amlodipine (5 mg, brand AMBES 5®) and amlodipine (10 mg, brand AMBES 10®, both made by the same manufacturer) (Supapaan TS, Songmuang A, et al., 2024) (see **Figure 6**). The cartons also start with the letter A and have virtually the same labels and color schemes; the only obvious difference is the declared strength.

Figure 6. Secondary packaging confusion between amlodipine 5 mg (AMBES-5®) and amlodipine 10 mg (AMBES-10®)

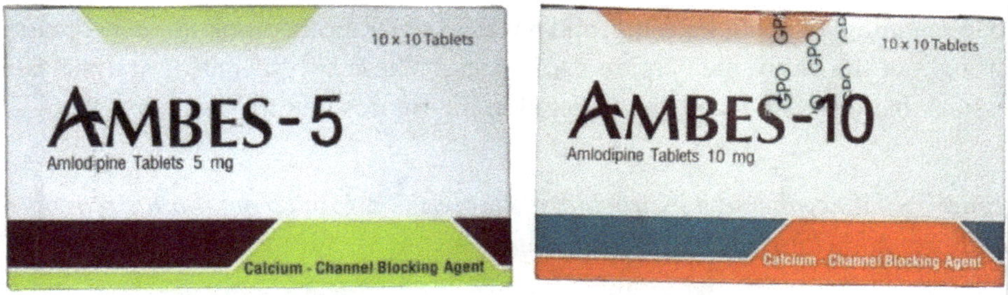

Images obtained from https://drugiden2.ubu.ac.th/ and used with permission

Appearance Confusion

The confusion of appearance refers to the state where drugs resemble each other in appearance (e.g., in shape, size, color, etc.) and are thus confused with each other. This similarity may overcome time-crossing double checks and result in incorrect drug or incorrect drug administration in fast-paced clinical settings (Cohen & Smetzer, 2015; World Health Organization, 2023). Tablets and capsules are particularly risky, as they are available in an infinite number of variations in shape, size, and color.

Examples of appearance confusion:

- Trihexyphenidyl tablets, 2 mg and 5 mg: 2 mg and 5 mg doses of the same drug, are small, white, round tablets that have been placed in the same white HDPE bottles. After we pour the tablets into unit-dose cups, the only difference is a small, embossed code of strength that is unemphasized. The two strengths may be mixed, leading to a fivefold overdose and causing anticholinergic toxicity. This mix-up is prevented with the assistance of segregated storage and barcode checks at dispensing (**Figure 7**) (Supapaan TS, Songmuang A, et al., 2024).
- Chlorpheniramine vs. folic acid: Chlorpheniramine maleate tablets (4 mg) and folic acid tablets (5 mg) appear nearly the same; they are small, yellow, and round. A mistake can occur in outpatient pharmacies that provide visual inspection of any item where excess chlorpheniramine (causing sedation) could be given or folic acid therapy could be overlooked. Blister foil color-coded and tall man printing on the labels of the bins are recommended protective measures (**Figure 8**) (Supapaan TS, Songmuang A, et al., 2024).

These examples demonstrate that appearance confusion is not restricted to look-alike vials but also impacts solid oral dosage forms in most therapeutic classes. To minimize this error and ensure patient safety, it is important to consistently use bar-code scanning, tall man lettering, and physical separation of look-alike medications throughout the entire medication-use process. These two scenarios and the safety lessons that they can teach are depicted in the figures that follow.

Figure 7. Trihexyphenidyl hydrochloride tablets, 2 mg and 5 mg. Both strengths are small, round, white tablets

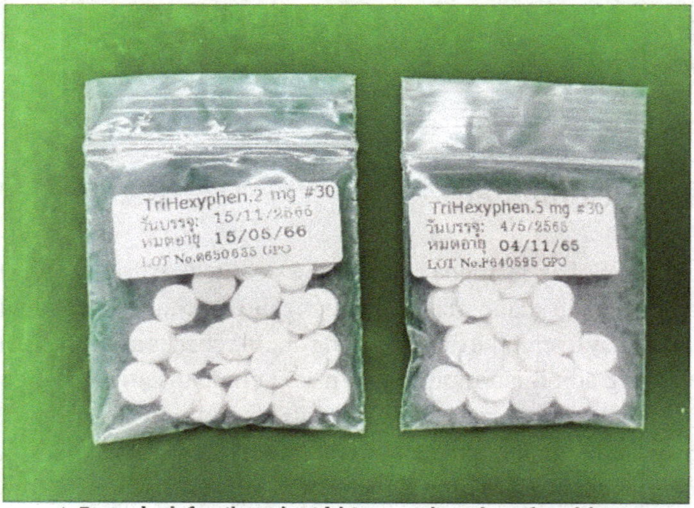

A. Prepack—left: trihexyphenidyl 2 mg; right: trihexyphenidyl 5 mg

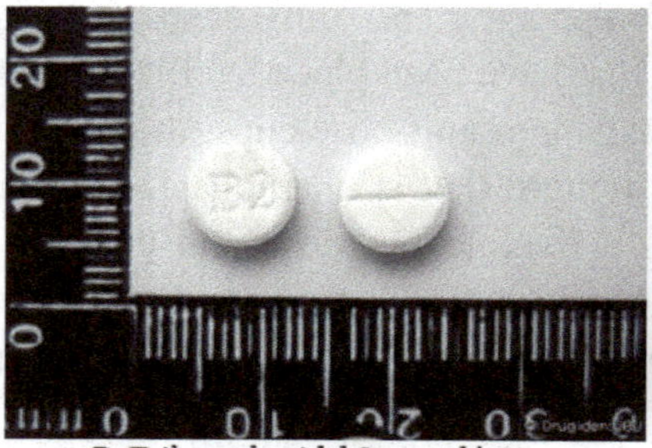

B. Trihexyphenidyl 2 mg tablets

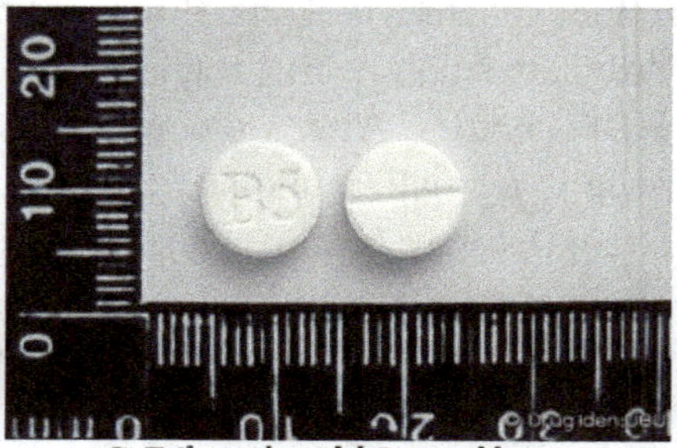

C. Trihexyphenidyl 5 mg tablets

Figure 8. Prepack 4 mg of chlorpheniramine and 5 mg of folic acid tablets. Both products are small, yellow, and round tablets

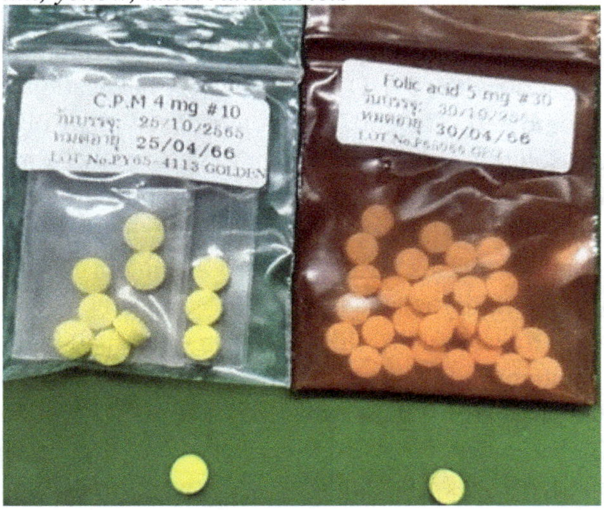

EXPLORING LASA MEDICATIONS

LASA may not be a complex word, but it has a significant effect on healthcare. This section examines the definition of an LASA drug, the psychology of human error in the use of these drugs, and why they are so problematic even for well-experienced medical practitioners. Medication errors may include the occurrence of similar-sounding or similar-looking names of drugs, which is, unfortunately, a widespread case. There are also errors that are related to such medications (Hughes & Blegen, 2008).

Consider the drugs "Celebrex®" (celecoxib, a nonsteroidal anti-inflammatory agent), "Celexa®" (citalopram, a selective serotonin reuptake inhibitor), and "Cerebyx®" (fosphenytoin, an antiseizure medication) (Cohen, 1999). Their names are easily mixed up when pronounced. This pronunciation resemblance has been attributed to some recorded cases of medication errors that have led to patient harm (Roy, 2001). Another example involves mixtures of Zyrtec® (cetirizine), which is an antihistamine, and Zyprexa® (olanzapine), an antipsychotic medication (NBC News, 2005; The Associated Press, 2005). Accidental consumption of Zyprexa® when Zyrtec® is intended can lead to dizziness and potential falls, whereas taking Zyrtec® instead of Zyprexa® may cause a relapse in mental health conditions (NBC News, 2005; The Associated Press, 2005).

The World Health Organization (WHO) has been actively developing and implementing strategies to minimize the risks posed by LASA medications. These efforts aim to reduce medication errors that stem from confusion between drugs with similar names or appearances (World Health Organization, 2023).

This section describes the WHO's major LASA medication safety initiatives and milestones (**Figure 9**). The 2007 creation of the WHO Collaborating Centre for Patient Safety Solutions began a program to reduce LASA medication errors. Pharmaceutical name screening was an early step to prevent the approval of confusing new drugs (World Health Organization, 2007). The WHO launched the third global patient safety challenge, "Medication Without Harm," in 2017 to reduce severe, avoidable medication-related harm by 50% globally within five years. This challenge encouraged lists of look-alike drug names and tall-man lettering to differentiate them to minimize LASA medication errors (International Pharmaceutical Federation (FIP), 2020; World Health Organization, 2017).

The WHO Global Patient Safety Action Plan 2021–2030 emphasized the need to aid in reducing LASA medication errors to prevent needless healthcare harm. The promotion of medication safety and LASA medication errors can be regarded as priorities of the plan (World Health Organization, 2021).

In 2022, World Patient Safety Day focused on the topic of medication without harm, which emphasized the need to continue pursuing medication safety and LASA-related error prevention in particular. This focus revealed the progress achieved and the areas that still need refinement with respect to medication safety (World Health Organization, 2023).

The WHO Patient Safety Flagship emphasized LASA medication safety in October 2023. The misinterpretation of drug names was a primary cause of drug name confusion. The WHO has been working gradually to prevent such errors and make the patient experience across the globe safer by targeting LASA medicines (World Health Organization, 2023). Since its initial awareness, there has been a push by the WHO to focus on medication safety in the current year, 2023, concerning LASA medicines. These efforts have led to medication-related harm reduction and patient safety worldwide.

Figure 9. Timeline of WHO initiatives for LASA medication safety

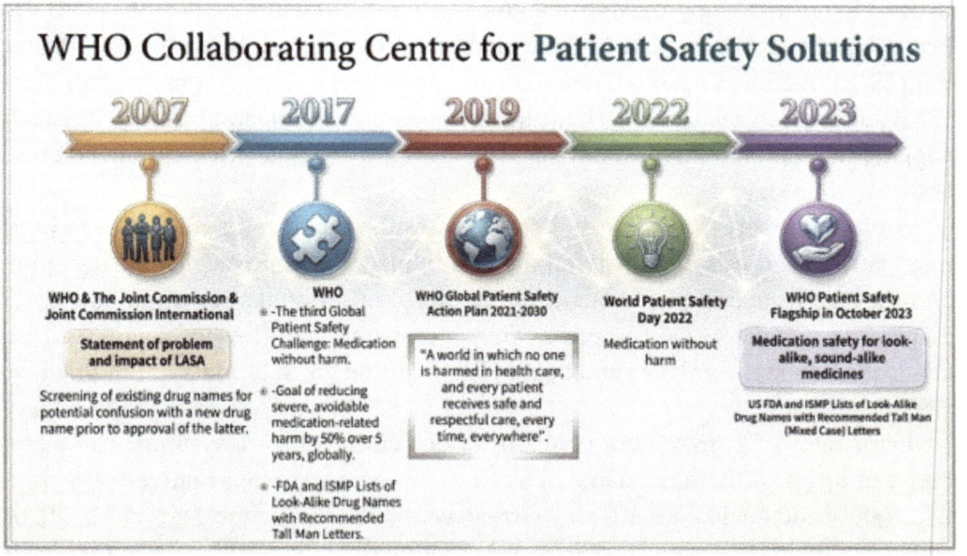

(World Health Organization, 2007, 2014, 2017, 2021, 2022, 2023)

The Institute of Safe Medication Practices (ISMP) is the organization to consider when addressing medication errors that took place with LASA drugs. ISMP's work has been at the forefront of defining, examining, and providing methods for curbing the risks associated with LASA errors in medication. The ISMP seeks to enhance medication safety through multiple initiatives, including the Medication Error Reporting Program, the release of a list of confusable drug names, the promotion of tall-man lettering, and the establishment of best practice guidelines. The ISMP has played an important role in international efforts to minimize medication-related injuries in cooperation with other organizations, such as the World Health Organization (WHO). The proposed collaborative effort will focus on standardizing drug nomenclature, educating more people about LASA medication hazards, and promoting policy changes prioritizing medication safety. The ISMP and its collaborators strive to diminish medication errors and improve patient safety globally through reporting initiatives, educational resources, advocacy, and policy formulation (Cohen, Domizio, et al., 2007; Cohen & Smetzer, 2017; Grissinger et al., 2007; The Institute for Safe Medication Practices (ISMP), 2023b).

The Institute for Safe Medication Practices (ISMP) has enumerated many means of controlling and preventing LASA medication errors (Cohen, Domizio, et al., 2007; The Institute for Safe Medication Practices (ISMP), 2023a, 2023b). These are not only specific but also systemic measures that these professionals can implement to reduce the risk of LASA errors in regard to the storage (in storage facilities), dispensing, and administration of medication. The US FDA has provided an alphabetized list of FDA-approved drug names with tall letters to support these efforts. For voluntary use by healthcare providers, the FDA provides a list of drug names with ISMP-recommended tall man letters. Several key organizations, including the ISMP, Joint Commission, WHO, and International Medication Safety Network, support this collaborative initiative (The Institute for Safe Medication Practices (ISMP), 2023a).

An ISMP report from August 2023 explains the tragic cesarean birth of a pregnant patient who was administered digoxin in place of BUPivacaine during spinal anesthesia. An anesthetist brought the wrong 2 mL ampule out of an automated dispensing cabinet (ADC) in error. They were similar in their packaging. Errors can lead to apnea, paralysis, and death (The Institute for Safe Medication Practices (ISMP), 2023c).

Error rates of LASA are a concern for current healthcare systems. Confusion between drugs of the same name or similar appearances may negatively affect patient safety and healthcare efficacy (Bryan et al., 2021b; Lizano-Díez et al., 2020).

One of the most serious problems is LASA medication errors between prescriptions and drug administration (Ostini et al., 2012). These errors frequently occur because of the similarity of medication names or packaging and the common use of generic and multi-indication medications, posing a significant threat to patients. Therefore, all medication details should be verified. The data in **Figure 10** illustrate how LASA errors can occur during prescription, transcription, dispensing, and administration, posing a threat to patient safety.

Figure 10. LASA medication errors in the medication use process. The figure shows how look-alike, sound-alike medication errors may occur at each stage of the process, including prescribing, transcription, dispensing, and administration, potentially resulting in patient harm

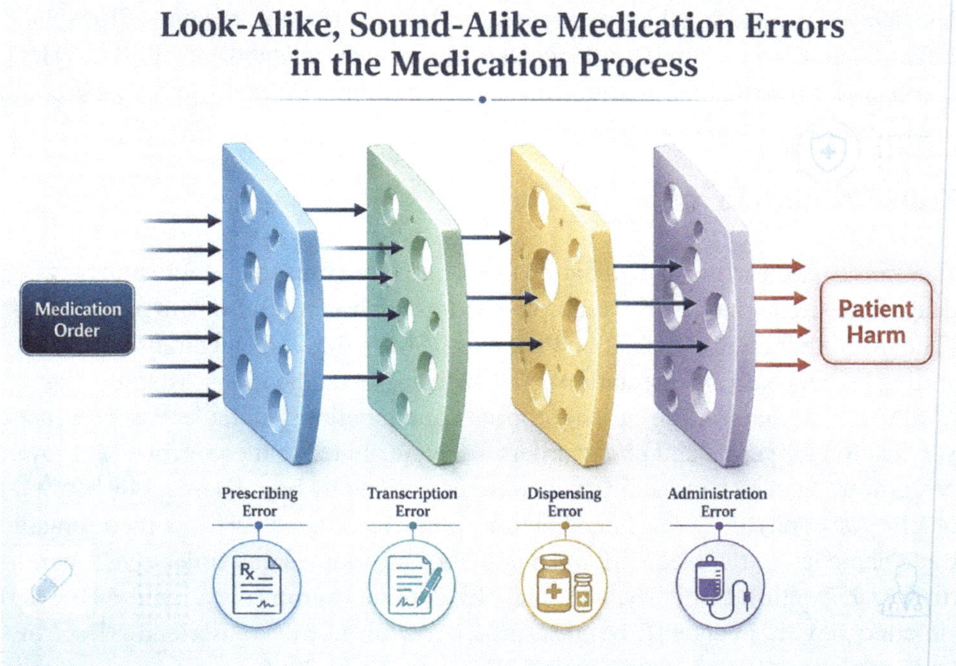

Prescribing Error

This type of error can occur when medications with similar names or appearances are confused with one another during the prescribing phase. All prescriptions should be viewed with caution. In the past few years, numerous new drugs have been released, and generic drugs with close names have been poured into the marketplace. In addition to these names being similar, a number of the medicines also have multiple applications and other nams. Failure to state the diagnosis of the prescription poses the risk of the drug being used for too long or not enough time. The proliferation of numerous new generics with similar names significantly heightens the risk of error. To address the issue of unintentional drug substitution, the U.S. Pharmacopeia has enumerated the names of look-alike medicines, and the ISMP has created a list of the most commonly misinterpreted abbreviations (Cohen,

Domizio, et al., 2007; Cohen & Smetzer, 2017; Grissinger et al., 2007; Supapaan TS, Somsorn S, et al., 2024; Tariq et al., 2021).

For example, after being diagnosed with hypokalemia, a patient was prescribed Slow-K but was mistakenly prescribed Slow-Na instead because of an error in selecting from a software drop-down list. A mistake was made before the patient, who had delayed completing the prescription for financial reasons, obtained Slow-Na. If left untreated, hypokalemia could result in arrhythmias, metabolic acidosis, skeletal myopathy, and acute kidney injury, and elevated sodium intake from Slow-Na could affect mental status (Naunton et al., 2015).

Transcription Error

Transcription errors in medication orders are often caused by confusion between drugs with similar names. For example, prednisone was confused with prednisolone (The Institute for Safe Medication Practices (ISMP), 2019) during transcription, resulting in incorrect documentation and dispensing of medications. Mistranscription of LASA drug names, use of inappropriate abbreviations, and a lack of read-back verification for verbal and phone orders also contributed to these errors. Moreover, errors were made when medications were prescribed by brand name. For example, Nuelin® (theophylline) was intended to be prescribed, but an error in recording the trade name led to the medication being incorrectly copied and ordered as Neurontin® (gabapentin). Similarly, although Berclomine® syrup (dicyclomine HCl and simethicone) was intended to be prescribed, it was mistakenly transcribed as Bactrim® (sulfamethoxazole and trimethoprim) (Puttilerpong C, 2006).

Reports concerning LASA in high-alert drugs have also been published. *"E. KCl 30 ml O q 6 hr"* was added. However, it was unclear, and the transcription was misread as "KCl 30 ml IV drip q 6 hr." An investigation revealed that there was uncertainty about what "E" referred to, and the handwriting for "O" (oral) was misinterpreted as "IV." Fortunately, no harm was caused to the patient (Puttilerpong C, 2006).

In another instance, a transcription error led to a patient's prescription for the antibiotic meropenem (Meronem®) being incorrectly copied as an order for Melperon, a low-potency antipsychotic. This mistake occurred when the drug was copied to the medication chart. Before the wrong drug was given, the error was captured and fixed, preventing a fatal outcome (Heck et al., 2020).

An 80-year-old patient received 75 mg of clozapine instead of clopidogrel. After incorrect intake, the patient was unconscious and taken to the ICU. Owing to time pressure in a noisy workplace, the medication prescription was "skimmed" rather than read. This life-threatening confusion between the two drugs was resolved, and the patient recovered without complications (Heck et al., 2020).

Dispensing Error

Drug dispensing errors can occur before and during patient administration. Drug selection and preparation errors differ from dispensing errors, which occur during patient administration. These errors are caused by look-alike drug names, packaging, and poor drug strength. Look-like drug pairs such as Amaryl/Amtrel, calcium acetate/calcium citrate, Concor/Cozaar, and Concor/Crestor often cause dispensing errors. Ineffective treatment and patient harm can result from such errors (Tseng et al., 2018).

Dispensing Lamictal (lamotrigine), an epilepsy and bipolar disorder medication, instead of Lamisil® (terbinafine), an antifungal, can occur. This error can cause treatment failure and patient harm (Medscape, 2000).

Similar packaging and color coding of insulin products, especially between rapid-acting and intermediate-acting insulin, can cause medication errors. Additionally, insulin glargine (300 IU/3 mL), INSULIN Mixtard HM Penfill®, and INSULIN NPH Penfill® have similar names, which can cause confusion. Owing to their similar names and shelf proximity, Mixtard® insulin was mistakenly dispensed instead of Mixtard Penfill®. These errors can lead to inappropriate treatment and adverse drug events (Department of pharmacy of Bueng Kan hospital, 2023; Puttilerpong C, 2006; Senior Care Consultant Group (SCCG), 2006).

Owing to their similar names, hydroxyzine, an antihistamine, is dispensed instead of hydralazine, an antihypertensive (Chanakit et al., 2013; Naunton et al., 2015; The Institute for Safe Medication Practices (ISMP), 2019). Owing to their similar names and packaging, 30 mg of morphine (MST Continus 30 mg®) and 10 mg were confused (**Figure 11**) (Department of pharmacy of Bueng Kan hospital, 2023).

Figure 11. Photograph showing 30 mg of morphine (MST Continus® 30 mg) and 10 mg of morphine (MST Continus® 10 mg), illustrating how similar their names and packaging appear

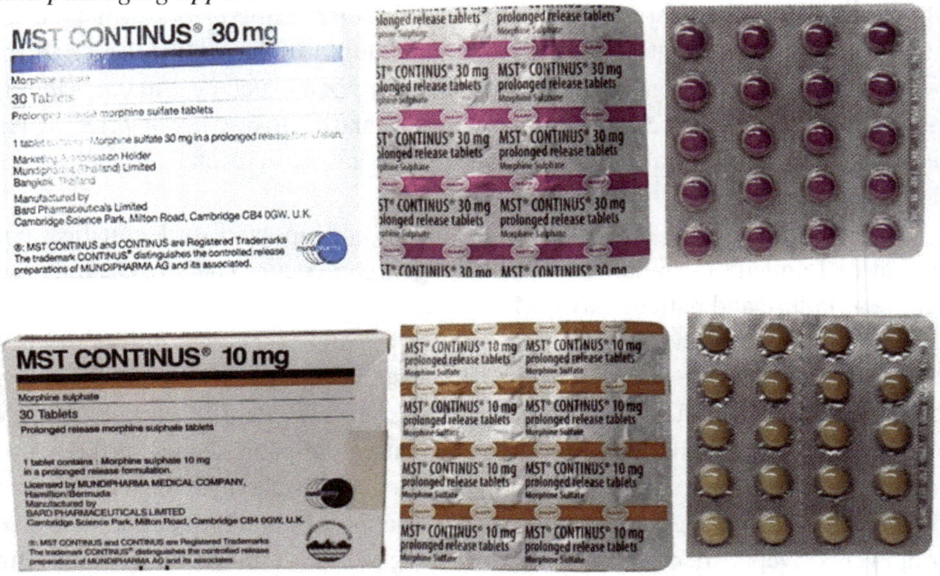

Administration Error

Uncertain administration instructions, failure to double-check the order, and failure to monitor the patient after administration can cause errors. LASA drugs exacerbate these issues. Similarities in drug names and packaging can lead to confusion, increasing the risk of administering the wrong medication. Such errors can result in significant issues in the administration and monitoring of medication, potentially leading to ineffective treatment and harm to the patient (World Health Organization, 2023).

PREVALENCE OF LASA MEDICATION ERRORS

Similarly, LASA medication errors are critical global issues that compromise patient safety across all healthcare settings. A comprehensive review revealed that LASA errors accounted for 6.2% to 14.7% of medication error events and ranged from 0.00003% to 0.0022% of prescriptions, highlighting the significant prevalence variation depending on healthcare context and reporting mechanisms (Bryan et al.,

2021a). Various studies have documented the frequency and clinical context of LASA error incidence globally (Table 3).

Table 3. Overview of LASA medication error prevalence

Setting	Prevalence of LASA Errors	Details/Examples of LASA Errors	Reference
Secondary-care hospital, Karachi	19% of 200 prescriptions	LASA errors split among orthographic (50%), phonetic (7.8%), and visual read-alike (42.1%). Most errors stemmed from poor differentiation in drug names and inadequate verification steps.	Zafar and Raza (2020)
Multiple clinical settings	0.00003–0.0022% of prescriptions; 6.2–14.7% of all medication errors	Demonstrated broad variability by institution. LASA issues were noted across all stages, with significant underreporting in outpatient contexts.	Bryan et al. (2021a)
Pediatric ER network (PECARN)	36% of incorrect medication events were associated with look-alike/sound-alike errors	Among 597 reported medication errors, 36% of incorrect medications were due to confusion involving LASA drugs. Reported incidents included administration of intravenous fluids when oral formulations were intended. The study highlights the susceptibility of pediatric ED settings to LASA-related errors, exacerbated by human factors such as procedural noncompliance, stress, and distractions.	Shaw et al. (2013)
Near-miss event review	7% of 2044 near-miss events	The overall error rate for analgesic prescriptions was 2.87 per 1,000 orders, with pediatric patients experiencing more than twice the error rate of adults. Sound-alike drug names were a significant factor, contributing to 7% (143 out of 2,044) of the near-miss prescribing errors evaluated.	Smith and Lesar (2011).
National error reporting system	6% of 5,003 reports	In 2011, the Medication Error Reporting System reported Madopar-Methyldopa, Lovastatin-Loratadine, Chlorpromazine-Carbamazepine, Cotrimoxazole-Cltrimazole, Carbimazole-Cotrimoxazole, Amlodipine-Felodipine, Difflam-Daflon, Enalapril-Perindopril, Neurobion-Neurontin, and Cycloserine-Cyclosporine. Standardized national alert systems were recommended.	Pharmaceutical Services Division (2012).

continued on following page

Table 3. Continued

Setting	Prevalence of LASA Errors	Details/Examples of LASA Errors	Reference
MEDMARX database for reports involving outpatient vaccinations (N = 465)	Highest prevalence in the tetanus group (Td, Tdap, DTaP, DT) 34 (36%). Pneumococcal group (PCV, PPV) had 13 (29%) incidence. Influenza group (Hib, TIV) had 27 (23%). Hepatitis group (HepA, HepB) had 15 (17%).	Highest error frequency among Td and Tdap. Errors frequently stemmed from selecting the wrong vial due to similar labels in the vaccine storage system.	Bundy et al. (2009).
Community pharmacies, UK	Similar names: 16.8%; Similar packaging: 7.6%	Most common causes: misreading handwriting (24.5%), selecting wrong drug strength/dose from records (11.4%), and confusing packaging. Uniform packaging increased risk.	Ashcroft et al. (2005)
Two tertiary hospitals (11 units, 6 months)	Not quantified	Identified 334 medication errors, with 264 preventable ADEs. A significant portion resulted from LASA-related failures in drug identity checks, especially at dispensing and administration stages.	Leape et al. (1995).
200-bed general hospital, Thailand	Not quantified	A total of 46 pairs of LASA drugs were identified, involved in 65 LASA-related events. The most frequently confused drugs were simvastatin 10 mg and 20 mg, implicated in 30 separate incidents, largely due to their nearly identical names and appearances. The majority of errors were attributed to drug name similarity (64.62%), followed by packaging resemblance (24.61%), and visual similarity form (10.77%). These errors typically occurred during periods of high workload and were primarily categorized as Category B (near-miss) events, although some did result in actual patient harm.	Supapaan TS, Songmuang A, et al. (2024)
128 hospitals in Thailand	Not quantified	Identified 2,510 LASA drug pairs: 66.69% tablets/capsules (simvastatin 10 mg/20 mg most frequent), 17.01% injections (ceftriaxone/ceftazidime), 3.39% liquids, 2.95% inhalers, 1.95% topicals, 1.12% powders. Most common similarity was in names/pronunciation. Category B (near-miss) errors were most frequent.	Supapaan et al. (2024)

In a detailed study from a secondary-care hospital in Karachi, LASA errors were observed in 19% of 200 prescriptions. These errors were caused primarily by the orthographic (50%), phonetic (7.8%), and visual (42.1%) similarities in drug names (Zafar & Raza, 2020). Similarly, a 2024 investigation in a 200-bed general hospital in Thailand reported that 7.4% of medication errors were LASA related, with drug name confusion (64.6%) being the most common cause. This study identified 46 LASA drug pairs, including 10 mg and 20 mg simvastatin, and revealed that these errors occurred during busy periods. Some of the proposed mitigation measures include improved workforce allocation, tall man lettering, and LASA labeling (Supapaan TS, Songmuang A, et al., 2024). LASA mistakes are a significant threat to children, and pediatricians could recognize LASA drug substitutions that might lead to injuries (Basco et al., 2016). According to the Pediatric Emergency Care Applied Research Network (PECARN), more than one-third of incorrect medication events are associated with LASA errors (Shaw et al., 2013).

Ashcroft et al. (2005) reported that 16.8% of incidents in UK community pharmacies were related to drugs with similar names and that 7.6% were due to similar packaging.(Ashcroft et al., 2005) Bundy et al. (2009) reported 465 instances of incorrect vaccine administration, with the highest prevalence of look-alike/sound-alike (LASA) errors found in the "tetanus" group (Td, Tdap, DTaP, DT), where 36% of the errors were due to this type of confusion. The "pneumococcal" group (PCV, PPV) had a 29% incidence of LASA errors, followed by the "influenza" group (Hib, TIV) with 23% and the "hepatitis" group (HepA, HepB) with 17% (Bundy et al., 2009).

CONCLUSION

Patient safety remains threatened by LASA medication errors. Although LASA pairs make up only a small fraction of the global inventory of medicines, they account for a disproportionately large share of wrong drug incidents, often between six and fifteen percent of all reported medication errors, because similarities in names, labels, or packaging exploit well-known human cognitive limits. These errors can occur during prescription, transcription, dispensing, and bedside administration, and many of them remain unreported, owing to which their actual impact is not seen. The name confusion, similar packaging, and similar appearance are three overlapping mechanisms that form the underlying hazards. The wrong choices are promoted by presenting orthographically similar names of drugs on the same list of electronic pick lists, placing almost identical cartons or vials on the same shelf, or by physically similar-looking tablets and syringes under the pressure of time. A good example of how these risks intersect in practice can be seen in the occurrence of insulin mix-ups and morphine–hydromorphone confusion. Efforts by international organizations such as the World Health Organization and Institute of Safe Medication Practices have promoted LASA prevention as a national health issue. The main recommendations involve the establishment of national LASA watchlists, the use of tall man lettering in all cases, uniform high-contrast labeling, and the incorporation of barcode verification and clinical decision support in daily operations. New technologies such as machine-learning warning systems and ADCs are built upon this safety net, but only with human-centered design and well-trusted work processes.

REFERENCES

Ashcroft, D. M., Quinlan, P., & Blenkinsopp, A. (2005). Prospective study of the incidence, nature and causes of dispensing errors in community pharmacies. *Pharmacoepidemiology and Drug Safety, 14*(5), 327–332. DOI: 10.1002/pds.1012 PMID: 15386722

Basco, W. T.Jr, Garner, S. S., Ebeling, M., Freeland, K. D., Hulsey, T. C., & Simpson, K. (2016). Evaluating the potential severity of look-alike, sound-alike drug substitution errors in children. *Academic Pediatrics, 16*(2), 183–191. DOI: 10.1016/j.acap.2015.06.014 PMID: 26946271

Bryan, R., Aronson, J. K., ten Hacken, P., Williams, A., & Jordan, S. (2015). Patient safety in medication nomenclature: Orthographic and semantic properties of International Nonproprietary Names. *PLoS One, 10*(12), e0145431. DOI: 10.1371/journal.pone.0145431 PMID: 26701761

Bryan, R., Aronson, J. K., Williams, A., & Jordan, S. (2021a). The problem of look-alike, sound-alike name errors: Drivers and solutions. *British Journal of Clinical Pharmacology, 87*(2), 386–394. DOI: 10.1111/bcp.14285 PMID: 32198938

Bryan, R., Aronson, J. K., Williams, A. J., & Jordan, S. (2021b). A systematic literature review of LASA error interventions. *British Journal of Clinical Pharmacology, 87*(2), 336–351. DOI: 10.1111/bcp.14644 PMID: 33197079

Bundy, D. G., Shore, A. D., Morlock, L. L., & Miller, M. R. (2009). Pediatric vaccination errors: Application of the "5 rights" framework to a national error reporting database. *Vaccine, 27*(29), 3890–3896. DOI: 10.1016/j.vaccine.2009.04.005 PMID: 19442422

Carter, D., & Sooknanan, D. (2024). *Long-acting oral opioids (MS Contin™, Oxycontin™)*. Retrieved 4 June from https://pain.ucsf.edu/opioid-analgesics/long-acting-oral-opioids-ms-contin%E2%84%A2-oxycontin%E2%84%A2

Chanakit, T., Napaporn, J., Chiempattanakajohn, T., Sangkhawan, S., & Wichakot, S. (2013). The survey of look alike/sound alike (LASA) drugs available in hospitals in Thailand. *African Journal of Pharmacy and Pharmacology, 7*(6), 227–239. DOI: 10.5897/AJPP11.812

Cohen, M. (1999). Celebrex, celexa, cerebyx. *Nursing, 29*(7), 14. DOI: 10.1097/00152193-199907000-00006

Cohen, M. R. (2006). Maalox brand name extension causes confusion near sight/ sound dead hit! omacor–amicar look-alike tylenol packets. *Hospital Pharmacy, 41*(1), 13–16. DOI: 10.1310/hpj4101-13

Cohen, M. R. (2007). The role of drug packaging and labeling in medication errors. In Cohen, M. R. (Ed.), *Medication Errors* (2nd ed., pp. 111–152). The American Pharmacists Association. https://doi.org/doi:10.21019/9781582120928.ch7

Cohen, M. R., Domizio, G. D., & Lee, R. E. (2007). The role of drug names in medication errors. In Cohen, M. R. (Ed.), *Medication Errors* (2nd ed., pp. 87–110). The American Pharmacists Association. https://doi.org/doi:10.21019/9781582120928.ch6

Cohen, M. R., & Smetzer, J. L. (2007). Preventing dispensing errors. In *Medication Errors* (2nd ed.). The American Pharmacists Association. DOI: 10.21019/9781582120928.ch10

Cohen, M. R., & Smetzer, J. L. (2015). No unlabeled containers anywhere, ever! where did this come from? *Hospital Pharmacy, 50*(3), 185–188. DOI: 10.1310/hpj5003-185 PMID: 26405305

Cohen, M. R., & Smetzer, J. L. (2017). ISMP medication error report analysis. *Hospital Pharmacy, 52*(6), 390–393. DOI: 10.1177/0018578717715346 PMID: 29276260

Cohen, M. R., Smetzer, J. L., Tuohy, N. R., & Kilo, C. M. (2007). High-alert medications: safeguarding against errors. In Cohen, M. R. (Ed.), *Medication Errors* (2nd ed., pp. 317–412). The American Pharmacists Association. DOI: 10.21019/9781582120928.ch14

Department of Pharmacy, Bueng Kan Hospital. (2023). *Look alike sound alike drug*. Retrieved 22 May from https://bkh.moph.go.th/bkhweb/uploads/media/202303310725123_4.LASA_update-_2566.pdf

Department of Pharmacy, Srinagarind Hospital. (2022a). *Medication error due to LASA mix-up on the shelf: levetiracetam vs hydrocortisone*. Retrieved 02 June from https://pharm.md.kku.ac.th/post/14

Department of Pharmacy, Srinagarind Hospital. (2022b). *Medication error due to LASA mix-up on the shelf: zinforo inj vs zavicefta inj*. Retrieved 02 June from https://pharm.md.kku.ac.th/post/13

Devine, E. B., Wilson-Norton, J. L., Lawless, N. M., Hazlet, T. K., Hansen, R., Kelly, K., . . . Wong, C. (2005). Preparing for ambulatory computerized prescriber order entry by evaluating preimplementation medication errors. In Henriksen K, Battles JB, Marks ES, et al. (eds.) Advances in Patient Safety: From Research to Implementation (Vol. 2: Concepts and Methodology). Rockville (MD): Agency for Healthcare Research and Quality (US); 2005 Feb. Available from: https://www.ncbi.nlm.nih.gov/books/NBK20508/

Grissinger, M., Cohen, H., & Vaida, A. J. (2007). Using rechnology to prevent medication errors. In *Medication Errors* (2nd ed.). The American Pharmacists Association. DOI: 10.21019/9781582120928.ch15

Heck, J., Groh, A., Stichtenoth, D. O., Bleich, S., & Krause, O. (2020). Look-alikes, sound-alikes: Three cases of insidious medication errors. *Clinical Case Reports*, *8*(12), 3284–3287. DOI: 10.1002/ccr3.3409 PMID: 33363919

Hughes, R. G., & Blegen, M. A. (2008). Medication administration safety. In Hughes, R. G. (Ed.), *Patient safety and quality: An evidence-based handbook for nurses*. Agency for Healthcare Research and Quality. https://www.ncbi.nlm.nih.gov/books/NBK2656/

Ibrahim, O. M., Ibrahim, R. M., Meslamani, A. Z. A., & Mazrouei, N. A. (2020). Dispensing errors in community pharmacies in the United Arab Emirates: Investigating incidence, types, severity, and causes. *Pharmacy Practice*, *18*(4), 2111. DOI: 10.18549/PharmPract.2020.4.2111 PMID: 33149793

Institute for Safe Medication Practices (ISMP). (2015). Open the bag to catch errors at the point-of-sale. *ISMP Medication Safety Alert! Community. Ambulatory Care*, *14*(7), 1–2.

International Pharmaceutical Federation (FIP). (2020). *Pharmacists' Role in Medication Without Harm*. The Hague. International Pharmaceutical Federation.

Lambert, B. L., Galanter, W., Liu, K. L., Falck, S., Schiff, G., Rash-Foanio, C., Schmidt, K., Shrestha, N., Vaida, A. J., & Gaunt, M. J. (2019). Automated detection of wrong-drug prescribing errors. *BMJ Quality & Safety*, *28*(11), 908–915. DOI: 10.1136/bmjqs-2019-009420 PMID: 31391313

Leape, L. L., Bates, D. W., Cullen, D. J., Cooper, J., Demonaco, H. J., Gallivan, T., & Edmondson, A. (1995). Systems Analysis of Adverse Drug Events. *Journal of the American Medical Association*, *274*(1), 35–43. DOI: 10.1001/jama.1995.03530010049034 PMID: 7791256

Levine, S., & Cohen, M. R. (2007). Preventing medication errors in pediatric and neonatal patients. In Cohen, M. R. (Ed.), *Medication Errors* (2nd ed., pp. 469–492). The American Pharmacists Association. DOI: 10.21019/9781582120928.ch17

Lizano-Díez, I., Figueiredo-Escribá, C., Piñero-López, M., Lastra, C. F., Mariño, E. L., & Modamio, P. (2020). Prevention strategies to identify LASA errors: Building and sustaining a culture of patient safety. *BMC Health Services Research, 20*(1), 63. DOI: 10.1186/s12913-020-4922-3 PMID: 31996197

Lowe, A., Hamilton, M., Greenall, B. M. J., Ma, J., Dhalla, I., & Persaud, N. (2017). Fatal overdoses involving hydromorphone and morphine among inpatients: A case series. *CMAJ Open, 5*(1), E184–e189. DOI: 10.9778/cmajo.20160013 PMID: 28401133

Medscape. (2000). *Prescribing alert sent to pharmacists about lamictal and lamisil.* Retrieved 22 May from https://www.medscape.com/viewarticle/411972?form=fpf

National Coordinating Council for Medication Error Reporting and Prevention (NCC MERP). (2022). *Types of Medication Errors*. Retrieved 11 Oct from https://www.nccmerp.org/types-medication-errors

Naunton, M., Gardiner, H. R., & Kyle, G. (2015). Look-alike, sound-alike medication errors: A novel case concerning a Slow-Na, Slow-K prescribing error. *International Medical Case Reports Journal, 8*, 51–53. DOI: 10.2147/IMCRJ.S78637 PMID: 25733932

News, N. B. C. (2005). *Zyprexa, Zyrtec similarities causing confusion*. Retrieved 15 Apr from https://www.nbcnews.com/health/health-news/zyprexa-zyrtec-similarities-causing-confusion-flna1c9439578

Ostini, R., Roughead, E. E., Kirkpatrick, C. M., Monteith, G. R., & Tett, S. E. (2012). Quality use of medicines—Medication safety issues in naming; look-alike, sound-alike medicine names. *The International Journal of Pharmacy Practice, 20*(6), 349–357. DOI: 10.1111/j.2042-7174.2012.00210.x PMID: 23134093

Pharmaceutical Services Division. M. o. H. M. (2012). *Guide on handling look alike, sound alike medications*. Retrieved 25 May from https://pharmacy.moh.gov.my/sites/default/files/document-upload/guide-handling-lasa.pdf

Pollak, P. T., Pierce, S., & Cooke, C. (1998). Amrinone and amiodarone: Serious confusion in the intravenous line. *Archives of Internal Medicine, 158*(2), 193–194. DOI: 10.1001/archinte.158.2.193 PMID: 9448563

Puttilerpong, C. (2006). System approach to resolve and prevent mediation error: experience of Prachuapkhirikhan hospital. In Chulavatnatol S, Montakantikul P, Chindavijak B, Suksomboon N, & S. T (Eds.), *Pharmacist and quality medication system* (pp. 38-61). The Association of Hospital Pharmacist (Thailand).

Rodziewicz, T. L., Houseman, B., & Hipskind, J. E. (2023). Medical error reduction and prevention. StatPearls Publishing. https://www.ncbi.nlm.nih.gov/books/NBK499956

Roy, P. K. (2001). To err is human, negligence is sin. *Medical Journal, Armed Forces India, 57*(4), 326–328. DOI: 10.1016/S0377-1237(01)80015-0 PMID: 27365633

Sakai, T., & Morimoto, Y. (2022). The history of infectious diseases and medicine. *Pathogens (Basel, Switzerland), 11*(10), 1147. Advance online publication. DOI: 10.3390/pathogens11101147 PMID: 36297204

Samaranayake, N. R., Cheung, D. S., Lam, M. P., Cheung, T. T., Chui, W. C., Wong, I. C., & Cheung, B. M. (2014). The effectiveness of a 'Do Not Use' list and perceptions of healthcare professionals on error-prone abbreviations. *International Journal of Clinical Pharmacy, 36*(5), 1000–1006. DOI: 10.1007/s11096-014-9987-9 PMID: 25098946

Senior Care Consultant Group (SCCG). (2006). *Appendix* 17: *sound alike/look alike medications*. Retrieved 22 May from http://mysccg.com/generalDocuments/Look%20and%20Sound%20Alike%20Meds.pdf

Shaw, K. N., Lillis, K. A., Ruddy, R. M., Mahajan, P. V., Lichenstein, R., Olsen, C. S., & Network, P. E. C. A. R. (2013). Reported medication events in a pediatric emergency research network: Sharing to improve patient safety. *Emergency Medicine Journal : EMJ, 30*(10), 815–819. DOI: 10.1136/emermed-2012-201642 PMID: 23117714

Smith, H. S., & Lesar, T. S. (2011). Analgesic prescribing errors and associated medication characteristics. *The Journal of Pain, 12*(1), 29–40. DOI: 10.1016/j.jpain.2010.04.007 PMID: 21187270

Supapaan, T. S., Napaporn, J., Ruthirakanok, R., Srichathum, S., Songmuang, A., & Pitchayajittipong, C. (2024). Look-alike sound-alike (LASA) medication errors in Thai hospitals. *Pharmacy Practice, 22*(1), 2886.

Supapaan, T. S., Somsorn, S., Saensupha, N., Songmuang, T., Songmuang, A., Jaturapattarawong, A., & Napaporn, J. (2024). Development of drug information and drug images identification database for supporting the medical management system at Warinchamrab hospital. *Pharmacy Practice*, *22*(4). Advance online publication. DOI: 10.18549/PharmPract.2024.4.3057

Supapaan, T. S., Songmuang, A., Napaporn, J., Sangsukwow, P., Boonrod, P., Intarapongsakul, P., Jaturapattarawong, A., & Pitchayajittipong, C. (2024). Look-alike/sound-alike medication errors: An in-depth examination through a hospital case study. *Pharmacy Practice*, *22*(2), 2959. DOI: 10.18549/PharmPract.2024.2.2959

Tariq, R. A., Vashisht, R., Sinha, A., & Scherbak, Y. (2021). Medication dispensing errors and prevention. In *StatPearls*. StatPearls Publishing.

The Academy of Managed Care Pharmacy (AMCP). (2019). *Medication errors*. Retrieved 16 Apr from https://www.amcp.org/about/managed-care-pharmacy-101/concepts-managed-care-pharmacy/medication-errors

The Associated Press. (2005). *Zyprexa, Zyrtec similarities causing confusion*. Retrieved 8 Feb from https://www.nbcnews.com/health/health-news/zyprexa-zyrtec-similarities-causing-confusion-flna1c9439578

The Institute for Safe Medication Practices Canada (ISMP Canada). (2016). *Drug labeling and the application of TALLman lettering project report*. Retrieved 15 June from https://www.ismp-canada.org/download/TALLman/TALLmanLettering-ProjectReport.pdf

The Institute for Safe Medication Practices (ISMP). (2011). *ISMP list of high-alert medications in community/ambulatory healthcare*. Retrieved 20 March from https://www.ismp.org/sites/default/files/attachments/2017-11/highAlert-community.pdf

The Institute for Safe Medication Practices (ISMP). (2015). *ISMP's list of confused drug names*. Retrieved 16 Apr from https://www.ismp.org/sites/default/files/attachments/2017-11/confuseddrugnames%2802.2015%29.pdf?

The Institute for Safe Medication Practices (ISMP). (2019). *ISMP list of confused drug names*. Retrieved 11 Oct from https://www.ismp.org/recommendations/confused-drug-names-list

The Institute for Safe Medication Practices (ISMP). (2023a). *FDA and ISMP lists of look-alike drug names with recommended tall man (mixed case) letters*. Retrieved 16 Apr from https://www.ismp.org/system/files/resources/2023-01/ISMP_Tallman_Letters_012523_MS5087%20%282%29.pdf

The Institute for Safe Medication Practices (ISMP). (2023b). *List of confused drug names*. Retrieved 16 Apr from https://www.ismp.org/recommendations/confused-drug-names-list

The Institute for Safe Medication Practices (ISMP). (2023c). *Obstetrical patient receives ampule of digoxin instead of BUPivacaine for spinal anesthesia*. Retrieved 05 Sep from https://www.ismp.org/resources/obstetrical-patient-receives-ampule-digoxin-instead-bupivacaine-spinal-anesthesia

The Institute for Safe Medication Practices (ISMP). (2024). *ISMP list of error-prone abbreviations, symbols, and dose designations*. Retrieved 12 April from https://www.ismp.org/recommendations/error-prone-abbreviations-list?check_logged_in=1

The Pennsylvania Patient Safety Advisory. (2004). Medication errors linked to drug name confusion. *PA PSRS Patient Saf Advis*, *1*(4), 7–8.

The Pennsylvania Patient Safety Advisory. (2005). Complexity of insulin therapy. *PA PSRS Patient Saf Advis*, *2*(2), 30–31.

The Pennsylvania Patient Safety Advisory. (2006). hydrOXYzine and hydrALAzine mix-ups. *PA PSRS Patient Saf Advis*, *3*(2), 21.

The Pennsylvania Patient Safety Advisory. (2007). Inadvertent mix-up of morphine and hydromorphone: A potent error. *PA PSRS Patient Saf Advis*, *4*(3), 86–88.

Tseng, H. Y., Wen, C. F., Lee, Y. L., Jeng, K. C., & Chen, P. L. (2018). Dispensing errors from look-alike drug trade names. *European Journal of Hospital Pharmacy : Science and Practice*, *25*(2), 96–99. DOI: 10.1136/ejhpharm-2016-001019 PMID: 31156995

U.S. Department of Health and Human Services Food and Drug Administration. (1999). *Guidance for industry: container closure systems for packaging human drugs and biologics*. Retrieved 11 July from https://www.fda.gov/media/70788/download

U.S. Department of Health and Human Services Food and Drug Administration. (2022). *Safety considerations for container labels and carton labeling design to minimize medication errors guidance for industry*. Retrieved 11 July from https://www.fda.gov/media/158522/download

Wheeler, A. J., Scahill, S., Hopcroft, D., & Stapleton, H. (2018). Reducing medication errors at transitions of care is everyone's business. *Australian Prescriber*, *41*(3), 73–77. DOI: 10.18773/austprescr.2018.021 PMID: 29922001

Wongboonnak, P. (2018). Look-alike sound-alike drugs situation in Thailand. *HCU Journal of Health Science*, *22*, 205–216.

World Health Organization. (2007). *WHO launches 'Nine patient safety solutions'.* Retrieved 12 Aug from https://www.who.int/news/item/02-05-2007-who-launches-nine-patient-safety-solutions

World Health Organization. (2014). *Reporting and learning systems for medication errors: the role of pharmacovigilance centers.* Retrieved 19 June from https://iris.who.int/bitstream/handle/10665/137036/9789241507943_eng.pdf?sequence=1

World Health Organization. (2017). *Medication without harm.* Retrieved 10 Feb from https://www.who.int/initiatives/medication-without-harm

World Health Organization. (2021). Toward eliminating avoidable harm in health care. *Global patient safety action plan*, 2030.

World Health Organization. (2022). *WHO launches' Nine patient safety solutions'.* Retrieved 2 July from https://www.who.int/news/item/02-05-2007-who-launches-nine-patient-safety-solutions

World Health Organization. (2023). *Medication safety for look-alike, sound-alike medicines.* World Health Organization. Retrieved 3 June from https://iris.who.int/bitstream/handle/10665/373495/9789240058897-eng.pdf?sequence=1

Zafar, R., & Raza, M. L. (2020). Assessment of look-alike, sound-alike and read-alike (LASARA) medicine-errors in pharmacy. *Journal of the College of Physicians and Surgeons—Pakistan : JCPSP, 30*(4), 425–428. DOI: 10.29271/jcpsp.2020.04.425 PMID: 32513366

ABBREVIATIONS

ADC: Automated Dispensing Cabinet
ADR: Adverse Drug Reaction
CPOE: Computerized Provider Order Entry
CR: Controlled-Release Formulation
e-MAR: Electronic Medication Administration Record
e-Rx: Electronic Prescription
GI: Gastrointestinal
H_2-blocker: Histamine-2 Receptor Antagonist
ICU: Intensive Care Unit
ISMP: Institute for Safe Medication Practices
LASA: Look-Alike, Sound-Alike
μ-opioid/κ- opioid: Mu-/Kappa-Opioid Receptor Agonist Subclasses
NSAID: Non-Steroidal Anti-Inflammatory Drug

OR: Operating Room
PA-PSRS: Pennsylvania Patient Safety Reporting System
PPSA: Pennsylvania Patient Safety Authority
SSRI: Selective Serotonin-Reuptake Inhibitor
WHO: World Health Organization

Chapter 2
Integrated Strategies for Preventing Look–Alike Sound–Alike (LASA) Medication Errors

ABSTRACT

Look-alike sound-alike (LASA) medication errors continue to pose a risk to patients. A multipronged prevention strategy should incorporate regulatory protection, technological measures, and humanistic practices. To minimize risks, before products are put on the market, regulators and manufacturers are required to apply name screening algorithms, tall man lettering, and unique packaging. Midstream healthcare protection is provided with electronic prescribing alerts, barcode verification, and orchestrated double checks. Patients should be empowered to avoid making mistakes beyond the clinical setting by using clear labeling, mobile applications, and health literacy programs. Real-world evidence and international guidelines aid in harmonized practices and constant monitoring. The cooperation of regulators, manufacturers, healthcare professionals, and patients is the key to reducing the harm associated with LASA medication errors.

INTRODUCTION

A multifaceted approach to regulation and an attitude of a manufacturer could help to avoid LASA errors. LASA control is also revealed and mitigated by regulatory authorities, such as the FDA, which leads to the need to unite on a global scale to develop distinct names for new medicines and consistent safe standards (Lizano-Díez et al., 2020; Marovino et al., 2022). Manufacturing companies should use tall

DOI: 10.4018/979-8-3373-5478-1.ch002

man lettering, color coding, and barcoding to distinguish similar drug names and packaging (Bryan et al., 2021a; Siddiqui, 2020).

Regulators such as the FDA must insist on premarket reviews to eliminate drug name confusion prior to launching a product (Trbovich & Hyland, 2017). Barcode systems and e-prescriptions minimize LASA dispensing and administration errors as well (Mulac et al., 2021; Sriboonruang & Rattanamahattana, 2022). Dispensing errors have been linked to similar packaging, so manufacturers should redesign it to reduce confusion (Mulac et al., 2021; Rider et al., 2019; U.S. Department of Health and Human Services Food and Drug Administration (FDA), 2015; U.S. Department of Health and Human Services Food and Drug Administration, 2016).

Healthcare providers should also be taught about LASA drug risks and preventive measures (World Health Organization, 2023). A comprehensive list of LASA drug pairs, with their generic names, therapeutic classes, and FDA-approved indications, can aid in their differentiation and minimize errors (Bryan et al., 2015; World Health Organization, 1997, 2017b, 2023). Close interactions between regulatory authorities, pharmaceutical companies, and clinicians play a crucial role in minimizing the risks of LASA medications and enhancing patient safety (Lizano-Díez et al., 2020; Rodziewicz et al., 2023).

Objectives of the Chapter

The aims of this chapter are as follows:

(1) To characterize regulatory and manufacturer prestream controls, such as name-screening algorithms, tall man lettering, unique packaging, and barcoding standards that help eliminate LASA errors prior to the medicines entering clinical practice.
(2) To evaluate interventions in health systems and the workforce to reduce LASA errors in the prescribing, transcribing, dispensing, and administration of medications, including electronic prescribing notifications, double checks, and barcode verification.
(3) To facilitate poststream measures, which include patient-centered programs, labeling, mobile applications, health literacy interventions, and shared incident reporting networks to ensure vigilance and enhance LASA safety following dispensing.

Organization of the Chapter

This chapter discusses LASA medication errors' global impact and the need for an integrated safety framework. It then discusses regulatory and manufacturer-level interventions such as name screening algorithms, tall man lettering, distinctive packaging, and barcoding to reduce LASA risks before medications enter the clinical setting. Medical systems use mid-stream safeguards such as electronic prescribing alerts, pharmacist verification, and bedside barcode scanning to prevent errors during prescribing, transcribing, dispensing, and administration. Thereafter, the chapter discusses poststream safety strategies such as patient-centered labeling, mobile apps, health literacy programs, and shared incident reporting networks. The chapter summarizes key takeaways and emphasizes the need for regulators, manufacturers, healthcare

BUILDING BLOCKS OF LASA SAFETY: THE PRE-, MID-, AND POST-STREAM MODEL

The medication use process can be divided into three simple phases: before a product enters clinical use (prestream), during prescription and administration (midstream), and after the patient receives the medication (poststream), as shown in Figure 1.

Prestream Controls

Prior to market release, regulatory and manufacturer measures identify and mitigate LASA risk. Name screening algorithms such as the FDA's Phonetic and Orthographic Computer Analysis tool flag high-risk look-alike or sound-alike name pairs (Larmené-Beld et al., 2018; U.S. Department of Health and Human Services Food and Drug Administration (FDA), 2021).

Tall-man lettering (for example, predniSONE versus predniSOLONE) is used to emphasize visual differences (Grissinger, 2012; Iglesias Gomez et al., 2022). Differentiation is also enhanced by unique packaging attributes (e.g., color codes and special vial shape). Standardized barcode requirements: The barcode requirements require that each unit has a distinct machine-readable identifier.

Midstream Safeguards

In medical practice, computerized provider order entry systems have built-in LASA alerts prescribers to verify orders that are similar to other drug names (Davis & Cohen, 1995; Devine et al., 2005; Galanter et al., 2014). The use of the double checks only means that the second clinician should verify the prescriptions at the pharmacy and at the bedside. With respect to dispensing and administration, barcode checking is used to compare the scanned products with electronic orders to identify discrepancies in real time.

Poststream Strategies

Self-verification is empowered by clear, patient-friendly labeling (both tall men and full generic names) after patients have left care facilities.

Mobile health applications provide notifications and interactive learning to support proper usage. Health literacy programs recommend materials according to different reading levels. Real-world LASA events are captured by shared incident reporting networks, which result in continuous improvement (Grissinger, 2012, 2013; Lizano-Díez et al., 2020; Supapaan et al., 2023; Veronin, 2011).

Figure 1. Three-stage LASA error prevention model: prestream measures, midstream controls, and poststream plans

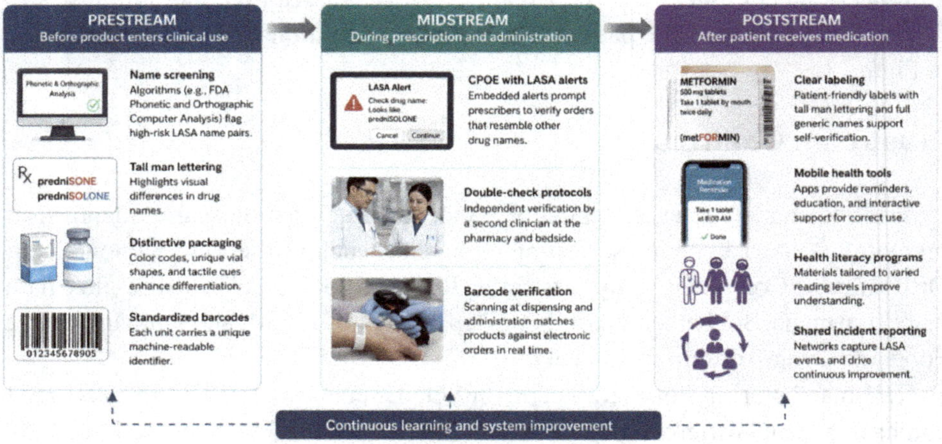

PRE-STREAM: REGULATORY AND MANUFACTURER LEVEL

The rising rate of LASA medication errors is a worldwide issue that is becoming more pronounced because of the ever-growing and diversifying pharmaceutical market. Patient safety is at stake, as these errors are made when medications with similar names or appearances are mixed together. To address this issue, regulators worldwide have taken their drug registration work more seriously, with particular emphasis on issues such as drug names, appearances, and packs. These rules, however, may differ in their size and urgency in different countries (Bryan et al., 2015; Bryan et al., 2021a; Bryan et al., 2021b; Cohen et al., 2007).

Regulatory Approaches

LASA medical errors require excellent regulation and coordinated approaches in place. Drug naming and labeling should be standardized to reduce misconfusion and to improve patient safety via International Nonproprietary Names (INNs), according to the WHO. The names of NNs must be specific and unambiguous in terms of their sounding and orthography (reflection of pharmacological classes via standardized stems, e.g., cephalosporins, cef-; local anesthetics, and -caine) and have no unreserved meaning (World Health Organization, 1997, 2017a).

Another important strategy is tall man lettering, which capitalizes on certain letters to make a difference between similar names of drug names (e.g., hydrOXYzine vs. hydrALAzine). Most of the leading organizations, including the WHO, the Food and Drug Administration (FDA), the European Medicines Agency (EMA) and the Institute for Safe Medication Practices (ISMP) of the U.S. and Canada, advocate this practice (European Medicines Agency (EMA), 2021; The Institute for Safe Medication Practices (ISMP), 2023a, 2023b, 2024; The Institute for Safe Medication Practices Canada (ISMP Canada), 2016; U.S. Department of Health and Human Services Food and Drug Administration (FDA), 2020). The ISMP suggests that drug prescribing, dispensing, and administration should be made safer and that comes with the use of tall man lettering lists.

Countries have implemented different strategies to curb LASA errors:

In Malaysia, the Ministry of Health has implemented some of these measures, including tall man lettering, adding more warning labels to look-alike drugs, and updating the LASA drug lists frequently (Pharmaceutical Services Division, 2012). These measures assist health care providers and patients in differentiating between closely related drugs, thus minimizing the risk of mistakes.

Canada has a rigorous, multistage review process of brand names with Health Canada. This comprises parallel evaluations, market research, and evidence-based reviews. In Canada, special packaging design and the need to report incidents are also obligatory and result in the constant enhancement of medication safety (Government of Canada, 2014; Health Canada, 2014; Marilyn Schwartz, 2007; The Institute for Safe Medication Practices Canada (ISMP Canada), 2016).

To ensure that the drug names are not confusing, the Pharmaceuticals and Medical Devices Agency (PMDA) of Japan has carried out comprehensive scrutiny of drug names submitted by pharmaceutical companies. The PMDA reinforces transparent labeling and packaging to enhance patient safety. Pharmaceutical companies are required to submit detailed records and reasons for their proposed drug names (Pharmaceuticals and Medical Devices Agency (PMDA), 2014, 2017, 2024).

The Central Drugs Standard Control Organization (CDSCO) in India encourages unique drug names in the approval process and emphasizes pharmacovigilance and legible prescriptions. The country is, however, affected by issues such as poor enforcement, lack of awareness, and a prevalence of similar brand names. To eliminate these gaps, specialists suggest more frequent enforcement of guidelines, the implementation of public awareness campaigns, the use of technologies such as computerized provider order entry (CPOE) and the bar-code medication administration (BCMA), and the strengthening of cooperation between stakeholders to improve the pharmacovigilance system (Neelakantan et al., 2024; Thakur DS & Prashant RT, 2024).

A national LASA list was compiled in 2023 by the Ministry of Public Health (MoPH) of Lebanon and was compiled in collaboration with marketing authorization holders (MAHs). The publicly reflected list is on the MoPH site, and any stakeholders, including healthcare professionals or pharmacovigilance units, can comment on such a list to amend it. This program highlights Lebanon's commitment to transparency, safety, and the continuous advancement of medication practices (Ministry of Public Health Republic of Lebanon, 2024). .

These international cases justify the importance of governance principles and permanent monitoring in the erosion of LASA mistakes. Regulatory bodies can significantly increase the safety of drugs through the introduction of standardized names, distinctive packaging, and close focus, which can help prevent patients from being harmed by manageable errors (World Health Organization, 2023).

Manufacturer Level

Manufacturers contribute greatly to LASA medication error prevention. Manufacturers can minimize such errors by making strategic decisions. Manufacturer perspectives and regulatory collaboration are covered in this section.

1. Proactive Name Selection and Testing
    - Phonetic and orthographic analysis: Manufacturers should use phonetic and orthographic computer analysis tools for drug naming. These tools examine the similarities of proposed drug names to already invented drug names on the basis of visual appearance and sound as a way of detecting LASA errors. Such a preventive initiative is needed not to have confusing drug names approved and marketed (Karet, 2023; Shah et al., 2017; U.S. Department of Health and Human Services Food and Drug Administration (FDA), 2020, 2021).

- International collaboration: Cooperation with other international/global naming organizations such as the WHO International Nonproprietary Names (INNs) initiative can help to avoid confusing names. Collaboration helps develop drug names that are not similar to existing names (Gopakumar KM & Syam N, 2007; World Health Organization, 2017a, 2023).

2. Packaging and Labeling Innovations
   - Tall man lettering (TML): Capitalizes letters in drug names to distinguish between similar names. This method reduces LASA errors and should be used on product labels, especially for high-risk medications identified as LASA pairs (Bryan et al., 2015; Filik et al., 2004; The Institute for Safe Medication Practices (ISMP), 2023a; The Institute for Safe Medication Practices Canada (ISMP Canada), 2016).
   - Distinctive packaging designs: Manufacturers should develop original packaging designs to distinguish products through their appearance. To minimize dispensing mistakes, the names of drugs together with their degree of strength must be clearly labeled (Cohen, 2007b; Emmerton & Rizk, 2012; Endestad et al., 2016; Filik et al., 2006).
   - Clear labeling and information: Have clear labeling and information, including brand and generic names with the right differentiation. Instructions on how to use the drug and warnings against LASA errors in relation to healthcare professionals and patients should also be outlined in the packaging (Cohen, 2007a, 2007b).
3. Regulatory Compliance and Standards
   - Adherence to guidelines: Manufacturers should be guided by the regulation directions of health agencies such as the U.S. FDA, EMA, and WHO. In some cases, drug naming, drug labeling, and drug packaging guidelines may incorporate LASA error prevention to reduce the occurrence of errors (European Medicines Agency (EMA), 2021; U.S. Department of Health and Human Services Food and Drug Administration (FDA), 2014; U.S. Department of Health and Human Services Food and Drug Administration, 2016; US Food and Drug Administration (US FDA), 2015).
   - Continuous monitoring and reporting: Postmarketing surveillance is necessary to record actual LASA errors. Manufacturers must possess effective medication error-related data collection and analysis systems and collaborate with regulatory bodies to address this problem (Jarernsiripornkul et al., 2009; Srisuriyachanchai et al., 2023).
4. Education and Training

- Healthcare professional training: Manufacturers can play a role in eliminating LASA errors by training healthcare professionals about the risks and possible prevention strategies of medication. This also incorporates TML utilization and reading of training labels (Rahman & Parvin, 2015; WHO Collaborating Centre for Patient Safety Solutions, 2007; World Health Organization, 2023).
- Patient engagement: Patients should be aware of their medications and the risks of LASA, and this helps raise their awareness (Supapaan et al., 2023; World Health Organization, 2024). Pharmaceutical companies contribute to patient education in the use of drug verification/LASA alerts (Jitanapakarn P et al., 2023; Khumsikiew et al., 2023; Sharma et al., 2018; World Health Organization, 2023).

5. Collaboration with Regulatory Bodies
   - Development and implementation of tools: Manufacturers should collaborate with regulatory authorities to develop and use tools such as phonetic and orthographic computer analysis (POCA). This tool measures the phonetic and orthographic similarities between proposed brand names and existing names to avoid LASA drugs (Karet, 2023; Rider et al., 2019; U.S. Department of Health and Human Services Food and Drug Administration (FDA), 2021).
   - Regulatory reviews: Monitoring trademark search reports with regulatory bodies prevents misleading brand names from being approved. This collaboration is based on high drug naming standards and LASA error reduction. Manufacturers are encouraged to endorse and use international standards with regard to drug labeling and packaging to lessen LASA mistakes. Playing an important role in international regulatory deliberations and the best practices implementation of medication safety (Cohen, 2007b, 2007c; Cohen & Davis, 1994a; Cohen et al., 2007; Cohen & Smetzer, 2018; Kalola & Dean, 2019).
   - Global standards and practices: Working with regulators and implementing targeted strategies can significantly reduce LASA errors. Medication safety requires regulators, healthcare providers, and manufacturers to work together (WHO Collaborating Centre for Patient Safety Solutions, 2007; World Health Organization, 2017b, 2023).

Manufacturer-level LASA prevention incorporates proactive name testing, distinctive labeling and packaging, and ongoing safety monitoring, as depicted in Figure 2.

Figure 2. Preventing LASA errors: strategic plans for drug manufacturers

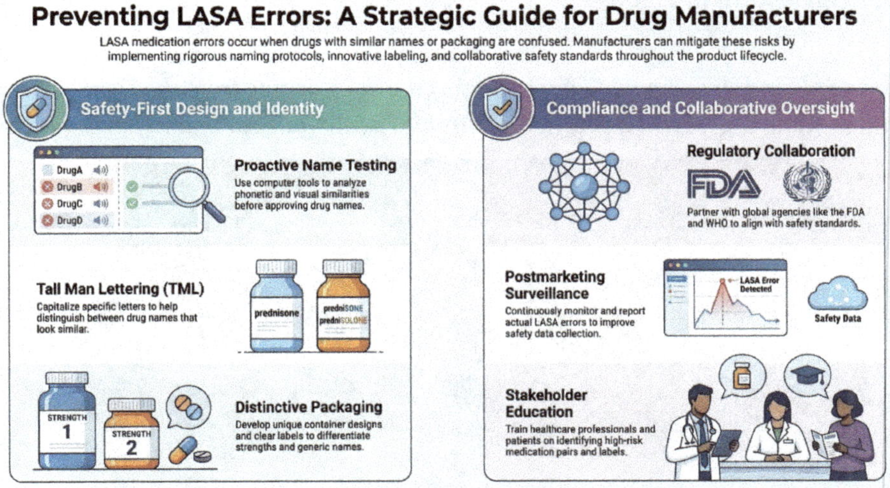

This figure describes the manufacturer-level approaches to prevent LASA medication errors, such as proactive testing of drug names on the basis of phonetic and orthographic analysis, the use of tall man lettering, and the design of unique packaging and labeling. It also emphasizes the need to collaborate to ensure the ongoing safety monitoring of products through regulatory collaboration, postmarketing surveillance, and stakeholder education.

Importance of Postmarketing and Pharmacovigilance in Preventing LASA Medication Errors

Pharmacovigilance and postmarketing surveillance are essential to the safety and efficacy of drugs after they hit the market. These processes are crucial for identifying and preventing LASA medication errors, which can harm patients (Jarernsiripornkul et al., 2009; Jeetu & Anusha, 2010; Raj et al., 2019; Rodziewicz et al., 2023; Srisuriyachanchai et al., 2023; World Health Organization, 2023).

A northeastern Thai survey of 330 households addressed the sampling of three type 1 drug stores, one type 2 drug store and 28 retail stores on LASA drugs. The findings demonstrated that most LASA drugs were harmful because of their appearance. The most frequent medications were medications of the same companies with similar names and a look at the packaging but varying strengths and doses. The findings indicated that LASA drugs in the community pose similar problems to those in hospitals because of the design of drug names, labels, and packaging

(Khontum & Chanthapasa, 2021). Examples of LASA drugs in community pharmacies are shown in Figure 3.

Figure 3. Examples of name and/or packaging similarities from the same company with the same ingredient but different strengths found in community pharmacies.

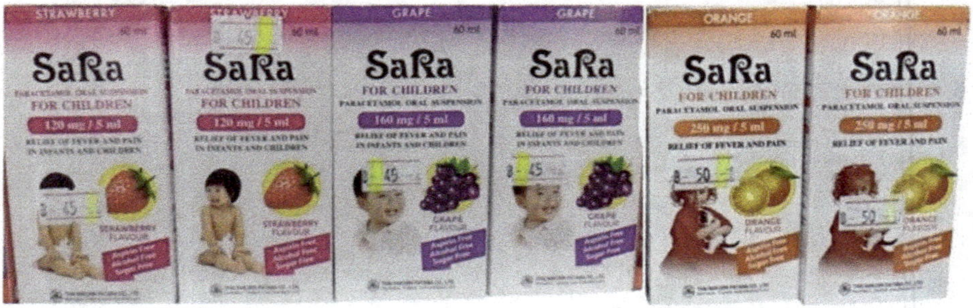

A. Paracetamol oral suspension in different flavors and strengths for children.

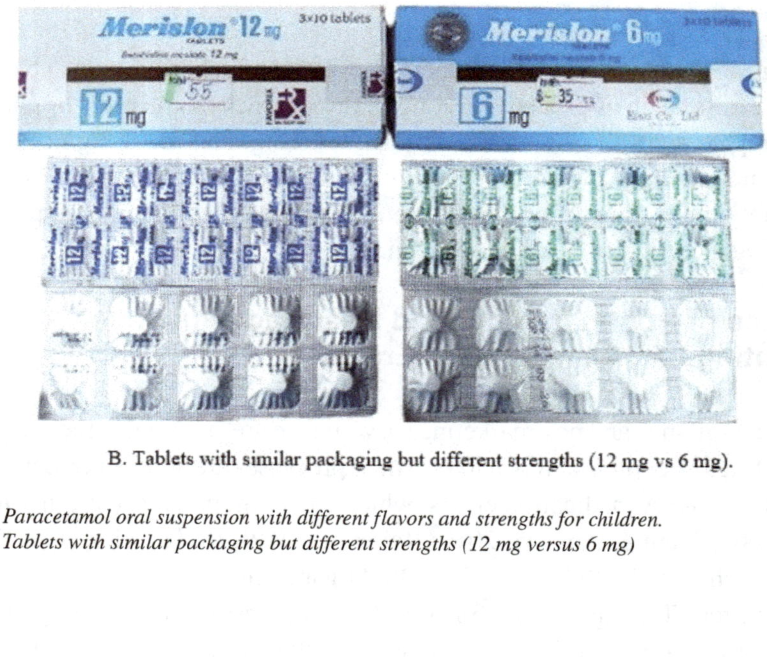

B. Tablets with similar packaging but different strengths (12 mg vs 6 mg).

A. Paracetamol oral suspension with different flavors and strengths for children.
B. Tablets with similar packaging but different strengths (12 mg versus 6 mg)

MID-STREAM: HEALTHCARE SYSTEM AND PERSONNEL

Responsibility and Accountability in Medication Management

Healthcare professionals across all units involved in the medication process, from prescribing to monitoring patient outcomes, are crucial in preventing medication errors. Physicians assess and review patient history, medication use, and allergies before they prescribe medications. They are responsible for ensuring that prescriptions are clear and appropriate and use computerized systems to eliminate errors in transcription (Rodziewicz et al., 2023; World Health Organization, 2023).

Pharmacists play a critical role in purchasing, storing, preparing, and dispensing medications. They evaluate the appropriateness of prescriptions, especially when there are concerns about dosage, method of administration, or potential allergic reactions. Pharmacists ensure that all medications are checked for accuracy and safety before being provided to the patient (Sinha, 2014).

To verify the drugs dispensed against physician orders, nurses adhere to the following 10 rights of medication administration: the right patient, right drug, right dose, right route, right time, right documentation, right reason, right response, right education, and right to refuse. It has a systematic design that minimizes mistakes in the administration process and strengthens accountability. Nurses monitor patients' adverse reactions and promptly report them to prescribers, facilitating timely interventions (Vaismoradi et al., 2020). The remaining healthcare personnel should follow the established rules and procedures to provide proper and full-fledged communication and transfer of medication-related data (World Health Organization, 2023).

Medication Management and LASA Drug Safety

Between the initial electronic order placed by the physician and the last scan on the bedside by the nurse, a medication undergoes four closely connected workflows: prescribing, transcribing, dispensing, and administering. Failures at any stage allow LASA products to pass, adding to the number of thousands of avoidable adverse events worldwide (World Health Organization, 2023). Thus, best-practice guidance layer technology (e.g., CPOE with LASA alerts and barcode checks) is superior to human double checks and environmentally quiet zones (American Society of Health-System Pharmacists, 2009, 2011; Galanter et al., 2014; The Institute for Safe Medication Practices (ISMP), 2022).

Table 1 offers a systematic description of the important LASA safety controls at each step in the process of medication use. It describes the necessary measures, the relevant system-wide protection, and a feasible LASA-specific precaution in prescribing, transcribing, dispensing, and administering LASA. This matrix is to be placed on clinical dashboards, embedded in hospital policy manuals, and in medication preparation areas so that LASA safety is visible and a constant reminder.

Table 1. Significant LASA safety measures throughout the medication-use process

Medication-use stage	Key action	System-level safeguard	LASA-specific tip
Prescribing	Standardized electronic orders	CPOE with embedded LASA alerts; direct link to the hospital formulary	Apply tall man lettering in order sets
Transcribing	Double-entry or Electronic Medication Administration Record (e-MAR) import	Autoprompt for a second checker before final save	Flag orders when names share ≥ 3 letters *and* identical strength
Dispensing	Barcode and image match verification	Split-shelf storage; color-coded shelf labels	Mark LASA items with red trays or shelf flags
Administration	Ten Rights with bedside barcode scan	"Quiet zone" plus buddy check for high-alert drugs	Wristband scan flashes extra LASA alert

(American Society of Health-System Pharmacists, 2009, 2011; The Institute for Safe Medication Practices (ISMP), 2022)

To support this process visually, Figure 4 depicts the funnel-shaped bands of sequential safeguards along the medication-use continuum, representing how several interventions, acting together, decrease the risk of prescription-to-administration error. In addition, Figure 5 addresses a LASA prescribing safety pyramid, which focuses on the tiered approach, beginning with regulatory underpinnings and progressing to real-time clinical decision support and, finally, the role of layered and proactive defenses in medication safety.

Figure 4. Funnel-based bands show step-by-step defenses along the medication-use continuum—prescribing (standardized electronic orders and alerts), transcribing (checking with two entries), dispensing (barcode and image match), and administration (bedside barcode scan)

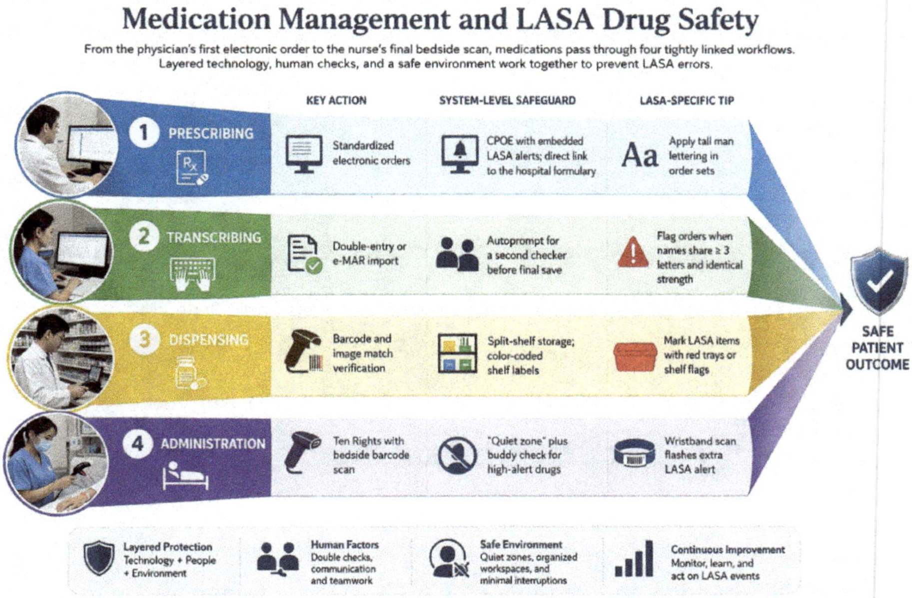

Medication Management and LASA Drug Safety
From the physician's first electronic order to the nurse's final bedside scan, medications pass through four tightly linked workflows.
Layered technology, human checks, and a safe environment work together to prevent LASA errors.
KEY ACTION
SYSTEM-LEVEL SAFEGUARD
LASA-SPECIFIC TIP
1 PRESCRIBING
Standardized electronic orders
CPOE with embedded LASA alerts; direct link to the hospital formulary
Aa
Apply tall man lettering in order sets
2 TRANSCRIBING
Double-entry or e-MAR import
Autoprompt for a second checker before final save
Flag orders when names share ≥ 3 letters and identical strength
3 DISPENSING
Barcode and image match verification
Split-shelf storage; color-coded shelf labels
Mark LASA items with red trays or shelf flags
4 ADMINISTRATION
Ten Rights with bedside barcode scan
"Quiet zone" plus buddy check for high-alert drugs
Wristband scan flashes extra LASA alert
SAFE PATIENT OUTCOME
Layered Protection
Technology + People + Environment
Human Factors
Double checks, communication and teamwork
Safe Environment
Quiet zones, organized workspaces, and minimal interruptions
Continuous Improvement
Monitor, learn, and act on LASA events

Figure 5. Safety pyramid for prescribing LASA medications

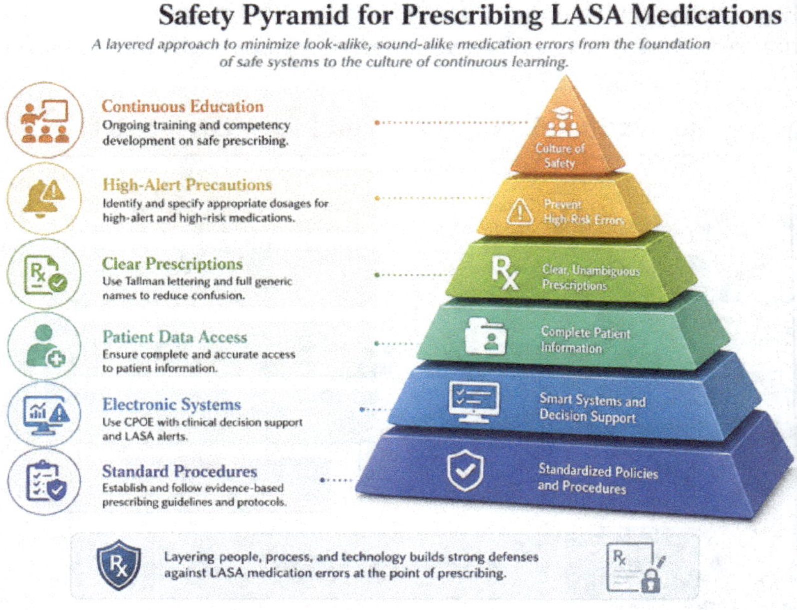
Safety Pyramid for Prescribing LASA Medications
A layered approach to minimize look-alike, sound-alike medication errors from the foundation of safe systems to the culture of continuous learning.
Continuous Education
Ongoing training and competency development on safe prescribing.
High-Alert Precautions
Identify and specify appropriate dosages for high-alert and high-risk medications.
Clear Prescriptions
Use Tallman lettering and full generic names to reduce confusion.
Patient Data Access
Ensure complete and accurate access to patient information.
Electronic Systems
Use CPOE with clinical decision support and LASA alerts.
Standard Procedures
Establish and follow evidence-based prescribing guidelines and protocols.
Culture of Safety
Prevent High-Risk Errors
Clear, Unambiguous Prescriptions
Complete Patient Information
Smart Systems and Decision Support
Standardized Policies and Procedures
Layering people, process, and technology builds strong defenses against LASA medication errors at the point of prescribing.

Tables 2–5 provide an overview of LASA-specific safeguards in every phase of the medication workflow. Table 2 is concerned with safeguarding prescriptions such as standard procedures, large fonts, full access to patient information, and clear written prescriptions to minimize ambiguity and thus appropriate selection. The safeguards in transcription, such as electronic systems, staff training, standard terminology, and peer review, are discussed in Table 3 to identify errors at the initial stages. Table 4 presents dispensing protection measures such as barcode scanning, systematized storage, verification measures, and employee training so that the right medication is given to the right patient. Table 5 details administration protection, such as real-time bedside scanning, the Ten Rights of Administration, silent workspaces, and nursing verification checks, to detect errors prior to reaching the patient. The combination of interventions presented in Tables 3-5 and Figures 6-8 can be viewed as a system-wide intervention that minimizes the number of LASA errors and improves the safety of patients during the care process.

A brief overview of transcription safeguards is provided in Figure 6, with key measures to minimize errors associated with LASAs during the transcription process. The reduction in LASA errors in dispensing involves a combination of verification and environmental and inventory control measures (Figure 7). Finally, Figure 8 illustrates the administrative safeguards needed to reduce LASA errors during administration.

Table 2. Prescribing safeguards for LASA drugs

Details	Hospital System Corrections and Prevention Strategies	LASA Drug Precautions
Standardized prescribing protocols	Use digital order systems (e.g., CPOE) with clinical decision support and tall man lettering. Train physicians on formulary use, abbreviations, and LASA risks.	Prescriptions should include brand and generic names, indication, and use decision support alerts for allergies, interactions, and LASA risks.
Complete patient data access	Ensure prescribers can view allergy history, diagnoses, and prior drug use.	Activate alerts for high-risk drugs and conditions (e.g., G6PD deficiency).
Verify patient identity	Confirm correct patient details before prescribing.	Use clear labels and flag LASA drugs in records.
Clear, complete prescription entries	Use e-prescribing or preprinted systems. Avoid verbal orders; complete all fields including drug, dose, form, and route.	Apply tall man lettering (e.g., hydrOXYzine vs. hydrALAZINE); update and share LASA drug lists regularly.
High-alert drug precautions	Clearly, specify dosing (e.g., mg/week for warfarin).	Provide specific training for high-alert and LASA drugs.
Indications and patient-specific info	Include diagnosis, patient weight, age, and allergies in prescriptions.	—
Decimal and unit precision	Use leading zeros (e.g., 0.1) and avoid trailing zeros (e.g., 1.0).	Write all doses in metric units. Avoid nonstandard abbreviations.
Avoid unsafe abbreviations/trade names	Standardize approved terms; prohibit unsafe short forms or brand-only use.	Conduct regular audits and feedback on LASA errors.
Order documentation and review	Maintain duplicate order sheets and sign all written orders promptly.	Ensure double-checks by pharmacists or other providers.
Physician accountability	Review all prescriptions before finalizing and remain available for clarification.	—

(ASHP; Cohen & Davis, 1993a, 1993b, 1994b; Davis & Cohen, 1994; Lizano-Díez et al., 2020; Puttilerpong C, 2006; World Health Organization, 2023)

Table 3. Transcribing safeguards for LASA drugs

Details	Hospital System Corrections and Prevention Strategies	LASA Drug Precautions
Transcribing errors refer to the discrepancies in the medication transcription process, leading to patients receiving medications that do not match the original prescriber's orders.	Adopt e-prescriptions to reduce human error in prescriptions. Implement computerized physician order entry (CPOE) systems that have in-built error-checking functionality to avoid errors. Regularly audit transcribed orders to quickly point out and address discrepancies.	Look at LASA drugs when checking transcription to ensure that the similar-sounding or similar-looking drug names are not mixed, and the chances of making serious errors are reduced.
Regularly train staff in accurate transcription procedures	Conduct regular training and competency tests for all healthcare personnel involved in the transcription process to guarantee high quality of accuracy and observance of best practices.	Incorporate specific modules on LASA drug transcription, highlighting the importance of precise transcription and verification processes.
Implement double-checking systems for transcribed orders	Create a system that would ensure that transcribed orders are reviewed at least by two qualified healthcare professionals, particularly high-risk medications and LASA drugs, prior to being processed and given to patients.	Use peer-review systems to verify transcriptions of LASA drugs, ensuring an additional layer of safety by having multiple checks before final approval.
Use of standardized terminology and abbreviations in transcriptions	Standardize medical abbreviations and terminologies and enforce the use of the same across all departments to avoid misinterpretation and transcription errors. Keep and distribute a general list of the acceptable abbreviations.	Strictly control the use of abbreviations for LASA drugs, promoting the use of full drug names wherever possible to avoid confusion.

(ASHP; Cohen & Davis, 1993a, 1993b, 1994b; Davis & Cohen, 1994; Lizano-Díez et al., 2020; Puttilerpong C, 2006; World Health Organization, 2023)

Figure 6. Concise overview of transcribing safeguards for LASA drugs

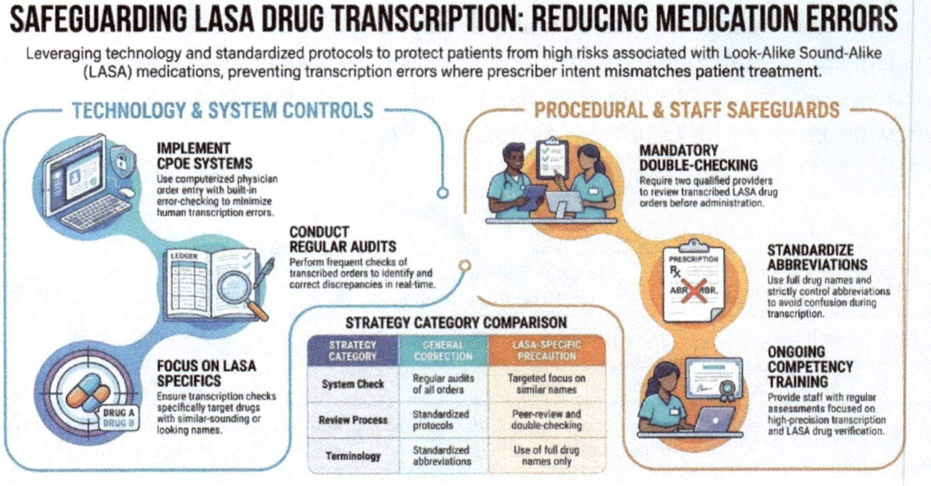

This figure presents key safeguards to reduce transcription-related errors involving look-alike, sound-alike (LASA) medications, combining technology-driven controls (e.g., CPOE systems, audits, and targeted LASA checks) with procedural strategies (e.g., mandatory double-checking, standardized terminology, and staff competency training).

Figure 7. Critical dispensing safeguards for LASA medications

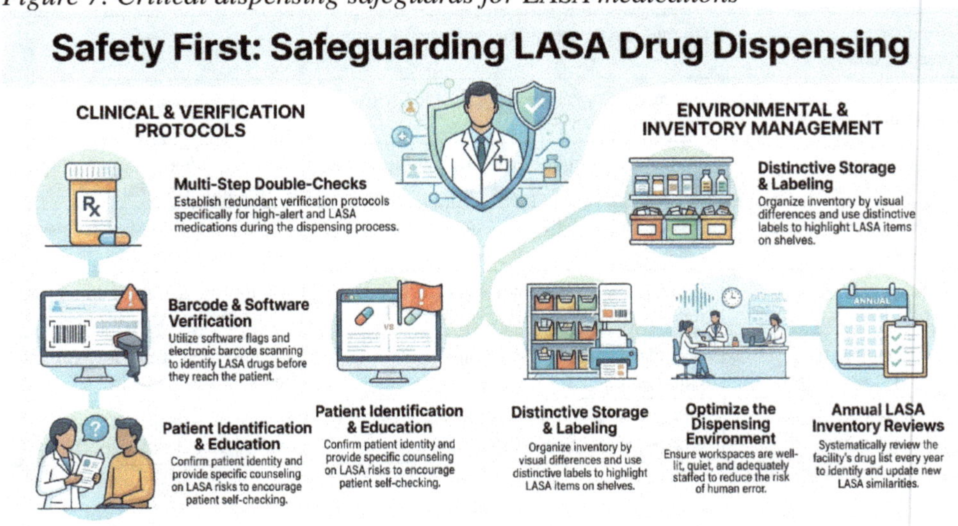

This image captures key dispensing safeguards for look-alike, sound-alike (LASA) medications, combining clinical verification systems (e.g., multistep double checks, barcode matching, and patient identification) with environmental and stock management strategies (e.g., distinctive packaging, workspace optimization, and periodic reviews of LASA medications). These measures complement system-based prevention strategies to prevent medication errors.

Table 4. Dispensing safeguards for LASA drugs

Details	Hospital System Corrections and Prevention Strategies	LASA Drug Precautions
Understand hospital med-use system	Ensure pharmacists are trained on hospital policies, ordering systems, and distribution processes.	Establish double-check protocols for LASA drugs.
Access complete patient data	Provide pharmacists with real-time access to full patient medication profiles.	Use software that flags LASA drugs during dispensing.
Review prescriptions thoroughly	Verify drug choice and dosage; consult prescriber if unclear.	Use barcode and electronic verification for LASA drugs.
Verify patient identity	Confirm patient identity before dispensing.	—
Maintain drug knowledge	Encourage continuous pharmacist education and access to updated resources.	—
Optimize dispensing environment	Ensure well-lit, quiet, organized spaces with adequate staffing.	Use distinctive packaging and labeling for LASA items.
Organize and label inventory clearly	Store medications based on visual/label differences; conduct regular checks.	Review LASA inventory routinely to prevent mix-ups.
Outpatient and inpatient procedures	Use queue systems, allergy checks, and summary stickers for verification.	Apply multistep verification for LASA drugs.
Predispensing verification	Double-check drug name, dose, and labeling.	—
Annual LASA inventory review	Systematically review drug list for LASA similarities each year.	Maintain and update a dedicated LASA list.
Ensure accurate medication delivery	Implement multiple verification points prior to dispensing.	Add redundant checks for high-alert and LASA drugs.
Educate patients and providers	Provide clear medication info and counseling at the point of dispensing.	Highlight LASA-specific risks and identification tips.
Track and learn from errors	Maintain dispensing error logs and review trends regularly.	Monitor LASA-related incidents for continuous improvement.
Store temperature-sensitive drugs properly	Monitor conditions and communicate storage requirements.	Ensure stability of temperature-sensitive LASA meds.
Manage returns and recalls safely	Follow protocols for handling and disposal of returned or recalled drugs.	Prevent reissuance of LASA items without full inspection.

continued on following page

Table 4. Continued

Details	Hospital System Corrections and Prevention Strategies	LASA Drug Precautions
Conduct daily shelf checks	Perform daily spot-checks to detect misplaced medications.	Prioritize LASA drugs during inspections.
Promote self-checking by patients	Educate patients to verify their meds by name, appearance, and dosage.	Reinforce LASA awareness and encourage questions.

(ASHP; Cohen & Davis, 1993a, 1993b, 1994b; Davis & Cohen, 1994; Lizano-Díez et al., 2020; Puttilerpong C, 2006; World Health Organization, 2023)

Table 5. Administration safeguards for LASA drugs

Details	Hospital System Corrections and Prevention Strategies	LASA Drug Precautions
Train in critical administration systems	Train staff on protocols for high-risk drugs, allergy prevention, and standard cycles.	Reinforce double-checking patient and drug information before administration.
Access full patient and treatment info	Ensure access to complete medication profiles and treatment plans.	Use EHRs to flag LASA-specific risks during prep and administration.
Clear, complete labeling	Label multidose meds with patient name, drug, concentration, and expiration.	Standardize labeling across all units to reduce errors.
Double-checks during prep	Require second nurse to verify med name, dose, and route before admin.	Use a buddy system for LASA and high-alert drugs.
Follow the 10 Rights	Apply the "10 Rights" of medication administration rigorously.	Emphasize LASA safety within this framework.
Distraction-free environment	Maintain quiet, organized spaces for medication handling.	Dedicate zones for LASA drug preparation and administration.
Coordinate across teams	Encourage nurse communication with physicians and pharmacists.	Strengthen interprofessional collaboration on LASA issues.
Verify orders before first dose	Cross-check pharmacy-prepared meds with original order.	Involve multiple providers for LASA order verification.
Match patient and med	Confirm patient identity before each administration.	Use wristbands and barcode scanning for LASA verification.
Monitor and report outcomes	Track treatment response and any adverse effects.	Establish systems for rapid LASA-related incident reporting.
Verify dosage calculations	Require a second nurse to confirm complex calculations.	Mandatory double-check for LASA dose accuracy.
Timely documentation	Administer on schedule and record in real-time.	Use eMAR and reminders for LASA drugs.

continued on following page

Table 5. Continued

Details	Hospital System Corrections and Prevention Strategies	LASA Drug Precautions
No med sharing between patients	Prohibit reuse or borrowing of leftover drugs.	Enforce tracking systems specific to LASA medications.
Question unusual doses	Confirm abnormal doses with pharmacist or prescriber.	Require consultation for high LASA doses.

(ASHP; Cohen & Davis, 1993a, 1993b, 1994b; Davis & Cohen, 1994; Lizano-Díez et al., 2020; Puttilerpong C, 2006; World Health Organization, 2023)

Figure 8. Critical safeguards for administering LASA drugs

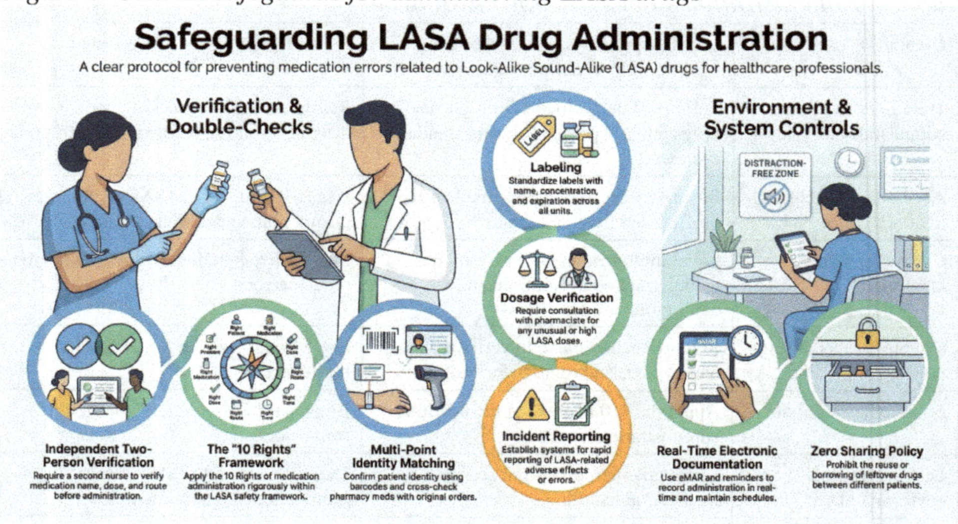

This figure outlines key safeguards during medication administration, including system controls, standard processes, and LASA-specific measures.

Strategies Designed to Reduce LASA Errors

Medication safety is a critical concern in healthcare, with LASA medications presenting significant risks owing to their potential to cause medication errors. This section integrates various strategies and educational initiatives designed to mitigate these risks (ASHP; Ryan et al., 2024).

Staff Training and Continuous Education

Continuous education is essential in combating medication errors, particularly those associated with LASA drugs. Regular training sessions, held monthly or quarterly, ensure that healthcare staff remain informed about the latest LASA issues, significantly reducing the incidence of errors. Simulation-based training programs, which utilize real-life scenarios, have proven especially effective. These programs not only enhance decision-making and situational awareness but also improve the skills of healthcare providers in managing medications under pressure. The implementation of such training in emergency healthcare settings has led to substantial reductions in the number of medication errors, including incorrect medication types, dosages, and administration times. This training approach ensures accurate dosing and minimizes the risk of dangerous drug interactions, thereby enhancing the competence of healthcare providers in emergency situations and improving the overall safety and efficacy of medication administration. This makes continuous education and training a critical component for healthcare staff to effectively mitigate LASA-related errors (Condren & Desselle, 2015; Ehsani et al., 2013; Grant et al., 2020; Hajibeglou et al., 2018; Institute of Medicine Committee on Quality of Health Care in, 2000; Khari & Pazokian, 2022; Pervanas et al., 2016; Siebert et al., 2017; World Health Organization, 2023).

Technology Integration and Human-Cantered Solutions

The integration of human-centered design and advanced technologies plays a vital role in reducing LASA medication errors. Tall-man lettering, which emphasizes specific letters within drug names, helps distinguish similar-sounding or similar-looking medications, reducing misidentification risks during various medication processes (Filik et al., 2004; Grissinger, 2012; The Institute for Safe Medication Practices (ISMP), 2023a; The Institute for Safe Medication Practices Canada (ISMP Canada), 2016).

Color-coding strategies further aid in distinguishing high-risk medications by assigning distinct colors to labels, packaging, and storage areas, allowing healthcare providers to quickly identify LASA drugs and prevent mix-ups (Filiatrault P, 2009; Larmené-Beld et al., 2018; Tariq et al., 2021). An example of LASA alert labeling on yellow storage bins is shown in Figure 9, with alphanumeric shelf addresses used to flag and separate these medications.

Figure 9. LASA alerts labeling on storage bins

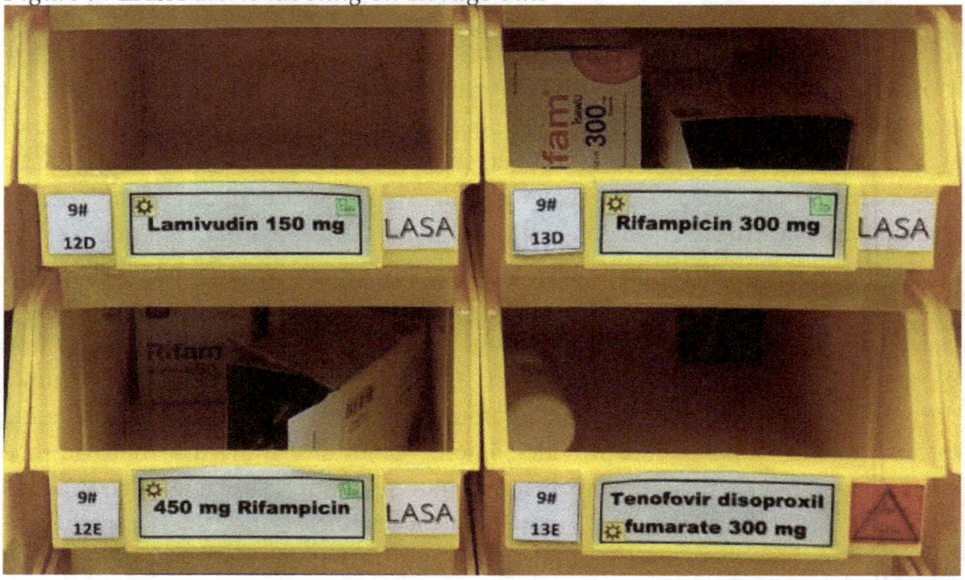

Certain yellow bins have labels with alphanumeric shelf addresses, labeled LASA, to indicate look-alike, sound-alike medications and aid in safe segregation.

Another safety measure is the medication address system, where each drug is given a special location code in the form of A-123-B, which identifies the particular section, shelf, and bin in which the medication is stored (The Australian Commission on Safety and Quality in Health Care, 2020). This system ensures that medication can be readily picked and retrieved quickly and lowers the chances of the wrong product being picked due to similar packaging. This address label, as shown in Figures 10 and 11, is printed on the actual medication package and is matched by the systematic shelving in the pharmacy. This approach enables effective work processes and reduces visual clutter.

Figure 10. The medication address system for drug labels provides an address to each drug stock location on the shelf. To illustrate, A-123-B could refer to a given medicine that is kept in section A, shelf 123, and bin B. The light navigation system may also use red light to guide the users to the right place on the shelf

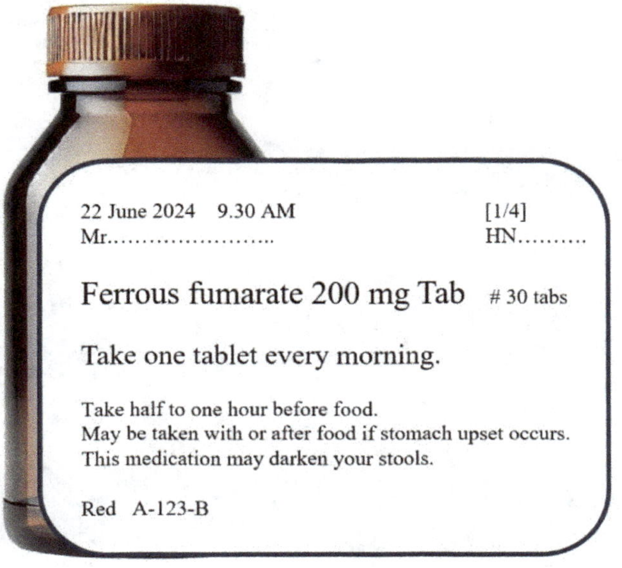

Figure 11. The drug labels have a medication address system that assigns each stock of medication on shelves a unique address. As an example, the name of the atropine sulfate injection is 9#02A

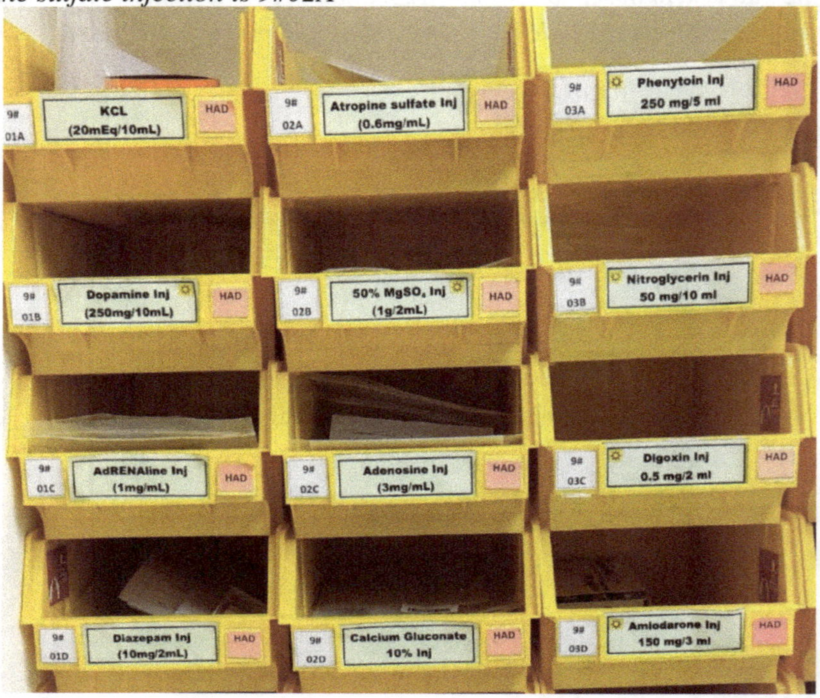

The light navigation system adds a visual aid to support this system. Once a certain drug is chosen in the system, LED lights help healthcare workers locate the exact shelf bin, which lights the way in real time. This is especially applicable to high-alert/risk medications. The ability of light-guided shelving systems to minimize the number of selection errors is shown in Figure 12, which illustrates the precise location of the medication and accelerates and improves the speed of the selection process.

Figure 12. Light-guided medication shelving

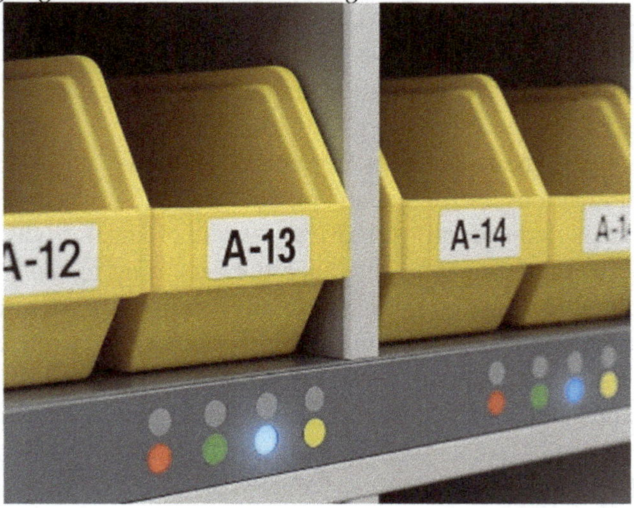

An LED displayed below bins A-12 to A-15 light up as an order is chosen; this lights in the order of the choice, leading the healthcare worker directly to the proper spot on the shelf.

Combined, the strategies introduced and illustrated in Figures 7 to 10 show how technological innovations may be combined with design innovations to improve the safety of LASA medication management. Implementing these tools in everyday clinical practice will allow healthcare organizations to foster a high-reliability culture, ongoing learning, and error prevention, which leads to the provision of safer patient outcomes (World Health Organization, 2024).

Examples of Abbreviations Used in the Hospital

The List of Error-Prone Abbreviations, Symbols, and Dose Designations included in the ISMP lists some of the most frequently misconstrued abbreviations and symbols that have resulted in the adverse medication errors documented via the ISMP National Medication Errors Reporting Program (ISMP MERP). They should not be used in any type of medical communication, such as verbal, electronic, or handwritten communication. They can be present in internal communications, prescriptions, medication labels, drug storage labels, and other medication management systems (The Institute for Safe Medication Practices (ISMP), 2024).

Abbreviations and dose names often cause considerable errors, although they are convenient. In one case, the Pennsylvania Patient Safety Reporting System (PA-PSRS) has reported more than 200 instances where such shorthands created confusion. Examples are U, which is read as 0 or 4 and causes overdoses; and QD, which is read as "daily" and is confused with QID, which means "four times a day," which causes the wrong dosing times. Furthermore, the use of symbols such as less than (<) and greater than (>) has resulted in the incorrect use of medications (The Pennsylvania Patient Safety Advisory, 2005).

To address these risks, the Joint Commission advised hospitals to eliminate hazardous abbreviations in all documentation and prescriptive systems. Some important tactics include adopting preprinted sets of orders, introducing electronic prescribing alerts, enforcing zero-tolerance policies, training staff regularly, and modeling best practices by designing physician champions. System-level solutions (e.g., modifying EMRs to highlight unsafe abbreviations and using clearly labeled storage labels) also complement these efforts. Compliance must be maintained through continuous education, visual reminders, and pharmacy-led interventions (The Institute for Safe Medication Practices (ISMP), 2024; The Joint Commission, 2016, 2024; The Pennsylvania Patient Safety Advisory, 2005). The similarity in packaging can lead to visual confusion, as demonstrated in Figure 13. The labeling of prazosin tablets of 1 mg and 2 mg strengths is almost identical, posing a greater risk of selection error. Removable ambiguous abbreviations and better labeling can prevent some LASA errors from being avoided.

Figure 13. Prazosin 1 mg and 2 mg tablets: examples of look-alike labeling. The label design and packaging are almost the same, and the only difference is in the numerical strength, which poses a risk of selection mistakes

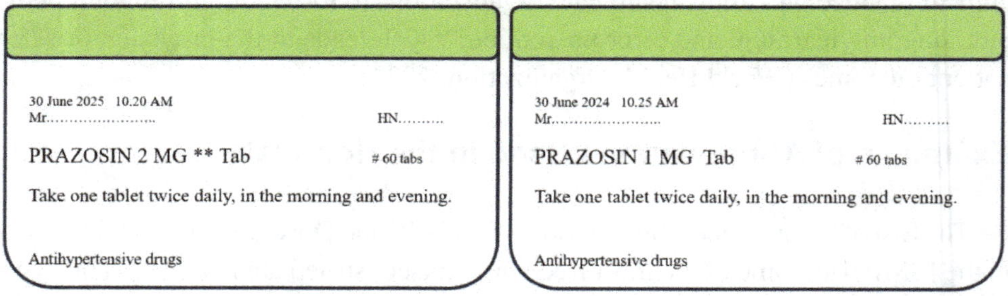

POST-STREAM: PATIENT EDUCATION AND COLLABORATIVE APPROACHES

Patient Education

Healthcare professionals must ensure that patients receive thorough education on the appropriate use of their medications as a fundamental component of any error prevention strategy. Proper education enables patients to actively participate in their healthcare and protect themselves against errors. Enhanced health literacy helps patients understand their medications better, fostering increased awareness, understanding, and rational behavior regarding drug use (Khumsikiew et al., 2023; Supapaan et al., 2023; World Health Organization, 2023).

Healthcare professionals should increase patients' understanding of potential LASA medication errors to aid in their prevention. Creating an environment where health and care workers listen to patients and their caregivers share details about medication management is key to mitigating LASA errors (Academy of Managed Care Pharmacy (AMCP), 2023; The Academy of Managed Care Pharmacy (AMCP), 2019).

To include patients and their families, healthcare workers should do the following:

1. Inform the patients, families, and caregivers about the danger of LASA errors and the importance of ensuring to check the names of their medications two times (Lizano-Díez et al., 2020).
2. Advise using TML on medication labels to differentiate between similar names outside of healthcare (Grissinger, 2012, 2013).
3. Presenting a patient with full details of medication is critical toward having comprehensive treatment management. The brand and generic names and the purpose each medication should be provided. Through smartphones or tablets, healthcare providers can enhance medical knowledge, medication or treatment plan adherence, patient satisfaction, and clinical outcomes of the patients. This method is also cost-effective in the healthcare sector (Mosa et al., 2012; Rameshkumar et al., 2022; Timmers et al., 2020).
4. Promote open communication with patients about medication concerns or changes (Kvarnström et al., 2021).
5. Educate the patients about the dangers of LASA drugs and inform the population about authoritative sources, in particular, the ones that are freely available online or offered in retail stores (Almohammed et al., 2023).
6. Urge the patients to speak with a healthcare provider about the medications and keep the list up-to-date to avoid LASA errors (Garfield et al., 2020; World Health Organization, 2023).

7. The patient is encouraged to read about drugs, do not share them but instead check expiration dates, dispose of expired medications, strictly follow storage guidelines, handle medications safely to a child does not touch them, and be aware of both possible warnings and interactions (Garfield et al., 2020; Manias et al., 2015; World Health Organization, 2023).

Not only do health practitioners and systems have a responsibility to halt errors in medication but also patients. The last line of defense in the healthcare system could be patients themselves, who assume that they possess sufficient knowledge about their medications, such as why they were taking them, when they needed to take them, and how much they needed to take them. The list of medications is very important, especially in cases of emergencies or when patients are incapacitated. This active interaction goes a long way in preventing cases of miscommunication or misinformation, thus preventing many possible errors (Khumsikiew et al., 2023; Supapaan et al., 2023; World Health Organization, 2023). The most critical aspects of patient training that may help prevent LASA medication errors are represented in Figure 14. It reveals important strategies that enable patients to be in control of ensuring that their medication is safe.

Figure 14. Enhancing patient safety by educating patients. The figure presents patient-oriented training techniques that help prevent LASA medication errors, including medication name-two-verification generic and brand name identification, use of tall-man letters, up-to-date medication lists, effective communication with healthcare providers, and medication handling safety

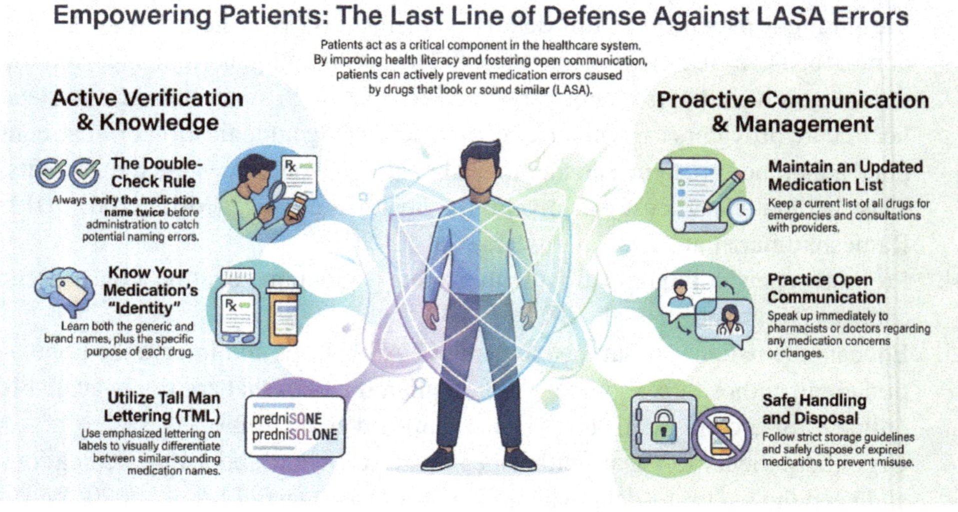

Collaborative Approaches

LASA medication errors must be addressed through patient education and stakeholder collaboration. To develop comprehensive error prevention strategies, these collaborative efforts should strengthen systems, foster partnerships, and promote global knowledge sharing (World Health Organization, 2014, 2023).

Monitoring and reporting medication errors, including LASA errors and near misses, are crucial for pharmacovigilance programs and patient safety organizations. Empowering these entities will enable healthcare systems to determine LASA error patterns and trends to provide interventions and make changes in the systems. The cultivation of the culture of healthcare professionals to report LASA errors and near misses can expand a database that can be studied and applied to prevent them (Lizano-Díez et al., 2020; World Health Organization, 2014, 2023).

Partnerships with Universities

Academic-practice partnerships are important because they equip healthcare organizations with emerging methods of LASA risk reduction. Further studies are necessary to find new ways of addressing this dilemma at the system level, including the identification of high-risk LASA drugs, the development of specific interventions and educational modules, testing new technologies, and error analysis. Such aspects can assist future studies in creating holistic LASA medication error prevention and patient safety strategies (Nyström et al., 2018; World Health Organization, 2017b, 2023).

Global LASA Conferences

LASA medication error events are held globally, where healthcare professionals exchange insights, best practices, and research. These conferences foster international guidelines and standards, knowledge sharing, innovation, networking, and collaboration. Such gatherings encourage the world to work together to create evidence-based and comprehensive LASA medication error interventions (Abdel-Latif, 2016; World Health Organization, 2023).

To prevent LASA medication errors and enhance patient safety, it is necessary to educate patients, establish pharmacovigilance, and form partnerships with academic institutions and global knowledge sharing (Bryan et al., 2015; Bryan et al., 2021a; Bryan et al., 2021b; Khoo et al., 2023; World Health Organization, 2023).

CONCLUSION

LASA medication errors put patients at risk during medication use. Tall man lettering, barcode scanning, clearly labeled, organized storage, and medication address systems increase the accuracy and workflow. Safety is facilitated by simulation training, lifelong learning, and the removal of abbreviations that are prone to errors. Collectively, these factors help reduce LASA risk and enhance medication management.

REFERENCES

Abdel-Latif, M. M. (2016). Knowledge of healthcare professionals about medication errors in hospitals. *Journal of Basic and Clinical Pharmacy*, *7*(3), 87–92. DOI: 10.4103/0976-0105.183264 PMID: 27330261

Academy of Managed Care Pharmacy (AMCP). (2023). *Medication errors*. Retrieved 16 Mar from https://www.amcp.org/about/managed-care-pharmacy-101/concepts-managed-care-pharmacy/medication-errors

Almohammed, O. A., Alnogaidan, R. A., Ghannam, F. O., Alqahtani, R. S., Aloraini, S. K., & Abanmy, N. O. (2023). Public awareness of online pharmacies, consumers' motivating factors, experience and satisfaction with online pharmacy services, and current barriers and motivators for non-consumers: The case of Saudi Arabia. *Saudi Pharmaceutical Journal : SPJ : The Official Publication of the Saudi Pharmaceutical Society*, *31*(8), 101676. DOI: 10.1016/j.jsps.2023.06.009 PMID: 37576852

American Society of Health-System Pharmacists. (2009). ASHP statement on bar-code-enabled medication administration technology. *American Journal of Health-System Pharmacy*, *66*(6), 588–590. DOI: 10.2146/ajhp080414 PMID: 19265189

American Society of Health-System Pharmacists. (2011). ASHP statement on bar-code verification during inventory, preparation, and dispensing of medications. *American Journal of Health-System Pharmacy*, *68*(5), 442–445. DOI: 10.2146/sp100012 PMID: 21330687

ASHP. *ASHP guidelines on preventing medication errors in hospitals*. Retrieved 12 May from https://www.ashp.org/-/media/assets/policy-guidelines/docs/guidelines/preventing-medication-errors-hospitals.ashx

Bryan, R., Aronson, J. K., ten Hacken, P., Williams, A., & Jordan, S. (2015). Patient safety in medication nomenclature: Orthographic and semantic properties of International Nonproprietary Names. *PLoS One*, *10*(12), e0145431. DOI: 10.1371/journal.pone.0145431 PMID: 26701761

Bryan, R., Aronson, J. K., Williams, A., & Jordan, S. (2021a). The problem of look-alike, sound-alike name errors: Drivers and solutions. *British Journal of Clinical Pharmacology*, *87*(2), 386–394. DOI: 10.1111/bcp.14285 PMID: 32198938

Bryan, R., Aronson, J. K., Williams, A. J., & Jordan, S. (2021b). A systematic literature review of LASA error interventions. *British Journal of Clinical Pharmacology*, *87*(2), 336–351. DOI: 10.1111/bcp.14644 PMID: 33197079

Cohen, M. R. (2007a). Causes of medication errors. In Cohen, M. R. (Ed.), *Medication Errors* (2nd ed., pp. 55–66). The American Pharmacists Association. DOI: 10.21019/9781582120928.ch4

Cohen, M. R. (2007b). The role of drug packaging and labeling in medication errors. In Cohen, M. R. (Ed.), *Medication Errors* (2nd ed., pp. 111–152). The American Pharmacists Association. https://doi.org/doi:10.21019/9781582120928.ch7

Cohen, M. R. (2007c). Preventing prescribing errors. In *Medication Errors* (2nd ed.). The American Pharmacists Association. https://doi.org/doi:10.21019/9781582120928.ch9

Cohen, M. R., & Davis, N. M. (1993a). Preventing errors: Errors caused by medical office personnel. *American Pharmacy*, *33*(7), 18. DOI: 10.1016/S0160-3450(15)30726-1 PMID: 8342489

Cohen, M. R., & Davis, N. M. (1993b). Preventing errors: Mixups with Norvasc and Navane. *American Pharmacy*, *33*(8), 26. DOI: 10.1016/S0160-3450(15)30717-0 PMID: 8213467

Cohen, M. R., & Davis, N. M. (1994a). Confusing name; tips for storing drugs. *American Pharmacy*, *34*(2), 20–21. DOI: 10.1016/S0160-3450(15)30526-2 PMID: 8166041

Cohen, M. R., & Davis, N. M. (1994b). Preventing errors. *American Pharmacy*, *34*(12), 18–74. DOI: 10.1016/S0160-3450(15)30239-7 PMID: 7856504

Cohen, M. R., Domizio, G. D., & Lee, R. E. (2007). The role of drug names in medication errors. In Cohen, M. R. (Ed.), *Medication Errors* (2nd ed., pp. 87–110). The American Pharmacists Association. https://doi.org/doi:10.21019/9781582120928.ch6

Cohen, M. R., & Smetzer, J. L. (2018). ISMP medication error report analysis. *Hospital Pharmacy*, *53*(4), 217–219. DOI: 10.1177/0018578718771814 PMID: 30038436

Condren, M. E., & Desselle, S. P. (2015). The fate of pediatric prescriptions in community pharmacies. *Journal of Patient Safety*, *11*(2), 79–88. DOI: 10.1097/PTS.0b013e3182948a7d PMID: 25996644

Davis, N. M., & Cohen, M. R. (1994). Preventing errors. *American Pharmacy*, *34*(10), 17–72. DOI: 10.1016/S0160-3450(15)30294-4 PMID: 7992786

Davis, N. M., & Cohen, M. R. (1995). Preventing errors: Computer-generated prescription orders. *American Pharmacy, 35*(9), 10. DOI: 10.1016/S0160-3450(15)30081-7 PMID: 7484808

Devine, E. B., Wilson-Norton, J. L., Lawless, N. M., Hazlet, T. K., Hansen, R., Kelly, K., . . . Wong, C. (2005). Preparing for ambulatory computerized prescriber order entry by evaluating preimplementation medication errors. Advances in Patient Safety: From Research to Implementation (Vol. 2). Concepts and Methodology.

Ehsani, S. R., Cheraghi, M. A., Nejati, A., Salari, A., Esmaeilpoor, A. H., & Nejad, E. M. (2013). Medication errors of nurses in the emergency department. *Journal of Medical Ethics and History of Medicine, 6*(11). PMID: 24427488

Emmerton, L. M., & Rizk, M. F. (2012). Look-alike and sound-alike medicines: Risks and 'solutions'. *International Journal of Clinical Pharmacy, 34*(1), 4–8. DOI: 10.1007/s11096-011-9595-x PMID: 22193703

Endestad, T., Wortinger, L. A., Madsen, S., & Hortemo, S. (2016). Package design affects accuracy recognition for medications. *Human Factors, 58*(8), 1206–1216. DOI: 10.1177/0018720816664824 PMID: 27591209

European Medicines Agency (EMA). (2021). *Recommendations on medication errors*. Retrieved 01 August from https://www.ema.europa.eu/en/human-regulatory/post-authorisation/pharmacovigilance/medication-errors/recommendations-medication-errors

Filiatrault, P., & Hyland, S. (2009). Does color-coded labeling reduce the risk of medication errors? *The Canadian Journal of Hospital Pharmacy, 62*(2), 154–156. DOI: 10.4212/cjhp.v62i2.446 PMID: 22478883

Filik, R., Purdy, K., Gale, A., & Gerrett, D. (2004). Drug name confusion: Evaluating the effectiveness of capital ("Tall Man") letters using eye movement data. *Social Science & Medicine, 59*(12), 2597–2601. DOI: 10.1016/j.socscimed.2004.04.008 PMID: 15474212

Filik, R., Purdy, K., Gale, A., & Gerrett, D. (2006). Labeling of medicines and patient safety: Evaluating methods of reducing drug name confusion. *Human Factors, 48*(1), 39–47. DOI: 10.1518/001872006776412199 PMID: 16696255

Galanter, W. L., Bryson, M. L., Falck, S., Rosenfield, R., Laragh, M., Shrestha, N., Schiff, G. D., & Lambert, B. L. (2014). Indication alerts intercept drug name confusion errors during computerized entry of medication orders. *PLoS One, 9*(7), e101977. DOI: 10.1371/journal.pone.0101977 PMID: 25025346

Garfield, S., Furniss, D., Husson, F., Etkind, M., Williams, M., Norton, J., Ogunleye, D., Jubraj, B., Lakhdari, H., & Franklin, B. D. (2020). How can patient-held lists of medication enhance patient safety? A mixed-methods study with a focus on user experience. *BMJ Quality & Safety*, *29*(9), 764–773. DOI: 10.1136/bmjqs-2019-010194 PMID: 31949006

Gopakumar, K. M., & Syam, N. (2007). A study on the use of International Non-proprietary Names in India. New Delhi: Centre for Trade & Development (Centad), in collaboration with the WHO India Country Office.

Government of Canada. (2014). *Guidance document for industry - review of drug brand names*. Retrieved 6 August from https://www.canada.ca/en/health-canada/services/drugs-health-products/reports-publications/medeffect-canada/guidance-document-industry-review-drug-brand-names.html

Grant, M., Remines, J., Nadpara, P., & Goode, J. K. R. (2020). Impact of live training on medication errors in a community-based pharmacy setting. *Innovations in Pharmacy*, *11*(3), 11. Advance online publication. DOI: 10.24926/iip.v11i3.3291 PMID: 34007633

Grissinger, M. (2012). Tall man letters are gaining wide acceptance. *P&T : a Peer-Reviewed Journal for Formulary Management*, *37*(3), 132–148. PMID: 22605902

Grissinger, M. (2013). Multiple brand names for the same generic drug can cause confusion. *P&T : a Peer-Reviewed Journal for Formulary Management*, *38*(6), 305. PMID: 23946623

Hajibeglou, A., Zagheri Tafreshi, M., Kamrani, F., & Nasiri, M. (2018). The impact of training on medication error rate of the emergency department in hospitals affiliated to Golestan University of Medical Sciences. *Advances in Nursing & Midwifery*, *27*(4), 32–36.

Health Canada. (2014). *Guidance document: review of drug brand names* Government of Canada, Department of Health. Retrieved 04 Mar from https://www.canada.ca/content/dam/hc-sc/migration/hc-sc/dhp-mps/alt_formats/pdf/pubs/medeff/guide/2014-review-examen_drug-medicament_names-marques/2014-review-examen_drug-medicament_names-marques-eng.pdf

Iglesias Gomez, R., Font Noguera, I., Correa Ballester, M., Ruiz Caldes, M. J., & Poveda Andres, J. L. (2022). Tall man lettering application in medication information systems as a quality and safety strategy in hospital organization. *Journal of Clinical Pharmacy and Therapeutics*, *47*(10), 1570–1575. DOI: 10.1111/jcpt.13703 PMID: 35641241

Institute of Medicine Committee on Quality of Health Care in. A. (2000). To err is human: building a safer health system. In L. T. Kohn, J. M. Corrigan, & M. S. Donaldson (Eds.). National Academies Press (US). DOI: 10.17226/9728

Jarernsiripornkul, N., Chaisrisawadsuk, S., Chaiyakum, A., & Krska, J. (2009). Patient self-reporting of potential adverse drug reactions to non-steroidal anti-inflammatory drugs in Thailand. *Pharmacy World & Science*, *31*(5), 559–564. DOI: 10.1007/s11096-009-9310-3 PMID: 19575308

Jeetu, G., & Anusha, G. (2010). Pharmacovigilance: A worldwide master key for drug safety monitoring. *Journal of Young Pharmacists : JYP*, *2*(3), 315–320. DOI: 10.4103/0975-1483.66802 PMID: 21042493

Jitanapakarn, P., Khunawaradisai, N., & Supapaan, T. (2023). Outcomes of medication reconciliation at patient ward in a community hospital in the Northeast. *Thai J Pharm Pract*, *15*(4), 1003–1014.

Kalola, A. S., & Dean, R. (2019). The United States Food and Drug Administration and Prescription Drug Promotion. *The Journal of Innovations in Cardiac Rhythm Management*, *10*(3), 3588–3591. DOI: 10.19102/icrm.2019.100305 PMID: 32477722

Karet, G. B. (2023). Linguistic analysis of generic-generic drug name pairs prone to wrong-drug errors for which tall-man lettering is recommended. *Therapeutic Innovation & Regulatory Science*, *57*(4), 751–758. DOI: 10.1007/s43441-023-00526-0 PMID: 37171707

Khari, S., & Pazokian, M. (2022). Simulation of training solution for the prevention of medication errors in the emergency ward. *Pharmacy Education*, *22*(1), 492–497. DOI: 10.46542/pe.2022.221.492497

Khontum, A., & Chanthapasa, K. (2021). Perceptions of communities regarding Look-Twin Sound-Twin drugs: A case study of a sub-district in the Northeastern Region of Thailand. *Risk Management and Healthcare Policy*, *14*, 2345–2355. DOI: 10.2147/RMHP.S303899 PMID: 34113190

Khoo, Y. K., Lim, J., Tan-Koi, W., Kitikiti, N., & Sim-Devadas, A. (2023). Promoting collaboration of regulators and patients in improving drug safety and regulatory decision making. *Drug Safety*, *47*(3), 217–225. DOI: 10.1007/s40264-023-01385-2 PMID: 38082120

Khumsikiew, J., Sripa, S., Moolasarn, S., Toh, L. S., Anderson, C., & Supapaan, T. (2023). Facilitators and barriers of the rational drug use hospital program in Thailand. *Pharmacy Practice*, *21*(3), 1–11. DOI: 10.18549/PharmPract.2023.3.2815

Kvarnström, K., Westerholm, A., Airaksinen, M., & Liira, H. (2021). Factors contributing to medication adherence in patients with a chronic condition: A scoping review of qualitative research. *Pharmaceutics, 13*(7), 1100. Advance online publication. DOI: 10.3390/pharmaceutics13071100 PMID: 34371791

Larmené-Beld, K. H. M., Alting, E. K., & Taxis, K. (2018). A systematic literature review on strategies to avoid look-alike errors of labels. *European Journal of Clinical Pharmacology, 74*(8), 985–993. DOI: 10.1007/s00228-018-2471-z PMID: 29754215

Lizano-Díez, I., Figueiredo-Escribá, C., Piñero-López, M., Lastra, C. F., Mariño, E. L., & Modamio, P. (2020). Prevention strategies to identify LASA errors: Building and sustaining a culture of patient safety. *BMC Health Services Research, 20*(1), 63. DOI: 10.1186/s12913-020-4922-3 PMID: 31996197

Manias, E., Rixon, S., Williams, A., Liew, D., & Braaf, S. (2015). Barriers and enablers affecting patient engagement in managing medications within specialty hospital settings. *Health Expectations : An International Journal of Public Participation in Health Care and Health Policy, 18*(6), 2787–2798. DOI: 10.1111/hex.12255 PMID: 25186633

Marilyn Schwartz. (2007). *Look-Alike/Sound-Alike (LASA) drug names - review update -Health Canada's Perspective*. Retrieved 14 April from https://capra.ca/_uploads/archive/presentations/14-MarilynSchwartz-LA-SAGuidanceUpdate.pdf

Marovino, E., Morgillo, A., Mancino, N., Di Feo, V., & Genito, E. (2022). Therapeutic error: Types and prevention strategies and focus about" Look Alike/Sound Alike" and" High Risk" drugs. *Journal of Pharmaceutical Research International, 34*(48A), 9–16. DOI: 10.9734/jpri/2022/v34i48A36409

Ministry of Public Health Republic of Lebanon. (2024). *Look alike sound alike medicines*. Retrieved 15 June from https://www.moph.gov.lb/en/view/68527/look-alike-sound-alike-medicines

Mosa, A. S., Yoo, I., & Sheets, L. (2012). A systematic review of healthcare applications for smartphones. *BMC Medical Informatics and Decision Making, 12*(1), 67. DOI: 10.1186/1472-6947-12-67 PMID: 22781312

Mulac, A., Mathiesen, L., Taxis, K., & Gerd Granås, A. (2021). Barcode medication administration technology use in hospital practice: A mixed-methods observational study of policy deviations. *BMJ Quality & Safety, 30*(12), 1021–1030. DOI: 10.1136/bmjqs-2021-013223 PMID: 34285114

Neelakantan, M., Sharma, P., & Kulkarni, A. (2024). Look-alike, sound-alike (LASA) drugs in India. *The Lancet Regional Health. Southeast Asia*, *26*, 100425. DOI: 10.1016/j.lansea.2024.100425 PMID: 38798984

Nyström, M. E., Karltun, J., Keller, C., & Andersson Gäre, B. (2018). Collaborative and partnership research for improvement of health and social services: Researcher's experiences from 20 projects. *Health Research Policy and Systems*, *16*(1), 46. DOI: 10.1186/s12961-018-0322-0 PMID: 29843735

Pervanas, H. C., Revell, N., & Alotaibi, A. F. (2016). Evaluation of medication errors in community pharmacy settings: A retrospective report. *The Journal of Pharmacy Technology : jPT : Official Publication of the Association of Pharmacy Technicians*, *32*(2), 71–74. DOI: 10.1177/8755122515617199 PMID: 34861023

Pharmaceutical Services Division. Ministry of Health Malaysia. (2012). *Guide on handling look alike, sound alike medications*. Retrieved 25 May from https://pharmacy.moh.gov.my/sites/default/files/document-upload/guide-handling-lasa.pdf

Pharmaceuticals and Medical Devices Agency (PMDA). (2014). *Medication errors in prescription orders*. Retrieved 15 June from https://www.pmda.go.jp/files/000153905.pdf

Pharmaceuticals and Medical Devices Agency (PMDA). (2017). *Mix-up of drugs due to similarity of nonproprietary names* Retrieved 15 June from https://www.pmda.go.jp/files/000220148.pdf

Pharmaceuticals and Medical Devices Agency (PMDA). (2024). *Profile of services*. Retrieved 15 June from https://www.pmda.go.jp/files/000241469.pdf

Puttilerpong, C. (2006). System approach to resolve and prevent mediation error: experience of Prachuapkhirikhan hospital. In Chulavatnatol S, Montakantikul P, Chindavijak B, Suksomboon N, & S. T (Eds.), *Pharmacist and quality medication system* (pp. 38-61). The Association of Hospital Pharmacist (Thailand).

Rahman, Z., & Parvin, R. (2015). Medication errors associated with look-alike/sound-alike drugs: A brief review. *J Enam Med Col*, *5*(2), 110–117. DOI: 10.3329/jemc.v5i2.23385

Raj, N., Fernandes, S., Charyulu, N. R., & Dubey, A., G, S. R., & Hebbar, S. (. (2019). Postmarket surveillance: A review on key aspects and measures on the effective functioning in the context of the United Kingdom and Canada. *Therapeutic Advances in Drug Safety*, *10*, 2042098619865413. DOI: 10.1177/2042098619865413 PMID: 31384423

Rameshkumar, T., Haputhanthrige, I. U., Misbahunnisa, M. Y., & Galappatthy, P. (2022). Patients' knowledge about medicines improves when provided with written compared to verbal information in their native language. *PLoS One*, *17*(10), e0274901. DOI: 10.1371/journal.pone.0274901 PMID: 36315507

Rider, B. B., Mehta, H., & Merchant, L. (2019). Special considerations for proprietary name review: Focus on products that may be prescribed "As Directed". *Therapeutic Innovation & Regulatory Science*, *53*(3), 381–386. DOI: 10.1177/2168479018782669 PMID: 29929377

Rodziewicz, T. L., Houseman, B., & Hipskind, J. E. (2023). Medical error reduction and prevention. [Updated 2024 Feb 12]. StatPearls Publishing. Retrieved 22 May from https://www.ncbi.nlm.nih.gov/books/NBK499956/

Ryan, A. N., Robertson, K. L., & Glass, B. D. (2024). Look-alike medications in the perioperative setting: Scoping review of medication incidents and risk reduction interventions. *International Journal of Clinical Pharmacy*, *46*(1), 26–39. DOI: 10.1007/s11096-023-01629-2 PMID: 37688737

Shah, M. B., Merchant, L., Chan, I. Z., & Taylor, K. (2017). Characteristics that may help in the identification of potentially confusing proprietary drug names. *Therapeutic Innovation & Regulatory Science*, *51*(2), 232–236. DOI: 10.1177/2168479016667161 PMID: 30231718

Sharma, A. E., Rivadeneira, N. A., Barr-Walker, J., Stern, R. J., Johnson, A. K., & Sarkar, U. (2018). Patient engagement in health care safety: An overview of mixed-quality evidence. *Health Affairs (Project Hope)*, *37*(11), 1813–1820. DOI: 10.1377/hlthaff.2018.0716 PMID: 30395509

Siddiqui, D. E. (2020). Minimizing medication errors by triangle check of look-alike sound-alike medications from crash cart of gynecology and obstetrics in emergency. *Innovations in Pharmacy*, *11*(4), 18. Advance online publication. DOI: 10.24926/iip.v11i4.3480 PMID: 34007659

Siebert, J. N., Ehrler, F., Combescure, C., Lacroix, L., Haddad, K., Sanchez, O., Gervaix, A., Lovis, C., & Manzano, S. (2017). A mobile device App to reduce time to drug delivery and medication errors during simulated pediatric cardiopulmonary resuscitation: A randomized controlled trial. *Journal of Medical Internet Research*, *19*(2), e31. DOI: 10.2196/jmir.7005 PMID: 28148473

Sinha, H. K. (2014). Role of pharmacists in retailing of drugs. *Journal of Advanced Pharmaceutical Technology & Research*, *5*(3), 107. DOI: 10.4103/2231-4040.137383 PMID: 25126530

Sriboonruang, P., & Rattanamahattana, M. (2022). Barcode scanning technology to improve pre-dispensing errors. *Greater Mekong Subregion Medical J*, *3*(1), 7–12.

Srisuriyachanchai, W., Cox, A. R., Kampichit, S., & Jarernsiripornkul, N. (2023). Severity and management of adverse drug reactions reported by patients and healthcare professionals: A cross-sectional survey. *International Journal of Environmental Research and Public Health*, *20*(4), 3725. Advance online publication. DOI: 10.3390/ijerph20043725 PMID: 36834422

Supapaan, T. S., Low, B. Y., Anderson, C., Boonlue, T., Puripunyavanich, N., Khumsikiew, J., & Poonphol, P. (2023). Evaluation of the rational drug use (RDU) literacy among undergraduate students. *Pharmacy Practice*, *21*(4), 2867.

Tariq, R. A., Vashisht, R., Sinha, A., & Scherbak, Y. (2021). Medication dispensing errors and prevention. [Updated 2024 Feb 12]. StatPearls Publishing. Retrieved 22 May from https://www.ncbi.nlm.nih.gov/books/NBK519065/

Thakur, D. S., & Prashant, R. T. (2024). *India's problem — different drugs, identical brand names*. Retrieved 15 June from https://www.thehindu.com/opinion/op-ed/indias-problem-different-drugs-identical-brand-names/article67773569.ece

The Academy of Managed Care Pharmacy (AMCP). (2019). *Medication errors*. Retrieved 16 Apr from https://www.amcp.org/about/managed-care-pharmacy-101/concepts-managed-care-pharmacy/medication-errors

The Australian Commission on Safety and Quality in Health Care. (2020). *Principles for the safe selection and storage of medicines: guidance on the principles and survey tool*. Retrieved 22 June from https://www.safetyandquality.gov.au/sites/default/files/resources/attachments//survey_tool_-_principles_for_safe_selection_and_storage_of_medicines_-_final.pdf

The Institute for Safe Medication Practices Canada (ISMP Canada). (2016). *Drug labeling and the application of TALLman lettering project report*. Retrieved 15 June from https://www.ismp-canada.org/download/TALLman/TALLmanLettering-ProjectReport.pdf

The Institute for Safe Medication Practices (ISMP). (2022). *Adopt strategies to manage look-alike and/or sound-alike medication name mix-ups*. Retrieved 11 July from https://www.ismp.org/sites/default/files/newsletter-issues/20220602.pdf

The Institute for Safe Medication Practices (ISMP). (2023a). *FDA and ISMP lists of look-alike drug names with recommended tall man (mixed case) letters*. Retrieved 16 Apr from https://www.ismp.org/system/files/resources/2023-01/ISMP_Tallman_Letters_012523_MS5087%20%282%29.pdf

The Institute for Safe Medication Practices (ISMP). (2023b). *List of confused drug names*. Retrieved 16 April from https://www.ismp.org/recommendations/confused-drug-names-list

The Institute for Safe Medication Practices (ISMP). (2024). *ISMP list of error-prone abbreviations, symbols, and dose designations*. Retrieved 12 April from https://www.ismp.org/recommendations/error-prone-abbreviations-list?check_logged_in=1

The Joint Commission. (2016). *Managing Health Information: use of abbreviations, acronyms, symbols and dose designations - understanding the requirements*. Retrieved 19 May from https://www.jointcommission.org/standards/standard-faqs/hospital-and-hospital-clinics/information-management-im/000001457/

The Joint Commission. (2024). *Managing Health Information: use of abbreviations, acronyms, symbols and dose designations - understanding the requirements*. Retrieved 12 May from https://www.jointcommission.org/standards/standard-faqs/hospital-and-hospital-clinics/information-management-im/000001457/

The Pennsylvania Patient Safety Advisory. (2005). Abbreviations: A shortcut to medication errors. *PA PSRS Patient Saf Advis*, *2*(1), 19–21.

Timmers, T., Janssen, L., Kool, R. B., & Kremer, J. A. (2020). Educating patients by providing timely information using smartphone and tablet Apps: Systematic review. *Journal of Medical Internet Research*, *22*(4), e17342. DOI: 10.2196/17342 PMID: 32281936

Trbovich, P., & Hyland, S. (2017). Responding to the challenge of look-alike, sound-alike drug names. *BMJ Quality & Safety, 26*(5), 357-359. https://qualitysafety.bmj.com/content/26/5/357

U.S. Department of Health and Human Services Food and Drug Administration. C. f. D. E. a. R. C. (2016). *Safety considerations for product design to minimize medication errors: guidance for industry*. Retrieved 8 June from https://www.fda.gov/files/drugs/published/Safety-Considerations-for-Product-Design-to-Minimize-Medication-Errors-Guidance-for-Industry.pdf

U.S. Department of Health and Human Services Food and Drug Administration (FDA). (2014). *Nonproprietary naming of biological products guidance for industry*. Retrieved 15 June from https://www.fda.gov/files/drugs/published/Nonproprietary-Naming-of-Biological-Products-Guidance-for-Industry.pdf

U.S. Department of Health and Human Services Food and Drug Administration (FDA). (2020). *FDA name differentiation project*. Retrieved 06 Aug from https://www.fda.gov/drugs/medication-errors-related-cder-regulated-drug-products/fda-name-differentiation-project

U.S. Department of Health and Human Services Food and Drug Administration (FDA). (2021). *Phonetic and Orthographic Computer Analysis (POCA) Program*. Retrieved 13 June from https://www.fda.gov/drugs/resources-drugs/phonetic-and-orthographic-computer-analysis-poca-program

U.S. Department of Health and Human Services Food and Drug Administration (FDA), Center for Drug Evaluation and Research (CDER). (2015). *Size, shape, and other physical attributes of generic tablets and capsules*. Retrieved 10 Jan from https://www.fda.gov/files/drugs/published/Size--Shape--and-Other-Physical-Attributes-of-Generic-Tablets-and-Capsules.pdf

US Food and Drug Administration. (US FDA). (2015). *FDA Drug Safety Communication: FDA warns about prescribing and dispensing errors resulting from brand name confusion with antidepressant Brintellix (vortioxetine) and antiplatelet Brilinta (ticagrelor)*. Retrieved 10 Feb from https://www.fda.gov/drugs/drug-safety-and-availability/fda-drug-safety-communication-fda-warns-about-prescribing-and-dispensing-errors-resulting-brand-name

Vaismoradi, M., Jordan, S., Vizcaya-Moreno, F., Friedl, I., & Glarcher, M. (2020). PRN medicines optimization and nurse education. *Pharmacy (Basel, Switzerland)*, *8*(4), 201. Advance online publication. DOI: 10.3390/pharmacy8040201 PMID: 33114731

Veronin, M. (2011). Packaging and labeling of pharmaceutical products obtained from the internet. *Journal of Medical Internet Research*, *13*(1), e22. DOI: 10.2196/jmir.1441 PMID: 21324833

WHO Collaborating Centre for Patient Safety Solutions. (2007). *Look-alike, sound-alike medication names*. Retrieved 9 August from https://cdn.who.int/media/docs/default-source/patient-safety/patient-safety-solutions/ps-solution1-look-alike-sound-alike-medication-names.pdf?sfvrsn=d4fb860b_8

World Health Organization. (1997). *Guidance on INN*. Retrieved 24 Dec from https://www.who.int/medicines/services/inn/innquidance/en/

World Health Organization. (2014). *Reporting and learning systems for medication errors: the role of pharmacovigilance centers*. Retrieved 19 June from https://iris.who.int/bitstream/handle/10665/137036/9789241507943_eng.pdf?sequence=1

World Health Organization. (2017a). *Guidance on the use of International Non-proprietary Names (INNs) for pharmaceutical substances*. Retrieved 16 June from https://cdn.who.int/media/docs/default-source/international-nonproprietary-names-(inn)/who-pharm-s-nom-1570.pdf

World Health Organization. (2017b). *Medication without harm*. Retrieved 10 Feb from https://www.who.int/initiatives/medication-without-harm

World Health Organization. (2023). *Medication safety for look-alike, sound-alike medicines*. World Health Organization. Retrieved 3 June from https://iris.who.int/bitstream/handle/10665/373495/9789240058897-eng.pdf?sequence=1

World Health Organization. (2024). *Promoting rational use of medicines*. Retrieved 6 Mar from https://www.who.int/activities/promoting-rational-use-of-medicines

ABBREVIATIONS

BCMA: Bar-Code Medication Administration
CDSCO: Central Drugs Standard Control Organization
CPOE: Computerized Provider Order Entry
e-MAR: Electronic Medication Administration Record
EMA: European Medicines Agency
FDA: Food and Drug Administration
INNs: International Nonproprietary Names
ISMP: Institute for Safe Medication Practices
LASA: Look-Alike Sound-Alike
MAR: Medication Administration Record
MAH: Marketing Authorization Holder
MoPH: Ministry of Public Health
PA-PSRS: Pennsylvania Patient Safety Reporting System
PMDA: Pharmaceuticals and Medical Devices Agency
POCA: Phonetic Orthographic Computerized Analysis
TML: Tall man lettering
WHO: World Health Organization
XL: Extended-release

Chapter 3
Challenges in Drug Identification and LASA Errors

ABSTRACT

Accurate drug identification is essential for preventing medication errors, particularly those involving look alike sound alike (LASA) drugs. This chapter explores the challenges of identifying medications in both clinical and community settings, focusing on visual similarity, labeling limitations, and the absence of standardized identifiers. In Thailand and similar contexts, repackaged or unlabeled medications such as Yaa Chud further complicate the verification process. The chapter reviews current identification tools, including imprint codes, packaging cues, and AI driven systems, and evaluates their limitations in real world practice. A multidisciplinary framework is proposed to strengthen drug identification and reduce LASA related harm.

INTRODUCTION

The process of drug identification has become increasingly complicated because of the rapid globalization of the pharmaceutical sector and the growth of generic drugs. A single active ingredient may be in various branded or generic forms and may vary greatly in color, form, size, and imprinting, even within a single nation. Such aesthetic differences make easy identification of drugs challenging, as they confuse healthcare practitioners and patients (World Health Organization, 2024).

Proper identification of drugs is crucial throughout the medication use process. In daily clinical practice, pharmaceutical products usually lose their original identifiers. As an example, tablets are normally extracted from blister packs and repackaged into

DOI: 10.4018/979-8-3373-5478-1.ch003

single, unlabeled bags and then dispensed in hospitals. In care units, medications can be mixed unintentionally with other medications and then given to the patient, whereas patients may arrive with them or have them repackaged by relatives, which may cause confusion during medication administration.

Australian and Canadian data support the LASA burden. According to national medication error reports, 60–65% of LASAs are the result of drug name errors, and 20–25% are the result of visual similarity to packaging or pills (Australian Commission on Safety and Quality in Health Care (ACSQHC), 2012; Larmené-Beld et al., 2018).

According to the report given by the Australian Commission on Safety and Quality in Health Care (ACSQHC), LASA drug names have resulted in numerous medical errors in Australia because of their similarity. They also proposed using tall man lettering for drug names that are considered high risk (Australian Commission on Safety and Quality in Health Care (ACSQHC), 2024). Similarly, Health Canada in Canada has enhanced pre- and postmarketing name screening policies to minimize errors that occur as a result of confusing product names and packaging (Health Canada, 2004).

When the appearance was altered by generic substitutions, 21% of the patients were concerned that they received another drug, and 8% of the patients discontinued or switched their treatment (Sarpatwari et al., 2019). One French survey, which included 768 patients, 345 physicians, and 198 pharmacists, revealed that 30% of the patients feared confusing the tablets because of their similarities, but physicians and pharmacists thought that patients did not highly depend on looking and feeling, which is a difference between the perception of the providers and actual patient behavior (Tranchard et al., 2019).

Thailand is a mirror of these global challenges but has context-specific limitations. The Thai Food and Drug Administration (Napaporn J et al., 2023; Supapaan TS, Kamnuek J, et al., 2024; Thailand Food and Drug Administration) cites more than 60% of all registered drugs in Thailand in the form of tablets and capsules.

Nevertheless, limited and incomplete drug identification resources are available for drugs produced locally. Although MIMS Thailand, Medilet® (Mahidol University), and the Ubon Ratchathani University Drug Identification Database are available, they are limited in scope of coverage and depend on human-error-prone manual searches based on imprint, shape, or color. A study at a local hospital revealed that *64.6%* of LASA mistakes in Thailand were due to drug name confusion, *24.6%* were due to similarity of packaging, and *10.8%* were due to similarity of the tablet/capsule, which are similar to international trends (Supapaan TS, Songmuang A, et al., 2024).

Additional data are provided by the Drug Information Services (DIS) in Thailand. Nationally, 575 out of the 1,336 hospitals surveyed (43 percent) responded, and 22.97 percent of all the questions sent to hospital DIS centers were drug identification queries. This was second only to adverse drug reaction (ADR) questions (28.85%), and questions about therapeutic effectiveness were third (16.53%) (Chanakit et al., 2009).

This observation demonstrates that drug identification has a significant burden on clinical information services, which means that, over time, it is difficult to achieve correct drug identification at all levels of the supply chain. The key issues and remedies presented in this chapter are presented in Figure 1.

Figure 1. Principal issues of drug identification and LASA mistakes

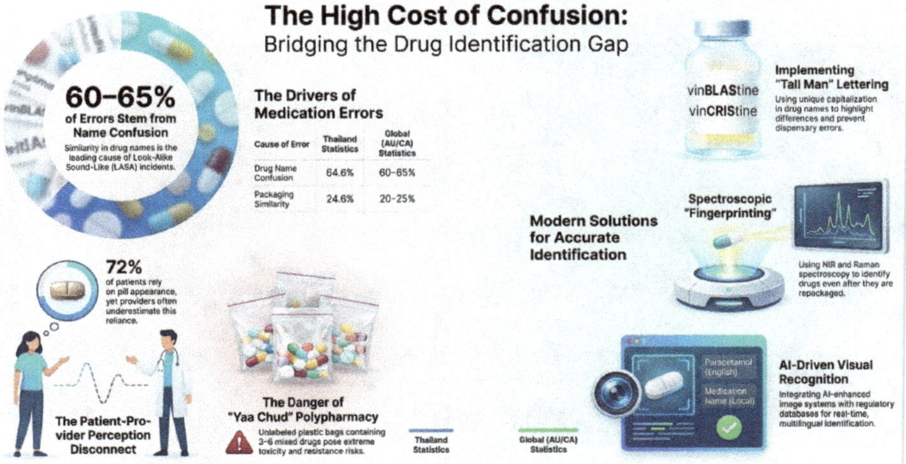

The figure summarizes major causes of medication errors, such as drug name confusion, similarity in packaging, perception gaps between patients and providers, repackaged medication, and new solutions, such as tall man lettering, spectroscopic identification, and AI-based visual recognition.

Community pharmacists in Thailand frequently have to address unlabeled or repackaged medicines submitted by patients to identify or continue taking them. These include Yaa Chud polypharmacy packets and tablets, which lack labels. Yaa Chud is a mixture of 3-6 drugs sold in small plastic bags by unregulated dealers, neighborhood grocery stores, and street markets. Common antibiotics include corticosteroids, painkillers, antihistamines, and muscle relaxants. None are marked with names, strengths, expiration dates, or manufacturer details (Newton et al., 2008; Sunpuwan et al., 2019).

Yaa Chud is affordable, appears to be effective, and is easy to obtain; this attribute makes it a common drug used in underserved regions of Thailand despite the Drug Act (Sunpuwan et al., 2019). Two kinds of packets are depicted in Figure 2:

1. Yaa Chud is dry-packed with low-quality or expired drugs in full sets.
2. Fresh-packed Yaa Chud: Prepared on order by symptom description, drugs are dispensed out of bulk containers without being properly documented.

Figure 2. Example of Yaa-Chud polypharmacy packs or tablets lacking identifying imprints

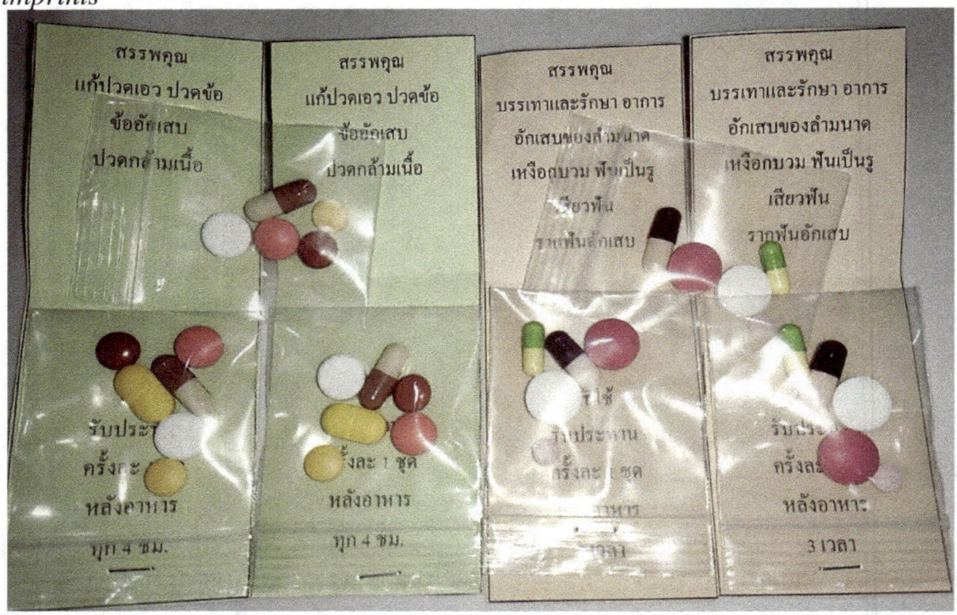

The safety issues associated with the use of such unidentifiable packets are serious concerns when they are raised in clinical practice, e.g., in the emergency or outpatient clinic. A lack of pill imprinting or original packaging poses major obstacles to the verification of the drug, putting the patient at serious risk of incorrect dosage, drug duplication, adverse interactions, and errors. Public health authorities have attributed the use of Yaa Chud to steroid toxicity, antimicrobial resistance, and treatment failure (Manager Online, 2018; Newton et al., 2008).

To overcome such challenges, community pharmacists are inclined to rely on a combination of individual clinical experience, peer consultation, and local resources. A qualitative study of 20 pharmacists revealed that in particular cases, most of them turned to public-access databases when unknown drugs were identified (Pornwattanakavee et al., 2021). Pharmacists were fond of tools that were simple to use, had wide local drug coverage, had visual references, and had no subscription charges. However, such systems are not as efficient in cases where high-resolution images or large datasets are not available.

A study in Mueang Chonburi District also revealed that pharmacists either relied on manual resources, e.g., the MIMS book, or relied on professional judgment, especially because of the limited offers in the Thai language in international drug databases such as Pillbox or RxList (Sangsuriyan et al., 2018).

Even though some of the tools (via the UBU Drug Identification database) could prove handy, they failed to meet the needs of front-line pharmacy services, especially in the accurate identification of less well-known drugs such as Yaa Chud that are common on the market.

The availability of Yaa Chud and other drugs that cannot be identified is still high, and this is a sign of the need to develop more effective drug recognition methods in the Thai context. It includes image recognition algorithms, which can be AI-based; multilingual databases; and other methods of analysis, such as grid factor analysis (GFA), that are functional without typical labeling or manufacturer identifiers (Manager Online, 2018).

The natural intricacy of hospital medicine management contributes to these challenges. Medicines undergo various processes in a complex workflow that starts with procurement and continues through to patient administration, all while ensuring a secure workflow. Pharmacies in hospitals regularly repackage large-volume drugs into unit-dose quantities to distribute them to wards.

During this process, crucial labeling information, such as the international nonproprietary name (INN), strength, lot number, and expiry date, can be incomplete or vague, which can be dangerous and may confuse similar-looking products (Reallon et al., 2021). Precision in drug identification at the intermediate stage is key to avoiding serious administration errors and ensuring patient safety, as the French MIND (Medicine Identification New Database) project identifies.

Packaging and serialization systems enhance the traceability of supply chains but cannot guarantee the accuracy of identification when tablets have been removed from their original blisters. At this stage, visual confusion between similar-looking medications continues to be one of the most frequent reasons for medication errors, and the look-alike, sound-alike product is one of the most frequent sources of preventable harm (Reallon et al., 2021).

To close this gap, new sophisticated nondestructive analytical methods have been developed to provide quick and trustworthy medical identification. Attenuated total reflectance Fourier transform infrared (ATR/FT-IR), near-infrared (NIR), and Raman spectroscopy methods can distinguish between oral solid dosage forms with high reproducibility and repeatability—even between similar active ingredients or excipients. These technologies enable tablet authentication, finding fake or damaged products, and confirming quality without damaging the integrity of medicines. Portable NIR spectrometers also facilitate rapid onsite screening and enhance throughput in terms of quality control and patient safety, in addition to aiding pharmacy technicians' training in the creation of personal pill organizers. The Medicine Identification New Database (MIND) in France demonstrates the usefulness of integrating spectroscopy analysis with a centralized database. It allows rapid recognition of medicines when they are repackaged, when patients enter the facility, in the care unit, or when they are suspected of being counterfeit or damaged due to improper storage. MIND eliminates a severe lack of medication workflow in hospitals since it guarantees proper identification beyond traditional packaging (Reallon et al., 2021).

Patients remain highly concerned about the appearance of medications, and healthcare professionals are facing increasing challenges because of the similarities in the appearance of generic drugs. To fill these gaps, countries with comparable limitations need to have a multifunctional, AI-based, image-based system of drug identification, which can be combined with regulatory data and have a multilingual interface. This would help minimize LASA errors and improve the quality and responsiveness of drug information services, enable patients to take care of their drugs safely, and serve as a model for other regions of Southeast Asia and other parts of the world.

Objectives of the Chapter

The aims of this chapter are as follows:

(1) To define drug identification and its relevance to LASA medication safety.
(2) To examine common challenges in identifying unlabeled, repackaged, or visually similar drugs.
(3) To review current drug identification tools and technologies
(4) To propose strategies that support accurate drug recognition in clinical and community contexts.

Organization of the Chapter

This chapter presents a Thai and worldwide overview of drug identification and its utmost importance in avoiding LASA mistakes. This highlights the issue of look-alike generics, informal drugs such as Yaa Chud, and the physical similarity of oral solid dosage forms. Further sections provide a review of global and local identification tools, physical properties of tablets and capsules, patient-centered strategies, and regulatory frameworks. The chapter ends with the presentation of grid factor analysis (GFA), a systematic framework to evaluate LASA risk under different drug attributes and conditions.

DRUG IDENTIFICATION SYSTEMS WORLDWIDE

Medication misidentification is a significant safety concern in all parts of the world and is predetermined by the visual similarity of drugs and fragmented identification systems. The subsequent review looks at patient-level practices, international databases, AI-supported technologies, and low-resource issues. Indications of improvement and remaining gaps are noted.

Perceptions of Patients and Health Care Providers on Drug Identification

The identification of medication is a joint responsibility of patients and healthcare professionals. Nevertheless, they have different perceptions, especially in relation to visual and name-based recognition, which leads to medication errors in LASA.

Patients are used to verifying medications on the basis of their visual properties, color, shape, size, and imprints. In a national survey of 814 adults conducted in the U.S., 72 percent of the respondents used the appearance of a pill as the main method of confirmation. As part of this group, 21% felt that they had been given the incorrect medication when it appeared different, and 8% made changes or stopped taking it without seeking medical advice. Even though 86% of the respondents preferred to be notified by pharmacists of the changes in appearance, only 37% of them remembered being notified.

Preferences for consistency were high: 72% for color, 71% for shape, and 75% for size, yet 58% would not pay even a small premium for such consistency (Sarpatwari et al., 2019).

Beyond the survey data, a cohort of 11,513 post-myocardial infarction patients revealed that 29% experienced changes in pill appearance. These changes significantly increased treatment nonpersistence, with color changes increasing by 34% (OR 1.34) and shape changes by 66% (OR 1.66) (Kesselheim et al., 2014). In response, the FDA recommends that generic manufacturers maintain a consistent tablet appearance to support adherence and patient trust (Munesh & Bhavaraju, 2024; U.S. Department of Health and Human Services Food and Drug Administration (FDA), 2015; US Food and Drug Administration (US FDA), 2024).

A systematic review of ten international studies confirmed that appearance changes were associated with lower adherence in seven of those studies. These changes were also linked to poorer clinical outcomes, such as hypertension control, and increased switching back to brand-name drugs because of patient distrust (Lumbreras et al., 2022).

Providers, however, often underestimate these concerns. A French study involving 768 patients, 345 physicians, and 198 pharmacists revealed perceptual gaps. While 50% of patients identified medications by brand name and 21% by generic name, only 16% cited packaging, and 7% cited tablet appearance. However, 28% of patients reported fearing confusion due to pill appearance, even more so than name similarity. Physicians and pharmacists underestimated patients' use of names (46% and 26%, respectively) and overestimated confusion caused by appearance (74% and 83%, respectively), whereas 61% of patients reported this concern (Tranchard et al., 2019).

Similar findings emerged in a U.S. survey of more than 1,000 patients and 710 pharmacists. While 51% of patients experienced pill appearance changes and 82% wanted notification, only 36% recalled verbal communication, and 45% reported sticker notification. In contrast, 47% of pharmacists reported such changes occurring six or more times monthly and reported that they notified patients in 88% of cases verbally and 77% via stickers—revealing a major communication gap (Barenie et al., 2020).

In Thailand, patients frequently bring in unlabeled medications obtained from informal vendors, markets, or leftover hospital supplies, including the well-known Yaa Chud packets. These are medications not dispensed by licensed pharmacies, and pharmacists have little alternative but use visual identification, peer consultation, experience, and printed Thai-language sources. Global pill identification tools are not as useful in such settings because of language barriers and a lack of local product visualization, which leads to the need to switch to more localized and trustworthy tools (Pornwattanakavee et al.).

In low- and middle-income nations (LMICs), the appearance of medicines can influence the perception and use of medications. In Laos, Ghana, Mozambique, and Vietnam, patients and informal suppliers commonly name antibiotics by capsule shape or color (e.g., red and yellow capsules) instead of name or indication. Such misidentification creates a mix of antibiotics and painkillers, increasing the likelihood of them being used inappropriately. A cross-country study of six LMICs, Thailand, revealed that physical appearance, as opposed to formal name, could be a significant factor in defining the classification of drugs in communities. The authors support the idea of the standard visual characteristics of antibiotics as a community health intervention, particularly in conditions of low literacy (Monnier et al., 2023).

These differences in perception between a patient and a healthcare professional indicate an international weakness in the practice of drug identification. Patients are guided by what they can visualize and touch, whereas health care systems focus on nomenclature, labeling, and barcoding. It is necessary to bridge this perceptual divide with standardized pill appearance, effective interaction with patients, and locally specific drug identification aids to reduce LASA-related errors and enhance medication safety in all care settings. The disparities in the identification of medicines and responses to alterations in pill appearance among patients and healthcare providers are shown in Table 1. As shown in Figure 3, visual drug identification can be a good method for reducing medication errors that are linked to LASA.

Table 1. Comparison of patient and provider perspectives on drug identification

Aspect of Drug Identification	Patient Perspective	Provider Perspective	Reference
Reliance on pill appearance	72% rely on appearance; 51% experienced changes	Providers assume reliance on names over visual cues	Barenie et al. (2020); Sarpatwari et al. (2019)
Reaction to appearance changes	21% believed wrong drug; 8–12% reduced or stopped use	Often unaware of adherence impact due to visual changes	Barenie et al. (2020); Sarpatwari et al. (2019)
Notification preferences vs. recall	86% want to be notified; only 36–37% recall notification	Report high notification rates verbally or via sticker despite low recall	Barenie et al. (2020); Sarpatwari et al. (2019)
Frequency of appearance changes	51% experienced at least one change during therapy	47% of pharmacists report ≥6 such changes monthly	Barenie et al. (2020)
Identification by brand vs generic name	50% identify by brand, 21% by generic; only <16% mention visual cues	Underestimate name-based identification (physicians 46%, pharmacists 26%)	Tranchard et al. (2019)
Perception of LASA confusion	28% fear look-alike pills; 31% cite name similarity	Overemphasize appearance risk (physicians 74%, pharmacists 83%)	Tranchard et al. (2019)
Impact of visual changes on adherence	Color change: +34% nonpersistence; shape change: +66%	Providers often do not consider visual variability a major adherence risk	Kesselheim et al. (2014)
Identification tools in community setting	Reliance on visual recognition, peer consultation; global apps limited	Pharmacists use self-reference, books, and peer help; visual ID is routine	(Pornwattanakavee et al., 2021)

Figure 3. Visual drug identification and medication safety. This number demonstrates the dependency of patients on the use of pills to determine medicines, how visual manipulations can lead to misunderstanding and noncompliance, and how AI-based and localized drug recognition systems can be used to minimize LASA-associated medication errors

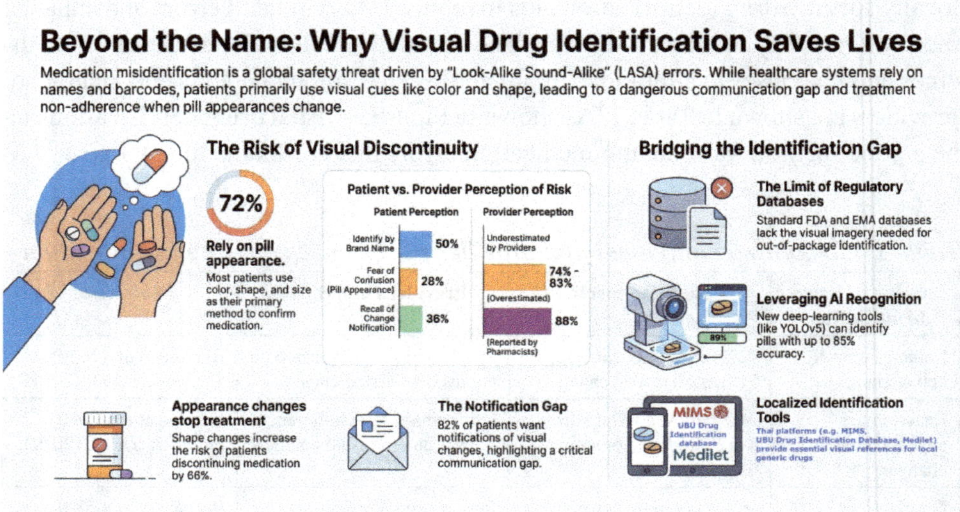

Drug Identification Databases and Platforms with Costs and Comparative Analysis

Drug identification tools are very important for preventing LASA medication errors. These systems, regulatory databases, public tools, commercial subscription platforms, and emerging AI-powered apps have different levels of coverage, functionality, accessibility, and cost. These systems are summarized in Table 2.

Regulatory systems such as the U.S. FDA's National Drug Code (NDC), RxNorm, the EMA Medicine Database, and national registries such as Health Canada's Drug Product Database offer reliable drug metadata for interoperability with electronic health records. However, they lack any visual identification capabilities, which limits their usefulness when tablets are out of labeled packaging (The Institute for Safe Medication Practices (ISMP), 2023a; U.S. Department of Health and Human Services Food and Drug Administration (FDA), 2024; US Food and Drug Administration (US FDA), 2024).

Public pill identifier tools, including Drugs.com (Figure 4, Figure 5), RxList, and Medscape Pill Identifier, allow end-users to search by color, shape, and imprint (Drug.com, 2025; RxList, 2025).

Figure 4. The screen of the Pill Identification Wizard on Drugs.com, displaying the terms of use and instructions for identifying pills on the basis of imprint, shape, or color. The tool guides users to search using visual characteristics to access drug information from its database

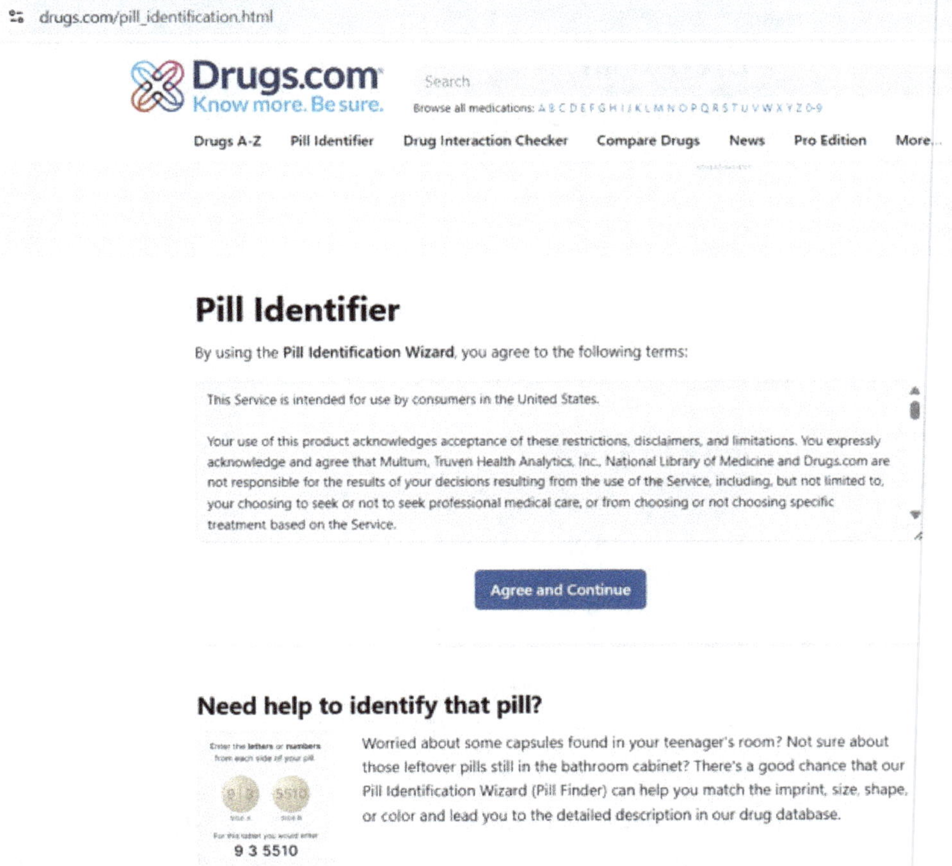

Drugs.com (2025)

Figure 5. Pill identification results for imprint code "A 112" on Drugs.com, showing a white, round 7 mm tablet identified as Indapamide 2.5 mg. The tool provides physical attributes, imprints, and pharmacological information to assist users in visual drug identification

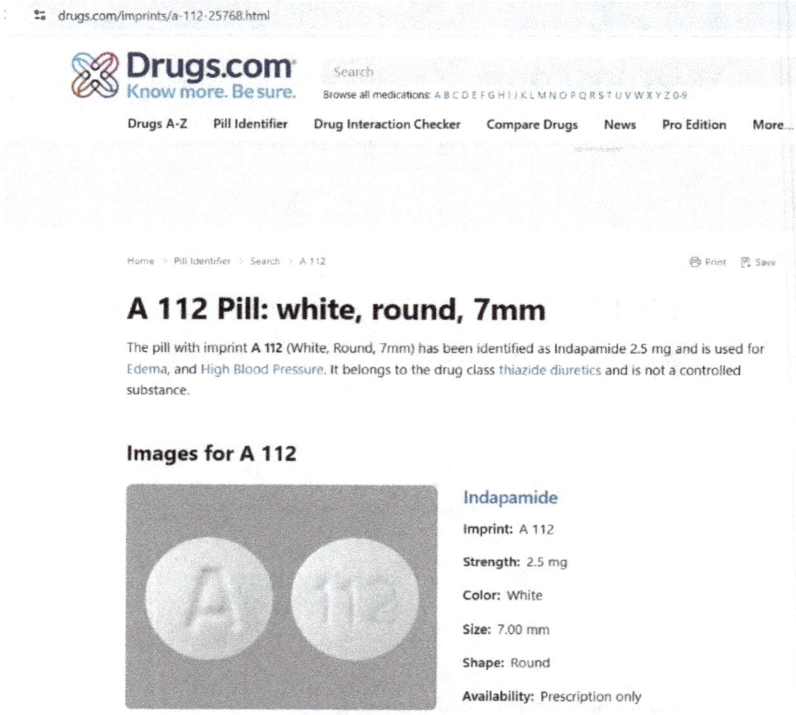

Drugs.com (2025, https://www.drugs.com/imprints/a-112-25768.html)

Micromedex®, Lexicomp®, Medi-Span®, and First Databank (FDB) are commercial clinical decision support platforms that offer comprehensive drug monographs, LASA alerts, and computerized provider order entry (CPOE) and eMAR system integration (see Table 2). They are typically applied to institutions in high-income countries but are prohibitively expensive for many LMICs.

Pill recognition is improved with AI and visual recognition. Heo et al. (2023) created a deep learning-based system with You Only Look Once version 5 (YOLOv5) for object detection and Residual Network-32 (ResNet-32) for feature extraction, as well as imprint recognition and correction to address ambiguous imprints. In an evaluation of Korean and U.S. pill image data, the system recorded top-1 accuracies of 85.65% and 74.46%, respectively, because of design and imprint standard variations in the U.S. (Heo et al., 2023). Similarly, Cunha et al. (2014) developed HelpMePills, an older adult-friendly mobile application, to detect oral solid medications using smartphones or tablets. The app used shape, size, and color analysis from a database and was offline and designed for the elderly in resource-poor environments. Nevertheless, in the prototype stage, mobile health (mHealth) apps can enhance medication safety in vulnerable groups at risk for LASA errors (Cunha et al., 2014).

Locally developed drug identification tools in Thailand are important for assisting in safe medication usage and minimizing LASA errors. MIMS Thailand provides pill identifiers, therapeutic categories, and prescribing information adapted to local healthcare providers and patients (MIMS Thailand, 2025; Thaipharmaitem, 2025). Furthermore, Thai-language interfaces such as the Medilet 2 (Figures 6-7) by Mahidol University and the UBU Drug Identification Database (Figures 8-9) by the Faculty of Pharmaceutical Sciences at Ubon Ratchathani University enable users to search a database by physical properties, such as imprint codes, shape, and color. Such publicly available systems are particularly interested in generic formulations and are useful tools for healthcare practitioners and the general population to verify medications and avoid errors (Faculty of Pharmaceutical Sciences, 2022; Mahidol University, 2025; Monthly Index of Medical Specialties (MIMS) Thailand, 2025; Thaipharmaitem, 2025).

Special clinical applications of Raman and near-infrared (NIR) spectroscopy-based devices, such as the MIND database in France, have been applied in special clinical settings to identify repackaged or counterfeit drugs in hospitals. They require specific equipment and technical expertise (Reallon et al., 2021), which may limit their accessibility and effectiveness in various healthcare settings.

Despite their merits, none of the systems are able to comprehensively combat global LASA. Commercial platforms work well in resource-intensive hospital settings; lay visuals are utilized, and local databases in underserved communities are employed, but gaps remain in terms of integration, cost, language, and coverage. Next-generation development should be based on AI-based, multilingual systems with regulatory metadata and local drug images. The possibility of introducing scalable and inexpensive instruments that can be implemented in hospitals and communities and are sensitive to linguistic and regional specifics is vital to reducing LASA risk at the global level.

Table 2. Examples of drug identification databases and platforms

Database/ Platform	Ownership	Country/ Region	Access Model	Content Coverage	Website/Link	Reference
Micromedex® (Merative)	Private (IBM Watson Health)	Global	Subscription	Drug monographs, LASA alerts, limited pill images	https://www.merative.com/clinical-decision-support/micromedex	Merative (2025)
Lexicomp®	Private (Wolters Kluwer)	Global	Subscription	Hospital-grade drug info, LASA alerts, pill images, eMAR integration	https://www.wolterskluwer.com/solutions/lexicomp	Lexicomp (2024)
Medi-Span®	Private (Wolters Kluwer)	Global	Subscription	Drug IDs, interactions, pricing; limited images	https://www.wolterskluwer.com/en/solutions/medi-span	Wolters Kluwer (2025)
MedSnap® ID	Private	US/EU	Subscription	AI-based visual pill recognition	https://medsnap.com	MedSnap (2025)
MIMS Thailand	Private	Thailand/ SE Asia	Subscription	Thai drug monographs, pill images; manual search	https://www.mims.com/thailand	Monthly Index of Medical Specialties (MIMS) Thailand (2025)
Drugs.com	Private (Drugsite Trust)	Global	Free	Consumer-friendly monographs, basic pill ID, interaction checker	https://www.drugs.com	Drug.com (2025)

continued on following page

Table 2. Continued

Database/ Platform	Ownership	Country/ Region	Access Model	Content Coverage	Website/Link	Reference
RxList.com	Private (WebMD)	Global	Free	Consumer drug index, monographs, pill identifier	https://www.rxlist.com	RxList (2025)
Regulatory databases (FDA NDC, RxNorm, EMA, PMDA Japan, Health Canada, Thai FDA NDI	Public	US/EU/ Japan/ Canada	Free	Standard metadata	Various official agency websites	European Medicines Agency (EMA) (2025); Health Canada (2025); (Pharmaceuticals and Medical Devices Agency (PMDA), 2025; Thai Food and Drug Administration, 2025); U.S. Food and Drug Administration (2025); U.S. National Library of Medicine (2025)
MIND (France)	Public/ Private partnership	France	Free for hospitals	Spectroscopy-based pill authentication for repackaged meds	https://www.spectroscopyeurope.com	Reallon et al. (2021)

continued on following page

Table 2. Continued

Database/ Platform	Ownership	Country/ Region	Access Model	Content Coverage	Website/Link	Reference
Medilet®	Public/Academic	Thailand	Free	Thai pill database (imprint/shape)	https://pharmacy.mahidol.ac.th/medilet/	Mahidol University (2025)
UBU Drug ID Database	Public/Academic	Thailand	Free	Thai generic pill images; manual input	https://drugiden2.ubu.ac.th/	Faculty of Pharmaceutical Sciences Ubon Ratchathani University (2025)

Figure 6. The Medilet online drug identification system developed by Mahidol University features search functions based on physical characteristics, imprint codes, and therapeutic categories.

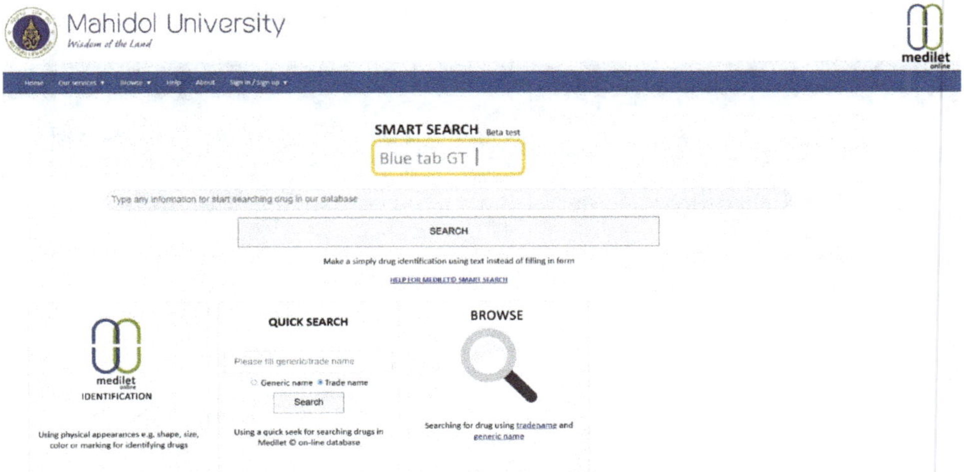

The platform is publicly accessible online and intended for healthcare professionals and the general public in Thailand (https://pharmacy.mahidol.ac.th/medilet/)

Figure 7. A Medilet online drug identification system developed by Mahidol University illustrates the use of "smart search" on the basis of physical characteristics. Users can enter traits such as dosage form (tablet/capsule), color (multiple selections allowed), shape, and imprint text to retrieve potential matches.

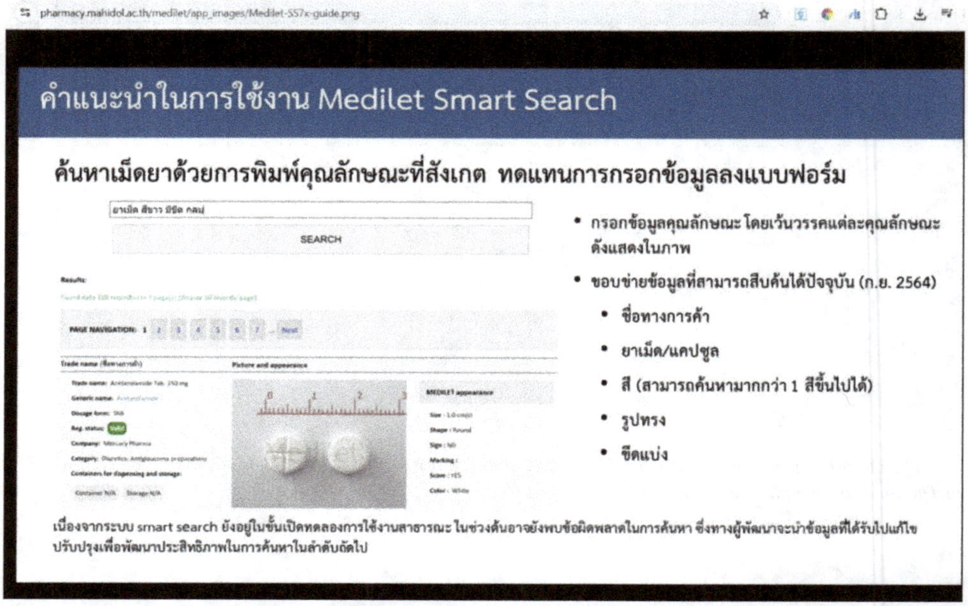

This search method replaces the manual form input and is publicly accessible online (https://pharmacy.mahidol.ac.th/medilet/app_images/Medilet-SS7x-guide.png)

Figure 8. Home page of the drug identification database developed by the Faculty of Pharmaceutical Sciences, Ubon Ratchathani University, Thailand.

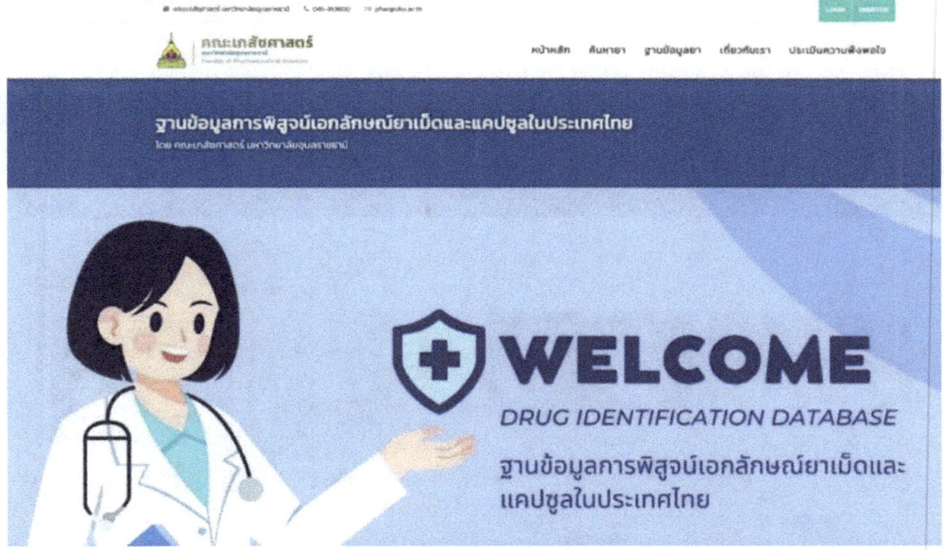

The platform is publicly available online and free of charge for all users, aiming to support safe medication use and drug identification nationwide (https://drugiden2.ubu.ac.th/)

Figure 9. Search results page for chlorpheniramine in the Ubon Ratchathani University drug identification database, showing visual references and drug information

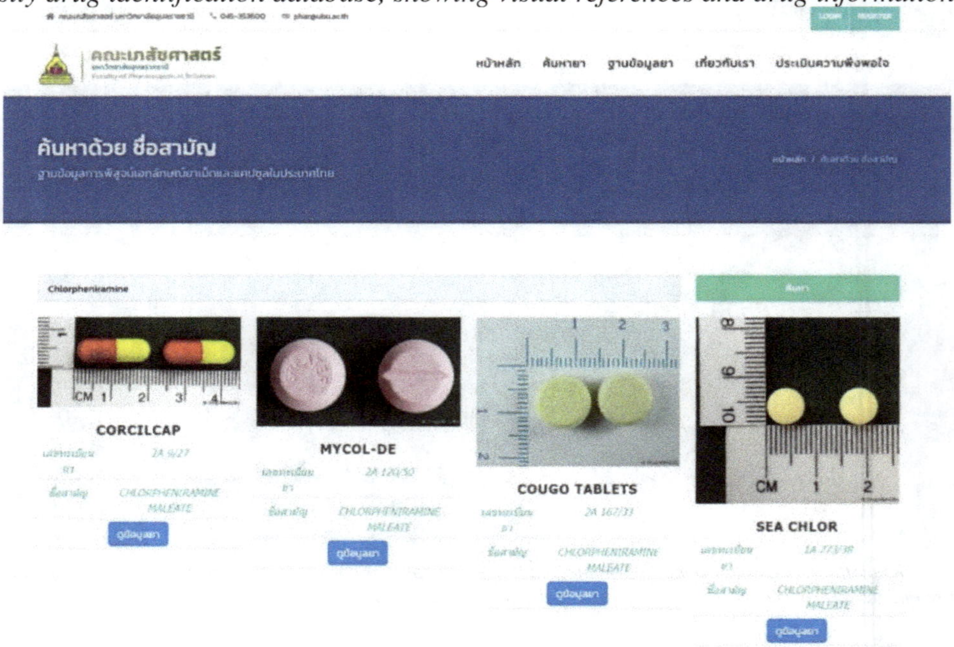

(https://drugiden2.ubu.ac.th/iden-genericname)

THE REGULATORY FRAMEWORK AND THE HUMAN FACTOR INVOLVED IN DRUG IDENTIFICATION ARE BOTH CRUCIAL

Effective drug identification is subject not only to technology or pharmaceutical data systems but also to regulatory structures and human cognitive constraints. In most countries, regulatory bodies have recognized that physical drug properties, including the size, shape, color, imprint, labeling, and packaging of tablets, are critical for either preventing or causing medication errors. However, in most areas, regulatory advice is not binding. This situation leads to differences among pharmaceutical companies and healthcare systems in the way that human factors are integrated into the drug product design and identification process. Consequently, patients and health practitioners are susceptible to the same medication errors.

Regulatory Guidance on Physical Drug Attributes

The Food and Drug Administration issued guidance in the United States entitled "Size, Shape, and Other Physical Attributes of Generic Tablets and Capsules" (U.S. Department of Health and Human Services Food and Drug Administration (FDA), 2015). As highlighted in this document, small differences in branded and generic drugs, including a change in the size of a tablet or its coating, may impact patient confidence, decrease adherence, and cause medication errors. The FDA suggests that generic pills or capsules must not be more than 20 percent in any one dimension or 40 percent in volume relative to the reference drug listed, particularly those that are less than 17 millimeters.

The Medicines and Healthcare Products Regulatory Agency in the United Kingdom proposed the use of user-centered design in labeling and packaging, especially when the drug is highly dangerous when it is used improperly, e.g., as an opioid or injectable drug. This suggestion highlights the font size, regularity of design, and visual clarity as factors in reducing the probability of confusion in clinical practice (Medicines and Healthcare products Regulatory Agency (MHRA), 2020).

These issues were also brought up by the National Patient Safety Agency in their designation Design for Patient Safety: A Guide to the Labeling and Packaging of Injectable Medicines (National Patient Safety Agency: Patient Safety Division, 2008). This report explains how poorly designed labels, unorganized ampoule layouts, and overcrowded packages can contribute to the risk of drug selection errors in emergency, anesthesia, and critical care settings (National Patient Safety Agency: Patient Safety Division, 2008).

A study conducted by Momtahan and colleagues in a Canadian hospital reviewed the quality of the design of injectable medicine labels used in clinical practice. The evaluation resulted in the identification of recurring problems such as small fonts and inconsistent positioning of details and other visual appeal hindering proper detection of drugs. These findings suggest that enforceable human-centered labeling standards should be used to increase safety in drug identification (Momtahan et al., 2008).

Human Factors in Drug Identification and LASA Errors

Human factor engineering is the study of the interaction of people with tools, systems, and environments. Human factor studies can assist researchers in examining the ways in which LASA errors occur and the ways in which their prevalence could be decreased by design, workflow streamlining, and environmental control of medication safety. In the case of two drugs that are packaged similarly or are in the form of a similar tablet, a stressed healthcare provider can easily confuse the two. Verbal or phone errors can occur when there is phonetic similarity between the names of drugs, e.g., dopamine and dobutamine, in a high-noise or high-stress clinical environment (Woods et al., 2017).

The environment influences drug identification rather than cognitive processes. Intensive care units, crisis rooms, and operating rooms are usually under time pressure, noisy, poorly lit, and interrupted. Mental workload makes healthcare workers less likely to recheck labels or ask questions on defaults. Various distractions and multitasking affect attention and memory, increasing drug selection errors (Carayon et al., 2014; Carayon et al., 2020).

Drug identification and verification are also influenced by the organizational culture and the way in which medication use systems are designed. LASA errors are exacerbated because of poor storage, overcrowded medication drawers, intermittent use of barcodes, and the absence of standard dispensing practices. Having similar products that are not separated or color-coded alerts may lead to mix-ups every day.

A reporting and reflection culture following near misses reinforces the mechanisms at the system level, such as an automated warning, tall typing, and standardized storage (Cohen MR et al., 2021; Institute for Safe Medication Practices (ISMP), 2021).

These examples suggest that drug verification systems must consider cognitive impairment and organizational and environmental factors. It is important to design safer labels, packages, and imprint codes to create a safe context for drug verification. A user-friendly approach, environmental considerations, and systems thinking will help reduce LASA errors and enhance medication safety. Safe drug identification, as depicted in Figure 10, requires a bridge between regulatory requirements on physical product characteristics and human-factor controls that consider the risks related to the cognitive, environmental, and workflow factors.

Figure 10. Protecting drug identification through regulation and human factors

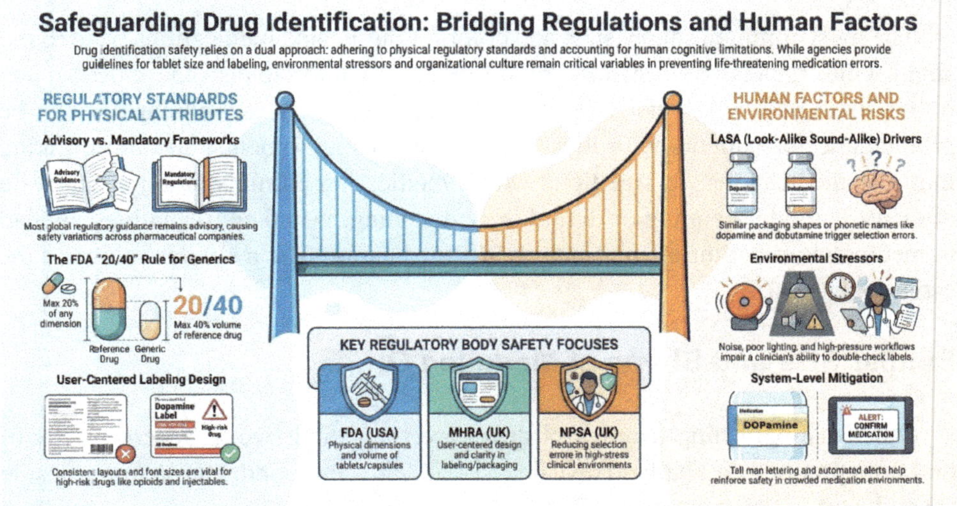

This value is a generalization of the way regulatory advice on physical drug characteristics, labeling, packaging, and product design needs to be merged with human-factor approaches to lessen LASA medication errors in clinical practice settings

PHYSICAL ATTRIBUTES OF ORAL TABLETS AND CAPSULES IN DRUG IDENTIFICATION

Physical attributes of oral solid dosage forms, such as tablets and capsules, are key means of drug identification for healthcare professionals and patients. In real-life situations, these characteristics are crucial in high-risk medication contexts and multiple drug regimens, where the potential for LASA medication errors is high. The physical characteristics of color, shape, size, imprint, texture, and packaging affect medication adherence and patient perceptions and play a role in the safety of medication dispensing, administration, and self-administration.

Color Similarity and LASA Risk

Visual features such as color are among the most prominent characteristics of medications. However, the frequent occurrence of certain colors, such as white, yellow, and pink, has been associated with an increased risk of LASA. A recent study of 2,837 registered oral tablets and capsules in Thailand revealed that one-third were white, followed by yellow (13.8%) and pink (8.96%), suggesting a risk of visual confusion in scenarios where color is used as the main identifier (Napaporn J et al., 2023).

The most common shape, size, and color for duplicated medications were round small white tablets (457 entries), round medium white tablets (253 entries), and round small yellow tablets (178 entries), respectively. These similarities can be problematic for patients with low literacy, vision impairments, and those taking multiple medications. In situations where medication administration systems do not have barcode scanning or digital drug matching, visual confirmation can lead to medication substitution, particularly if a medication is of a similar color and the same package size.

Similar Size and Shape of Marketed Drugs

Other distinguishing features of drugs are shape and size. A recent survey of oral drug products in Thailand revealed that 52.7% were round, 18.6% were capsule shaped, and 12.1% were oval. Almost 90% of the tablets were considered medium (1.0–2.0 cm) or small (<1.0) in size. The common shape of small, round, and white tablets, comprising more than 16% of the sample, illustrates the issue of identifying medications on the basis of their physical appearance (Napaporn J et al., 2023).

This similarity greatly increases the risk of medication errors in the outpatient environment, where medications are repackaged or stored in unlabeled containers. In elderly individuals or those with cognitive impairment, these similarities can result in confusion, medication errors, or omitted doses, particularly when two or more medications are similar in shape, size, and color.

Orthographic and Brand Name Similarity with Physical Look-Alike Risk

In addition to physical appearances, brand naming activities cause LASA events. A retrospective study of 18,108 registered Thai brand names revealed that two-thirds had been registered by the same firm under other registration numbers, and they often looked very similar. Different companies registered one-third of the names, some of which had completely different active ingredients, but a similar brand name was used (Napaporn et al., 2022; Supapaan TS, Kamnuek J, et al., 2024).

The fact that other products containing different APIs (or therapeutic purposes) contain similar word roots (e.g., "AMINE," "HYDRO," or even just the word "prednis") contributes to confusion as well. These roots of words have been generally associated with orthograph error. Such word roots have frequently been involved in spelling errors. In other cases, such as the brand name "GEMZIL," one and the same name was assigned to gemfibrozil and captopril in other pharmaceutical companies, which created a necessity to regulate brand names (Napaporn et al., 2022; Supapaan et al., 2024).

Drug name and tablet shape/appearance mismatches lead to exponential medication errors. Without tablet imprinting or labels, it is difficult to distinguish "PREDNISOLONE" from another tablet with a similar name and appearance.

Integration of the Hospital Information System's Drug Images

Using drug images in computerized drug information systems is vital for enhancing hospital visual identification. Warinchamrab Hospital in Thailand was the first hospital to use a drug image-integrated database throughout the hospital for drug management. This system has a web platform with searchable drug photos by shape, color, dosage form, and therapeutic class (Supapaan T et al., 2024).

Pharmacists use a Type 1 visual report with generic/trade names and tablet/capsule photos to dispense medication. These images are used to verify that prepared medications match the prescriber's intent before being given to patients or sent to wards. Type 2 and 3 reports are used for patient-specific education, especially in drug brand changes or emergencies such as COVID-19 mail-order refills.

This image-enabled verification process reduces visual similarity-related dispensing errors, especially when drugs have similar packaging or form factors. It also empowers patients to self-identify medications, improving adherence and reducing pill misidentification. Such reports with the dosage indicated, image of the drug, and usage warnings enhance patient awareness and confidence ((Supapaan TS, Somsorn S, et al., 2024).

Overall satisfaction was high among the hospital pharmacy teams with respect to user interface image quality, convenience of search, and ease of use, demonstrating that drug image integration in hospital IT infrastructure is possible. Such a model is emerging as a Thai hospital network best practice that can possibly be scaled at the national level.

Regulatory and System-Level Packaging Guidance

To counter these obstacles, regulatory bodies in such nations as the MHRA in the UK and the FDA in the U.S. have developed detailed packaging and labeling guidelines. They are the need to show the name of the drug, its strength, and the route of administration on the same visible panel; fonts and white space are required to be legible (Medicines and Healthcare products Regulatory Agency (MHRA), 2020). Tall-man lettering is another strategy that is encouraged by regulatory agencies and the Institute of Safe Medication Practices (Institute for Safe Medication Practices (ISMP) Canada, 2023; The Institute for Safe Medication Practices (ISMP), 2023b).

In this practice, letters in confusable drug names are selectively capitalized to make them visually distinct. Despite these recommendations, there is little implementation in Thai regulatory systems. Differences due to container design, lack of braille, low-contrast printing, and other factors still remain barriers to easy identification of drugs in a real-world environment, which can lead to medication errors and negatively impact patient safety.

Design of Blister Packs and Calendar Packs

The packaging design influences the identification of drugs at the point of use. Color differences in blister foils, font types, or the orientation of blisters among different manufacturers can mislead users, especially when the medications are not communicated to them during brand changes. Variations in imprinting or pill finish during generic substitution can affect patient confidence and compliance.

Blister calendar packs, which are commonly used with chronic medications, offer potential safety improvements. Evidently, day marks, the use of the same colors of pills depending on dose, and sequence indicators can decrease the chances of missed or repeated doses. On the other hand, calendars with poor designs can add to the confusion, particularly with elderly patients.

National Database, Visual Clustering, and Image-Based Research Findings

Recent efforts to create a digital repository of marketed oral dosage forms in Thailand have demonstrated widespread physical duplication. An examination of more than 2,800 products by high-resolution photography indicated that white, round tablets dominated, regardless of therapeutic class. In numerous situations, tablets can be visually clustered and not differentiable without imprint data or packaging information (Napaporn et al., 2022).

Structural analysis of the images revealed that the most frequent forms were medium-sized white round tablets (n=253) and small-sized white round tablets (n=457).

The standardized photography protocols and the use of colorimetric tools such as the Pantone Matching System have shown that there is a large overlap in appearance, which in most cases makes medications visually indistinct over brands and APIs (Napaporn J et al., 2023; Napaporn et al., 2022) (see Figure 11).

Physical properties are still the backbone of drug identification, especially when there are no digital tools for verification. Nonstandardized naming and packaging procedures, however, can turn them into a source of medication error instead of protection when combined. The existing information demonstrates the existence of visual and orthographic duplication in the Thai pharmaceutical environment, which imposes the need to change the structure of the policy and increase the level of design. In the future, visual design, regulatory police, and AI-enhanced technologies will be crucial elements in guaranteeing the safe use of oral tablets and capsules.

Figure 11. Images of white, round tablets in the Ubon Ratchathani University Drug Identification Database. Although the active ingredients and therapeutic groups may vary, many tablets may be similar in size, color, and shape; hence, there is a risk of visual confusion and therapeutic duplication, especially in the case of no clear imprint codes

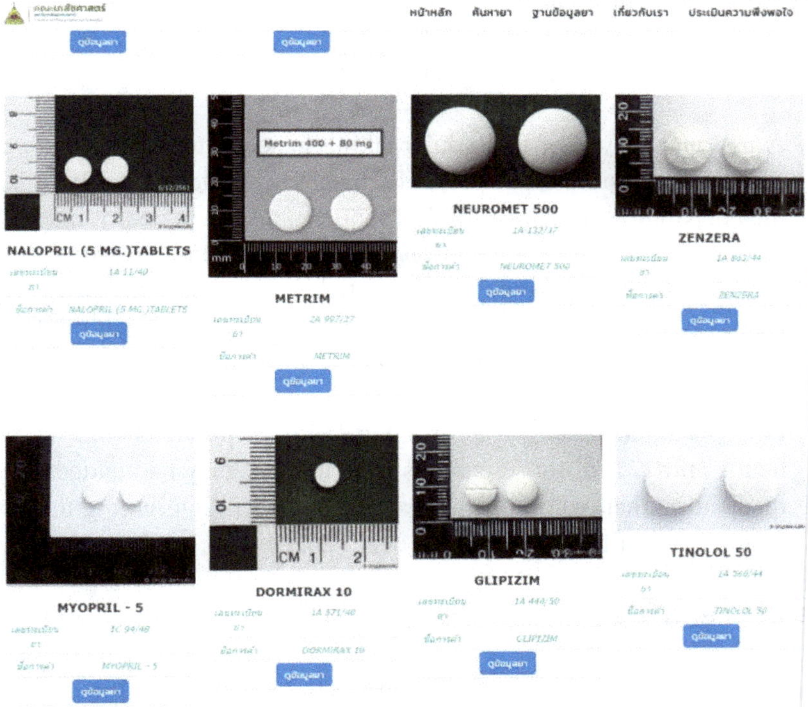

Faculty of Pharmaceutical Sciences, Ubon Ratchathani University (2022)

PATIENT-CENTERED MEDICATION IDENTIFICATION STRATEGIES

Despite the development of packaging technology, pill databases, and barcode scanning, patients remain the ultimate decision makers in ensuring medication safety. This role is vital, especially in drug identification, where a LASA error of similar-appearing or similar-sounding products may cause fatality.

Challenges in Patient Drug Identification

Despite improvements in the packaging, barcoding, and consistency of generic drugs, patients play a crucial role in identifying their medications, particularly in preventing LASA medication errors.

Reliance on Pill Appearance and Patient Confusion

- A national survey of 814 adults taking generics to treat chronic conditions (i.e., hypertension, diabetes, and epilepsy) revealed that 72% of them used the appearance of the pills (color, shape, and size) to determine whether they were taking the right medication. Nevertheless, only 37% remembered pharmacist notification (verbal or via a sticker) when it changed its appearance, and 21% felt that they had been given the wrong drug. Additionally, 8% discontinued or decreased their use because of the change (Sarpatwari et al., 2019).
- Pill appearance changes were reported in the previous year by 51% of patients, and 12% of those patients reported that they had ended up using less medication than before the appearance change, highlighting the risk of confusion in identification (Barenie et al., 2020).

Health Literacy and Label Comprehension

- A 2007 systematic review by Shrank et al. revealed that the features of label design, which are a larger font, definite headings, white space, and simplified text, have a significant positive effect on understanding, although there is a relative lack of evidence to support how design affects clinical outcomes (Shrank et al., 2007).
- Patients with low literacy were significantly more likely to misinterpret prescription drug warning labels and thus misidentify or misuse medications. In one structured interview study of adults reading at or below the sixth-grade level, the interpretation accuracy for eight commonly used warning labels

ranged from 0% to 78.7%, and low-literacy patients were 3.4 times less likely to interpret labels correctly than those with higher literacy (Davis et al., 2006).

Evidence-Based Patient Tools for Drug Identification

- Pictograms and visual aids: In a randomized controlled study in South Africa, pictographic medication labels significantly improved understanding from 69.5% to 95.2% and adherence from 71.5% to 89.6% among low-literacy patients. High adherence (>90%) occurred in 54% of the pictogram group compared with only 2% of the control group (Dowse & Ehlers, 2005).
- A controlled usability study revealed that 63 % of users were willing to photograph their pills daily, and 92.9 % believed that the app would improve medication adherence and ease identification. A higher level of compliance with prescribed regimens was observed among those participants who took pills every day (Babigumira & Lewis, 2020).
- Brown-bag medication review is a pharmacist-led medication review conducted by the patient during a health care visit in which the patient brings all their current medications and the pharmacist and patient reconciles them. Such meetings tend to unearth unrecognized, duplicate, or unnecessary drugs, especially in patients who have to manage multiple prescriptions. In one of the studies in which a structured brown-bag review tool was introduced, the number of drug therapy problems identified by the pharmacist increased significantly, and the medication regimen changes doubled after the intervention, which also indicated that previously unknown or misdiagnosed medications were widespread (Weiss et al., 2016).

Moreover, medication reconciliation by the pharmacist has proven effective in resolving patient medication claims and clinical intent. In a meta-analysis, compared with standard care, pharmacists decreased the number of medication discrepancies by 68% and the overall discrepancy by 88% (Choi & Kim, 2019). Makes in drug name recognition, confusion in drug name appearance, and the use of outdated regimens are frequent.

A different study carried out in a hospital indicated that 21–42% of pharmacist-led review conflicts were clinically significant, which demonstrates the risks of misidentified medications, particularly similar-named medications or similar packaging (Studer et al., 2023). Brown-bag sessions are good for assessing the appearance of pills, labeling, and understanding of the patient, particularly with repackaged or unlabeled medications. An overview of patient-level barriers and tools for locating them is presented in Figure 12.

Figure 12. Centered approaches to helping patients identify their medications

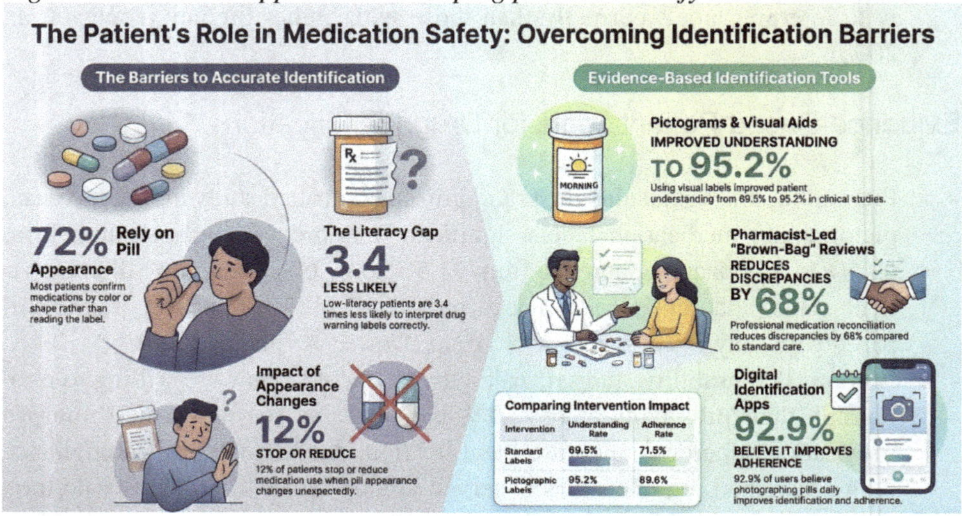

The figure shows the aspects that complicate the process of patients finding the appropriate medication and enumerating effective tools such as pictograms, brown-bag reviews under the leadership of pharmacists, and digital medication identification applications.

Quick Response Code (QR Code) and Global Standard One (GS1) Barcoded Packaging for Drug Identification

Quick response (QR) codes and Global Standard One (GS1) barcodes improve medication identification and reduce confusion, especially in the context of LASA drug errors. QR-coded medication bottles improved users' ability to identify and self-administer medications in a randomized controlled trial in the U.S. QR technology helps patients verify drug identity and understand instructions, regardless of age (Svensk & McIntyre, 2021). Participants who used QR code–linked information gave more correct responses in the simulated medication-use scenarios.

The Japanese Pharmaceutical and Medical Device Act now requires drug packaging to have GS1 barcodes for smartphone access to electronic package inserts. These digital inserts have real-time updates, multilingual instructions, and visual identifiers. Self-medication and over-the-counter drug users reported increased confidence in identifying their medications with GS1 barcode access (Hatabu et al., 2025). Although professional pill identification requires imprint codes, these digital innovations improve patient accessibility and clarity, promote safe medication use and reduce misidentification.

Label Design, Cultural Sensitivity and Interpretation

Effective labeling of medication is vital in the process of having the drug be identified accurately and limiting the LASA errors associated with drugs. According to a systematic review of a study conducted by Shrank et al., patient-centered label design components such as increased font size, plain language, clear headings, logical layout, and the usage of white spaces significantly increase readability and understanding, especially in the case of both older people and those with low health literacy. Although there is a relative paucity of data linking these design features to clinical safety outcomes, they are consistently associated with enhanced patient comprehension and thus provide a rationale to incorporate them into label development (Shrank et al., 2007). A panacea is needed to address the problem of auxiliary warning stickers that are commonly pasted on prescription bottles or into blister packs. It was found that such labels are often printed in small fonts, in hard-to-read positions (e.g., at a vertical angle or around corners), often inconsistent, unstandardized usage of colors. Injuries to patients with low literacy or sighted patients are far less likely to correctly interpret the intended warnings efficiently, in part because of such design flaws (Davis et al., 2006).

GRID FACTOR ANALYSIS (GFA): A MUITIDIMENSIONAL APPROACH TO LASA RISK EVALUATION

Grid factor analysis (GFA) is a comparison of two products based on spelling, pronunciation, formulation, packaging, and therapeutic use. In comparison to single-metric models, GFA considers visual and contextual effects that lead to LASA errors in the process of prescribing, dispensing, and self-administration.

Health Canada has developed the GFA to support its own proprietary name review process and has been supported by frameworks in Australia and the U.S. It has been scaled to hospital formularies, regulatory approvals, and risk assessment at the pharmacy level (Emmerton et al., 2020; Marilyn Schwartz, 2007; U.S. Department of Health and Human Services Food and Drug Administration (FDA), 2019, 2020). This instrument is especially applicable in environments where generic replacements, repackaging, or unit-dose dispensing hides the labels of original drugs—circumstances that make it more likely to mix up.

Attributes are rated on the basis of how much they have the potential to contribute to a LASA error with the following scoring levels (Table 3):

- High: The feature is almost the same or closely similar to the comparator. This is likely confusing unless it is alleviated.

- Moderate: There is a minor visual, phonetic, or contextual overlap; in some situations, confusion may arise.
- Low: There are clear distinctions in spelling, pronunciation, form, or labeling, which minimizes the risk of confusion.

Identical: Applied to nondifferentiating attributes (e.g., same dose, group of patients) that do not directly cause harm but can combine with other high-risk factors to increase risk.

Once each factor has been scored, the reviewer establishes the cumulative LASA risk on the basis of the number and severity of the high and moderate scores:

- When 3 or more high-risk factors are detected, the couple is said to have a high cumulative LASA risk.
- If the pair scores are predominantly moderate with a small number of high scores, further mitigation can be required (e.g., the use of auxiliary labels and barcode scanning).
- In the case that all the scores are low or the same, the LASA risk is minimal.

This method of expert judgment offers the flexibility to use contextual information of clinical experience, e.g., whether a drug is used in high-risk transitions (e.g., during night shifts) or in vulnerable groups.

Table 3. Grid factor analysis example for drug name similarity

Factor Category	Drug A: Prednoral	Drug B: Prenoral	Risk Score
Brand name spelling	Similar letter sequence	Similar start and ending	High
Generic name (INN)	Prednisolone	Prenisolone	Moderate
Sound-alike pronunciation	/ˈprɛd.nə.rɔːl/	/ˈprɛn.ə.rɔːl/	High
Dosage form	Oral tablet	Oral tablet	High
Strength available	5 mg, 10 mg	5 mg	Moderate
Indication overlap	Autoimmune conditions	Autoimmune conditions	High
Packaging & color scheme	White/red blister strip	White/pink blister strip	Moderate
Label font and layout	Red sans-serif font	Red serif font	Moderate
Patient group	Adults	Adults	Identical
Daily dosing schedule	Once daily	Once daily	Identical
Cumulative LASA Risk			High

Note: Prednoral and Prenoral are fictional names that are used only to demonstrate.

Grid factor analysis has been adopted by national health authorities and hospital systems that are focused on preventing LASA-related incidents. Health Canada, as an example, employs GFA to evaluate proprietary drug name submissions, especially in cases where new entrants are similar to existing products (Schwartz, 2007). (Marilyn Schwartz, 2007). The POCATool is a phonetic and orthographic similarity tool used by the U.S. FDA to measure preapproval risk (U.S. Department of Health and Human Services, Food and Drug Administration (FDA), 2021). Hospitals are able to customize GFA (Generic Formulary Assessment) scoring matrices to local scripts, language, and patient populations. The tool, when incorporated into electronic health records (EHRs) or pharmacy information systems, may result in alerts when faced with a high-risk prescribing or dispensing situation, thereby improving medication safety processes.

CONCLUSION

To prevent LASA medication errors, identifying drugs is important. This chapter discussed the issue of visually similar or repackaged or unlabeled drugs. Although assistance is provided with the help of tools such as imprint codes, AI-based recognition, and drug image systems, gaps still exist regarding the availability, uniformity, and usability of these tools for patients. It is essential to have an integrated solution that involves regulatory supervision, user-centered design, and patient education. Healthcare systems can mitigate the risks of misidentification through enhancing both system-level protection and patient-facing initiatives to ensure medication safety in clinical and community environments.

REFERENCES

Australian Commission on Safety and Quality in Health Care (ACSQHC). (2012). *Consultation on labelling and packaging of medicines: Submission to the consultation on theTGA Medicine Labelling and Packaging Review* Retrieved 24 July from https://www.tga.gov.au/sites/default/files/consult-labelling-packaging-review-120524-submission-acsqhc.pdf?

Australian Commission on Safety and Quality in Health Care (ACSQHC). (2024). *National mixed-case lettering list*. ACSQHC. Retrieved 18 March from https://www.safetyandquality.gov.au/sites/default/files/2024-04/national_mixed-case_lettering_list.pdf

Barenie, R. E., Kesselheim, A. S., Gagne, J. J., Lu, Z., Campbell, E. G., Dutcher, S. K., & Sarpatwari, A. (2020). Preferences for and experiences with pill appearance changes: National surveys of patients and pharmacists. *The American Journal of Managed Care*, *26*(8), 340–347. DOI: 10.37765/ajmc.2020.44070 PMID: 32835461

Carayon, P., Wetterneck, T. B., Rivera-Rodriguez, A. J., Hundt, A. S., Hoonakker, P., Holden, R., & Gurses, A. P. (2014). Human factors systems approach to healthcare quality and patient safety. *Applied Ergonomics*, *45*(1), 14–25. DOI: 10.1016/j.apergo.2013.04.023 PMID: 23845724

Carayon, P., Wooldridge, A., Hoonakker, P., Hundt, A. S., & Kelly, M. M. (2020). SEIPS 3.0: Human-centered design of the patient journey for patient safety. *Applied Ergonomics*, *84*, 103033. DOI: 10.1016/j.apergo.2019.103033 PMID: 31987516

Chanakit, T., Kumpalum, D., Kunwaradisai, N., Swatwongchai, Y., & Ragsawong, N. (2009).. . *Characteristics of Drug Information Service in Thailand Thai Pharmaceutical and Health Science Journal*, *4*(4), 490–499.

Choi, Y. J., & Kim, H. (2019). Effect of pharmacy-led medication reconciliation in emergency departments: A systematic review and meta-analysis. *Journal of Clinical Pharmacy and Therapeutics*, *44*(6), 932–945. DOI: 10.1111/jcpt.13019 PMID: 31436877

Cohen, M. R., Harris, D., Zanoletty, A., & Linvill-Neal, D. (2021). *The inside track on drug naming safety standards*. Retrieved 15 June from https://www.ismp.org/sites/default/files/attachments/2021-07/The%20Inside%20Track%20on%20Drug%20Naming%20Standards-%20Handouts.pdf

Cunha, A., Adão, T., & Trigueiros, P. (2014). HelpmePills: A Mobile Pill Recognition Tool for Elderly Persons. *Procedia Technology*, *16*, 1523–1532. DOI: 10.1016/j.protcy.2014.10.174

Davis, T. C., Wolf, M. S., Bass, P. F.III, Middlebrooks, M., Kennen, E., Baker, D. W., Bennett, C. L., Durazo-Arvizu, R., Bocchini, A., Savory, S., & Parker, R. M. (2006). Low literacy impairs comprehension of prescription drug warning labels. *Journal of General Internal Medicine*, *21*(8), 847–851. DOI: 10.1111/j.1525-1497.2006.00529.x PMID: 16881945

Dowse, R., & Ehlers, M. (2005). Medicine labels incorporating pictograms: Do they influence understanding and adherence? *Patient Education and Counseling*, *58*(1), 63–70. DOI: 10.1016/j.pec.2004.06.012 PMID: 15950838

Drug.com. (2025). *Pill Identifier*. Retrieved 30 July from https://www.drugs.com/pill_identification.html

Emmerton, L., Curtain, C., Swaminathan, G., & Dowling, H. (2020). Development and exploratory analysis of software to detect look-alike, sound-alike medicine names. *International Journal of Medical Informatics*, *137*, 104119. DOI: 10.1016/j.ijmedinf.2020.104119 PMID: 32172184

European Medicines Agency (EMA). (2025). *Medicines*. Retrieved 31 July from https://www.ema.europa.eu/en/medicines

Faculty of Pharmaceutical Sciences. U. R. U. (2022). *Drug identification database*. Retrieved 11 Oct from https://drugiden.ubu.ac.th/

Faculty of Pharmaceutical Sciences Ubon Ratchathani University. (2025). *Drug Identification Database, Ubon Ratchathani University*. Retrieved 31 July from https://drugiden2.ubu.ac.th/

Health Canada. (2004). *ARCHIVED - Issue analysis summary: Look-alike Sound-alike (LA/SA) health product names: the development of a comprehensive policy recommendation for Look-alike Sound-alike (LA/SA) health product names*. Retrieved 15 June from https://www.canada.ca/en/health-canada/services/drugs-health-products/biologics-radiopharmaceuticals-genetic-therapies/look-alike-sound-alike/issue-analysis-summary-look-alike-sound-alike-health-product-names-development-comprehensive-policy-recommendation-look-alike-sound-alike.html

Health Canada. (2025). *Drug Product Database (DPD)*. Retrieved 31 July from https://health-products.canada.ca/dpd-bdpp/index-eng.jsp

Heo, J., Kang, Y., Lee, S., Jeong, D. H., & Kim, K. M. (2023). An Accurate Deep Learning-Based System for Automatic Pill Identification: Model Development and Validation. *Journal of Medical Internet Research*, *25*, e41043. DOI: 10.2196/41043 PMID: 36637893

Institute for Safe Medication Practices (ISMP). (2021). *ISMP targeted medication safety best practices for hospitals.* Retrieved 31 July from https://www.ismp.org/sites/default/files/attachments/2020-02/2020-2021%20TMSBP-%20FINAL_1.pdf

Institute for Safe Medication Practices (ISMP) Canada. (2023). *Reported Concerns with Labeling and Packaging of High-Alert Medications in Vials and Ampoules: A Multi-Incident Analysis.* Retrieved 25 Feb from https://ismpcanada.ca/wp-content/uploads/ISMPCSB2023-i2-Label-Package-High-Alert-Meds.pdf

Kesselheim, A. S., Bykov, K., Avorn, J., Tong, A., Doherty, M., & Choudhry, N. K. (2014). Burden of changes in pill appearance for patients receiving generic cardiovascular medications after myocardial infarction: Cohort and nested case–control studies. *Annals of Internal Medicine, 161*(2), 96–103. DOI: 10.7326/M13-2381 PMID: 25023248

Larmené-Beld, K. H. M., Alting, E. K., & Taxis, K. (2018). A systematic literature review on strategies to avoid look-alike errors of labels. *European Journal of Clinical Pharmacology, 74*(8), 985–993. DOI: 10.1007/s00228-018-2471-z PMID: 29754215

Lexicomp. (2024). *Metformin: Drug information.* UpToDate. Retrieved 10 Fwb from https://www-uptodate-com

Lumbreras, B., Sanz-Valero, J., & López-Pintor, E. (2022). Impact of Variation in Pill/Package Appearance of Drugs on Patients' Behavior: A Systematic Review. *Journal of Patient Safety, 18*(4), 310–317. DOI: 10.1097/PTS.0000000000000941 PMID: 35452203

Mahidol University. (2025). *Medilet: Thailand drug database by Faculty of Pharmacy, Mahidol University.* Retrieved 31 July from https://pharmacy.mahidol.ac.th/medilet/

Manager Online. (2018). *Yaa Chud is dangerous! Thai FDA warns it can be fatal due to lack of control and regulation.* Retrieved 28 July from https://mgronline.com/onlinesection/detail/9680000053297

Marilyn Schwartz. (2007). *Look-Alike/Sound-Alike (LASA) drug names - review update -Health Canada's Perspective.* Retrieved 14 April from https://capra.ca/_uploads/archive/presentations/14-MarilynSchwartz-LA-SAGuidanceUpdate.pdf

Medicines and Healthcare products Regulatory Agency (MHRA). (2020). *Best practice guidance on the labeling and packaging of medicines. Medicines and Healthcare products Regulatory Agency.* Retrieved 13 July from https://assets.publishing.service.gov.uk/media/5fe09fa48fa8f51489f14374/Best_practice_guidance_labelling_and_packaging_of_medicines.pdf

MedSnap. (2025). *MedSnap: Mobile drug verification using computer vision.* Retrieved 31 July from https://medsnap.com

Merative. (2025). *Micromedex: Clinical decision support.* Retrieved 31 July from https://www.merative.com/clinical-decision-support/micromedex

Momtahan, K., Burns, C. M., Jeon, J., Hyland, S., & Gabriele, S. (2008). Using human factors methods to evaluate the labeling of injectable drugs. *Healthc Q*, 11(3 Spec No.), 122-128. DOI: 10.12927/hcq.2013.19598

Monnier, A. A., Do, N. T. T., Asante, K. P., Afari-Asiedu, S., Khan, W. A., Munguambe, K., Sevene, E., Tran, T. K., Nguyen, C. T. K., Punpuing, S., Gómez-Olivé, F. X., van Doorn, H. R., Caillet, C., Newton, P. N., Ariana, P., Wertheim, H. F. L., Wertheim, H. F. L., Monnier, A. A., Newton, P. N., & van Doorn, H. R. (2023). Is this pill an antibiotic or a painkiller? Improving the identification of oral antibiotics for better use. *The Lancet. Global Health, 11*(8), e1308–e1313. DOI: 10.1016/S2214-109X(23)00258-9 PMID: 37474237

Monthly Index of Medical Specialties (MIMS) Thailand. (2025). *Pill identifier.* Retrieved 31 July from https://www.mims.com/thailand/image/advancedsearch

Munesh, G., & Bhavaraju, M. L. R. (2024). Regulatory framework for USFDA regulated drug product labeling update. *Pharmaceutical Sciences Asia*, 51(1), 10–18

Napaporn, J., Buakaew, P., Suksakornthanawat, P., Sripa, S., Jinatongthai, P., & Supapaan, T. (2022). Analogous comparison of registered brand name drugs of tablets and capsules commercially available in Thailand: A retrospective study. *PLoS One, 17*(10), e0276321. DOI: 10.1371/journal.pone.0276321 PMID: 36260612

Napaporn, J., Supapaan, J., Jinathongthai, P., Sripa, S., Kamnuek, J., Khakaew, C., & Pitchayajittipong, C. (2023). Analysis of similarity of physical appearances of pills in the forms of tablets and capsules commercially available in Thailand. *Thai J Pharm Pract, 15*(4), 1060–1070.

National Patient Safety Agency. Patient Safety Division. (2008). *Design for patient safety: a guide to labeling and packaging of injectable medicines.* Retrieved 31 July from https://www.intmedsafe.net/wp-content/uploads/2014/01/0592_InjectablesBookV9_Web1.pdf

Newton, P. N., Hampton, C. Y., Alter-Hall, K., Teerwarakulpana, T., Prakongpan, S., Ruangveerayuth, R., White, N. J., Day, N. P. J., Tudino, M. B., Mancuso, N., & Fernández, F. M. (2008). Characterization of "Yaa Chud" Medicine on the Thailand-Myanmar border: Selecting for drug-resistant malaria and threatening public health. *The American Journal of Tropical Medicine and Hygiene*, *79*(5), 662–669. DOI: 10.4269/ajtmh.2008.79.662 PMID: 18981500

Pharmaceuticals and Medical Devices Agency (PMDA). (2025). *PMDA English website*. Retrieved 31 July from https://www.pmda.go.jp/english/

Pornwattanakavee, S., Petchsomrit, A., Methaneethorn, J., & Leelakanok, N. (2021). How to Know the Unknown Drugs: A Qualitative Study for Drug Identification Tools Used in Thai Community Pharmacies. *Teikyo Medical Journal*, *44*(3), 849–858.

Prokop, D., Babigumira, J., & Lewis, A. (2020). Pill Identification using a Mobile Phone App for Assessing Medication Adherence and Post-Market Drug Surveillance. *arXiv preprint arXiv:*2004.11479.

Reallon, E., Yailian, A.-L., Marchand, C., Filali, S., Merienne, C., Pivot, C.,...Pirot, F. (2021). Medicine Identification New Database (MIND): A quick, simple and accurate tool for the identification of unlabeled medication in hospital pharmacies. *Spectroscopy Europe*, 33(6). https://doi.org/10.1255/sew.2021.a27

RxList. (2025). *RxList Pill Identification Tool*. Retrieved 30 July from https://www.rxlist.com/pill-identification-tool/article.htm

Sangsuriyan, S., Duangkhan, S., Anekprasongkul, W., & Leelakanok, N. (2018). *Drug identification tools in pharmacies*. Faculty of Pharmaceutical Sciences, Burapha University.

Sarpatwari, A., Gagne, J. J., Lu, Z., Campbell, E. G., Carman, W. J., Enger, C. L., Dutcher, S. K., Jiang, W., & Kesselheim, A. S. (2019). A Survey of Patients' Perceptions of Pill Appearance and Responses to Changes in Appearance for Four Chronic Disease Medications. *Journal of General Internal Medicine*, *34*(3), 420–428. DOI: 10.1007/s11606-018-4791-1 PMID: 30632102

Shrank, W., Avorn, J., Rolon, C., & Shekelle, P. (2007). Effect of content and format of prescription drug labels on readability, understanding, and medication use: A systematic review. *The Annals of Pharmacotherapy*, *41*(5), 783–801. DOI: 10.1345/aph.1H582 PMID: 17426075

Studer, H., Imfeld-Isenegger, T. L., Beeler, P. E., Ceppi, M. G., Rosen, C., Bodmer, M., Boeni, F., Hersberger, K. E., & Lampert, M. L. (2023). The impact of pharmacist-led medication reconciliation and interprofessional ward rounds on drug-related problems at hospital discharge. *International Journal of Clinical Pharmacy*, *45*(1), 117–125. DOI: 10.1007/s11096-022-01496-3 PMID: 36327045

Sunpuwan, M., Punpuing, S., Jaruruengpaisan, W., Kinsman, J., & Wertheim, H. (2019). What is in the drug packet?: Access and use of non-prescribed poly-pharmaceutical packs (Yaa Chud) in the community in Thailand. *BMC Public Health*, *19*(1), 971. DOI: 10.1186/s12889-019-7300-5 PMID: 31331304

Supapaan, T., Pitchayajittipong, C., Sonrasawan, K., Chittawee, C., & Napaporn, J. (2024). Development of the database for look-alike, sound-alike drugs in Thailand. *Thai J Pharm Pract*, *16*(1), 112–125.

Supapaan, T. S., Kamnuek, J., Khakaew, C., Jungsuwadee, T., Songmuang, A., Saksit, S., & Napaporn, J. (2024). Assessment of look-Alike, Sound-Alike similarities among brand names of tablets and capsules: A cross-sectional survey in Thailand. *Pharmacy Practice*, *22*(3), 2955. DOI: 10.18549/PharmPract.2024.3.2955

Supapaan, T. S., Napaporn, J., Ruthirakanok, R., Srichathum, S., Songmuang, A., & Pitchayajittipong, C. (2024). Look-alike sound-alike (LASA) medication errors in Thai hospitals. *Pharmacy Practice*, *22*(1), 2886.

Supapaan, T. S., Somsorn, S., Saensupha, N., Songmuang, T., Songmuang, A., Jaturapattarawong, A., & Napaporn, J. (2024). Development of drug information and drug images identification database for supporting the medical management system at Warinchamrab hospital. *Pharmacy Practice*, *22*(4). Advance online publication. DOI: 10.18549/PharmPract.2024.4.3057

Supapaan, T. S., Songmuang, A., Napaporn, J., Sangsukwow, P., Boonrod, P., In-tarapongsakul, P., Jaturapattarawong, A., & Pitchayajittipong, C. (2024). Look-alike/sound-alike medication errors: An in-depth examination through a hospital case study. *Pharmacy Practice*, *22*(2), 2959. DOI: 10.18549/PharmPract.2024.2.2959

Svensk, J., & McIntyre, S. E. (2021). Using QR Code Technology to Reduce Self-Administered Medication Errors. *Journal of Pharmacy Practice*, *34*(4), 587–591. DOI: 10.1177/0897190019885245 PMID: 31835959

Thai Food and Drug Administration. (2025). *National Drug Information (NDI) database*. Retrieved 31 July from https://ndi.fda.moph.go.th/

Thailand Food and Drug Administration. (2025). *Public pharmaceutical regulatory information: Details of medicinal product.* Retrieved 3 April from Thaipharmaitem. (2025). *Pill identifier.* Retrieved 31 July from https://thaipharmaitem.com/en/drug-identification-pill-identifier/

The Institute for Safe Medication Practices (ISMP). (2023a). *FDA and ISMP lists of look-alike drug names with recommended tall man (mixed case) letters.* Retrieved 16 Apr from https://www.ismp.org/system/files/resources/2023-01/ISMP_Tallman_Letters_012523_MS5087%20%282%29.pdf

The Institute for Safe Medication Practices (ISMP). (2023b). *List of confused drug names.* Retrieved 16 Apr from https://www.ismp.org/recommendations/confused-drug-names-list

Tranchard, F., Gauthier, J., Hein, C., Lacombe, J., Brett, K., Villars, H., Sallerin, B., Montastruc, J.-L., & Despas, F. (2019). Drug identification by the patient: Perception of patients, physicians and pharmacists. *Thérapie*, *74*(6), 591–598. DOI: 10.1016/j.therap.2019.03.003 PMID: 31014975

U.S. Department of Health and Human Services Food and Drug Administration (FDA). (2019). *Procedures for handling requests for nonproprietary name suffix review for biological products newly licensed under section* 351*of the PHS Act.* Retrieved 15 June from https://www.fda.gov/media/123894/download

U.S. Department of Health and Human Services Food and Drug Administration (FDA). (2020). *FDA name differentiation project.* Retrieved 06 Aug from https://www.fda.gov/drugs/medication-errors-related-cder-regulated-drug-products/fda-name-differentiation-project

U.S. Department of Health and Human Services Food and Drug Administration (FDA). (2024). *Medication errors related to CDER-regulated drug products.* Retrieved 13 June from https://www.fda.gov/drugs/drug-safety-and-availability/medication-errors-related-cder-regulated-drug-products

U.S. Department of Health and Human Services Food and Drug Administration (FDA), Center for Drug Evaluation and Research (CDER). (2015). *Size, shape, and other physical attributes of generic tablets and capsules.* Retrieved 10 Jan from https://www.fda.gov/files/drugs/published/Size--Shape--and-Other-Physical-Attributes-of-Generic-Tablets-and-Capsules.pdf

US Food and Drug Administration. (US FDA). (2024). *Utilizing Generic Drug Awareness to Improve Patient Outcomes with Dr. Sarah Ibrahim.* Retrieved 25 July from https://www.fda.gov/drugs/news-events-human-drugs/utilizing-generic-drug-awareness-improve-patient-outcomes-dr-sarah-ibrahim?

U.S. Food and Drug Administration. (2025). *National Drug Code Directory*. Retrieved 31 July from https://www.accessdata.fda.gov/scripts/cder/ndc/index.cfm

U.S. National Library of Medicine. (2025). *RxNorm overview*. https://www.nlm.nih.gov/research/umls/rxnorm/

Weiss, B. D., Brega, A. G., LeBlanc, W. G., Mabachi, N. M., Barnard, J., Albright, K., Cifuentes, M., Brach, C., & West, D. R. (2016). Improving the Effectiveness of Medication Review: Guidance from the Health Literacy Universal Precautions Toolkit. *Journal of the American Board of Family Medicine : JABFM*, *29*(1), 18–23. DOI: 10.3122/jabfm.2016.01.150163 PMID: 26769873

Wolters Kluwer. (2025). *Medi-Span: drug data for clinical and business decision support*. Retrieved 31 July from https://www.wolterskluwer.com/en/solutions/medi-span

Woods, D., Dekker, S., Cook, R., Johannesen, L., & Sarter, N. (2017). *Behind human error*. CRC Press. DOI: 10.1201/9781315568935

World Health Organization. (2024). *Medication safety: WHO webinar on the Global Patient Safety Challenge Medication Without Harm*. Retrieved 24 July from https://cdn.who.int/media/docs/default-source/integrated-health-services-%28ihs%29/psf/medication-without-harm/medication-safety-who-webinar-7march2024.pdf

ABBREVIATIONS

ACSQHC: Australian Commission on Safety and Quality in Health Care
ADR: Adverse Drug Reaction
AI: Artificial Intelligence
BCMA: Barcode Medication Administration
GFA: Grid Factor Analysis
COVID-19: Coronavirus Disease of 2019
CPOE: Computerized Provider Order Entry
DIS: Drug Information Services
DPD: Drug Product Database
e-MAR: Electronic Medication Administration Record
EHR: Electronic Health Record
FDB: First Databank
ISMP: Institute for Safe Medication Practices
LASA: Look-Alike, Sound-Alike
MIMS Thailand: Monthly Index of Medical Specialties (MIMS) Thailand

NDC: U.S. FDA's National Drug Code
PMDA: Pharmaceuticals and Medical Devices Agency
ResNet-32: Residual Network-32
YOLOv5: You Only Look Once version 5
WHO: World Health Organization

Chapter 4
Addressing LASA Medication Errors Through Improved Drug Packaging and Labeling

ABSTRACT

Look-alike, sound-alike (LASA) medication errors have continued to pose a great challenge to patient safety across the globe. This chapter discusses the role of drug packaging and labeling as systems of active safety with respect to LASA error prevention. It evaluates and examines typography, color coding, tall man lettering, barcode validation, and trade dress in ophthalmic, pediatric, anesthetic, and injectable products depending on human factors engineering, regulatory frameworks, and international standards. Reviewed case studies and international recommendations from the FDA, WHO, MHRA, ISO, and ADA are used to demonstrate how the cognitive load reduction and enhancement of medication safety can be achieved through structured design and technological integration.

INTRODUCTION

Look-Alike, Sound-Alike (LASA) medication errors, caused by drug packaging and labeling similarities, threaten patient safety (Cohen, 2007; WHO Collaborating Centre for Patient Safety Solutions, 2007). Improved drug packaging and labeling can reduce LASA errors and prevent adverse events (Ciociano & Bagnasco, 2014; Ciociano et al., 2013; Ostini et al., 2012). This chapter introduces LASA drug packaging and labeling errors, a complex topic. Similarities in these areas can cause LASA medication errors (Dsouza & Kulkarni, 2017; Merry et al., 2011; Ryan et al.,

DOI: 10.4018/979-8-3373-5478-1.ch004

2024). Name confusion accounts for 25% of medication errors, and packaging and labeling confusion accounts for 33% (Berman, 2004; Estock et al., 2018). LASA drugs pose a significant risk. Ashcroft et al. reported that similar medication packaging causes 7.6% of dispensing errors(Ashcroft et al., 2005). Look-alike labels and drug packaging designs can cause medication errors (Momo et al., 2019; Ryan et al., 2024). In one of the tertiary care hospitals supported by the government, midazolam, heparin, and rocuronium vials were mixed accidentally (Gangakhedkar et al., 2019).

Although automated dispensing cabinets (ADCs) are created to increase medication safety, they fail to fully eradicate the LASA error probability, particularly when several LASA medicines are placed in a single compartment (Ruutiainen et al., 2021). High workloads aggravate this issue, and the use of generic brands with a similar outlook, which, despite being economically beneficial, may cause confusion and underdose, has been brought up in the case of opioids as post-operative analgesia (Schnoor et al., 2015).

The importance of being alert in avoiding such errors is paramount, as a case example where a dispensing error by packaging confusion was well explored to avoid repetition (Shao et al., 2018). These errors are caused by environmental factors, which include distractions at the time of dispensing, and technological solutions, including font variations, automated notifications, barcode scanning, and real-time reporting during dispensing. Software is suggested to reduce such risks (Emmerton & Rizk, 2012).

The equal coloring of drug labels, identical packaging, word positioning and word color have also been found to be major contributors to medication errors, especially during the dispensing, storage and administration stages (de Almeida Lopes et al., 2012; Dsouza & Kulkarni, 2017).

The Institute for Safe Medication Practices (ISMP) stresses the importance of addressing these issues to ensure medication safety (WHO Collaborating Centre for Patient Safety Solutions, 2007; World Health Organization, 2007). Financial constraints and local setups often prevent full security implementation even with extensive LASA error prevention recommendations (Schnoor et al., 2015). (Schnoor et al., 2015). The Institute of Medicine's "Crossing the Quality Chasm" report recommends a systems approach to improve patient safety in the healthcare industry, which lags behind manufacturing (Rastogi, 2012). The Joint Commission required identifying and annually reviewing a list of LASA drugs and proactively implementing safety strategies in 2005 (Rastogi, 2012). LASA medication errors indicate that hospitals, the medical industry, and regulatory authorities must work together to prevent look-alike packaging and ensure medication safety (Schnoor et al., 2015; Shao et al., 2018).

Objectives of the Chapter

The aims of this chapter are as follows:

(1) To explain how to use the color, font, layout and container shape could help healthcare professionals and patients recognize medicines and prevent LASA errors.
(2) To demonstrate this difference, tall man lettering and the use of color coding can make labels more readable and differentiate between look-alike products and names.
(3) To analyze and compare the labeling and packaging of safety requirements established by the FDA, WHO, MHRA, ISO and ADA.
(4) To explain how barcodes and RFID can enhance the safety of injectable medicine at the point of care, which is the bedside.
(5) To discuss the role of international standards of packaging and labeling of medication in decreasing confusion and enhancing the medication safety rate across healthcare systems.

Organization of the Chapter

This chapter introduces look-alike sound-alike (LASA) medication errors and emphasizes how packaging and labeling protect patients. Packaging design principles, including container shape, typography, layout, and visual cues to differentiate drugs, are then discussed. Next, the chapter discusses how tall man lettering, color coding, and standardized key information placement improve readability and reduce confusion. Ophthalmic eye-drop cap color standards, local anesthetic cartridge banding, and anesthesia syringe labels are then examined. Barcodes, and RFID enable real-time verification and traceability in high-risk environments. Afterward, the FDA, WHO, MHRA, ISO, and ADA regulatory frameworks and safety standards are reviewed. Case studies and best practices constitute the last part of the chapter, as they demonstrate how packaging has played a part in the reduction of LASA errors in hospitals and pharmacies. Integration and future directions underline how consideration of design, digital solutions, and standardization at the global level can make packaging an active safety tool and provide practice and policy suggestions.

MEDICATION PACKAGING AS A SAFETY SYSTEM

LASA confusion is most likely when containers and labels become mixed on a crowded shelf. Distinctive, clear packaging ruptures that chain, as it enables every user, pharmacist, nurse, patient, or caregiver to recognize the appropriate product with just one look (Estock et al., 2018; Lizano-Díez et al., 2020; World Health Organization, 2023).

The WHO suggests mapping known LASA pairs, restricting the strength of a product, and ensuring that each strength appears visually different (World Health Organization, 2023).

It has been reported that one-third of medication errors are associated with confusing packaging and labeling, with almost 30% of the reported lethal errors (Berman, 2004). In numerous instances, the name of the drug and its strength were not well defined, the fonts were too small, and the vials of dissimilar medications resembled each other. To avoid this, the FDA and ISMP suggest that clutter should be avoided, important details should be placed at the forefront, and corporate logos should be kept to a minimum, which may divert attention to important information. The basic strategies that have been effective in reducing the LASA risk are as follows:

1. A high-contrast font with bold letters that are easy to read for the generic name and the strength.
2. Unified color systems for high-alert areas such as anesthetics, eye drops, and emergency drugs.
3. Selections were checked twice using automated identifiers, barcodes, quick response (QR) codes, and radio-frequency identification (RFID) tags.
4. Unit-dose and unit-of-use designs that do not require multistrength look-alike vials.
5. Bright warning signs indicating concentrated or high-risk drugs.
6. Easy-to-understand patient labels in plain language and pictograms.

The possibility of an extremely similar neuromuscular blocker and a sedative being mixed in nearly identical vials in an ICU is a tragic reminder (Cohen, 2007). The same mistakes were made with vials of potassium chloride that resembled saline, and the FDA had to add black caps and warning labels of MUST BE DILUTED to avoid mistakes. These illustrations demonstrate the need to design packaging in a manner that minimizes visual and cognitive overload (Cohen, 2007; Monnier et al., 2023).

These broad principles are translated in the following sections to three main design areas that promote safety: standardization to minimize visual noise, visual differentiation to promote clarity, and inclusive and accessible design for all users.

Standardization to Reduce Visual Noise

Standardization reduces variability in packaging so that any anomaly is easier to detect. The WHO recommends limiting each concentration to one container size and one cap color to avoid strength-stacking errors (World Health Organization, 2023). The US FDA encourages avoiding unnecessary vial sizes and keeping design elements consistent across product lines (U.S. Department of Health and Human Services Food and Drug Administration, 2022). Berman also reported that aligning the volume of a vial with drug strength decreases the patient's cognitive load (Berman, 2004).

Strategies include the following:

- Assigning one bottle size, cap color, and closure style per strength.
- Aligning volume increments with strength increments (e.g., 1 mg/1 mL, 5 mg/5 mL).
- Printing the generic name and strength on all sides of vials or ampoules.
- Removing distracting logos or graphics (U.S. Department of Health and Human Services Food and Drug Administration, 2022).

For example, in 2006 and 2007, nine neonates received 1,000-fold heparin overdoses because 10 units/mL and 10,000 units/mL vials were packaged in nearly identical 1-mL vials with nondistinct look-alike labels. Three infants in Indiana died, while three in California survived after intensive care. Investigators identified multiple contributing factors, including look-alike vial sizes, inadequate label differentiation, and stocking errors in automated dispensing cabinets. To prevent recurrence, high-strength vials were removed and replaced with unit-dose prefilled syringes, barcode verification was introduced, and the manufacturer redesigned the labels to emphasize concentration differences. After these interventions, no further LASA errors occurred (Arimura et al., 2008).

Visual Differentiation to Improve Clarity

Even with standardized packaging, products must remain unmistakable at a glance. The FDA (2022) recommends high-contrast fonts, clear hierarchies, and sufficient white space (U.S. Department of Health and Human Services Food and Drug Administration, 2022). The WHO (2023) encourages the use of distinct shapes and textures for high-risk drugs to improve tactile recognition (World Health Organization, 2023).

The following design approaches can be used:

- Bold sans serif fonts, high contrast color bands, and abundant white space. The guidance of the FDA also emphasizes having a clear hierarchy of layouts and avoiding clutters (U.S. Department of Health and Human Services Food and Drug Administration, 2022).
- The brand name is written below the generic name, which is based on a user-centric design to emphasize the importance of core information (The Institute for Safe Medication Practices (ISMP), 2022; U.S. Department of Health and Human Services Food and Drug Administration, 2022).
- Tall man lettering is used for similar-sounding drug names (e.g., DOPamine vs. DOBUTamine). Tall man is officially supported by the FDA and the Institute for Safe Medication Practices (ISMP) to lessen name confusion, and it was supported by eye-tracking research (Cohen, 2001; Filik et al., 2004; Otero López et al., 2011; The Institute for Safe Medication Practices Canada (ISMP Canada), 2007).
- Unique blister pack layouts and tactile caps provide shape and touch cues for users who are under stress or who are experiencing low vision.

In a neonatal intensive care unit (NICU), researchers evaluated how human-centered design (HCD) labels improve medication safety using the Human Error Assessment and Reduction Technique (HEART). Redesigned labels featured a clear layout hierarchy, emphasis on generic name and strength, simplified information, and reduced visual clutter. Compared with standard look-alike labels, HCD labels reduced the human error probability by up to 56%, and the contribution of label design to overall unreliability decreased by more than 40%. Clinicians reported that the redesigned labels were easier to read under stress and improved reliability in high-risk environments (Aceves-Gonzalez et al., 2024).

Inclusive and Accessible Design for all Users

Medication packaging must be usable by all stakeholders, including older adults, caregivers with limited literacy, and healthcare workers with color vision deficiencies. FDA guidelines suggest working with at least 12-point sans-serif fonts, nonglare or matte surfaces to minimize reflections, and clear layouts with a minimum amount of clutter (U.S. Department of Health and Human Services Food and Drug Administration, 2022). Similarly, the WHO emphasizes the need to use plain language, pictograms, and multilingual labeling to enhance patient-centered communication (World Health Organization, 2023).

The key elements of inclusive design are as follows:

- Large, clear sans-serif fonts (at least 12 points) on patient labels.

- Matte or low-glare surfaces to make text easier to read in any light.
- Raised symbols or embossed warnings for high-alert medicines.
- Easy-to-open caps for patients with arthritis or weak grip.

Research on human factors highlights that tactile cues and ergonomic packaging improve usability in low-light or high-stress clinical environments, further enhancing medication safety (Berman, 2004). Standardization minimizes visual overload, visual differentiation enhances readability, and inclusive design safeguards every user. These measures are in line with the recommendations provided by the WHO (2023) and the FDA (2022), who do not consider packaging a mere container but an active safety system (U.S. Department of Health and Human Services Food and Drug Administration, 2022; World Health Organization, 2023).

LABELING STRATEGIES FOR LASA RISK REDUCTION

Effective labeling is among the most significant and changeable variables for preventing look-alike, sound-alike (LASA) medication errors. The intuitive labels help to decrease the cognitive load, allowing healthcare providers and patients to locate medications quickly and correctly. According to the World Health Organization (WHO), poorly differentiated labels are well-known causes of dispensing and administration errors (World Health Organization, 2023). The U.S. Food and Drug Administration (FDA) suggests focusing on the generic name, using a clear layout hierarchy, and not being cluttered so that vital information can be easily identified (U.S. Department of Health and Human Services Food and Drug Administration, 2022).

Typography and Tall Man Lettering

Typography serves as a crucial tool for distinguishing between similar drug names. Both the FDA and the Institute for Safe Medication Practices (ISMP) support tall man lettering, i.e., selective capitalization of dissimilar parts of LASA names (e.g., DOPamine vs. DOBUTamine). Experimental and eye-tracking experiments have shown that lettering by tall man enhances name differentiation and minimizes selection errors, especially when under time pressure (Filik et al., 2004, 2006). One simulation revealed a 23-percentage-point advantage of tall man lettering in choosing the correct drug, and this effect was greatest in high-alert LASA pairs (Filik et al., 2004). The WHO now includes tall man lettering as a core typographic safety measure for high-risk medications (Estock et al., 2018; Filik et al., 2004; World Health Organization, 2023).

Color and Contrast Rules

Anesthetic classes have particular colors of syringe sleeves, which are defined by ISO26825 (Boaden, 2022; Fasting & Gisvold, 2000). Color coding has been extensively applied in anesthesia to aid in the differentiation of high-risk medications, yet it has been revealed to have certain advantages and shortcomings. ISO 26825 sets the standard colors for syringe sleeves so that they all look the same. In a prospective study of 55,426 anesthesia procedures, drug errors were reported in 0.11% of the cases. These errors were 44% attributed to syringe swaps, which are typically made with muscle relaxants. The ampoule swap rate decreased significantly after plain white labels were changed to color-coded syringe labels with staff education ($p = 0.04$). Nevertheless, the total rate of drug errors did not decrease significantly (40 errors in 28,971 cases vs. 23 errors in 26,455 cases; $p = 0.07$), which means that color was not sufficient to reduce syringe swaps (Fasting & Gisvold, 2000).

These findings support the WHO warning that color should not become the only distinguishing factor, as it may not work in low-light settings or with staff members with color-blind issues (World Health Organization, 2023). FDA guidelines (2022) propose the use of color and clear text, tactile shapes, and barcodes to produce redundant cues. Color might be used to make labels easier to identify, although it must not substitute for the adequate reading of the drug name (U.S. Department of Health and Human Services Food and Drug Administration, 2022).

Warning Statements and Symbols

Easy identification of high-alert drugs is promoted through clear warning statements and uniform symbols, but this issue is of particular concern during stressful or high-pressure situations. The World Health Organization emphasizes the use of bold, unambiguous warnings placed prominently near the drug name and strength to reduce the chance of oversight (World Health Organization, 2023). Similarly, the U.S. FDA recommends incorporating signal words such as *"High Alert"* or *"Dilute Before Use"* in high-contrast fonts and ensuring their consistent placement across all packaging(U.S. Department of Health and Human Services Food and Drug Administration, 2022; U.S. Department of Health and Human Services Food and Drug Administration (FDA), 2005).

REGULATORY AND STANDARDS LANDSCAPE

Global Requirements

Medication labeling regulations around the world share the goal of ensuring the clear, unambiguous identification of medicines and safe use instructions. The U.S. Food and Drug Administration (FDA) guidance (2023) requires that the established (generic) name be prominently displayed near the strength and dosage form, with minimal visual clutter, and that labels include machine-readable barcodes to support point-of-care verification (U.S. Department of Health and Human Services Food and Drug Administration, 2022). The Institute for Safe Medication Practices (ISMP) maintains a list of more than 40 look-alike, sound-alike (LASA) drug name pairs with recommended tall man lettering (e.g., *hydrOXYzine* vs. *hydrALAzine*), which has been shown in controlled studies to improve drug name differentiation and reduce selection errors (Filik et al., 2004; The Institute for Safe Medication Practices (ISMP), 2023).

The Medicines and Healthcare Products Regulatory Agency (MHRA) best practice guidance (2020) emphasizes that critical information—medicine name, strength, route of administration, warnings, and posology—should be colocalized in the same field of view, given greater prominence than noncritical elements, and appear on at least three nonopposing faces of the carton when space allows. For high-risk drug classes, such as cephalosporins, tall man lettering or other highlighting is mandated to aid correct selection (Medicines and Healthcare products Regulatory Agency (MHRA), 2020).

Impact of Risk-Based Name Approval and Labeling

The package and labeling of a drug depends on its proprietary name. Even with the best label design, a name that is too close to any other medication may lead to confusion. To minimize this, the FDA must review the proprietary name of a product before approving it, and it does so by testing orthographic and phonetic similarity, analyzing the risk of medication errors attached to that product, and simulating possible medication errors (Food and Drug Administration, 2020). Equivalent LASA confusion risk screening is applied in the European Medicines Agency (European Medicines Agency (EMA), 2009, 2023) to evaluate confusion in European prescribing and dispensing. The Medicines and Healthcare Products Regulatory Agency (MHRA) indicates that brand names that contain company identifiers or do not match the international nonproprietary name (INN) should be avoided because they can create inconsistency across other packaging aspects and make them visually confusing (European Medicines Agency (EMA), 2023). The

WHO has proposed the use of technology-based tools such as algorithmic checks of name similarity during such reviews to discourage similarly worded names prior to being put on the labels (World Health Organization, 2023).

Technological Features Embedded in Labels and Packaging

Many countries now require machine-readable codes to be printed directly on medical packaging. In the United States, the *Drug Supply Chain Security Act (DSCSA)* mandates that prescription drug packages carry a 2D GS1 DataMatrix barcode containing the global trade item number (GTIN), lot number, expiration date, and a unique serial number (U.S. Food and Drug Administration, 2023). In the European Union, the *Falsified Medicines Directive (Directive 2011/62/EU)* requires similar serialization and the use of GS1 DataMatrix standards to ensure interoperability between countries (European Medicines Agency (EMA), 2009; General Specifications Association Internationale Sans But Lucratif (GS1 AISBL), 2024). With the help of these codes, medicines can be traced and authenticated across the supply chain, counterfeiting can be avoided, and immediate recalls are possible.

With respect to packaging/labeling, barcode regulations influence the location and placement of information. The Medicines and Healthcare Products Regulatory Agency (MHRA) recommends that barcodes be placed in a prominent section of the label, with adequate white space and contrast, and that no graphics should be near the barcodes that may disorient scanning (Medicines and Healthcare products Regulatory Agency (MHRA), 2020). Codes must be on more than one side of a carton to be scanned in other settings.

Combined with bar-code medication administration (BCMA) systems in hospitals, properly designed barcodes on packaging serve as a final control measure at the bedside, which ensures the proper medicine, dose, route, and timing to the appropriate patient. In practice, the nurse reads the patient's identification band and the barcode on the medication package. If the scan data deviate from the order in the prescribed section of the electronic medication administration record (eMAR), the system alerts the administrator, and the administration cannot proceed until the discrepancy is corrected. Poon et al. (2010) evaluated 9 months of BCMA and eMAR in a large before-after study in two academic hospitals. The intervention decreased the rate of nontiming medication administration errors by 41.4 percent (11.5 percent to 6.8 percent) and the number of potential adverse drug events (ADEs) by 51 percent. Moreover, the problem of transcription errors, when nurses manually entered medication information, was eradicated on intervention units, which further confirms the importance of scanning directly out of the package label (Poon et al., 2010).

The quality and positioning of the barcode on the packaging is crucial to these benefits. Poorly positioned, low-contrast, or curved-surface barcodes can increase scan failure rates, prompting staff to bypass the system—commonly called "work-arounds." Findings show that workarounds reduce safety and create new risks when doses are given without barcode scanning or confirmation (Franklin et al., 2007; Patterson et al., 2002). Therefore, the layout of barcodes and their location in the given medication package should also ensure medication packaging safety, according to GS1 and regulatory design rules that enhance barcode scannability in clinical practice. In packaging and labeling, barcode regulations influence information placement. MHRA suggests placing barcodes at a visible location on the label with sufficient white space and contrast and without adjacent graphics that may hamper scanning (Medicines and Healthcare products Regulatory Agency (MHRA), 2020). Multiple carton sides should bear codes when there is sufficient space to ensure that they can be scanned in any setting.

IILUSTRATIVE CASE STUDIES

Illustrations of real-life situations that demonstrate how mixing between look-alike, sound-alike (LASA) medication errors can be minimized through labeling and packaging are provided. Examples of clinical and public health case studies include national versions of the antibiotic stewardship program, which is very specialized in areas such as ophthalmology and anesthesiology. In each case, visual markers, standardized color coding, and human factor-based design aspects are looked at in terms of their advantages and disadvantages. The authors demonstrate that specific packaging and label modifications can contribute to a decrease in LASA risk, but their effects are actually long term and require education and regulation and system seals.

AntiBiotic ACcess and USe (ABACUS) Project and Red Line Campaign Insights

The ABACUS Project shows how nonstandardized packaging and labeling cause LASA-related confusion, especially for antibiotics. ABACUS reported that health-care workers and patients in several low- and middle-income countries confused antibiotics with common analgesics and antipyretics on the basis of packaging color, shape, and size rather than label reading (Monnier et al., 2023). Similar packaging misled people who it was the actual thing, leading to improper use or not treating them at all.

In 2016, India introduced the Red Line Campaign to identify antibiotics and other high-risk prescription-only medicines, with a bold red line on the package label. This visual warning reminds pharmacists, prescribers, and patients who they should use the medicine only under medical supervision (Mathew et al., 2022; Monnier et al., 2024; Travasso, 2016). This red line is used to minimize look-alike errors in pharmacies and clinics where several types of drugs are stored.

The use of visual elements to distinguish between antibiotics and other similar-looking drugs is illustrated in Figure 1. This intervention is consistent with the LASA prevention theory (utilizing distinctive visual cues to identify high-risk drugs), but the campaign has significant drawbacks. Only 7 percent of healthcare professionals in Kerala were aware of the red line, whereas none of the patients were aware (Mathew et al., 2022; Monnier et al., 2023).

This observation can inform LASA reduction that visual cues will not work to avoid medication errors unless there is user education and regulatory enforcement. To achieve an effective distinction in the packaging of antibiotics and other LASA-prone drugs, it is necessary to implement standard labeling that includes the drug's name, dosage, and strength; provide education for both public and healthcare professionals on how to interpret visual cues; and ensure regulatory uniformity to ensure that manufacturers are consistent in their labeling practices. The Red Line Campaign shows that a single visual marker can reduce packaging confusion but requires systemic support to eliminate LASA errors, similar to other interventions such as tall man lettering and color coding in various drug classes (Estock et al., 2018; Lizano-Díez et al., 2020; World Health Organization, 2023).

Figure 1. Two antibiotic packages with a red line as a visual marker were used to prescribe only medications

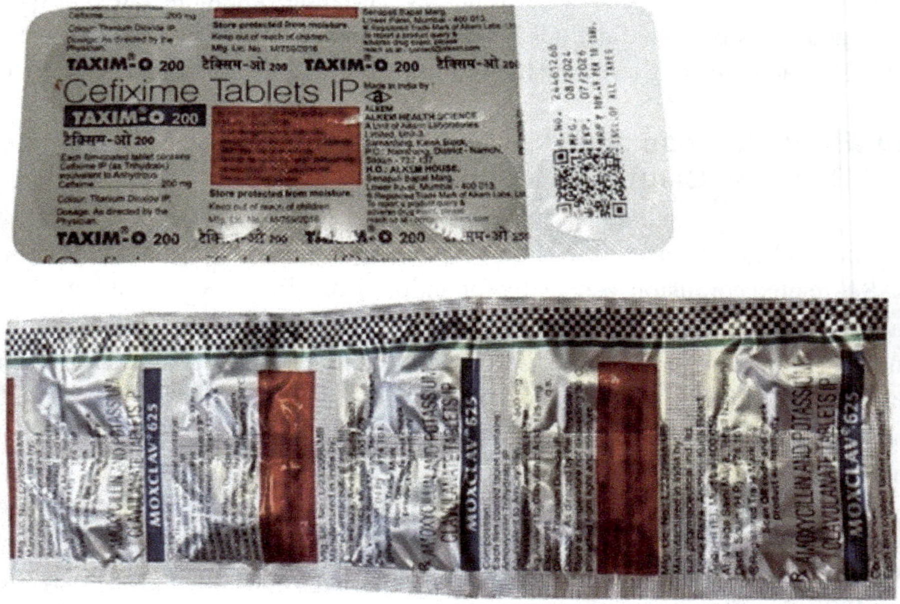

This figure does not depict a documented medication error involving this drug pair or their respective brands.

Pharmaceutical products are displayed solely for academic and educational purposes. Their inclusion does not constitute endorsement, promotion, or advertising of any specific manufacturer or brand.

Utilizing Color Coding for Medicine Identification

The use of color coding is an established method for differentiating between drugs and eliminating LASA errors. Drug class color coding or medicines are simply easier than taking the time to sound out the code as required in high-risk establishments such as hospitals and pharmacies (Filiatrault P, 2009).

Eye Drops: Standardized Color-Coding System for Ophthalmic Drugs

The color coding of topical ocular medication has long been advocated by the American Academy of Ophthalmology (AAO) to enhance safety. Since the mid-1990s, this system has labeled drug classes with Pantone colors according to therapeutic use, risks and mix-ups. This system is expected to enhance the recognition of medications, minimize errors and harmonize the packaging of medications used in ophthalmology (Mishra et al., 2022; The American Academy of Ophthalmology, 2015). Medical mishaps, particularly those of ophthalmology, can result in grave issues. The color-coded labeling of medications and caps provides patients and clinical professionals with a fast and effective technique for differentiating medicine types and minimizing the occurrence of medication errors. The AAO identifies Pantone colors to a therapeutic category so that they can be recognized easily.

By standardizing the identification of eye drop medications, this system plays a crucial role in enhancing patient safety and promoting medication adherence. (The American Academy of Ophthalmology, 2015) The recommended color codes from the American Academy of Ophthalmology, as proposed to the FDA and the pharmaceutical industry, are shown in Table 1.

Table 1. Standardized eye drop cap colors, pantone numbers, and corresponding therapeutic classes with examples

Cap color	Therapeutic class and examples
1. Light Green	Adrenergic agonist combinations: brinzolamide and brimonidine
2. Purple	Adrenergic agonists: brimonidine, dipivefrin HCI
3. Tan	Anti-infectives: azithromycin, besifloxacin, ciprofloxacin, erythromycin, gatifloxacin, levofloxacin, moxifloxacin, ofloxacin, tobramycin, and trimethoprim.

continued on following page

Table 1. Continued

Cap color	Therapeutic class and examples
4. Gray	Anti-inflammatory (nonsteroidal): bromfenac, diclofenac, ketorolac, nepafenac
5. Pink	Anti-inflammatory (steroids): dexamethasone sodium phosphate, difluprednate, fluorometholone, loteprednol, and prednisolone acetate
6. Olive Green	Anti-inflammatory (immunomodulators): methotrexate, voclosporin
7. Dark Blue	Beta-blocker combinations: brimonidine and timolol, dorzolamide and timolol
8. Yellow	Beta-blockers: betaxolol, timolol
9. Orange	Carbonic anhydrase inhibitors: brinzolamide, dorzolamide
10. Black	Cytotoxic agents: not available
11. Dark Green	Miotics: pilocarpine
12. Red	Mydriatics and cycloplegics: atropine, cyclopentolate, homatropine, phenylephrine, scopolamine, and tropicamide
13. Turquoise	Prostaglandin analogs: bimatoprost, latanoprost, tafluprost, and travoprost

(Allie, 2022; Amcon, 2025; Bradley, 2022; The American Academy of Ophthalmology, 2015)

This color-coding system is widely adopted to increase patient safety by minimizing the risk of administering incorrect medications. Patients are encouraged to familiarize themselves with these color codes to ensure proper usage of their prescribed eye drops, as illustrated with the examples in Figure 2 (Amcon, 2025; Hardy L, 2015; The American Academy of Ophthalmology, 2015).

Figure 2. Example of a standardized cap color-coding system for ophthalmic medications, with adrenergic agonists in purple and nonsteroidal anti-inflammatory drugs in gray, to reduce errors.

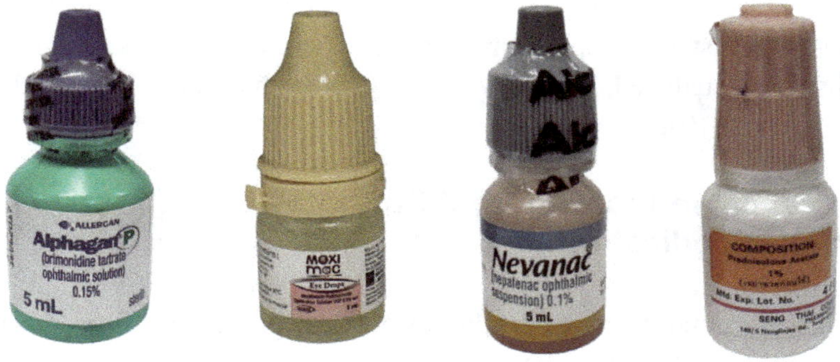

Adrenergic agonists: Brimonidine (purple cap)

Anti-infectives: Moxifloxacin (tan cap)

Anti-inflammatory (non-steroidal): Nepafenac (gray cap)

Anti-inflammatory (steroids): Prednisolone (pink cap)

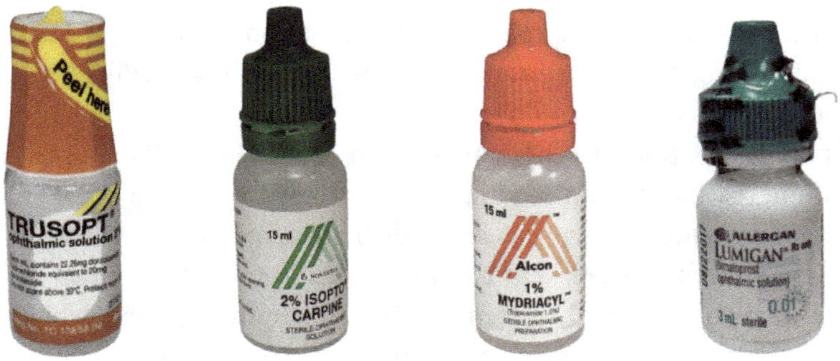

Carbonic anhydrase inhibitors: Dorzolamide (orange cap)

Miotics: Pilocarpine (dark green cap)

Mydriatics and cycloplegics: Tropicamide (red cap)

Prostaglandin analogues: Bimatoprost (turquoise cap)

Pharmaceutical products are displayed solely for academic and educational purposes. Their inclusion does not constitute endorsement, promotion, or advertising of any specific manufacturer or brand

Cap switching is remarkably common, where patients mistakenly place the wrong cap on a different bottle. This might cause confusion and inappropriate prescription use, especially when many eye drops are administered. Clearer labeling and packaging are needed to reduce the probability of such errors when drug identification is based solely on cap color (Mishra et al., 2022; The American Academy of Ophthalmology, 2015). In addition, not all manufacturers and countries follow the color coding method of the AAO. Labeling, bottle design, and cap colors might confuse patients, especially those who travel or switch brands. In the absence of a universal standard, ophthalmic medicine packaging is more complicated and prone to error. Although the color coding system has become very popular for enhancing patient safety by reducing the chances of patients receiving the wrong medications, difficulties still exist in its implementation and efficacy. Drug packaging in ophthalmology has been analyzed, and a few major concerns have been identified (Brandt, 2015; Kierstan, 2019).

Similar Packaging for Different Strengths of the Same Medication

One of the crucial problems in pharmaceutical packaging is the resemblance between the design of medications with various strengths from the same company. The close similarity of packaging between two or more strengths of a medication can pose a significantly high risk of medication error (Schnoor et al., 2015; Supapaan TS et al., 2024; Supapaan et al., 2024). Patients and healthcare providers might administer the medication improperly because of confusion caused by the almost identical packaging of two or more strengths of the same medication, leading to adverse outcomes.

Multiple reports point to the similarity in packaging between medications of varying strengths by the same company and the fact that they are placed close together in dispensing units as causes of dispensing errors, especially in hospitals where multiple strengths are kept together. Selection confusion can be caused in the case of medications that have almost the same bottle designs, labels, and color schemes, with some slight differences in the text or numbers.

Strength may be inappropriately prescribed, resulting in underdosing/overdosing or side effects. Color differences, bold type, and apparent labeling are visual identifiers that can be used to reduce such errors and enhance medication safety; therefore, such visual identifiers need to be standardized.

Industry professionals recommend color variance, large font shapes and clear marking that delineate drug strengths to reduce this risk.

The wrong strength can be administered, leading to underdose, overdose or side effects. To alleviate these mistakes and enhance drug safety, visual identifiers, such as color distinctions, bold font, and judicious labeling, must be standardized (Bryan et al., 2021a; Bryan et al., 2021b; Lambert et al., 1999; Phatak et al., 2005; World Health Organization, 2023).

One of the recommendations by industry professionals in regard to the use of color differences, bold font, and labeling is to alleviate such a risk. To enhance patient safety and to cause less confusion, the FDA and the WHO place requirements on standardized packaging (Health Canada, 2019; World Health Organization, 2023).

Design Human Factors

Elderly and visually impaired or motor-impaired individuals are underrepresented in ophthalmic drug packaging (Beckman et al., 2005; Dietlein et al., 2008). Presbyopia, cataracts, and macular degeneration make reading small labels and identifying similar containers difficult. It is well known that eyedrop bottles expel drops with age. Compared with 95% of younger patients, only 57% of those 80 years and older could self-administer eye drops from single-use vials (Dietlein et al., 2008).

Arthritis and Parkinson's illness can decrease hand function, making opening pharmaceutical packages difficult. Studies have shown that many people 81 years and older struggle with screw-cap bottles and other packaging types. Self-administering eye drops are further complicated by reduced grip strength and hand coordination, leading to uneven dosing and treatment failure (Beckman et al., 2005; Winfield et al., 1990.

Packaging should be performed in such a way that it is user friendly. This involves large and high-contrast letters, ergonomic bottle shapes to enable easier handling, and rugged markings, which assist in the identification of drugs. These modifications have the potential to improve patient treatment and prevent medication errors in the most vulnerable groups of the population (Gupta et al., 2023; Kowing & Kester, 2007; Mumani, 2018; U.S. Department of Health and Human Services Food and Drug Administration (FDA), 2020).

Global Standardization

The adoption of the AAO system worldwide is incomplete. Although the standard is common in the United States, some manufacturers and countries have not adopted it. To maximize the level of safety, color coding should be supplemented with large, high-contrast labels and tactile markers, and international regulations should be harmonized. A globally accepted system would enhance medication safety and cross-border continuity of care (Brandt, 2015; Mishra et al., 2022).

Anesthesia and Sedation

The other instance of a color-coding system is in the case of anesthesia drugs. According to the statement by the American Society of Anesthesiologists (ASA) on the labeling of drugs to be used in anesthesiology, the main aim of medication labeling is to minimize errors and provide safer patient care, especially in anesthesiology, where potent drugs are mostly used. The ASA promotes standardized labels in line with the American Society for Testing and Materials (ASTM) International, the International Organization of Standardization (ISO), and the Food and Drug

Administration (FDA) and Institute of Safe Medication Practices (ISMP) guidelines (Christie & Hill, 2002; Grissinger, 2012).

The labeling system specifies clear and legible text, including the generic name and concentration of the drug as the most prominent details. Additional information, such as the preparation date, time, and initials of the preparer, along with patient-specific details, is recommended for infusion bags and syringes.

The color coding of the syringes to identify drug classes helps in urgent moments (American Society of Anesthesiologists, 2020; Grissinger, 2012; The American Society for Testing and Materials (ASTM), 2022). In the operating room (OR), anesthesia providers can apply color-coded adhesive labels to syringes directly from labeled vials or ampules to identify the medication. This is useful since most providers tend to select only one drug per category to use in procedures, eliminating confusion. Color codes take less time to select drugs that are important in cases of emergency (Grissinger, 2012).

Opioids look blue and can therefore be easily identified. To highlight the importance and warning, the neuromuscular blockers are shown in fluorescent red. Yellow denotes induction agents, which are necessary for anesthesia. Orange symbolizes the tranquilizers, who act on the patients when they are anxious or sedated. Violet is applied to vasopressors, which maintain blood pressure during tasks. Finally, green is related to anticholinergics that control the type of secretions and heart rate. This color-coded system allows anesthesiology practitioners to identify and apply the correct medication in the operating room easily (The American Dental Association (ADA), 2023).

The ASA suggests labeling drugs with barcodes to limit the number of mistakes. Barcodes mechanize electronic record entry, validate drug identity and enhance workflow. Color coding is effective, but the ASA records its disadvantages, which include color blindness and darkness. Syringe gradations can also be blocked by improper label placement, causing dosing errors (American Society of Anesthesiologists, 2020; Thomas & Mollon, 2018).

This standard is exclusively for anesthesia practice and helps clinicians quickly and accurately and standardize drug administration in operating rooms and critical care areas. In the OR, anesthesia providers prepare medications themselves and label syringes with color-coded adhesive labels for easy identification (Fasting & Gisvold, 2000). Syringe swaps with identical-sized syringes and color alone remain issues. These issues require additional safety measures such as label reading and barcode scanning (Fasting & Gisvold, 2000; Grissinger, 2012).

There is hazard in color coding regardless of the advantages. In the case of misuse of safety checks, such as neglecting drug label reading, it is possible to misuse color as the only identifier; therefore, mistakes may occur. Poor label quality, fading colors, and relying on memory to associate colors with drug classes may also cause errors. The risk of choosing the wrong drug increases when multiple drugs in a class (e.g., morphine, fentanyl, and hydromorphone) are stored in the same color syringes (Fasting & Gisvold, 2000; Grissinger, 2012).

Nevertheless, this specification was later removed in 2022, indicating the continuous transformation of safety provisions in the world of anesthesiology (The American Society for Testing and Materials (The American Society for Testing and Materials (ASTM), 2022). Although it has been removed, the concepts that were presented in the standard still hold the truth to proper implementation and application to clinical practice.

Preventing medication errors requires well-designed labels with color coding, legible text, contrast, and barcodes, according to the FDA. Color coding helps to visually differentiate quickly, but it should be supplemented by detailed safety procedures to ensure that it is most effective and that the risks of overreliance are minimized (Fasting & Gisvold, 2000; U.S. Department of Health and Human Services Food and Drug Administration (FDA), 2005; U.S. Department of Health and Human Services Food and Drug Administration, 2016).

The current 2022 syringe labeling guidelines superseded the earlier advice given by the Association of Anesthetists as the new ISO standard BS ISO 26825:2020 became effective (Boaden, 2022). This new publication is a technical revision of the 2008 standard, which includes new safety measures that have been adopted to improve drug identification in anesthesia practice. The specifications of the syringe labels that are applied by users and mainly concentrate on color coding by the type of drug, the size of the label, the type of design and its durability, and readability requirements, such as font size, font contrast, and uniform spellings of drug names. This standard is unique to anesthesia practice, and it assists clinicians in rapidly and clearly identifying and standardizing the administration of drugs in operating rooms and critical care facilities. The standard is specifically anesthesia practice and can be used to find an easy and effective way to optimally discern syringe contents in a short period of time, thus minimizing drug error risks in intensive areas (Boaden, 2022). The benefits of uniform labeling concerning patient safety and ways to standardize the administration of drugs in operating rooms and critical care zones are shown in Figure 3 and Table 2.

Figure 3. Examples of syringe labels and corresponding ampoules for anesthesia and critical care medications. Standardized color-coded labels are shown for adrenaline (violet), diazepam (orange), and neostigmine (red striped)

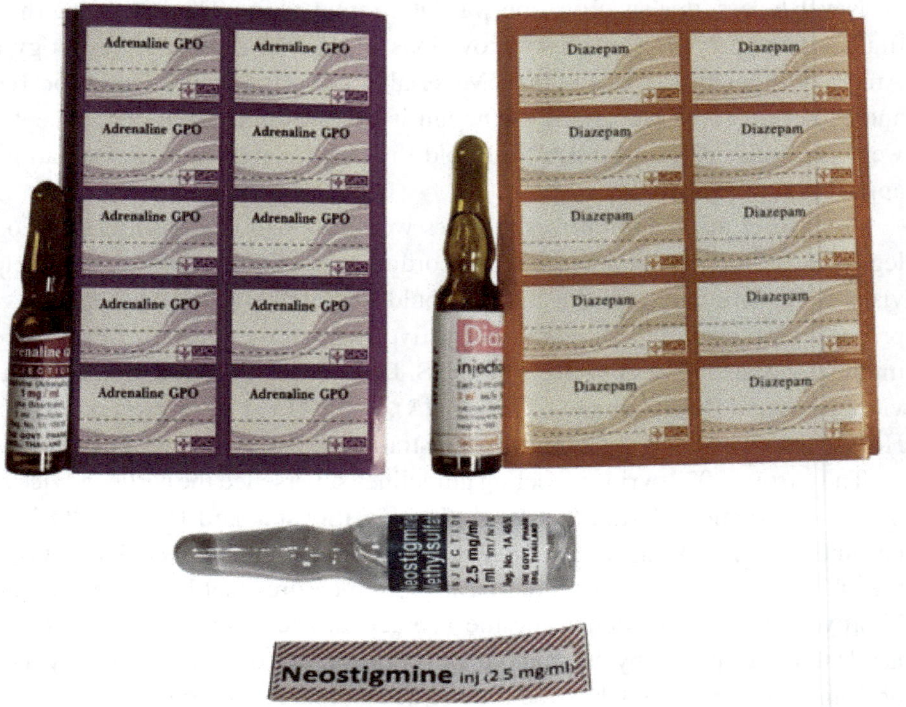

Pharmaceutical products are displayed solely for academic and educational purposes. Their inclusion does not constitute endorsement, promotion, or advertising of any specific manufacturer or brand.

Table 2. Recommended syringe label color codes for anesthesia and critical care drugs. Colors are intended only as guidance; every syringe must be labeled with the correct drug and concentration. Blank colored labels should be avoided to minimize confusion

Therapeutic class	Color	Examples	Label example
Anti-emetics and major tranquilizers: metoclopramide, tropisetron, ondansetron, droperidol, haloperidol	Salmon, Black	Metoclopramide ....mg/ml	Metoclopramide .... mg/ml
Anticholinergic drugs: atropine, glycopyrronium	Green, Black	Atropine ....mg/ml	Atropine .... mg/ml
Benzodiazepines and tranquilzers: diazepam, midazolam, phenytoin	Orange, White, Black	Diazepam ....mg/ml	Diazepam .... mg/ml
Benzodiazepine Antagonists: flumazenil	Orange, White, Black	Flumazenil ....mg/ml (Striped)	Flumazenil .... mg/ml
Induction drugs: thiopental, methohexitone, propofol, ketamine	Yellow, Black	Propofol ....mg/ml	Propofol .... mg/ml
Local anesthetics: procaine, lidocaine, bupivacaine, ropivacaine	Gray, Black	Lidocaine ....%	Lidocaine ... %
Miscellaneous drugs: 1.White, Black: heparin, protamine	White, Black	Heparin ....units/ml	Heparin .... units/ml
2. Black, White: other drugs (e.g., amoxicillin)	White, Black	Protamine ....mg/ml (Striped)	Protamine .... mg/ml
	Black, White	Amoxicillin	Amoxicillin ....
Muscle Relaxants: 1. Black, White, Warm Red: suxamethonium	Black, White, Warm Red	Suxamethonium ....mg/ml	Suxamethonium .....mg/ml
2. Warm Red, Black: pancuronium, (Cis) atracurium, vecuronium, rocuronium	Warm Red, Black	Vecuronium ....mg/ml	Vecuronium .... mg/ml
Muscle relaxant reversal : neostigmine, edrophonium, pyridostigmine, sugammadex	Warm Red, White, Black	Pyridostigmine ....mg/ml (Striped)	Pyridostigmine .... mg/ml
Opioids: fentanyl, meperidine, morphine, pethidine, remifentanil, sufentanil, tramadol	Blue, Black	Morphine	Morphine ......mg/ml
Opioid antagonists: naloxone	Blue, White, Black	Naloxone ....ug/ml	Naloxone ....µg/ml
Vasopressors: 1. Black, White, Violet: adrenaline	Black, White, Violet	Adrenaline ....mg/ml	Adrenaline ...... mg/ml
2. Violet, Black: Noradrenaline, ephedrine, phenylephrine, metaraminol, dopamine, dobutamine, milrinone	Violet, Black	Phenylephrine ....mg/ml	Phenylephrine .... mg/ml
Hypotensive drugs: nitroprusside, nitroglycerine, phentolamine, hydralazine	Violet, White, Black	Nitroglycerine ....mcg/ml (Striped)	Nitroprusside .... mcg/ml

(Boaden, 2022; Castro-Gómez, 2023)

Local Anesthetic Cartridges

To minimize the risk of medication errors in dental practice, the American Dental Association (ADA) established a standardized color-coding system for local anesthetic cartridges, first introduced in 2003 and formalized under ANSI/ADA Standard No. 190:2020. This standard—which is harmonized with ISO 11499—applies specifically to single-use dental cartridges containing local anesthetics and mandates the use of two permanently colored bands for each cartridge to indicate the drug identity and vasoconstrictor content (The American Dental Association (ADA), 2023).

The system requires two permanent color bands on each single-use cartridge:

Band 1: Anesthetic agent and concentration (The American Dental Association (ADA), 2023):

- 2% lidocaine: Red
- 3% lidocaine: Purple
- 2% mepivacaine: Brown
- 3% mepivacaine: Tan
- 3% prilocaine: Orange
- 4% prilocaine: Yellow
- 4% articaine: Gold
- 0.5% bupivacaine: Blue

Band 2: Vasoconstrictor type and concentration (The American Dental Association (ADA), 2023):

- White/blank: No vasoconstrictor
- Epinephrine
  - o <1:200,000 (very dilute epinephrine): Yellow)
    Example: epinephrine 1:250,000 or 1:300,000.
  - o <1:100,000 to 1:200,000 (moderate concentrations): Orange
  - o <1:50,000 to 1:100,000: Brown
  - o 1:50,000: Green
- Levonordefrin: Black
- Norepinephrine 1:100,000: Tan
- Norepinephrine 1:25,000: Purple
- Felypressin (octapressin): Blue

Placement and size requirements (The American Dental Association (ADA), 2023):

- Band 1: 3.0 ± 0.5 mm wide, placed 8–20 mm from the plunger end

- Band 2: 1.5 ± 0.5 mm wide, positioned 2 ± 0.5 mm from Band 1

Color coding is highly recommended for identifying local anesthetic cartridges, but dentists are highly encouraged to read the entire label to ensure that they are taking the right drug and dose. The use of color should not be used as a single identifier. In an attempt to reinforce safe practice, the ADA and several manufacturers have published visual instructions showing the standard configuration of the two bands on cartridges. An example of this is the popular preparation Lidocaine HCl 2% with Epinephrine 1:100,000, usually labeled with red for Band 1 (anesthetic agent) and brown for Band 2 (vasoconstrictor) according to the ANSI/ADA and ISO standards (Mohammed, 2022; Pierrel S.P.A., 2021). Conversely, single-color bands continue to be used with many products in routine use, as shown in Figure 4, which can result in inconsistency and LASA errors.

Figure 4. Single-color (e.g., blue with articaine 4% with epinephrine, green with 3% mepivacaine without a vasoconstrictor, and brown with 2% mepivacaine with a vasoconstrictor) local anesthetic cartridges. Such marks are advantageous for visualizing but do not align with ANSI/ADA Standard No. 190: 2020, a two-band system that limits LASA errors

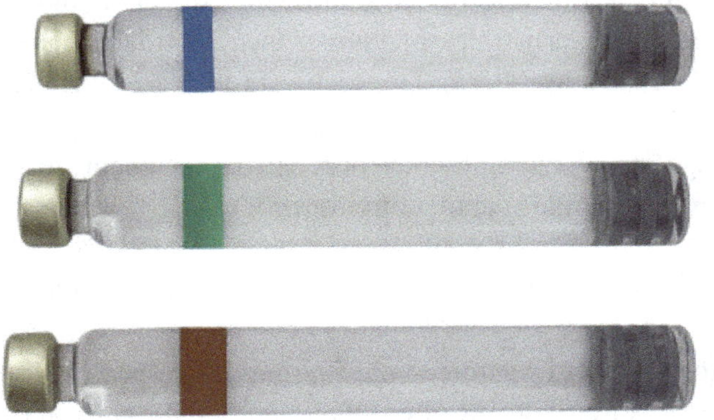

The American Dental Association (ADA) (2023).

Pharmaceutical products are displayed solely for academic and educational purposes. Their inclusion does not constitute endorsement, promotion, or advertising of any specific manufacturer or brand

Intramanufacturer Trade Dress Similarity

The literature on medication safety explains that the packaging of a brand family of medication within the same manufacturer may contribute to look-alike medication risks. Trade dress is what the product generally looks like or what is termed the total image of a product, which identifies the commercial origin of the product, the layout structure, color scheme, typography, graphic elements, and container arrangement (Bone, 2015; Dinwoodie & Janis, 2008). Applied to pharmaceutical products, trade dress therefore reflects the cumulative visual identity created by these elements.

Corporate identity continuity may facilitate brand awareness and promote lucidity. Nonetheless, studies of human factors have shown that clinicians often use rapid visual pattern recognition when they choose medicine, especially when they are under time pressure (Berman, 2004; Cohen, 2007). Structurally similar layout architecture, typography hierarchy, container morphology, and prevailing color themes across therapeutically differentiated products may result in less visual differentiation, which can increase vulnerability to selection.

The similarity of packaging has consistently been found in medication safety studies to be a factor in wrong-drug and wrong-strength errors (Cohen, 2007; Hicks et al., 2008; World Health Organization, 2023). The World Health Organization also identifies look-alike packaging and dependency on color as risk factors for LASA errors and recommends increasing the significance of active ingredient names and strengths and applying principles of human factors to label and package design (World Health Organization, 2023). This section provides only academic illustrations of structural design patterns discussed in the medication safety literature. They are not aimed at regulatory noncompliance or reporting the occurrence of documented error events for a particular manufacturer or product.

Example 1: Ophthalmic Products (Trade Dress Similarity)

No regulatory actions or enforcement findings have specifically implicated any individual manufacturer in terms of ophthalmic trade dress similarity. Ophthalmic products, as depicted in Figure 5, display the same brand-family packaging of therapeutically different agents.

It is proposed in the literature on medication safety that similarity in packaging and dependence on color differences can be a source of vulnerability to LASA, especially in settings where time pressure or cognitive load is present (Berman, 2004; Schnoor et al., 2015; World Health Organization, 2023). The example is made to be analyzed by scholars only and does not mean recorded instances of error in any particular product or manufacturer.

Figure 5. Example of intrameufacturer trade dress similarity among ophthalmic products

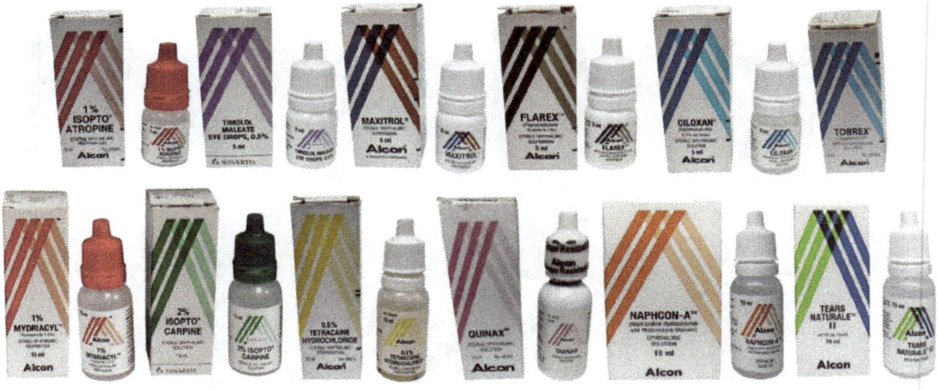

The image illustrates a consistent packaging architecture across therapeutically distinct ophthalmic agents and is presented for academic and educational purposes. The inclusion of these products does not imply the endorsement of any manufacturer or brand. Certain regions may no longer market some of the shown products, and availability may differ depending on the country and its regulatory status.

Example 2: "-Oph" Product Line

This trade dress is exhibited in the -Oph series. The common elements are a dark green central panel, vertical typography, a uniform location of Eye Drops STERILE, a standard lower panel (white), a similar bottle structure, and a common suffix (-Oph) (Figure 6). Even though the cap colors differ, the general scheme is structurally similar.

The similarity of orthography (similar suffix) and similarity of packaging can enhance visual similarity in the process of rapid selection. According to the literature, overlapping similarities in names and packaging may increase selection risk more than either of the two sources of risk does (Hicks et al., 2008; ISMP, 2020). This case is presented for an academic illustration of general LASA risk patterns and does not imply documented errors or regulatory concerns regarding any specific product.

Figure 6. Example of intrameufacturer trade dress similarity among ophthalmic products

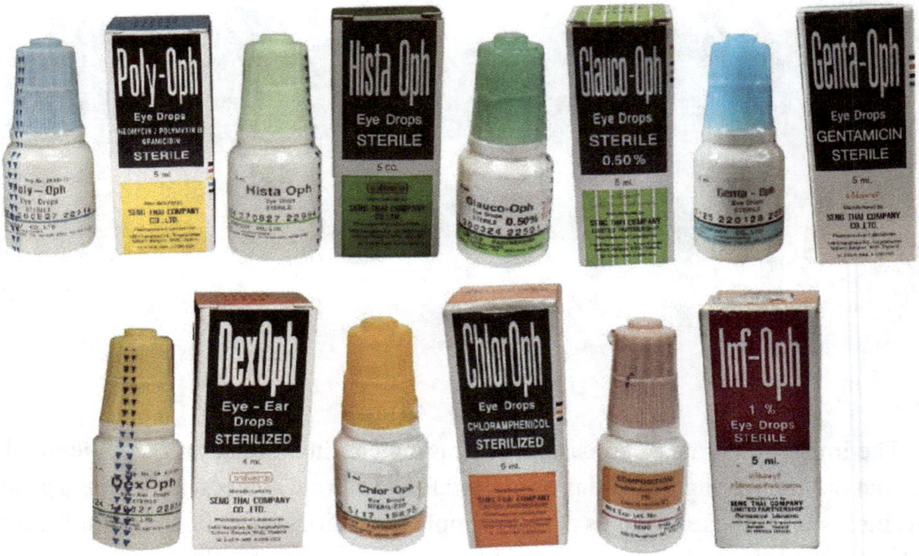

The image illustrates a consistent packaging architecture across therapeutically distinct ophthalmic agents and is presented for academic and educational purposes. The inclusion of these products does not imply the endorsement of any manufacturer or brand. Certain regions may no longer market some of the shown products, and availability may differ depending on the country and its regulatory status.

Example 3: Metered-Dose Inhaler (Several Strengths)

Several pressurized metered-dose inhalers (pMDIs) are available in several doses with a significantly high level of consistency in the packaging structure. The common characteristics can be the same carton color schemes and layout, typography and logo positioning, morphology of the device, and strength differentiation (Figure 7). The stereotypical look of devices can also promote the possibility of choosing the device according to the overall visual pattern but not by intentionally checking the strength. This case is given as an illustrative example of the general patterns of LASA risks and does not mean that any errors or issues concerning a particular product or manufacturer are reported.

Figure 7. Illustration of uniform packaging construction of numerous strengths of a pressurized metered-dose inhaler (pMDI)

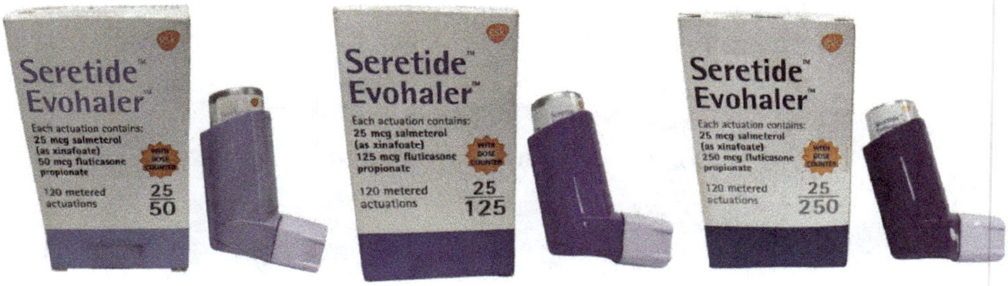

The picture has been provided as an academic demonstration of general LASA risk trends as outlined in the medication safety literature, and it does not suggest a reportable error occurrence or regulatory issues pertaining to some specific product or manufacturer.

Example 4: Pediatric Paracetamol Syrups

In terms of the availability of various concentrations of oral suspensions of paracetamol in bottles, the carton images, layout, bottle shape, and typography may be similar, with the only difference being a small numeric text (e.g., 120 mg/5 mL, 160 mg/5 mL, 250 mg/5 mL) and slight color differences. Owing to the weight-based dosing (mg/kg) of pediatric dosing, correct identification of the concentration is essential. The literature on medication safety suggests that the use of similar visual presentations of multiple strengths can impose a cognitive load on overall appearance, especially in caregiver administration dosing environments (The Institute for Safe Medication Practices (ISMP), 2011; World Health Organization, 2023; Yin et al., 2010).

This case has been introduced to illustrate the general LASA risk patterns conceptually and should not be considered the report of any particular product or manufacturer-related concerns.

Figure 8. Samples of comparable packaging structures of various concentrations of oral suspensions from children. The figure shows that the carton layout, imagery, type, and bottle presentation are consistent across various strength formulations, with the concentration mainly varying across numeric text and color accents

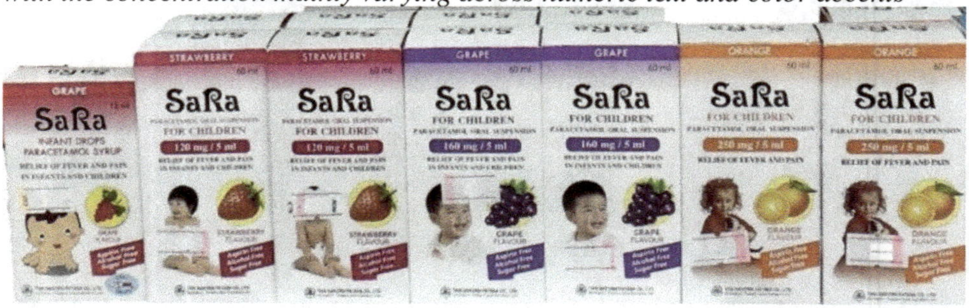

The picture is introduced as an academic example of general LASA risk patterns as outlined in the literature on medication safety and does not denote reported error incidences and issues in reference to a particular product or manufacturer.

REGULATORY AND INDUSTRY STANDARDS FOR INJECTABLE MEDICATION LABELING

Injectable medication labels are among the barriers to LASA errors on the front line. Governing bodies, including the U.S. Food and Drug Administration (FDA), the UK Medicines and Healthcare Products Regulatory Agency (MHRA), and the World Health Organization (WHO), stipulate that the necessary information has to be included on both secondary packages and containers on the outer display (Medicines and Healthcare products Regulatory Agency (MHRA), 2020; U.S. Department of Health and Human Services Food and Drug Administration, 2022; World Health Organization, 2023). These are the generic and brand names of the drug, the strength in total and per milliliter (e.g., "500 mg/5 mL; 100 mg/mL"), the route of administration, the lot number, the expiry date, and warnings (e.g., "For Intrathecal Use Only" (United States Pharmacopeia (USP), 2020)). The MHRA also recommends that such information should be displayed alongside without distracting logos or graphic elements and that even smaller containers (less than 10 mL) should maintain readability with all information being reinforced on the secondary package (Shrank et al., 2007).

One approach that has demonstrated an advantage in minimizing confusion of similar drug names in a drug label is tall-man lettering, emphasizing the dissimilar portions of the drugs (e.g., cefTAZidime vs. cefTRIAXone). Effective methods of enhancing recognition and reducing the error rate of Tallman lettering include lettering, particularly in simulation research and real-life circumstances, among nurses of critical care or pharmacists (Iglesias Gomez et al., 2022; Lohmeyer et al., 2023). In this strategy, hospital formularies and electronic prescribing systems enhance the visual salience of safer drug selection.

Furthermore, the readability of labels is important. Sans-serif fonts should be large and spaced well; no trailing zeros (2.5 mg vs. 2.50 mg) and spelling out of micrograms are recommended to prevent confusion. RFID tags and 2D DataMatrix barcodes on vials and ampoules and on their containers are used together to permit bedside real-time scanning of different drugs to prove their identity, batch information and expiry date. These FDA-required interventions decrease the incidence of high-alert medication dispensing errors and increase traceability (DeYoung et al., 2009; Food and Drug Administration, 2004).

ISMP, USP, NCC MERP, and The Joint Commission promote consistent, Humane labeling of injectable medication. Reducing brand clutter, labeling drug names and strengths on all sides of the containers and including frontline clinicians in the label codesign. In simulation studies, tall man lettering, simplification of layouts and high-contrast design increase recognition and decrease med errors in high-stakes places, such as operating rooms or intensive care units (Aceves-Gonzalez et al., 2024; Catchpole & McCulloch, 2010; Estock et al., 2018).

CONCLUSION

Packaging and labeling are safety tools that can prevent or cause errors. Standards such as clear font hierarchy, color coding, and tall man lettering are useful, but they must be combined with barcoding, RFID, and consistent key information placement. Label design and testing by frontline healthcare professionals is crucial. Usability and human factors improve recognition and reduce error, especially in high-pressure environments. In the future, it is vital to have global labeling harmonization medication packaging mitigate risks and prevent harm by being designed well and using digital tools, regulation, and clinician collaboration.

REFERENCES

Aceves-Gonzalez, C., Caro-Rojas, A., Rey-Galindo, J. A., Aristizabal-Ruiz, L., & Hernández-Cruz, K. (2024). Estimating the impact of label design on reducing the risk of medication errors by applying HEART in drug administration. *European Journal of Clinical Pharmacology, 80*(4), 575–588. DOI: 10.1007/s00228-024-03619-3 PMID: 38282080

Allie, J. (2022). *What different eye drop cap colors mean*. Retrieved 15 March from https://www.allaboutvision.com/treatments-and-surgery/drugs-medications/eye-drop-cap-color-meanings/

Amcon, T. E. S. C. (2025). *Know your ophthalmic eye drops by cap colors*. Retrieved 14 March from https://www.amconlabs.com/blog/why-ophthalmic-eye-drop-caps-colors/

American Society of Anesthesiologists. (2020). *Statement on Labeling of Pharmaceuticals for Use in Anesthesiology*. Retrieved 2024 from https://www.asahq.org/standards-and-practice-parameters/statement-on-labeling-of-pharmaceuticals-for-use-in-anesthesiology

Arimura, J., Poole, R. L., Jeng, M., Rhine, W., & Sharek, P. (2008). Neonatal heparin overdose-a multidisciplinary team approach to medication error prevention. *The Journal of Pediatric Pharmacology and Therapeutics: The Official Journal of PPAG, 13*(2), 96–98. DOI: 10.5863/1551-6776-13.2.96 PMID: 23055872

Ashcroft, D. M., Quinlan, P., & Blenkinsopp, A. (2005). Prospective study of the incidence, nature and causes of dispensing errors in community pharmacies. *Pharmacoepidemiology and Drug Safety, 14*(5), 327–332. DOI: 10.1002/pds.1012 PMID: 15386722

Beckman, A., Bernsten, C., Parker, M. G., Thorslund, M., & Fastbom, J. (2005). The difficulty of opening medicine containers in old age: A population-based study. *Pharmacy World & Science, 27*(5), 393–398. DOI: 10.1007/s11096-005-7903-z PMID: 16341746

Berman, A. (2004). Reducing medication errors through naming, labeling, and packaging. *Journal of Medical Systems, 28*(1), 9–29. DOI: 10.1023/B:-JOMS.0000021518.60670.10 PMID: 15171066

Boaden, B. (2022). *Syringe labeling in anesthesia and critical care areas: review 2022*. Retrieved 15 March from https://anaesthetists.org/Home/Resources-publications/Guidelines/Syringe-labelling-in-anaesthesia-and-critical-care-areas-review-2022

Bone, R. G. (2015). Trademark Functionality Reexamined. *The Journal of Legal Analysis*, *7*(1), 183–246. DOI: 10.1093/jla/lav002

Bradley, S. H. (2022). *Know Your Drops by Color*. Retrieved 15 March from https://www.aao.org/young-ophthalmologists/yo-info/article/know-your-drops-by-color

Brandt, J. D. (2015). Human Factors and Ophthalmic Drug Packaging: Time for a Global Standard. *Ophthalmology*, *122*(12), 2368–2370. DOI: 10.1016/j.ophtha.2015.08.035 PMID: 26592669

Bryan, R., Aronson, J. K., Williams, A., & Jordan, S. (2021a). The problem of look-alike, sound-alike name errors: Drivers and solutions. *British Journal of Clinical Pharmacology*, *87*(2), 386–394. DOI: 10.1111/bcp.14285 PMID: 32198938

Bryan, R., Aronson, J. K., Williams, A. J., & Jordan, S. (2021b). A systematic literature review of LASA error interventions. *British Journal of Clinical Pharmacology*, *87*(2), 336–351. DOI: 10.1111/bcp.14644 PMID: 33197079

Castro-Gómez, A. (2023). Labeling of medications in anesthesia: Colors and letters that save lives. *Revista Colombiana de Anestesiología*, *51*(2). Advance online publication. DOI: 10.5554/22562087.e1065

Catchpole, K., & McCulloch, P. (2010). Human factors in critical care: Toward standardized integrated human-centered systems of work. *Current Opinion in Critical Care*, *16*(6), 618–622. DOI: 10.1097/MCC.0b013e32833e9b4b PMID: 20736826

Christie, I. W., & Hill, M. R. (2002). Standardized color coding for syringe drug labels: a National Survey. *Anesthesia, 57*(8), 778-817. https://doi.org/10.1046/j.1365-2044.2002.02698_3.x

Ciociano, N., & Bagnasco, L. (2014). Look alike/sound alike drugs: A literature review on causes and solutions. *International Journal of Clinical Pharmacy*, *36*(2), 233–242. DOI: 10.1007/s11096-013-9885-6 PMID: 24293334

Ciociano, N., Saullo, F., Pacillo, M., Romano, F., & Bagnasco, L. (2013). GRP-020 Analysis of Italian Hospital Pharmacist Activities to Prevent LASA Drug Errors in Treatment: First Results. *European Journal of Hospital Pharmacy: Science and Practice*, *20*(Suppl 1), A7–A8. DOI: 10.1136/ejhpharm-2013-000276.020

Cohen, M. R. (2001). Another purpose for "purpose" look-alike unit-dose containers mixed up misinterpretation of sliding-scale insulin dose. *Hospital Pharmacy*, *36*(12), 1132–1133. DOI: 10.1177/001857870103601203

Cohen, M. R. (2007). The role of drug packaging and labeling in medication errors. In Cohen, M. R. (Ed.), *Medication Errors* (2nd ed., pp. 111–152). The American Pharmacists Association. https://doi.org/doi:10.21019/9781582120928.ch7

de Almeida Lopes, D. M., Rabelo Néri, E. D., Santos Madeira, L., de Souza Neto, P. J., Araújo Lélis, A. R., de Souza, T. R., de Oliveira, A. B., Oliveira Costa, L., & de França Fonteles, M. M. (2012). Análise da rotulagem de medicamentos semelhantes: Potenciais erros de medicação. *Revista da Associação Médica Brasileira*, *58*(1), 95–103. DOI: 10.1590/S0104-42302012000100021 PMID: 22392323

DeYoung, J. L., Vanderkooi, M. E., & Barletta, J. F. (2009). Effect of bar-code-assisted medication administration on medication error rates in an adult medical intensive care unit. *American Journal of Health-System Pharmacy*, *66*(12), 1110–1115. DOI: 10.2146/ajhp080355 PMID: 19498127

Dietlein, T. S., Jordan, J. F., Lüke, C., Schild, A., Dinslage, S., & Krieglstein, G. K. (2008). Self-application of single-use eyedrop containers in an elderly population: Comparisons with standard eyedrop bottle and with younger patients. *Acta Ophthalmologica*, *86*(8), 856–859. DOI: 10.1111/j.1755-3768.2007.01155.x PMID: 18494743

Dinwoodie, G. B., & Janis, M. D. (2008). *Trademark law and Theory: A handbook of contemporary research*. Edward Elgar Publishing. DOI: 10.4337/9781848441316

Dsouza, S., & Kulkarni, A. (2017). The hazards of look alike packaging in anesthesia practice. *Asian Journal of Anesthesiology*, *55*(4), 91–92. DOI: 10.1016/j.aja.2017.10.003 PMID: 29239830

Emmerton, L. M., & Rizk, M. F. (2012). Look-alike and sound-alike medicines: Risks and 'solutions'. *International Journal of Clinical Pharmacy*, *34*(1), 4–8. DOI: 10.1007/s11096-011-9595-x PMID: 22193703

Estock, J. L., Murray, A. W., Mizah, M. T., Mangione, M. P., Goode, J. S.Jr, & Eibling, D. E. (2018). Label Design Affects Medication Safety in an Operating Room Crisis: A Controlled Simulation Study. *Journal of Patient Safety*, *14*(2), 101–106. DOI: 10.1097/PTS.0000000000000176 PMID: 25760652

European Medicines Agency (EMA). (2009). *Guideline on the readability of the label and package leaflet of medicinal products for human use*. Retrieved 11 June from https://health.ec.europa.eu/system/files/2016-11/2009_01_12_readability_guideline_final_en_0.pdf

European Medicines Agency (EMA). (2023). *Guideline on the acceptability of names for human medicinal products processed through the centralized procedure - Scientific guideline*. https://www.ema.europa.eu/en/documents/scientific-guideline/guideline-acceptability-names-human-medicinal-products-processed-through-centralised-procedure-revision-7_en.pdf

Fasting, S., & Gisvold, S. E. (2000). Adverse drug errors in anesthesia, and the impact of colored syringe labels. *Canadian Journal of Anaesthesia = Journal Canadien d'Anesthésie*, *47*(11), 1060–1067. DOI: 10.1007/BF03027956 PMID: 11097534

Filiatrault, P., & Hyland, S. (2009). Does color-coded labeling reduce the risk of medication errors? *The Canadian Journal of Hospital Pharmacy*, *62*(2), 154–156. DOI: 10.4212/cjhp.v62i2.446 PMID: 22478883

Filik, R., Purdy, K., Gale, A., & Gerrett, D. (2004). Drug name confusion: Evaluating the effectiveness of capital ("Tall Man") letters using eye movement data. *Social Science & Medicine*, *59*(12), 2597–2601. DOI: 10.1016/j.socscimed.2004.04.008 PMID: 15474212

Filik, R., Purdy, K., Gale, A., & Gerrett, D. (2006). Labeling of medicines and patient safety: Evaluating methods of reducing drug name confusion. *Human Factors*, *48*(1), 39–47. DOI: 10.1518/001872006776412199 PMID: 16696255

Food and Drug Administration. (2004). Bar code label requirement for human drug products and biological products. Final rule. *Federal Register*, *69*(38), 9119–9171. PMID: 14986679

Food and Drug Administration. (2020). *Best Practices in Developing Proprietary Names for Human Prescription Drug Products; Guidance for Industry*. Retrieved 15 Aug from https://www.fda.gov/regulatory-information/search-fda-guidance-documents/best-practices-developing-proprietary-names-human-prescription-drug-products-guidance-industry

Franklin, B. D., O'Grady, K., Donyai, P., Jacklin, A., & Barber, N. (2007). The impact of a closed-loop electronic prescribing and administration system on prescribing errors, administration errors and staff time: A before-and-after study. *Quality & Safety in Health Care*, *16*(4), 279–284. DOI: 10.1136/qshc.2006.019497 PMID: 17693676

Gangakhedkar, G. R., Waghalkar, P. V., Shetty, A. N., & Dalvi, A. M. (2019). Look-Alike Drugs: Avoiding Potential Medical Errors. *International Journal of Preventive Medicine*, *10*(1), 9. DOI: 10.4103/ijpvm.IJPVM_331_18 PMID: 30774843

General Specifications Association Internationale Sans But Lucratif (GS1 AISBL). (2024). *GS1 General Specifications Standard*. Retrieved 15 Aug from https://ref.gs1.org/standards/genspecs/

Grissinger, M. (2012). Color-coded syringes for anesthesia drugs-use with care. *P&T : a Peer-Reviewed Journal for Formulary Management*, *37*(4), 199–201. PMID: 22593629

Gupta, P. K., Ishihara, R., Zhao, Z., Owji, S., Anyama, E., Schmitz-Brown, M., Chacin, A. C., Iyer, B., Friedman, D., & Ladki, M. S. (2023). Novel tactile bottle neck adaptor facilitates eye drop adherence in visually impaired patients. *BMJ Open Ophthalmology*, *8*(1), e001462. Advance online publication. DOI: 10.1136/bmjophth-2023-001462 PMID: 38154911

Hardy, L. (2015). *Name That Drop*. Retrieved 23 Nov from https://www.2020mag.com/article/name-that-drop

Health Canada. (2019). *Good label and package practices guide for prescription drugs*. Retrieved 15 March from https://www.canada.ca/en/health-canada/services/drugs-health-products/reports-publications/medeffect-canada/good-label-package-practices-guide-prescription-drugs-profile/guidance-document.html

Hicks, R., Becker, S., & Cousins, D. (2008). *MEDMARX data report. A report on the relationship of drug names and medication errors in response to the institute of Medicine's call for action*. Center for the Advancement of Patient Safey, US Pharmacopeia.

Iglesias Gomez, R., Font Noguera, I., Correa Ballester, M., Ruiz Caldes, M. J., & Poveda Andres, J. L. (2022). Tall man lettering application in medication information systems as a quality and safety strategy in hospital organization. *Journal of Clinical Pharmacy and Therapeutics*, *47*(10), 1570–1575. DOI: 10.1111/jcpt.13703 PMID: 35641241

Kierstan, B. (2019). *Eye medication mix-ups*. Retrieved 14 March from https://www.aao.org/eye-health/treatments/eye-medication-mix-ups

Kowing, D., & Kester, E. (2007). Keep an eye out for glaucoma. *The Nurse Practitioner*, *32*(7), 18–23. DOI: 10.1097/01.NPR.0000279566.70700.09 PMID: 17595584

Lambert, B. L., Lin, S. J., Chang, K. Y., & Gandhi, S. K. (1999). Similarity as a risk factor in drug-name confusion errors: The look-alike (orthographic) and sound-alike (phonetic) model. *Medical Care*, *37*(12), 1214–1225. DOI: 10.1097/00005650-199912000-00005 PMID: 10599603

Lizano-Díez, I., Figueiredo-Escribá, C., Piñero-López, M., Lastra, C. F., Mariño, E. L., & Modamio, P. (2020). Prevention strategies to identify LASA errors: Building and sustaining a culture of patient safety. *BMC Health Services Research*, *20*(1), 63. DOI: 10.1186/s12913-020-4922-3 PMID: 31996197

Lohmeyer, Q., Schiess, C., Wendel Garcia, P. D., Petry, H., Strauch, E., Dietsche, A., Schuepbach, R. A., Buehler, P. K., & Hofmaenner, D. A. (2023). Effects of tall man lettering on the visual behavior of critical care nurses while identifying syringe drug labels: A randomized in situ simulation. *BMJ Quality & Safety*, *32*(1), 26–33. DOI: 10.1136/bmjqs-2021-014438 PMID: 35260415

Mathew, P., Thomas, S. A., & Chandy, S. J. (2022). The role of Schedule H1 and Red Line campaign in improving antibiotic use in India. *Journal of Family Medicine and Primary Care*, *11*(6), 2656–2661. DOI: 10.4103/jfmpc.jfmpc_1811_21 PMID: 36119342

Medicines and Healthcare products Regulatory Agency (MHRA). (2020). *Best practice guidance on the labeling and packaging of medicines. Medicines and Healthcare products Regulatory Agency.* Retrieved 13 July from https://assets.publishing.service.gov.uk/media/5fe09fa48fa8f51489f14374/Best_practice_guidance_labelling_and_packaging_of_medicines.pdf

Merry, A. F., Shipp, D. H., & Lowinger, J. S. (2011). The contribution of labeling to safe medication administration in anesthetic practice. *Best Practice & Research. Clinical Anaesthesiology*, *25*(2), 145–159. DOI: 10.1016/j.bpa.2011.02.009 PMID: 21550540

Mishra, D., Kaur, K., Gurnani, B., Heda, A., & Dwivedi, K. (2022). Clinical and diagnostic color-coding in ophthalmology - An indispensable educational tool for ophthalmologists. *Indian Journal of Ophthalmology*, *70*(9), 3191–3197. DOI: 10.4103/ijo.IJO_442_22 PMID: 36018086

Mohammed, A. (2022). *Instruments of local anesthesia*. Retrieved 17 March from https://uomus.edu.iq/img/lectures21/MUCLecture_2022_3111211.pdf

Momo, K., Shimano, M., Kanezaki, Y., Minagawa, A., Takagi, A., Seino, T., & Koinuma, M. (2019). Assessment of. *Die Pharmazie-An International Journal of Pharmaceutical Sciences*, *74*(5), 310–312. PMID: 31109403

Monnier, A. A. C. S., Matin A, Kamath S, Sharmeen T, Khan WA, Bright HR, Mathew P, Wertheim HFL, (2024). What can be learned from Medicine Labeling Initiatives in Asia, with a focus on Antibiotics? *J Community Med Public Health, 8*(2), 432. https://doi.org/10.29011/2577-2228.100432

Monnier, A. A., Do, N. T. T., Asante, K. P., Afari-Asiedu, S., Khan, W. A., Munguambe, K., Sevene, E., Tran, T. K., Nguyen, C. T. K., Punpuing, S., Gómez-Olivé, F. X., van Doorn, H. R., Caillet, C., Newton, P. N., Ariana, P., Wertheim, H. F. L., Wertheim, H. F. L., Monnier, A. A., Newton, P. N., & van Doorn, H. R. (2023). Is this pill an antibiotic or a painkiller? Improving the identification of oral antibiotics for better use. *The Lancet. Global Health*, *11*(8), e1308–e1313. DOI: 10.1016/S2214-109X(23)00258-9 PMID: 37474237

Mumani, A. A. (2018). User-packaging interaction (UPI): A comprehensive research platform and techniques for improvement, evaluation, and design.

Ostini, R., Roughead, E. E., Kirkpatrick, C. M., Monteith, G. R., & Tett, S. E. (2012). Quality use of medicines—Medication safety issues in naming; look-alike, sound-alike medicine names. *The International Journal of Pharmacy Practice*, *20*(6), 349–357. DOI: 10.1111/j.2042-7174.2012.00210.x PMID: 23134093

Otero López, M. J., Martín Muñoz, R., Sánchez Barba, M., Abad Sazatornil, R., Andreu Crespo, A., Arteta Jiménez, M.,…Cajaraville Ordoñana, G. (2011). Development of a List of Look-alike Drug Names With Recommended Tall Man Letters. *Farmacia Hospitalaria, 35*(5), 225-235. DOI: 10.1016/j.farmae.2011.06.001

Patterson, E. S., Cook, R. I., & Render, M. L. (2002). Improving Patient Safety by Identifying Side Effects from Introducing Bar Coding in Medication Administration. *Journal of the American Medical Informatics Association*, *9*(5), 540–553. DOI: 10.1197/jamia.M1061 PMID: 12223506

Phatak, H. M., Cady, P. S., Heyneman, C. A., & Culbertson, V. L. (2005). Retrospective Detection of Potential Medication Errors Involving Drugs with Similar Names. *Journal of the American Pharmacists Association*, *45*(5), 616–624. DOI: 10.1331/1544345055001247 PMID: 16295648

Pierrel, S. P. A. (2021). *The mechanics of the dental anesthetic cartridge*. Retrieved 17 March from https://www.orabloc.com/wp-content/uploads/Clinical-Tips-The-Mechanics-of-the-Dental-Anesthetic-Cartridge.pdf

Poon, E. G., Keohane, C. A., Yoon, C. S., Ditmore, M., Bane, A., Levtzion-Korach, O., Moniz, T., Rothschild, J. M., Kachalia, A. B., Hayes, J., Churchill, W. W., Lipsitz, S., Whittemore, A. D., Bates, D. W., & Gandhi, T. K. (2010). Effect of Bar-Code Technology on the Safety of Medication Administration. *The New England Journal of Medicine*, *362*(18), 1698–1707. DOI: 10.1056/NEJMsa0907115 PMID: 20445181

Rastogi, S. (2012). Look alike sound alike drugs: From hospitals to homes. *Journal of Pediatric Intensive Care*, *1*(3), 125–126. DOI: 10.3233/PIC-2012-021 PMID: 31214397

Ruutiainen, H. K., Kallio, M. M., & Kuitunen, S. K. (2021). Identification and safe storage of look-alike, sound-alike medicines in automated dispensing cabinets. *European Journal of Hospital Pharmacy : Science and Practice*, *28*(e1, Suppl 2), e151–e156. DOI: 10.1136/ejhpharm-2020-002531 PMID: 33452109

Ryan, A. N., Robertson, K. L., & Glass, B. D. (2024). Look-alike medications in the perioperative setting: Scoping review of medication incidents and risk reduction interventions. *International Journal of Clinical Pharmacy*, *46*(1), 26–39. DOI: 10.1007/s11096-023-01629-2 PMID: 37688737

Schnoor, J., Rogalski, C., Frontini, R., Engelmann, N., & Heyde, C. E. (2015). Case report of a medication error by look-alike packaging: A classic surrogate marker of an unsafe system. *Patient Safety in Surgery*, *9*(1), 12. DOI: 10.1186/s13037-014-0047-0 PMID: 25767564

Shao, S. C., Lai, E. C., Owang, K. L., Chen, H. Y., & Chan, Y. Y. (2018). Look-Alike Medication Packages and Patient Safety. *Journal of Patient Safety*, *14*(3), e47–e48. DOI: 10.1097/PTS.0000000000000506 PMID: 29894438

Shrank, W., Avorn, J., Rolon, C., & Shekelle, P. (2007). Effect of content and format of prescription drug labels on readability, understanding, and medication use: A systematic review. *The Annals of Pharmacotherapy*, *41*(5), 783–801. DOI: 10.1345/aph.1H582 PMID: 17426075

Supapaan, T. S., Napaporn, J., Ruthirakanok, R., Srichathum, S., Songmuang, A., & Pitchayajittipong, C. (2024). Look-alike sound-alike (LASA) medication errors in Thai hospitals. *Pharmacy Practice*, *22*(1), 2886.

Supapaan, T. S., Songmuang, A., Napaporn, J., Sangsukwow, P., Boonrod, P., Intarapongsakul, P., Jaturapattarawong, A., & Pitchayajittipong, C. (2024). Look-alike/sound-alike medication errors: An in-depth examination through a hospital case study. *Pharmacy Practice*, *22*(2), 2959. DOI: 10.18549/PharmPract.2024.2.2959

The American Academy of Ophthalmology. (2015). *Color Codes for Topical Ocular Medications*. Retrieved 20 Nov from https://www.aao.org/about/policies/color-codes-topical-ocular-medications

The American Dental Association (ADA). (2023). *Anesthesia and Sedation: Color Coding of Local Anesthetic Cartridges*. Retrieved 23 Nov from https://www.ada.org/resources/ada-library/oral-health-topics/anesthesia-and-sedation

The American Society for Testing and Materials (ASTM). (2022). *Standard Specification for User Applied Drug Labels in Anesthesiology (Withdrawn 2022)*. Retrieved 21 Nov from https://www.astm.org/d4774-11r17.html

The Institute for Safe Medication Practices Canada (ISMP Canada). (2007). Patient Report of Insulin Mix-Up Shared. *ISMP Canada Safety Bulletin, 7*(6), 1–2.

The Institute for Safe Medication Practices (ISMP). (2011). *ISMP list of high-alert medications in community/ambulatory healthcare*. Retrieved 20 March from https://www.ismp.org/sites/default/files/attachments/2017-11/highAlert-community.pdf

The Institute for Safe Medication Practices (ISMP). (2022). *Adopt strategies to manage look-alike and/or sound-alike medication name mix-ups*. Retrieved 11 July from https://www.ismp.org/sites/default/files/newsletter-issues/20220602.pdf

The Institute for Safe Medication Practices (ISMP). (2023). *List of confused drug names*. Retrieved 16 Apr from https://www.ismp.org/recommendations/confused-drug-names-list

Thomas, P. B. M., & Mollon, J. D. (2018). Syringe labels seen through the eyes of the color-deficient clinician. *British Journal of Anaesthesia, 121*(6), 1370–1373. DOI: 10.1016/j.bja.2018.07.023 PMID: 30442268

Travasso, C. (2016). India draws a red line under antibiotic misuse. *BMJ (Clinical Research Ed.), 352*, i1202. DOI: 10.1136/bmj.i1202 PMID: 26926703

United States Pharmacopeia (USP). (2020). *General Chapter <7> Labeling. USP–NF*. Retrieved 22 Aug from https://www.uspnf.com/sites/default/files/usp_pdf/EN/USPNF/revisions/gc-7-ira-20200731.pdf?

U.S. Department of Health and Human Services Food and Drug Administration. "Center for Drug Evaluation and Research (CDER). (2016). *Safety considerations for product design to minimize medication errors: guidance for industry*. Retrieved 8 June from https://www.fda.gov/files/drugs/published/Safety-Considerations-for-Product-Design-to-Minimize-Medication-Errors-Guidance-for-Industry.pdf

U.S. Department of Health and Human Services Food and Drug Administration. (2022). *Safety considerations for container labels and carton labeling design to minimize medication errors guidance for industry*. Retrieved 11 July from https://www.fda.gov/media/158522/download

U.S. Department of Health and Human Services Food and Drug Administration (FDA). (2005). Use of Color on Pharmaceutical Product Labels, Labeling and Packaging; Public Hearing. *Federal Register, 70*(22), 5687–5689.

U.S. Department of Health and Human Services Food and Drug Administration (FDA). (2020). *FDA name differentiation project*. Retrieved 06 Aug from https://www.fda.gov/drugs/medication-errors-related-cder-regulated-drug-products/fda-name-differentiation-project

WHO Collaborating Centre for Patient Safety Solutions. (2007). *Look-alike, sound-alike medication names*. Retrieved 9 August from https://cdn.who.int/media/docs/default-source/patient-safety/patient-safety-solutions/ps-solution1-look-alike-sound-alike-medication-names.pdf?sfvrsn=d4fb860b_8

Winfield, A. J., Jessiman, D., Williams, A., & Esakowitz, L. (1990). A study of the causes of non-compliance by patients prescribed eyedrops. *The British Journal of Ophthalmology*, *74*(8), 477–480. DOI: 10.1136/bjo.74.8.477 PMID: 2390523

World Health Organization. (2007). *WHO launches 'Nine patient safety solutions'*. Retrieved 12 Aug from https://www.who.int/news/item/02-05-2007-who-launches-nine-patient-safety-solutions

World Health Organization. (2023). *Medication safety for look-alike, sound-alike medicines*. World Health Organization. Retrieved 3 June from https://iris.who.int/bitstream/handle/10665/373495/9789240058897-eng.pdf?sequence=1

Yin, H. S., Mendelsohn, A. L., Wolf, M. S., Parker, R. M., Fierman, A., van Schaick, L., Bazan, I. S., Kline, M. D., & Dreyer, B. P. (2010). Parents' medication administration errors: Role of dosing instruments and health literacy. *Archives of Pediatrics & Adolescent Medicine*, *164*(2), 181–186. DOI: 10.1001/archpediatrics.2009.269 PMID: 20124148

ABBREVIATIONS

project: ABACUS – AntiBiotic ACcess and USe
AAO: American Academy of Ophthalmology
ADA: American Dental Association
ADC: Automated Dispensing Cabinet
ADE: Adverse Drug Event
ANSI: American National Standards Institute
ASA: American Society of Anesthesiologists
ASTM: American Society for Testing and Materials
BCMA: Bar-Code Medication Administration
BS ISO: British Standard International Organization for Standardization
DSCSA: Drug Supply Chain Security Act
EMA: European Medicines Agency
eMAR: Electronic Medication Administration Record
FDA: U.S. Food and Drug Administration
GS1: General Specifications1
GTIN: Global Trade Item Number

HCD: Human-Centered Design
HEART: Human Error Assessment and Reduction Technique
ICU: Intensive Care Unit
INN: International Nonproprietary Name
ISMP: Institute for Safe Medication Practices
LASA: Look-Alike Sound-Alike
MHRA: Medicines and Healthcare products Regulatory Agency (UK)
NCC MERP: National Coordinating Council for Medication Error Reporting and Prevention
NICU: Neonatal Intensive Care Unit
OR: Operating Room
pMDI: Pressurized metered-dose inhaler
PMS: Pantone Matching System
QR: Quick Response (code)
RFID: Radiofrequency Identification
USP: United States Pharmacopeia
WHO: World Health Organization

Chapter 5
Look-Alike, Sound-Alike Medication Errors Caused by Drug Names

ABSTRACT

Look alike and sound alike medication errors threaten patient safety worldwide because drug names with similar spelling or pronunciation are confused. This chapter discusses the causes and clinical impacts of these errors as well as their prevention. International case studies have shown that morphine–hydromorphone and vinblastine–vincristine mixtures cause serious harm and death. Regulatory frameworks in the U.S., Canada, the UK, Thailand, and the WHO show how systematic name screening and standardized conventions reduce these risks. Hospitals use tall man lettering, electronic prescribing alerts, and clinician education. Overall, the chapter concludes that to prevent and reduce medication errors on a global scale, incorrect drug errors should be addressed in a multilayered manner.

INTRODUCTION

Medication safety depends on many small details, and one of the most important yet risky is the drug name itself. Look-alike, sound-alike (LASA) drug names, those that look or sound very similar, create hidden dangers that even careful healthcare professionals can miss. These are not just spelling or pronunciation similarities; they are safety risks built into the system of how medicines are named, prescribed, dispensed, and administered.

Although errors caused by name confusion are relatively rare in percentage terms, their impact is large. Research indicates that they occur in only a very small fraction of prescriptions (0.00003–0.0022%), yet they account for up to 7% of near

DOI: 10.4018/979-8-3373-5478-1.ch005

misses and as much as 14.7% of all reported medication errors (Bryan et al., 2015; Bryan et al., 2021a; Bryan et al., 2021b). When these errors reach the patient, the results can range from loss of treatment effectiveness to severe harm, including life-threatening complications. Wrong drug errors caused by name confusion have been linked to respiratory depression from morphine–hydromorphone mix-ups (Lowe et al., 2017; The Pennsylvania Patient Safety Advisory, 2007) and toxic chemotherapy overdoses from vinblastine–vincristine confusion (The Institute for Safe Medication Practices (ISMP), 2015). These are powerful reminders that every error matters.

Processing in the language brain is among the factors that cause such danger. It is not the fault of people to comprehend information by pattern recognition and mental shortcuts as they instinctively do in high-stress situations. Such a pattern has the potential to make clinicians believe that hydralazine is hydroxyzine or that dopamine is dobutamine. Laboratory experiments indicate that the names of drugs with similar lettering/sounding have more recognition mistakes. Notably, these laboratory error rates were correlated with community pharmacy database dispensing errors; thus, it is clear that controlled tests can be used to predict real-world risk (Schroeder et al., 2017).

Steps have also been taken by linking those elements of a group of charts that lend themselves especially to a linguistic design. Many drug names overlap in terms of prefixes, suffixes, or close lengths. Classic names that end in -pril in the case of ACE inhibitors or -mab in the case of a monoclonal antibody are useful in categorizing the drugs but are ineffective at distinguishing drugs within the category (Karet, 2019, 2023). Early computational research revealed how small drug name differences can cause confusion. In a landmark study, Lambert (1997) compared 969 name pairs with reported errors to 969 randomly selected controls. He reported that compared with controls, error pairs were more similar in terms of bigram, trigram, and Levenshtein distance. Pairs with similar scores above the thresholds were 25 to 500 times more likely to make an error. A Levenshtein distance test had 94% accuracy, 84% sensitivity, and 98.8% specificity in distinguishing confusing names from nonproblematic names (Lambert et al., 1999). These findings showed that even minor spelling errors can deceive clinicians under time pressure.

Drug name confusion is a challenge not only for linguistics but also at the environmental and psychological levels. Under pressure, action-based or memory-based lapses cause many errors (Aronson, 2009). Experimental evidence supports these mechanisms. Using eye-movement tracking, Filik et al. (2004) reported that look-alike names take longer to process and are more likely to be misread, especially in time-constrained tasks (Filik et al., 2004). Tall man lettering decreased but did not eliminate errors. Lizano-Díez et al. (2020) studied LASA name prevention strategies, such as tall man lettering, computerized alerts, and harmonized naming systems (Lizano-Díez et al., 2020). They reported that interruptions, multitasking, and cognitive overload create ideal LASA error conditions without safeguards. These data reveal that drug name mix-ups are not occasional clerical mistakes. Collectively, these findings emphasize that drug name confusion is not merely an infrequent technical error. It depicts the anticipated interrelationship between the actions of the human mind, environmental factors, and poor system protection capability and remains a serious threat to patient safety worldwide.

Objectives of the Chapter

The aims of this chapter are as follows:

(1) To explain chemical, nonproprietary, and brand drug nomenclature and their clinical relevance.
(2) To describe and define LASA medication errors and how orthographic and phonetic similarities hurt patients.
(3) To categorize international regulatory and institutional mechanisms to reduce LASA risk, examples will include the United States, Canada, the United Kingdom and Thailand, along with international structures.
(4) To provide a summary of approaches to reducing LASA errors throughout the drug life cycle, including name creation and regulatory approval, hospital-based interventions and pharmacovigilance.

Organization of the Chapter

A brief overview of drug nomenclature in clinical care and patient safety begins this chapter. Comparisons of chemical, nonproprietary, and brand names and their impact on medication errors follow. Orthographic and phonetic confusion that causes LASA errors are discussed next, with clinical examples and case reports. Hospital-based strategies and global error reduction initiatives follow international regulatory practices. This chapter underscores the importance of a multilayered (global) approach to drug name safety.

DRUG NAMING SYSTEMS

Physicians and patients know how a drug works and how it is used on the basis of the nomenclature. Systematic nomenclature improves clinical decision-making, medication errors and patient safety. (Karet, 2019; Pelletier-Dattu, 2017). The chemical, generic and brand names of new drugs. In several ways, the names communicate to clinicians and patients

Chemical Name

In accordance with IUPAC standards, drug chemical names describe the molecular structure, components, and stereochemistry of pharmaceutical substances, making them the most scientifically accurate. Research, regulatory filings, and patent documentation require these names because they clearly describe the compound's structure (International Union of Pure and Applied Chemistry, 2013). The painkiller aspirin is 2-(acetyloxy)benzoic acid. Cisplatin, an anticancer drug, is named cis-diamminedichloroplatinum(II), which describes its coordination geometry but is too complicated for clinical or patient communication (Serafini et al., 2021). Chemical names are rarely used in medicine because of their length and complexity. Their place is taken by generic (nonproprietary) names such as those from the WHO International Nonproprietary Names (INN) or USAN programs. While maintaining structural and pharmacological identity, these simplified names improve pronounceability, recognition, and safety (Cohen et al., 2007; Cohen & Smetzer, 2007; World Health Organization, 1997, 2017). The consistent use of nonproprietary names will alleviate some of the issues associated with LASA as the leading cause of medication dispensing errors of a drug. Karet (2023) reported that linguistic similarity between generic names can still cause confusion, emphasizing why USAN and INN authorities carefully manage naming conventions and use FDA tools such as the Phonetic and Orthographic Computer Analysis (POCA) tool to screen for similarity conflicts (Karet, 2023). Chemical names are important for drug discovery and regulation; generic and trade names are useful for medical practice (Cohen et al., 2007; Dunne & Dunne, 2015; Karet, 2019, 2023).

Nonproprietary Name

The official medical names for drug active ingredients are generic or nonproprietary. These names are assigned by the WHO's International Nonproprietary Names (INN) Programme or the USAN Council in the U.S. These systems standardize drug nomenclature globally and nationally, giving each active substance a unique, universal name. Standardization improves healthcare provider communication, reduces prescribing errors, and improves patient safety (Karet, 2019; World Health Organization, 2017).

Chemical nomenclatures are simplified into nonproprietary names for clinical use. They frequently have common stems that organize drugs by pharmacological class (e.g., "-olol" for drugs in the beta-blocker class and "-mab" for monoclonal antibodies), providing name recognition cues and therapeutic class prompts to health care practitioners. Most USANs are harmonized with INNs, but some are not due to linguistic or historical preferences. Acetaminophen is paracetamol under the INN, and acetaminophen under the USAN. In the US, salbutamol (INN) is an albuterol. While these naming differences are inconsequential, they can be confusing to patients and providers when they encounter the same drug by a different name in different regions (Cohen & Smetzer, 2007; Dunne & Dunne, 2015; Meredith, 1996).

The existence of numerous brand names for a single generic drug, such as Tylenol® for acetaminophen/paracetamol, highlights the need for generic nomenclature. Practitioners, pharmacists, and scientists alike need to become familiar with the INNs and USANs to ensure safe prescribing, clear communication, and universal pharmacovigilance. Nonproprietary names serve as a connector between complex chemical nomenclature and commercially motivated brand names and are therefore indispensable in drug identification (Serafini et al., 2021).

Brand Recognition

Brand names, or trade names, are proprietary names pharmaceutical companies select to improve the pronunciation, recognition, and memorability of drugs. Whereas generic names are standardized and international, trade names are covered by a trade mark, and essentially, their use is to distinguish a product from the competition on the market (Cohen et al., 2007; Cohen & Smetzer, 2007). By registering trademarks, firms protect the name of the brand from being utilized by other companies looking to use the same or similar naming conventions, maintaining the brand's commercial uniqueness.

A drug is generally recommended under a few brand names, even by different companies and in different forms. In contrast, a generic (nonproprietary) name is invariant, being a name assigned by an international or national naming authority such as the World Health Organization (WHO)'s International Nonproprietary Names (INN) Program or the United States Adopted Names (USAN) Council (Archambault, 1983; World Health Organization, 2017). For instance, acetaminophen (USAN)—an analgesic and antipyretic agent, internationally referred to as paracetamol—has been synthesized under several brand names globally—where the brand Tylenol® is known to the U.S. population (FDA, 2022). This redundancy of trade names highlights the potential for medication errors and patient confusion, especially if consumers come across the same generic medication on offer under several trade names differing between countries (Cohen et al., 2007; Cohen & Smetzer, 2007; Dunne & Dunne, 2015).

Regulatory Brand naming occurs as a concomitant procedure to protocols of universally standardized generic names, for example, the INN Naming system recommended by the WHO, as well as the USAN of the United States Adopted Names Council. The INN is an original generic name that is a unique name and belongs globally to only one active substance to ensure safe and rational prescription practices throughout the planet. Likewise, the USAN system contributes to the harmonization of drug nomenclature in the United States, in line with the INN conventions where practicable (World Health Organization, 1997, 2017). Both methods are essential for avoiding medication errors by minimizing ambiguity in drug designation, particularly in international healthcare and research environments.

Names may be chosen on the basis of how they evoke therapeutic use, clinical efficacy, or ease of administration but are often only unique identifiers without any direct relevance to the drug's pharmacology. This discrepancy highlights the need to avoid the use of chemical, generic and brand names interchangeably. It is important for clinicians, pharmacists and researchers to be aware of these differences to ensure safe prescribing and dispensing as well as patient education. Patients also profit from it, as it eliminates confusion and prompts higher compliance with changes from generic to branded versions and vice versa.

To demonstrate these differences, examples of frequently used drugs are shown in **Table 1**, where differences in chemical names, generic names and brand names between the WHO INN and USAN are given. These similarities illustrate the complexity of international drug naming systems and highlight the need for standardization to ensure patient safety (Cohen & Smetzer, 2017; World Health Organization, 2017).

Table 1. Comparison of drug nomenclature variations

	Chemical name (The International Union of Pure and Applied Chemistry (IUPAC) nomenclature standards)	Generic name		Brand Name(s) (country)
		The World Health Organization International Nonproprietary Names (INN)	United States Adopted Name (USAN)	
1	N-(4-hydroxyphenyl) acetamide	Paracetamol	Acetaminophen	Tylenol (USA), Panadol (Global)
2	4-[2-(tert-butylamino)-1-hydroxyethyl]-2-(hydroxymethyl)phenol	Salbutamol	Albuterol	Ventolin (USA), Proventil (USA)
3	(6R,7R)-7-[[(2R)-2-amino-2-phenylacetyl]amino]-3-methyl-8-oxo-5-thia-1-azabicyclo[4.2.0]oct-2-ene-2-carboxylic acid	Cefalexin	Cephalexin	Keflex (USA), Biocef (USA)
4	5-chloro-N-[2-[4-(cyclohexylcarbamoylsulfamoyl) phenyl]ethyl]-2-methoxybenzamide	Glibenclamide	glyBURIDE	Glynase (USA) Daonil (Australia)

continued on following page

Table 1. Continued

	Chemical name (The International Union of Pure and Applied Chemistry (IUPAC) nomenclature standards)	Generic name		Brand Name(s) (country)
		The World Health Organization International Nonproprietary Names (INN)	United States Adopted Name (USAN)	
5	ethyl 1-methyl-4-phenylpiperidine-4-carboxylate	Pethidine	Meperidine	Demerol (USA)
6	3-[(4-Methyl-1-piperazinyl) imino] methylrifamycin SV	Rifampicin	rifAMpin	Rifadin (USA), Rimactane (USA)
7	2-[1-(4-chlorobenzoyl)-5-methoxy-2-methylindol-3-yl]acetic acid	Indometacin	Indomethacin	Indocin (USA), Tivorbex (USA)
8	1-[4-(3-methylanilino)pyridin-3-yl]sulfonyl-3-propan-2-ylurea	Torasemide	Torsemide	Demadex (USA), Soaanz (USA)

(Cohen & Smetzer, 2017; National Center for Biotechnology Information, 2024a, 2024b, 2024c, 2024d, 2024e, 2024f, 2024g, 2024h)

DEFINING THE ISSUE: LASA ERRORS BY DRUG NAME

Confusion between drug names is the fundamental cause of LASA errors. The World Health Organization (WHO) has highlighted the importance of the need to address risks arising through the similarity of drug names or medication labels and has published safety solutions and lists of high-risk examples. Extending this model, the Institute for Safe Medication Practices (ISMP) has generated and circulated detailed lists of LASA pairs for use in clinical medicine. These names may have orthographic (look-alike) or phonetic similarity (sound-alike) (The Institute for Safe Medication Practices (ISMP), 2023b; World Health Organization, 2023).

Orthographic (Look-Alike) Confusion

Orthographic similarity occurs among drug names that share similar spelling patterns, letter sequences, or other identifier components, which may confuse them and lead to misreading at different points in the medication use system. This risk is also encountered in handwritten prescriptions because incorrect medication names resulting from indecipherable handwriting can be in close proximity to real medication names or in electronic systems in which names that are similar can be found adjacent to each other in an alphabetical list (The Pennsylvania Patient Safety Advisory, 2004). As shown in **Figure 1**, other factors that would compound the above are the visual similarity of drug names, the presence of frequently confused drug pairs, and the constraints of electronic support tools and numerical techniques, all of which further increase the level of risk.

Figure 1. Orthographic (look-alike) confusion

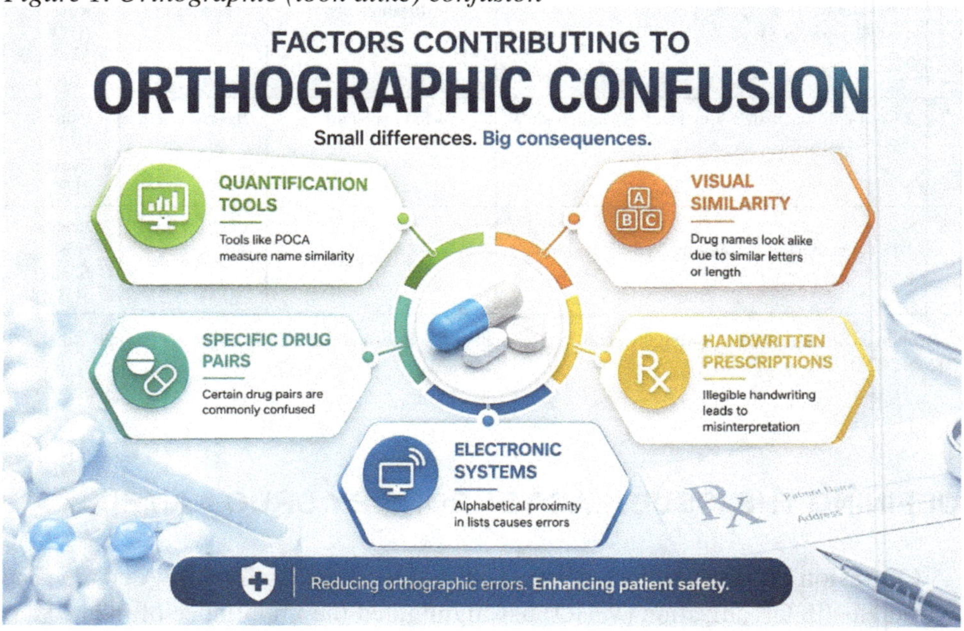

A classic example is the pair hydrALAZINE and hydrOXYzine (The Institute for Safe Medication Practices (ISMP), 2023b; The Pennsylvania Patient Safety Advisory, 2006). The first is an antihypertensive, and the second is an antihistamine. Confusion can cause serious hypotension, unattended allergic reactions or bronchospasm.

Another major risk is the similarity of Avandia® (rosiglitazone), which is used to treat diabetes, and Coumadin® (warfarin), which is utilized as a blood thinner. While treating completely different diseases, for reasons inexplicable to me other than their similar naming, these two brand names have been confused in handwritten scripts, particularly in cursive, and with dire consequences, including untreated diabetes or unintended excessive anticoagulation. The ISMP's "List of Confused Drug Names" specifically identifies Avandia and Coumadin as high risk, accordingly warranting increased attention to this issue (The Institute for Safe Medication Practices (ISMP),

2023b). This is reinforced by patient safety literature describing known instances where these misread prescriptions have resulted in significant negative patient outcomes, including stomach or gut bleeding needing surgery (Gaunt, 2007; The Institute for Safe Medication Practices (ISMP), 2023b).

Likewise, the chemotherapy drugs vinblastine and vincristine have a deadly LASA risk; they not only appear very similar in writing but also to be dosed in error can be deadly. Although not strictly a "tenfold dose difference," vincristine is at least an order of magnitude more neurotoxic and, when administered by the wrong route (i.e., the intrathecal route), can be nearly lethal. This pair appears in the tall-man lettering do not use an abbreviation list published by the FDA and ISMP (vinBLAStine vs. vinCRIStine), indicating the associated concern for medication error. In response, the ISMP and oncology safety groups have required measures such as only allowing vincristine to be dispensed in minibags while discouraging the use of syringes to avoid fatal mix-ups (ISMP, 2016; ISMP News/ECRI, 2020; Joint Commission International, 2017; The Institute for Safe Medication Practices (ISMP), 2023b; World Health Organization, 2023).

The degree of orthographic confusability can be calculated by computational means. For example, the FDA's Phonetic and Orthographic Computer Analysis (POCA) tool reports a composite similarity for each pair of 0 (no similarity) and to up to 100 (exact match) (Karet, 2023; Lambert, 1997; Lambert et al., 1999). A POCA orthographic score >70 is highly similar (Karet, 2023; Shah et al., 2017; U.S. Department of Health and Human Services Food and Drug Administration (FDA), 2021). In a pioneering study, a statistically significant increase in the odds of medication error of between 25 and 523 times was found among drug pairs with the highest orthographic scores compared with those with the lowest (Lambert, 1997). A Levenshtein distance test (which represents the number of alterations needed to transform one name to another) was also found to have 94% accuracy in detecting ambiguous names with true names (Lambert et al., 1999).

Phonetic (Sound-Alike) Confusion

Phonetic confusion arises from the acoustic similarity of drug names and is particularly hazardous in environments that rely on spoken communication, such as emergency departments and operating rooms (The Pennsylvania Patient Safety Advisory, 2004; World Health Organization, 2023). While this has most frequently been recorded within an anglophone context, such a challenge is of course global, as well as being informed in all locations by local language and nomenclature systems.

Highly publicized examples include Foradil® (formoterol, a bronchodilator) and Toradol® (ketorolac, a nonsteroidal anti-inflammatory drug, an NSAID). The Pennsylvania Patient Safety Authority has received reports where a written order for

Foradil® was read incorrectly as Toradol, which could have resulted in harm (The Pennsylvania Patient Safety Advisory, 2004). This pair is also cited as a look-alike error in the ISMP List of Confused Drug Names (The Institute for Safe Medication Practices (ISMP), 2023b).

Zyrtec® (cetirizine) vs Zyprexa® (olanzapine): Mixture of medications dispensed in error; despite actions by the FDA, the manufacturer and others, i.e., label re-design, this problem continued (NBC News, 2005; The Associated Press, 2005). Dopamine–dobutamine pairs Dopamine versus Dobutamine, mentioned in the same sound class, are high-alert, soundalike, lookalike pairs in verbal order confusion (The Institute for Safe Medication Practices (ISMP), 2023a).

Five thousand LASA drug pairs were identified in a national survey in Thailand spanning 128 hospitals, with name/pronunciation being the most prevalent class of similarity (Chanakit et al., 2013). One good example herein is the contrast between dopamine and dobutamine for injections—a common root of mistreatment between inpatients. Phonetic interventions extend beyond medicine. New names When Ya maa ("horse medicine") became a problem, the name of that offending drug was changed to Ya ba ("crazy medicine") in the 1990s. This was done to highlight its negative consequences (Cohen, 2014).

In Japan, LASA hazards are increased by the use of the Katakana script, which encourages sound-like errors to be made with drug names. One solution to this problem is "finger pointing and calling", which significantly decreases errors by directing attention toward the correct name (Mitobe & Higuchi, 2016). At the level of regulation, proposed drug names are screened for likeness in the Japan Pharmaceutical Information Center (JAPIC), especially the first three syllables of Katakana (Brand Institute, 2023). More recently, national efforts have been directed toward harmonizing terminology so that Japanese drug names can be cross-mapped to the RxNorm standard to support worldwide interoperability and limit international pharmacovigilance LASA risks (Kimura et al., 2025). As shown in **Figure 2**, phonetic confusion is the leading cause of LASA medication errors and has led to the development of several measures to minimize the risk in practical environments and regulatory frameworks.

Figure 2. Phonetic (sound-alike) drug name mixing and chosen risk-reduction approaches

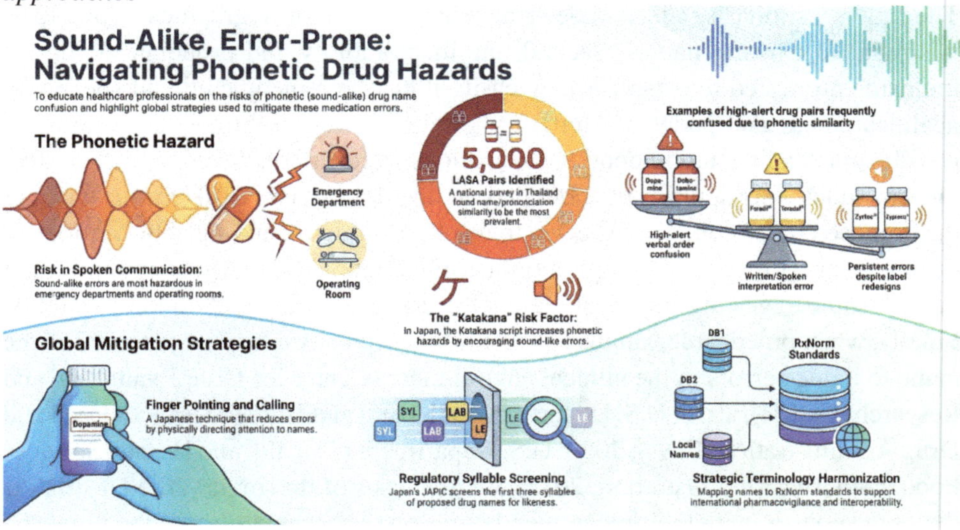

EXAMPLES OF DRUG NAME REGISTRATION

The United States

The United States has one of the strictest and most comprehensive drug approval regulations in the world, which is controlled by the U.S. FDA. A critical component in this process is ensuring that the names of new medicinal products are clear and acceptable and that LASA medication errors do not occur. In this part of the report, we looked at the path of new drug registration in the USA and focused on the contribution of the Division of Medication Error Prevention and Analysis (DMEPA) to limiting the number of LASA medication errors (World Health Organization, 2023).

Before a drug can be marketed in the U.S., it must undergo a stringent approval process that includes preclinical testing, clinical trials, and thorough evaluation by the FDA's Center for Drug Evaluation and Research (CDER). CDER reviews new drug applications (NDAs) to determine that the benefits of drug use outweigh its risks (U.S. Department of Health and Human Services Food and Drug Administration (FDA), 2024).

In this context, the Division of Medication Error Prevention and Analysis (DMEPA) has served to prevent LASA medication errors. One of its main tasks is reviewing proposed proprietary (brand) drug names for use prior to marketing. The intent is that these names are not confused with other products, which may then mitigate medication errors. The DMEPA review process includes several important steps. The first is a similarity check to determine how well an orthographically/phoneme is similar to existing names. Second, the memorability and pronounceability of the name are tested to establish how easily it can be remembered and spoken by healthcare staff and patients. Third, a phonological and orthographic analysis of possible misleading, ambiguous and suspicious words is conducted. Fourth, the review includes consideration of abbreviations and dosing risks to determine whether the proposed name could be expected to result in similar-sounding abbreviations or dosing errors. Fifth, there are promotional implications to consider in preventing names from suggesting improper claims for safety, efficacy and/or comparability. Finally, when practicable, simulation testing is used to evaluate the potential of the name to induce errors in the clinical environment (Center for Drug Evaluation and Research (CDER), 2016; U.S. Department of Health and Human Services Food and Drug Administration (FDA), 2020; U.S. Department of Health and Human Services Food and Drug Administration, 2016). On the basis of this review, the DMEPA is the drug sponsor, with their recommendations on the acceptability of the proposed proprietary name.

In addition to the safety review, the Division of Medication Error Prevention and Analysis (DMEPA) analyzes the misbranding potential of proposed proprietary names. This review is conducted in conjunction with the Office of Prescription Drug Promotion (OPDP) for prescription products and the Office of Nonprescription Drugs (ONPD) for nonprescription products. Misbranding considers whether the new name overstates effectiveness, understates risks, exceeds indications, does not meet claims of enhanced efficacy, or is otherwise false or misleading (Bai et al., 2021; Kalola & Dean, 2019; Nightingale, 1998). This iterative process is also reinforced by computational tools. The Phonetic Orthographic Computer Analysis (POCA) tool is used to calculate a similarity score between a proposed drug name and an existing drug name (Karet, 2019, 2023; Kondrak & Dorr, 2006; Rider et al., 2019; U.S. Department of Health and Human Services Food and Drug Administration (FDA), 2021). One such version in the cloud was introduced in 2020 by the FDA to make reporting easier for manufacturers.

As part of the drug approval process, the DMEPA works closely with drug sponsors (known as NDA applicants and as IND sponsors) to ensure that the submitted proprietary name is acceptable and that LASA medication errors are reduced. This "partnership" falls under the category of continuous, open communication, guidance, and feedback to help sponsors select appropriate names for their products. Sponsors may choose to incorporate their own evaluations with respect to an assessment, for example, name simulation studies or analyses using the POCA, in their proprietary name submission to the FDA (Shah et al., 2017; U.S. Department of Health and

Human Services Food and Drug Administration (FDA), 2022a, 2022b). In addition to reviewing proprietary names for biological products, the DMEPA is responsible for assigning suffixes for designated biological products to support pharmacovigilance and distinguish between biological products.

Suffix Review for Biological Products

In the case of biological products, the DMEPA has taken on the responsibility of deciding what that designated suffix in the proper name will be to support pharmacovigilance, to help prevent medication errors and to minimize the potential for accidental substitution. When proposed, the suffix shall be a unique string of four letters in lower case, nonproprietary, without meaning, and at least three of the four letters shall be different. A hypen should be used to connect it to the root name. The suffix should not be false or misleading, contain numbers or punctuations (with the exception of the hyphen), use common abbreviations, imply or refer to any drug substance or core name, look like any marketed product or the license holder's name, or be too similar to any other FDA-designated suffix (U.S. Department of Health and Human Services Food and Drug Administration (FDA), 2014, 2019).

Postmarketing Surveillance

The DMEPA continues to track the safety of drugs after they are released to the market in postmarketing surveillance. This includes an analysis of medication error reports, adverse event reports, and other information to identify any new issues that may have emerged involving LASA medication errors. If deemed necessary, the DMEPA may recommend label, packaging and even proprietary name changes to reduce the possibility of medication error (Aimette et al., 2007; Cohen et al., 2007).

Labels and Labeling Review

DMEPA reviews proposed labeling for new drugs to protect against legibility, readability, and comprehension failures that contribute to medication errors. The review of these combines considerations such as color differentiation and tall man lettering of textual portions and clarity of the content.

Education and Outreach

As part of its regulatory functions, the DMEPA has a long-term commitment to educating the public about safe medication use and preventing LASA errors. This includes partnerships with clinician organizations, patient safety advocacy groups, and industry to alert the health care community about LASA and share best practices to prevent errors (Cohen, 2007b; Cohen et al., 2007; Cohen & Smetzer, 2015, 2018). The new medical registration process in the U.S. is a complicated and strict system fueled first by patient safety. The Division of Medication Error Prevention and Analysis (DMEPA) is an integral part of this process, as it scrutinizes proposed proprietary names to prevent them from causing LASA errors. With its thorough review process, drug sponsor cooperation, postmarketing follow-up, and education and outreach activities, the DMEPA protects public health and ensures the safe use of drugs. Even with the addition of new drugs to the market, the efforts of the DMEPA remain essential for reducing the vulnerability of patients to LASA errors (Tu et al., 2012).

Canada

Health Canada is the federal department responsible for helping Canadians maintain and improve their health and contributes to minimizing the risk of LASA medication errors through the review of drug brand names. These errors occur when health care practitioners or patients confuse one drug name with another name because the names look alike, sound alike, or are packaged together and can result in serious adverse reactions (Government of Canada, 2014; Health Canada, 2004, 2014; Marilyn Schwartz, 2007).

During the submission of a new drug in Canada, one of the requirements for sponsors is to assess their proposed brand name for confusion risk with the drug names currently on the Canadian market. Health Canada's Guidance Document for Industry - Review of Drug Brand Names, 2014, details the requirements and process for such review (Government of Canada, 2014; Health Canada, 2014; Marilyn Schwartz, 2007).

The guidance requires that sponsors follow a series of steps to evaluate the potential for confusion between their proposed brand name and the names of authorized Canadian products. This systematic methodology, depicted in **Table 2**, is known as the "search, simulate, synthesize" approach, which consists of database searches, medication use process simulations and a synthesis of findings (Government of Canada, 2014). The review of the brand name step by step is as follows:

Step 1: Initial brand name review

The sponsor presubmits the proposed trade name to Health Canada. The application must include the proposed name, which must not be misleading, unsafe, or easily mistaken for another product. In case the name does not succeed the first review, the sponsor is required to provide another name (Government of Canada,

2014; Health Canada, 2004, 2014, 2019; The Institute for Safe Medication Practices Canada (ISMP Canada), 2016).

Step 2: LASA attribute testing

The name is then submitted to the LASA review: if the name is found to pass this review, it is subjected to a further, more in depth, LASA assessment through a three-stage process:

Step 2.1: Search

The sponsor must search the Health Canada Drug Product Database and Licensed Natural Health Products Database to find an existing name that has an orthographic and phonetic similarity score of 50% or more with that of the proposed name(Government of Canada, 2014; Health Canada, 2004, 2014, 2019; The Institute for Safe Medication Practices Canada (ISMP Canada), 2016).

Step 2.2: Simulate

The product sponsor creates process maps for med-use activities involving the product and runs simulations with HCPs and patients to identify potential failure modes related to the proposed proprietary name. These simulations challenge the name in clinical situations such as prescribing, transcribing, dispensing, and administering (Government of Canada, 2014; Health Canada, 2004, 2014, 2019; The Institute for Safe Medication Practices Canada (ISMP Canada), 2016).

Step 2.3: Synthesizing

The severity and detectability of potential failure modes that are discovered during the search and simulation steps are evaluated by the sponsor through failure mode and effects analysis (FMEA). They summarize the results in a full report and offer a justification for the acceptability of the proposed name (Government of Canada, 2014; Health Canada, 2004, 2014, 2019; The Institute for Safe Medication Practices Canada (ISMP Canada), 2016).

Step 3: Decision

Health Canada considers the sponsor's brand name evaluation, including the search, LASA, and FMEA findings, and may perform further searches or analyses prior to making a final decision. If the agency believes that the proposed name is likely to be mistaken for other health products or is not appropriate, it may refuse the name and request a new name (Government of Canada, 2014; Health Canada, 2004, 2014, 2019; The Institute for Safe Medication Practices Canada (ISMP Canada), 2016).

Health Canada's comprehensive process for reviewing brand names, in a systematic manner, to facilitate early identification and mitigation of risks associated with placement in the market of LASA drug products is the embodiment of a proactive approach and responsibility. By requiring sponsors to conduct comprehensive name reviews and detailed reviews, Health Canada seeks to reduce the risks of name confusion and keep the public safe during the drug review process.

Table 2. The health Canada brand name review process with illustrative examples

Step	Description	Example (Medicare vs Medicaid)
Step 1: Initial brand-name review	Health Canada scrutinizes the name for general safety considerations to make sure it is not misleading and cannot be confused with an existing product. If it does not pass, the sponsor needs to come up with a new name.	Medicare is raised in this first search as it is very similar to the target product Medicaid.
Step 2: Testing of proposed brand names for LASA attributes	A full LASA evaluation consists of three substeps: search, simulate, and synthesize, after (and only if) the name receives a pass in Step 1.	Medicare now progresses to full LASA assessment.
Step 2.1: Search	The sponsor searches Health Canada's Drug Product Database and Licensed Natural Health Products Database. All names for which the overall orthographic (and phonetic) similarity score is at least 50% are detected.	Meditation has a 60% resemblance to Medicare.
Step 2.2: Simulate	Medication-use process diagrams and simulations with physicians, pharmacists, nurses, and patients highlight a variety of failure modes during prescribing, transcribing, dispensing, and administration.	In simulated dispensing, many people mix up Medicare, Medicaid and choose the wrong product.
Step 2.3: Synthesize	In the execution of a Failure Mode and Effects Analysis (FMEA), the severity and detectability of all failure modes under consideration is evaluated and the sponsor produces a report demonstrating that (or that the name is not) acceptable.	The FMEA shows a substantial risk of dispensing errors with a Medicare approval, particularly on the pharmacy counter.
Step 3: Decision	Health Canada evaluates the available evidence (literature, search, simulation and the risk analysis) to make a decision and might in some cases perform additional analyses prior to the final decision. It is denied noting that the name seems to be misleading and confusing and an alternate one is sought for.	Health Canada refuses Medicare and asks the sponsor to provide an alternative name due to the potential for LASA errors.

(Government of Canada, 2014; Health Canada, 2014)

The United Kingdom

The registration of a new drug in the UK involves a number of very important steps, as described in the MHRA Guideline for the Naming of Medicinal Products and Braille Requirements for the Name on Label. First, a proposed name should not be too close to either the common name or proprietary name or give the impression that the drug has a therapeutic benefit while not implying composition or safety (Medicines and Healthcare products Regulatory Agency (MHRA), 2019).

Promotional terms and acronyms or initials are to be avoided along with proper names that are no more than an initial or code number. Every proposed name is assessed by the MHRA on its own merits to assess printing, handwriting or spoken similarity; the indication for use; the type of patient to receive the medicine; the pharmaceutical form; route of administration; strength; and dispensing route; and whether the medicine is prescription-only or available for sale over the counter.

For nonprescription medicines, the invented name should contain information about the strength and the pharmaceutical form, and claim indications for them (such as “fast acting” or “one-a-day”) should be justified on the basis of information in the Summary of Product Characteristics (SmPC) (Medicines and Healthcare products Regulatory Agency (MHRA), 2019).

Qualifiers or dosage-form suffixes should provide valuable information regarding a medicinal product or substantially differentiate a medicinal product from another. Single, individual letters or numbers are not recommended, unless required or critically necessary. For prolonged release and enteric formulations, established suffixes such as controlled-release (CR), long-acting (LA), prolonged-release (PR), sustained-action (SA), sustained-release (SR), extended-release (XL), enteric-coated (EC), and gastro-resistant (GR) methods may be used.

Umbrella labeling should be properly justified to avoid confusion and for reasons of safety where differentiation can be accomplished by packaging and labeling (European Medicines Agency (EMA), 2023; Medicines and Healthcare products Regulatory Agency (MHRA), 2019). The generic name should be as the INN lists, and this may be followed by strength and pharmaceutical form, while the MAH name is mentioned on the package. Both the name, strength, and the pharmaceutical form should be indicated in braille on the packaging, and short-term approval of the European Directorate for the Quality of Medicine & Health Care (EDQM) can be used when necessary (Council of Europe, 2024; European Medicines Agency (EMA), 2009).

Further considerations in this regard are the continuity of suppliers for “brand naming” or prescribing, especially that of substances with a narrow therapeutic range, or the fear of problems of interchangeability. Braille text should comply with European standards Marburg medium Braille font (Council of Europe, 2024;

European Commission, 2001; Pharmaceutical Braille, 2025), stipulating a consistent dot diameter, separation space, and character dimensions.

An example to highlight the importance of sensitively naming a new drug is the case of sound-alike names, mercaptamine and mercaptopurine, which led to pancytopenia following medication error in a 9-month-old child (Medicines and Healthcare products Regulatory Agency (MHRA), 2014a). It was also reported that interference resulted from confusion between medication names such as sulfadiazine and sulfasalazine, risperidone and ropinirole, and zuclopenthixol decanoate and zuclopenthixol acetate, where these errors were responsible for serious cases of medication errors (Medicines and Healthcare products Regulatory Agency (MHRA), 2014b).

Negative names could be refused by the MHRA for safety or efficacy reasons, or the option to appeal via Type II variations of new marketing applications could be permitted. Product name issues can be discussed in MHRA presubmission advice. By doing so, these practices are in line with guidance in the United Kingdom (UK) and will enable smooth registration of new medicinal products (Medicines and Healthcare products Regulatory Agency (MHRA), 2018, 2019).

Thailand

In Thailand, the process of drug regulation is regulated through the 1967 Drug Act and several good practice guidelines, particularly on how to prevent LASA medication errors (Prompradith V & Chimvong P, 2017). Although this regulation covers a broad range of principles for drug safety, including the power to not register a drug if it is considered unsafe, it does not specifically stipulate measures to mitigate the specific risks related to LASA medications, leaving a wide regulatory gap.

To address this gap, hospitals nationwide have adopted several risk mitigation plans. Various measures have been implemented in this regard, such as the segregation of drugs with similar physical characteristics (appearance, name or perceived sounds) and LASA alerts available on the electronic software, providing alerts when high-alert drugs with high-risk similar sounding letter combination names are prescribed. These local strategies are not only useful but also often inadequate alone. A more holistic, system-level strategy is needed to elucidate the causes of LASA errors (Chanakit et al., 2013; Supapaan TS, Songmuang A, et al., 2024; Wongboonnak P, 2017, 2018).

- Without focused national legislation targeting LASA drugs, risks go unchecked at the macro level. Patients routinely use visual attributes, such as shape, color, or labeling, to recognize medication, and this behavior increases the potential for LASA error. Moreover, marketing efforts that focus on "brands" serve only to confuse health care professionals and the public even more and worsen the risk of errors.

- To address these challenges, analysts have suggested a holistic approach that includes short-, medium-, and long-term measures:
- Short-term initiatives A national LASA working group consisting of members from regulatory agencies, healthcare professionals and patient groups. This committee should focus on high-risk LASA pairs and recommend immediate actions. Public health campaigns should also be implemented to educate consumers about LASA and the consequences of a failure to verify medication identification.
- Intermediate level: The focus is on the construction of national definite guidelines for the Thai context. Guidelines should include directions for medication naming, labeling and packaging and should utilize standardized computer programs that would allow us to standardize and potentially identify the level of potential LASA risk.
- The longer-term steps include enshrining this advice in ministerial regulations made under the 1967 Drug Act. The Department of the FDA should be the key player, along with a national pharmacovigilance center with regular audits and strong reporting channels, as well as a compulsory remedy for noncompliance (Wongboonnak P, 2017, 2018).

Chumchit et al. provided significant information on the problems and solutions of LASA errors in Thailand (Chumchit et al., 2015). More recently, Author et al. underscores the need for a LASA national database that captures high-risk medication pairs and enables the development of targeted interventions (Napaporn et al., 2022; Supapaan TS, Kamnuek J, et al., 2024; Supapaan TS, Songmuang A, et al., 2024; Supapaan et al., 2024; Treejan et al., 2022); (Napaporn J et al., 2023; Napaporn et al., 2022; Supapaan T et al., 2024).

Despite continuous work, LASA errors continue to occur among both inpatients and those receiving community care. In response, the author constructed a master LASA drug list as a starting point for a national LASA database (Supapaan T et al., 2024). This program requires cooperation among hospitals, drug regulators and professional organizations to gather, validate, and periodically exchange LASA data (Chumchit et al., 2015; Khontum & Chanthapasa, 2021; Supapaan T et al., 2024).

Despite continued attempts, LASA medication errors continue to be important health care problems in Thailand. In conclusion, an integrated national approach is needed to address these errors effectively. Regulatory, healthcare, and public health – urgent, intermediate and long-term actions are needed or should be implemented. With a unified dedication from healthcare providers, manufacturers, policy makers, and patients, Thailand has an opportunity to further develop its LASA safety infrastructure and to spearhead regional efforts to mitigate preventable harm (Chanakit et al., 2013; Jitruknatee et al., 2020; Khontum & Chanthapasa, 2021; Khumsikiew et al., 2023; Napaporn et al., 2022; Prompradith V & Chimvong P, 2017; Supapaan TS, Kamnuek J, et al., 2024; Tansuwannarat et al., 2022). Real-world data from both the Thai community and the hospital sector support the need for such an integrated approach.

International Approaches

Clinical LASA errors are a major issue affecting global patient safety, leading the regulatory counterparts of many countries to introduce stringent strategies at the time of drug approval and postmarketing. Common approaches include thorough examination of drug names and labeling, prioritization of unique and different drug names, use of clear labels, and encouragement of INNs and tall man lettering. In addition, many organizations promote the reporting and analysis of LASA-related mishaps to enhance continuous quality improvement (Bryan et al., 2015; Filik et al., 2004; The Institute for Safe Medication Practices (ISMP), 2023a; The Institute for Safe Medication Practices Canada (ISMP Canada), 2016; World Health Organization, 1997, 2017, 2023).

Prevention does start at the policy level, with Medicine Labeling rules requiring medicines to have titles that are not difficult to read or pronounce and not easily confused with anything else. Such a strong safety culture, which promotes the rapid and anonymous reporting of LASA events and near misses by health care providers, also promotes early risk identification. When these reports are reviewed as part of routine audits and feedback, they result in focused improvements in medication safety practices in healthcare organizations. Moreover, communication between front-line staff and manufacturers on labels and packaging is encouraged. By providing such proactive feedback, timely adjustments can prevent widespread damage or harm.

Finally, cooperation between countries is important for standard harmonization. Regulatory authorities can reduce heterogeneity across countries in terms of consistency and differences in contributing to LASA risk by establishing common principles for labeling, packaging, and nomenclature use (Cohen, 2001, 2007a, 2007b, 2007c; World Health Organization, 2023). These strategies, which include clear naming policies, transparent reporting systems, open lines of communication between healthcare and the pharmaceutical industry, and international cooperation, together constitute a solid global structure to help prevent LASA medication errors. Widespread implementation of these strategies could greatly improve medication safety and reduce the global burden of LASA-related episodes (Neelakantan et al., 2024; World Health Organization, 2023).

Automated dispensing machines (ADMs) are computerized systems for storing, dispensing, and recording the use of medications. Such machines operate on barcode technology and e-medication record systems that help in the right medication selection and supply. ADMs can be set up to trigger warnings to healthcare providers when LASA drugs are selected, which results in pharmacists performing a double-check of the medication before dispensing it. In addition, ADMs can be integrated with drug location systems and light navigation systems to further improve the precision and efficiency of drug withdrawal.

Moreover, by using the latest technologies such as robotics, IoT, and machine learning, automated medication management systems are advancing patient safety by handling the entire medication lifecycle turnout and improving accuracy from prescription to administration. These workflows improve accuracy and provide efficiency by combining barcode scanning, electronic medical records, and automated dispensing to guarantee that the appropriate drug is dispensed to the correct patient at the right time (Anand et al., 2021; Shermock et al., 2023). Their advanced safety mechanisms also help reduce the likelihood of human error and their efficiency in operation. As **Figure 3** illustrates, the registration of drug names and the use of look-alike sound-alike (LASA) risk mitigations differ across the United States, Canada, the United Kingdom, and Thailand and among international practices, but proactive name review, regulatory control, and system-based controls are considered to minimize medication errors.

Figure 3. Drug name registration and look-alike sound-alike (LASA) risk mitigation strategies in the United States, Canada, the United Kingdom, Thailand, and international practice

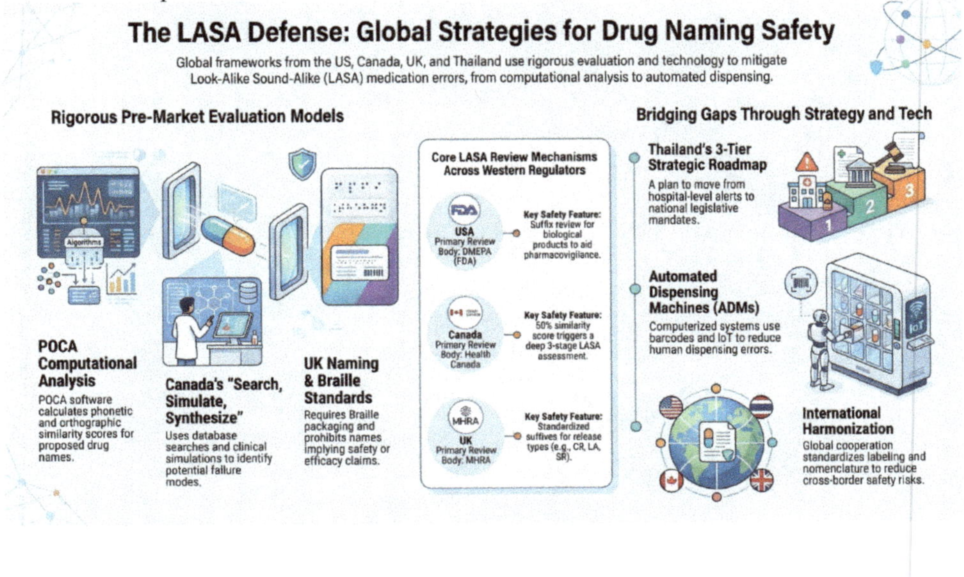

CONCLUSION

LASA drug errors threaten patient safety worldwide. The orthographic and phonetic similarity of drug names can lead to ineffective treatment and overdose deaths, as shown in this chapter. To manage these risks, the US FDA, Health Canada, UK MHRA, WHO, and Thailand's FDA use name screening tools and international standards. Hospitals also use tall man lettering, e-prescribing alerts, and automated dispensing safety. These tragedies can be prevented with strict regulation, institutional safety mechanisms, professional education, and patient awareness. Instead of one intervention, a multifactorial approach can significantly reduce the number of incorrect drug errors. Therefore, improving drug naming is a global regulatory priority and an ethical duty to protect patients from preventable harm.

REFERENCES

Aimette, S. A., Tuohy, N. R., & Cohen, M. R. (2007). The Patient's role in preventing medication errors. In *Medication Errors* (2nd ed.). The American Pharmacists Association. DOI: 10.21019/9781582120928.ch13

Anand, N., Prathibha, P., Purohit, P., Nalamitha, R., & Rajarao Padma, C. (2021). *Biometric enabled patient-centric automated medication dispenser using IoT*. Computer Networks and Inventive Communication Technologies. DOI: 10.1007/978-981-15-9647-6_43

Archambault, G. F. (1983). USAN and the USP dictionary of drug names—Who needs it? *Drug Intelligence & Clinical Pharmacy*, *17*(7-8), 608. DOI: 10.1177/106002808301700741 PMID: 6347600

Aronson, J. K. (2009). Medication errors: Definitions and classification. *British Journal of Clinical Pharmacology*, *67*(6), 599–604. DOI: 10.1111/j.1365-2125.2009.03415.x PMID: 19594526

Bai, H. K., Ahearn, J. D., & Bartlett, M. G. (2021). Over-the-counter drugs: Regulatory analysis of warning letters between fiscal years 2015-2019. *Therapeutic Innovation & Regulatory Science*, *55*(2), 426–436. DOI: 10.1007/s43441-020-00231-2 PMID: 33095420

Brand Institute, Inc. (2023). *Brand Institute's Vice President of Creative Nomenclature Explains the Pharmaceutical Brand Name Review Process Used by Japanese Regulators*. Retrieved 06 Sep from https://www.prnewswire.com/news-releases/brand-institutes-vice-president-of-creative-nomenclature-explains-the-pharmaceutical-brand-name-review-process-used-by-japanese-regulators-301734086.html

Bryan, R., Aronson, J. K., ten Hacken, P., Williams, A., & Jordan, S. (2015). Patient safety in medication nomenclature: Orthographic and semantic properties of International Nonproprietary Names. *PLoS One*, *10*(12), e0145431. DOI: 10.1371/journal.pone.0145431 PMID: 26701761

Bryan, R., Aronson, J. K., Williams, A., & Jordan, S. (2021a). The problem of look-alike, sound-alike name errors: Drivers and solutions. *British Journal of Clinical Pharmacology*, *87*(2), 386–394. DOI: 10.1111/bcp.14285 PMID: 32198938

Bryan, R., Aronson, J. K., Williams, A. J., & Jordan, S. (2021b). A systematic literature review of LASA error interventions. *British Journal of Clinical Pharmacology*, *87*(2), 336–351. DOI: 10.1111/bcp.14644 PMID: 33197079

Center for Drug Evaluation and Research (CDER). (2016). *Procedures for handling requests for proprietary name review*. Retrieved 15 June from https://www.fda.gov/files/about%20fda/published/Procedures-for-Handling-Requests-for-Proprietary-Name-Review.pdf

Chanakit, T., Napaporn, J., Chiempattanakajohn, T., Sangkhawan, S., & Wichakot, S. (2013). The survey of look alike/sound alike (LASA) drugs available in hospitals in Thailand. *African Journal of Pharmacy and Pharmacology*, *7*(6), 227–239. DOI: 10.5897/AJPP11.812

Chumchit, C., Amrumpai, Y., & Treesak, C. (2015). Recognition on medication safety and look-alike/sound-alike medication problems in Thai public hospitals. *Silpakorn U Science & Tech J*, *9*(2), 40–51.

Cohen, A. (2014). Crazy for Ya Ba: Methamphetamine use among northern Thai youth. *The International Journal on Drug Policy*, *25*(4), 776–782. DOI: 10.1016/j.drugpo.2014.06.005 PMID: 25067795

Cohen, M. R. (2001). Another purpose for "purpose" look-alike unit-dose containers mixed up misinterpretation of sliding-scale insulin dose. *Hospital Pharmacy*, *36*(12), 1132–1133. DOI: 10.1177/001857870103601203

Cohen, M. R. (2007a). Causes of medication errors. In Cohen, M. R. (Ed.), *Medication Errors* (2nd ed., pp. 55–66). The American Pharmacists Association. DOI: 10.21019/9781582120928.ch4

Cohen, M. R. (2007b). The role of drug packaging and labeling in medication errors. In Cohen, M. R. (Ed.), *Medication Errors* (2nd ed., pp. 111–152). The American Pharmacists Association. https://doi.org/doi:10.21019/9781582120928.ch7

Cohen, M. R. (2007c). Preventing prescribing errors. In *Medication Errors* (2nd ed.). The American Pharmacists Association. https://doi.org/doi:10.21019/9781582120928.ch9

Cohen, M. R., Domizio, G. D., & Lee, R. E. (2007). The role of drug names in medication errors. In Cohen, M. R. (Ed.), *Medication Errors* (2nd ed., pp. 87–110). The American Pharmacists Association. https://doi.org/doi:10.21019/9781582120928.ch6

Cohen, M. R., & Smetzer, J. L. (2007). Preventing dispensing errors. In *Medication Errors* (2nd ed.). The American Pharmacists Association. DOI: 10.21019/9781582120928.ch10

Cohen, M. R., & Smetzer, J. L. (2015). No unlabeled containers anywhere, ever! where did this come from? *Hospital Pharmacy*, *50*(3), 185–188. DOI: 10.1310/hpj5003-185 PMID: 26405305

Cohen, M. R., & Smetzer, J. L. (2017). ISMP medication error report analysis. *Hospital Pharmacy*, *52*(6), 390–393. DOI: 10.1177/0018578717715346 PMID: 29276260

Cohen, M. R., & Smetzer, J. L. (2018). ISMP medication error report analysis. *Hospital Pharmacy*, *53*(4), 217–219. DOI: 10.1177/0018578718771814 PMID: 30038436

Council of Europe. (2024). *European Directorate for the Quality of Medicines & Healthcare (EDQM)*. Retrieved 15 June from https://www.coe.int/en/web/civil-society/european-directorate-for-the-quality-of-medicines-healthcare-edqm-#:~:text=European%20Directorate%20for%20the%20Quality%20of%20Medicines%20%26%20Healthcare%20(EDQM),-Drugs%20and%20Addictions

Dunne, S. S., & Dunne, C. P. (2015). What do people really think of generic medicines? A systematic review and critical appraisal of literature on stakeholder perceptions of generic drugs. *BMC Medicine*, *13*(1), 173. DOI: 10.1186/s12916-015-0415-3 PMID: 26224091

European Commission. (2001). *Guidance concerning the Braille requirements for labeling and the package leaflet*. Retrieved 15 June from https://academy.gmp-compliance.org/guidemgr/files/BRAILLE_TEXT20050411.PDF

European Medicines Agency (EMA). (2009). *Guideline on the readability of the label and package leaflet of medicinal products for human use*. Retrieved 11 June from https://health.ec.europa.eu/system/files/2016-11/2009_01_12_readability_guideline_final_en_0.pdf

European Medicines Agency (EMA). (2023). *Guideline on the acceptability of names for human medicinal products processed through the centralized procedure - Scientific guideline*. Retrieved 11 June from https://www.ema.europa.eu/en/documents/scientific-guideline/guideline-acceptability-names-human-medicinal-products-processed-through-centralised-procedure-revision-7_en.pdf

Filik, R., Purdy, K., Gale, A., & Gerrett, D. (2004). Drug name confusion: Evaluating the effectiveness of capital ("Tall Man") letters using eye movement data. *Social Science & Medicine*, *59*(12), 2597–2601. DOI: 10.1016/j.socscimed.2004.04.008 PMID: 15474212

Gaunt, M. (2007). Error Trifecta: Avandia, Coumadin, and Cardura. *Pharmacy Times*, *73*(11), 53.

Government of Canada. (2014). *Guidance document for industry - review of drug brand names*. Retrieved 6 August from https://www.canada.ca/en/health-canada/services/drugs-health-products/reports-publications/medeffect-canada/guidance-document-industry-review-drug-brand-names.html

Health Canada. (2004). *ARCHIVED - Issue analysis summary: Look-alike Sound-alike (LA/SA) health product names: the development of a comprehensive policy recommendation for Look-alike Sound-alike (LA/SA) health product names*. Retrieved 15 June from https://www.canada.ca/en/health-canada/services/drugs-health-products/biologics-radiopharmaceuticals-genetic-therapies/look-alike-sound-alike/issue-analysis-summary-look-alike-sound-alike-health-product-names-development-comprehensive-policy-recommendation-look-alike-sound-alike.html

Health Canada. (2014). *Guidance document: review of drug brand names* Government of Canada, Department of Health. Retrieved 04 Mar from https://www.canada.ca/content/dam/hc-sc/migration/hc-sc/dhp-mps/alt_formats/pdf/pubs/medeff/guide/2014-review-examen_drug-medicament_names-marques/2014-review-examen_drug-medicament_names-marques-eng.pdf

Health Canada. (2019). *Good label and package practices guide for prescription drugs*. Retrieved 15 March from https://www.canada.ca/en/health-canada/services/drugs-health-products/reports-publications/medeffect-canada/good-label-package-practices-guide-prescription-drugs-profile/guidance-document.html

International Union of Pure and Applied Chemistry. (2013). *Nomenclature of Organic Chemistry. IUPAC Recommendationsand Preferred Names* 2013. Retrieved 06 Sep from https://iupac.qmul.ac.uk/BlueBook/PDF/2013BlueBook.pdf

ISMP. (2016). *FDA and ISMP lists of look-alike drug names with recommended tall man letters*. Retrieved 5 Sep from https://www.ismp.org/sites/default/files/attachments/2017-11/tallmanletters.pdf?

ISMP News/ECRI. (2020). *Due to ISMP Advocacy, VinCRIStine Labeling and Packaging Changed to Prevent Wrong Route Administration*. Retrieved 5 Sep from https://home.ecri.org/blogs/ismp-news/due-to-ismp-advocacy-vincristine-labeling-and-packaging-changed-to-prevent-wrong-route-administration?

Jitruknatee, A., Martro, J., Tosanguan, K., Doangjai, Y., & Theantawee, W. (2020). National drug policies in Thailand: Evolution and lessons for the future. *J Health Sci*, *29*(Special Issue), S3–S14.

Joint Commission International. (2017). *Quick Safety Issue* 37: *Eliminating vincristine administration events*. Retrieved 5 Sep from https://www.jointcommission.org/en/knowledge-library/newsletters/quick-safety/issue-37?

Kalola, A. S., & Dean, R. (2019). The United States Food and Drug Administration and Prescription Drug Promotion. *The Journal of Innovations in Cardiac Rhythm Management*, *10*(3), 3588–3591. DOI: 10.19102/icrm.2019.100305 PMID: 32477722

Karet, G. B. (2019). How do drugs get named? *AMA Journal of Ethics*, *21*(8), E686–E696. DOI: 10.1001/amajethics.2019.686 PMID: 31397664

Karet, G. B. (2023). Linguistic analysis of generic-generic drug name pairs prone to wrong-drug errors for which tall-man lettering is recommended. *Therapeutic Innovation & Regulatory Science*, *57*(4), 751–758. DOI: 10.1007/s43441-023-00526-0 PMID: 37171707

Khontum, A., & Chanthapasa, K. (2021). Perceptions of communities regarding Look-Twin Sound-Twin drugs: A case study of a sub-district in the Northeastern Region of Thailand. *Risk Management and Healthcare Policy*, *14*, 2345–2355. DOI: 10.2147/RMHP.S303899 PMID: 34113190

Khumsikiew, J., Sripa, S., Moolasarn, S., Toh, L. S., Anderson, C., & Supapaan, T. (2023). Facilitators and barriers of the rational drug use hospital program in Thailand. *Pharmacy Practice*, *21*(3), 1–11. DOI: 10.18549/PharmPract.2023.3.2815

Kimura, E., Kawakami, Y., Inoue, S., & Okajima, A. (2025). A dataset for mapping the Japanese drugs to RxNorm standard concepts. *Data in Brief*, *59*, 111418. DOI: 10.1016/j.dib.2025.111418 PMID: 40124300

Kondrak, G., & Dorr, B. (2006). Automatic identification of confusable drug names. *Artificial Intelligence in Medicine*, *36*(1), 29–42. DOI: 10.1016/j.artmed.2005.07.005 PMID: 16359851

Lambert, B. L. (1997). Predicting look-alike and sound-alike medication errors. *American Journal of Health-System Pharmacy*, *54*(10), 1161–1171. DOI: 10.1093/ajhp/54.10.1161 PMID: 9161623

Lambert, B. L., Lin, S. J., Chang, K. Y., & Gandhi, S. K. (1999). Similarity as a risk factor in drug-name confusion errors: The look-alike (orthographic) and sound-alike (phonetic) model. *Medical Care*, *37*(12), 1214–1225. DOI: 10.1097/00005650-199912000-00005 PMID: 10599603

Lizano-Díez, I., Figueiredo-Escribá, C., Piñero-López, M., Lastra, C. F., Mariño, E. L., & Modamio, P. (2020). Prevention strategies to identify LASA errors: Building and sustaining a culture of patient safety. *BMC Health Services Research*, *20*(1), 63. DOI: 10.1186/s12913-020-4922-3 PMID: 31996197

Lowe, A., Hamilton, M., Greenall, B. M. J., Ma, J., Dhalla, I., & Persaud, N. (2017). Fatal overdoses involving hydromorphone and morphine among inpatients: A case series. *CMAJ Open*, *5*(1), E184–e189. DOI: 10.9778/cmajo.20160013 PMID: 28401133

Marilyn Schwartz. (2007). *Look-Alike/Sound-Alike (LASA) drug names - review update -Health Canada's Perspective*. Retrieved 14 April from https://capra.ca/_uploads/archive/presentations/14-MarilynSchwartz-LA-SAGuidanceUpdate.pdf

Medicines and Healthcare products Regulatory Agency (MHRA). (2014a). *Mercaptamine and mercaptopurine: confusion between drug names*. Retrieved 15 June from https://www.gov.uk/drug-safety-update/mercaptamine-and-mercaptopurine-confusion-between-drug-names

Medicines and Healthcare products Regulatory Agency (MHRA). (2014b). *Recent drug-name confusion*. Retrieved 11 July from https://www.gov.uk/drug-safety-update/recent-drug-name-confusion

Medicines and Healthcare products Regulatory Agency (MHRA). (2018). *Drug-name confusion: reminder to be vigilant for potential errors*. Retrieved 15 June from https://www.gov.uk/drug-safety-update/drug-name-confusion-reminder-to-be-vigilant-for-potential-errors

Medicines and Healthcare products Regulatory Agency (MHRA). (2019). *MHRA guideline for the naming of medicinal products and Braille requirements for nme on lbel*. Retrieved 15 June from https://assets.publishing.service.gov.uk/media/5d0cb4dd40f0b620109f090c/MHRA_Guideline_for_the_Naming_of_Medicinal_Products_and_Braille_Requirements_for_Name_on_Label.pdf

Meredith, P. A. (1996). Generic drugs: Therapeutic equivalence. *Drug Safety*, *15*(4), 233–242. DOI: 10.2165/00002018-199615040-00001 PMID: 8905248

Mitobe, J., & Higuchi, T. (2016). Does finger pointing toward drug names prevent confusion between similar names during rapid search? *Psychologia*, *59*(1), 38–49. DOI: 10.2117/psysoc.2016.38

Napaporn, J., Buakaew, P., Suksakornthanawat, P., Sripa, S., Jinatongthai, P., & Supapaan, T. (2022). Analogous comparison of registered brand name drugs of tablets and capsules commercially available in Thailand: A retrospective study. *PLoS One*, *17*(10), e0276321. DOI: 10.1371/journal.pone.0276321 PMID: 36260612

Napaporn, J., Supapaan, T., Jinathongthai, P., Sripa, S., Kamnuek, J., Khakaew, C., & Pitchayajittipong, C. (2023). Analysis of similarity of physical appearances of pills in the forms of tablets and capsules commercially available in Thailand. *Thai J Pharm Pract*, *15*(4), 1060–1070.

National Center for Biotechnology Information. (2024a). *PubChem Compound Summary for CID* 1983, *Acetaminophen*. Retrieved 19 May from https://pubchem.ncbi.nlm.nih.gov/compound/Acetaminophen

National Center for Biotechnology Information. (2024b). *PubChem Compound Summary for CID* 2083, *Albuterol*. Retrieved 19 May from https://pubchem.ncbi.nlm.nih.gov/compound/Albuterol

National Center for Biotechnology Information. (2024c). *PubChem Compound Summary for CID* 3488, *Glyburide*. Retrieved 19 May from https://pubchem.ncbi.nlm.nih.gov/compound/Glyburide

National Center for Biotechnology Information. (2024d). *PubChem Compound Summary for CID* 4058, *Meperidine*. Retrieved 19 May from https://pubchem.ncbi.nlm.nih.gov/compound/Meperidine

National Center for Biotechnology Information. (2024e). *PubChem Compound Summary for CID* 27447, *Cephalexin*. Retrieved 19 May from https://pubchem.ncbi.nlm.nih.gov/compound/Cephalexin

National Center for Biotechnology Information. (2024f). *PubChem Compound Summary for CID* 41781, *Torsemide*. Retrieved 19 May from https://pubchem.ncbi.nlm.nih.gov/compound/Torsemide

National Center for Biotechnology Information. (2024g). *PubChem Compound Summary for CID* 135398735, *Rifampin*. Retrieved 19 May from https://pubchem.ncbi.nlm.nih.gov/compound/Rifampin

National Center for Biotechnology Information. (2024h). *ubChem Compound Summary for CID* 3715, *Indomethacin*. Retrieved 19 May from https://pubchem.ncbi.nlm.nih.gov/compound/Indomethacin

Neelakantan, M., Sharma, P., & Kulkarni, A. (2024). Look-alike, sound-alike (LASA) drugs in India. *The Lancet Regional Health. Southeast Asia*, *26*, 100425. DOI: 10.1016/j.lansea.2024.100425 PMID: 38798984

News, N. B. C. (2005). *Zyprexa, Zyrtec similarities causing confusion*. Retrieved 15 Apr from https://www.nbcnews.com/health/health-news/zyprexa-zyrtec-similarities-causing-confusion-flna1c9439578

Nightingale, S. L. (1998). Guidance on industry-supported scientific and educational activities. *Journal of the American Medical Association*, *279*(5), 346–346. DOI: 10.1001/jama.279.5.346-JFD81013-2-1 PMID: 9459455

Pelletier-Dattu, C. E. (2017). Pharmacologic Suffixes. In *Lange Smart Charts: Pharmacology, 2e*. McGraw-Hill Medical.

Pharmaceutical Braille. (2025). *Marburg medium Braille font standard*. Retrieved 11 July from https://www.pharmabraille.com/pharmaceutical-braille/marburg-medium-font-standard/

Prompradith, V., & Chimvong, P. (2017). *Drug regulation in Thailand*. Retrieved 14 April from https://nsp.mohw.org.tw/dl-34-960f0775f3234877a9cde3b445548c62.html

Rider, B. B., Mehta, H., & Merchant, L. (2019). Special considerations for proprietary name review: Focus on products that may be prescribed "As Directed". *Therapeutic Innovation & Regulatory Science*, *53*(3), 381–386. DOI: 10.1177/2168479018782669 PMID: 29929377

Schroeder, S. R., Salomon, M. M., Galanter, W. L., Schiff, G. D., Vaida, A. J., Gaunt, M. J., Bryson, M. L., Rash, C., Falck, S., & Lambert, B. L. (2017). Cognitive tests predict real-world errors: The relationship between drug name confusion rates in laboratory-based memory and perception tests and corresponding error rates in large pharmacy chains. *BMJ Quality &amp. Safety (Basel, Switzerland)*, *26*(5), 395–407. DOI: 10.1136/bmjqs-2015-005099 PMID: 27193033

Serafini, M., Cargnin, S., Massarotti, A., Tron, G. C., Pirali, T., & Genazzani, A. A. (2021). What's in a Name? Drug Nomenclature and Medicinal Chemistry Trends using INN Publications. *Journal of Medicinal Chemistry*, *64*(8), 4410–4429. DOI: 10.1021/acs.jmedchem.1c00181 PMID: 33847110

Shah, M. B., Merchant, L., Chan, I. Z., & Taylor, K. (2017). Characteristics that may help in the identification of potentially confusing proprietary drug names. *Therapeutic Innovation & Regulatory Science*, *51*(2), 232–236. DOI: 10.1177/2168479016667161 PMID: 30231718

Shermock, S. B., Shermock, K. M., & Schepel, L. L. (2023). Closed-loop medication management with an electronic health record system in U.S. and Finnish hospitals. *International Journal of Environmental Research and Public Health*, *20*(17), 6680. DOI: 10.3390/ijerph20176680 PMID: 37681820

Supapaan, T., Pitchayajittipong, C., Sonrasawan, K., Chittawee, C., & Napaporn, J. (2024). Development of the database for look-alike, sound-alike drugs in Thailand. *Thai J Pharm Pract*, *16*(1), 112–125.

Supapaan, T. S., Kamnuek, J., Khakaew, C., Jungsuwadee, T., Songmuang, A., Saksit, S., & Napaporn, J. (2024). Assessment of look-Alike, Sound-Alike similarities among brand names of tablets and capsules: A cross-sectional survey in Thailand. *Pharmacy Practice*, *22*(3), 2955. DOI: 10.18549/PharmPract.2024.3.2955

Supapaan, T. S., Napaporn, J., Ruthirakanok, R., Srichathum, S., Songmuang, A., & Pitchayajittipong, C. (2024). Look-alike sound-alike (LASA) medication errors in Thai hospitals. *Pharmacy Practice*, *22*(1), 2886.

Supapaan, T. S., Songmuang, A., Napaporn, J., Sangsukwow, P., Boonrod, P., Intarapongsakul, P., Jaturapattarawong, A., & Pitchayajittipong, C. (2024). Look-alike/sound-alike medication errors: An in-depth examination through a hospital case study. *Pharmacy Practice*, *22*(2), 2959. DOI: 10.18549/PharmPract.2024.2.2959

Tansuwannarat, P., Vichiensanth, P., Sivarak, O., Tongpoo, A., Promrungsri, P., Sriapha, C., Wananukul, W., & Trakulsrichai, S. (2022). Characteristics and consequences of medication errors in pediatric patients reported to Ramathibodi Poison Center: A 10-year retrospective study. *Therapeutics and Clinical Risk Management*, *18*, 669–681. DOI: 10.2147/TCRM.S363638 PMID: 35795851

The Associated Press. (2005). *Zyprexa, Zyrtec similarities causing confusion*. Retrieved 8 Feb from https://www.nbcnews.com/health/health-news/zyprexa-zyrtec-similarities-causing-confusion-flna1c9439578

The Institute for Safe Medication Practices Canada (ISMP Canada). (2016). *Drug labeling and the application of TALLman lettering project report*. Retrieved 15 June from https://www.ismp-canada.org/download/TALLman/TALLmanLettering-ProjectReport.pdf

The Institute for Safe Medication Practices (ISMP). (2015). *ISMP's list of confused drug names*. Retrieved 16 Apr from https://www.ismp.org/sites/default/files/attachments/2017-11/confuseddrugnames%2802.2015%29.pdf?

The Institute for Safe Medication Practices (ISMP). (2023a). *FDA and ISMP lists of look-alike drug names with recommended tall man (mixed case) letters*. Retrieved 16 Apr from https://www.ismp.org/system/files/resources/2023-01/ISMP_Tallman_Letters_012523_MS5087%20%282%29.pdf

The Institute for Safe Medication Practices (ISMP). (2023b). *List of confused drug names*. Retrieved 16 Apr from https://www.ismp.org/recommendations/confused-drug-names-list

The Pennsylvania Patient Safety Advisory. (2004). Medication errors linked to drug name confusion. *PA PSRS Patient Saf Advis*, *1*(4), 7–8.

The Pennsylvania Patient Safety Advisory. (2006). hydrOXYzine and hydrALAzine mix-ups. *PA PSRS Patient Saf Advis*, *3*(2), 21.

The Pennsylvania Patient Safety Advisory. (2007). Inadvertent mix-up of morphine and hydromorphone: A potent error. *PA PSRS Patient Saf Advis*, *4*(3), 86–88.

Treejan, K., Jinatongthai, P., Moolasarn, S., Low, B. Y., Anderson, C., & Supapaan, T. (2022). Self-health care behaviors and knowledge of youth living with HIV. *J Am Pharm Assoc (*2003), 62(4), 1249-1259.e1247. DOI: 10.1016/j.japh.2022.02.006

Tu, C.-M., Taylor, K., & Chai, G. (2012). Use of proprietary names by prescribers for discontinued brand drug products with existing generic equivalents. *Drug Information Journal*, *46*(6), 677–682. DOI: 10.1177/0092861512456282

U.S. Department of Health and Human Services Food and Drug Administration (FDA). (2014). *Nonproprietary naming of biological products guidance for industry*. Retrieved 15 June from https://www.fda.gov/files/drugs/published/Nonproprietary-Naming-of-Biological-Products-Guidance-for-Industry.pdf

U.S. Department of Health and Human Services Food and Drug Administration (FDA). (2019). *Procedures for handling requests for nonproprietary name suffix review for biological products newly licensed under section* 351*of the PHS Act*. Retrieved 15 June from https://www.fda.gov/media/123894/download

U.S. Department of Health and Human Services Food and Drug Administration (FDA). (2020). *FDA name differentiation project*. Retrieved 06 Aug from https://www.fda.gov/drugs/medication-errors-related-cder-regulated-drug-products/fda-name-differentiation-project

U.S. Department of Health and Human Services Food and Drug Administration (FDA). (2021). *Phonetic and Orthographic Computer Analysis (POCA) Program*. Retrieved 13 June from https://www.fda.gov/drugs/resources-drugs/phonetic-and-orthographic-computer-analysis-poca-program

U.S. Department of Health and Human Services Food and Drug Administration (FDA). (2022a). *Investigational New Drug (IND) Application*. Retrieved 15 June from https://www.fda.gov/drugs/types-applications/investigational-new-drug-ind-application

U.S. Department of Health and Human Services Food and Drug Administration (FDA). (2022b). *New Drug Application (NDA)*. Retrieved 15 June from https://www.fda.gov/drugs/types-applications/new-drug-application-nda

U.S. Department of Health and Human Services Food and Drug Administration (FDA). (2024). *Medication errors related to CDER-regulated drug products*. Retrieved 13 June from https://www.fda.gov/drugs/drug-safety-and-availability/medication-errors-related-cder-regulated-drug-products

U.S. Department of Health and Human Services Food and Drug Administration, Center for Drug Evaluation and Research (CDER). (2016). *Safety considerations for product design to minimize medication errors: guidance for industry*. Retrieved 8 June from https://www.fda.gov/files/drugs/published/Safety-Considerations-for-Product-Design-to-Minimize-Medication-Errors-Guidance-for-Industry.pdf

Wongboonnak, P. (2017). Resolving the problems on look-alike sound-alike drugs at the system level. *Thai J Pharm Pract*, *9*(1), 251–258.

Wongboonnak, P. (2018). Look-alike sound-alike drugs situation in Thailand. *HCU Journal of Health Science*, *22*, 205–216.

World Health Organization. (1997). *Guidance on INN*. Retrieved 24 Dec from https://www.who.int/medicines/services/inn/innquidance/en/

World Health Organization. (2017). *Guidance on the use of International Nonproprietary Names (INNs) for pharmaceutical substances*. Retrieved 16 June from https://cdn.who.int/media/docs/default-source/international-nonproprietary-names-(inn)/who-pharm-s-nom-1570.pdf

World Health Organization. (2023). *Medication safety for look-alike, sound-alike medicines*. World Health Organization. Retrieved 3 June from https://iris.who.int/bitstream/handle/10665/373495/9789240058897-eng.pdf?sequence=1

ABBREVIATIONS

ADM: Automated Dispensing Machines
CDER: Center for Drug Evaluation and Research
CPOE: Computerized Provider Order Entry

DMEPA: Division of Medication Error Prevention and Analysis
EMA: European Medicines Agency
FDA: U.S. Food and Drug Administration
FMEA: Failure Mode and Effects Analysis
IND: Investigational New Drug application
INN: International Nonproprietary Name (WHO)
ISMP: Institute for Safe Medication Practices
IUPAC: International Union of Pure and Applied Chemistry
JAPIC: Japan Pharmaceutical Information Center
LASA: Look-Alike, Sound-Alike
MHRA: Medicines and Healthcare products Regulatory Agency (UK)
NDA: New Drug Application
NSAIDs: Nonsteroidal Anti-Inflammatory Drugs
ONPD: Office of Nonprescription Drugs
OPDP: Office of Prescription Drug Promotion (FDA)
PA-PSRS: Pennsylvania Patient Safety Reporting System
POCA: Phonetic and Orthographic Computer Analysis
USAN: United States Adopted Name
WHO: World Health Organization

Chapter 6
Dealing With Look-Alike, Sound-Alike (LASA) Risks in Oncology Pharmacy

ABSTRACT

The oncology safety of medication is a complex issue that is dynamic and constantly changing, and it is tied to swift therapeutic innovations and further complications in the system. The narrow therapeutic index, toxicity, complexities of the treatment process, and growing drug formularies are the typical features of oncology drugs, making them even more harmful to patients in the case of an error. These risks share the most common one, the look-alike, sound-alike (LASA) medication error, which has long been a major hazard that has been repeatedly brought up in the history of different generations of cancer therapy. It has been demonstrated that the LASA risk is not unique to a particular group of drugs or a period of history but rather is a continuum driven by the development of drug-naming conventions, conventional practices involving the use of drugs, and clinical working processes.

INTRODUCTION

Oncology pharmacies are among the most complex and high-risk domains of healthcare practice. Cancer drugs provide a revolutionary treatment option but are riddled with proportions of error that are associated with high risk. There are few other specialties with narrower therapeutic margins and higher stakes when the wrong medications are mixed together.

Medication errors in chemotherapy drug use are well documented and may occur at any point in the medication-use process. Direct observation in a medical surgical intensive care setting revealed one preventable medication error in five doses ad-

DOI: 10.4018/979-8-3373-5478-1.ch006

ministered, and errors typically involved omissions, incorrect doses, wrong drugs, or administration technique failures (Kopp et al., 2006).

A literature review revealed that compared with intensive care units (0.82 per 100 patient days), hemato-oncology units had the highest medication error rate (2.48 per 100 patient days) (Lustig, 2000). In different investigations, the number of errors in the prescription of chemotherapy ranged from 0.1 to more than 9%, and errors in prescription, transcription, dispensing, and mainly in the administration process were identified (Fyhr & Akselsson, 2012; Schwappach & Wernli, 2010). This vulnerability in cancer patients stems, in part, from the nature of the anticancer drugs themselves, which have a small therapeutic window, are toxic at therapeutic doses, and are complex in dosing regimens, often involving multiple drugs (Eiland et al., 2018). Moreover, with the growing shift to outpatients and oral chemotherapy, new risks have been added, as the preparation or administration of the treatment is performed by patients or carers.

Drug names serve as a primary source of these risks. Confusion over drug names has been a long-known leading cause of medication errors, especially as identified by the World Health Organization (WHO, 2007; WHO, 2007 Patient Safety Solution No. 1). In oncology, classes of drugs have similar stems (-mab for monoclonal antibodies, -nib for tyrosine kinase inhibitors), which may not communicate differences adequately. Schulmeister (2006) also identified well-known LASA oncology examples such as carboplatin/cisplatin, paclitaxel/docetaxel, vincristine/vinblastine, and anthracycline susceptibility for mix-ups (doxorubicin/daunorubicin/idarubicin) (Schulmeister, 2006). Similar packaging as well as confirmation bias and the use of abbreviations contribute to the risk of error.

The value of complete LASA drug lists should not be underestimated in risk prevention. Research projects have used computational string similarity algorithms such as the Levenshtein distance, Bigrams, and Trigrams to rank LASA pairs for risk mitigation, such as tall man lettering (Nagamotoo et al., 2022). This kind of systematic triage focuses on safety efforts for the highest-risk pairs. In oncohematological pharmacies, such lists are reported for antineoplastics and associated drugs with evidence of confusion risk (Chanakit et al., 2013). Local data and historical incident reports should be added to national or public LASA lists as part of an individualized prevention strategy.

Four techniques were employed in a proactive review of the Alberta Oncology Formulary (81 medications; 3,320 pairs) to identify LASA risk: (1) Levenshtein distance (≤5 letter changes; 42 pairs, 1.3%); (2) Bigram similarity (two-letter overlap score ≥0.30; 186 pairs, 5.6%, increased to 367 with sensitivity analysis); (3) same first/last letter rule (75 pairs, 2.3%); and (4) Lexi-Comp alerts (38 pairs, 1.1%). All four methods identified only five pairs as the most dangerous combinations: vinblastine–vincristine, vinblastine–vinorelbine, daunorubicin–doxorubicin, sorafenib–sunitinib, and carboplatin–cisplatin (Kovacic & Chambers, 2011).

The effects of such mistakes can be devastating. Cisplatin has also been confused with carboplatin, with fatal overdoses as the result (Schulmeister, 2006). Among LASA-related errors in oncology, the most serious is the administration of vinca alkaloids via the wrong route, especially vincristine. When mistakenly administered intrathecally instead of intravenously, vincristine causes severe irreversible neurologic impairment and is virtually always fatal. Grissinger (2016) reported that these failures are among the most devastating in contemporary medicine and, despite generations of warnings, continue to occur around the world. In an effort to prevent this from occurring, safety organizations, such as the ISMP, the WHO, and the Joint Commission, require that vincristine should be given only in a minibag, never in a syringe, and must be marked as "FOR INTRAVENOUS USE ONLY-FATAL IF GIVEN BY OTHER ROUTES" (Grissinger, 2016; ISMP News/ECRI, 2020; The Joint Commission, 2023).

This change process has been identified as one of the simplest and most useful ways of avoiding recurrent errors worldwide. Close calls or adverse outcomes have been treated even with supportive care agents, such as epoetin and darbepoetin (Schulmeister, 2006).

The Swiss Cheese Model of accident causation (Reason, 2000) is a visual depiction of how these events occur: a series of fallible barriers that include vague naming, similar labeling, ineffective electronic alerts, and cognitive demands on staff at the time collide, and damage is inflicted on the patient (Elmzughi et al., 2025; Nchinech et al., 2023; Reason, 2000). These are heroic tragedies of humankind, other than systemic collapse. Families also experience avoidable mix-ups, leading to the loss of a loved one, and the healthcare providers involved tend to be long-term victims, who are the second victims (Wu, 2000).

The multilayered protections needed to prevent LASA risks in oncology include formulary reviews, tall man lettering, nonadjacent storage, computerized provider order entry (CPOE) alerts, bar code scanning, smart infusion pumps, double-check systems, and (possibly most importantly) patient activation. The WHO also emphasizes the need to update LASA lists annually, the need to reduce the utilization of verbal orders, and the need to have indications of prescriptions, including both generic and brand names (World Health Organization, 2007, 2023).

It focuses on LASA drugs in oncology, particularly in complicated patients. Important LASA pairs are characterized by systemic and technology-oriented prevention approaches; attentive involvement, training, and a balanced safety culture are suggested to bolster the defense. By integrating evidence, safety science, and the human experience, this discussion aims to address these gaps and provide oncology pharmacy practices with the means to avoid harm due to these so-called dangerous doubles.

Objectives of the Chapter

The aims of this chapter are as follows:

(1) To describe why oncology pharmacy practice is especially susceptible to medication errors in terms of drug toxicity, dosing complexity, and clinical processes.
(2) To define measures to prevent medication errors related to chemotherapy, which revolve mainly around system-based protection and professional practice guidelines.
(3) To determine common look-alike, sound-alike (LASA) drug pairs that are faced in oncology practice and explain how these errors occur.
(4) To examine LASA mistakes related to oncology drug name stems, including the importance of naming conventions in creating risky medications used in various therapeutic periods.

Organization of the Chapter

Chapter 6 introduces why oncology pharmacy practice is especially susceptible to drug errors, with a focus on high-risk chemotherapy, complicated regimens, and systemic factors. It then discusses major approaches to preventing chemotherapy-related errors and discusses common look-alike, sound-alike (LASA) drug pairs experienced in the practice of oncology. The chapter also discusses the LASA mistakes that are related to the oncology drug name stems, emphasizing the role of naming practices and therapeutic expansion as the source of continuing risk. The chapter ends with a synthesis of these findings to highlight the significance of system-based and integrated approaches for decreasing LASA-related harm in oncology care.

WHY ONCOLOGY PHARMACY IS VULNERABLE

Oncology pharmacies are especially prone to medication errors because of multiple compound risk factors (see Figure 1). High-alert medications such as vincristine leave almost no room for mistakes. For instance, intrathecally administering vincristine by accident has killed many people. In two instances in Thailand, where intravenous doses were intended but administered intrathecally, patients died despite efforts at lumbar puncture lavage (Chotsampancharoen et al., 2016). Parenteral formulations increase the risk: doxorubicin infusions are usually red, whereas cyclophosphamide infusions are clear. If the packaging or display is not clear, it can lead to incorrect drug selection. Furthermore, safety organizations have pushed for changes in practice, such as the "minibag-only" rule for vincristine, which means preparing vincristine in minibags instead of syringes to stop intrathecal injection (Joint Commission International, 2017; The Joint Commission, 2023).

Figure 1. Oncology's vulnerability to medication errors

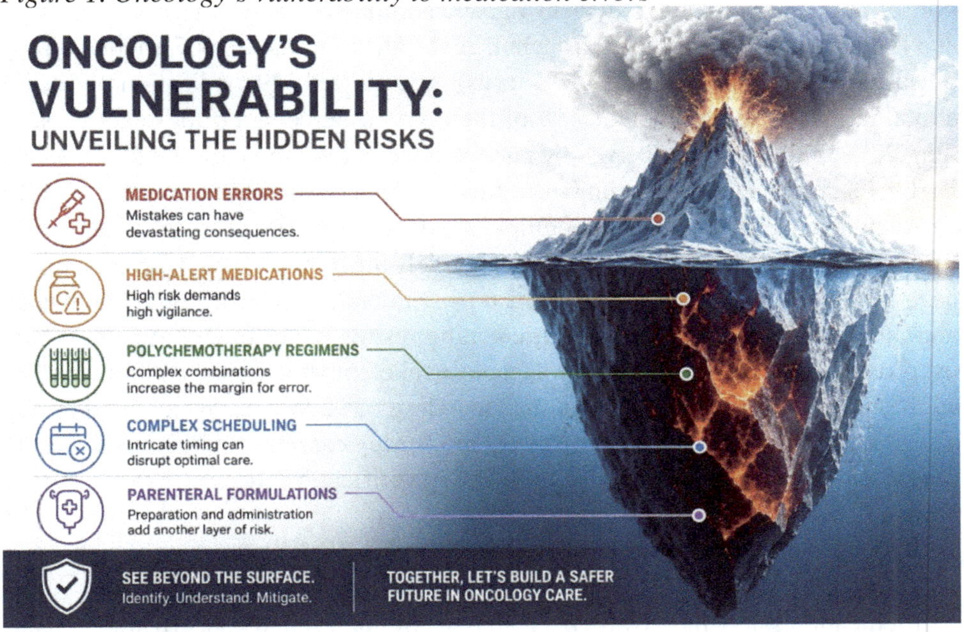

WHEN SYSTEMS FAIL: PATIENT AND CLINICIAN ARE INJURED

Because of the very narrow therapeutic index, precipitous toxicity profiles, and complexity of contemporary oncology regimens, medication-use system errors, specifically LASA errors, have grave, potentially irreversible impacts. The ideal sentinel event is intrathecal vincristine administration, which is virtually lethal because of incurable spinal neurotoxicity. More than one hundred such cases have been reported worldwide, leading to universal changes in the use of cytotoxic preparations and drug administration. Regulatory and professional organizations have also made it necessary that vinca alkaloids should be dispensed in minibags with a clear label of being used intravenously only, kept separate from intrathecal medicine, and under independent checks and balances before administration (American Society of Health-System Pharmacists (ASHP), 2018; ISMP News/ECRI, 2020; Noble & Donaldson, 2010; The Joint Commission, 2023).

The Scope of Chemotherapy System Failures

Despite discussions about these sentinel events, medication error penetration persists throughout the entire chemotherapy process, encompassing prescribing and transcription, compounding, dispensing, and administration. In a prospective study at a French university hospital, Ranchon et al. (2011) studied 6,607 chemotherapy prescriptions (approximately 22,138 doses) and reported 449 medication errors, for a total rate of 5.2. Even though 97% of them were intercepted prior to administration, 2.9% of them were received by patients, which is an indication that no system is 100% safe. An enormous number of them were created in the prescription stage and included incorrect dosages, incomplete orders, or incorrect choices of regimens. Professional evaluation indicated that when left unaddressed, 13.4 percent would have resulted in momentary damage, 2.6 percent ended up permanently damaged, and the other 2.6 percent had life-threatening results—four to eight possible fatal overdoses were prevented. There was a physical element to these near misses: 216 additional hospital days and an annual spending of 92,907 on avoidable damage. The results revealed that the safety of chemotherapy cannot be maintained without pharmacist intervention and multidisciplinary verification (Ranchon et al., 2011).

Safety in Ambulatory Chemotherapy Medication

Medication safety has always been an issue of interest and concern among pharmacists, but oncological treatment has been of special interest, as many cytotoxic regimens are given at the maximum tolerated dosage, leaving virtually no room to make mistakes. High-profile U.S. cancer centers have experienced disastrous chemotherapy drug errors, such as improper route administration and lethal overdoses (Kloth, 2002), indicating that extra systemic safeguarding is indeed necessary. The 1999 Institute of Medicine (IOM) report To Err Is Human: Building a Safer Health System made the ready occurrence of preventable adverse events in health care more evident and underscored prescribing as an important target for harm reduction. This led to policy and institutional reforms in the direction of safer medication use (Donaldson et al., 2000; Institute of Medicine Committee on Quality of Health Care in, 2000).

Before the mid-2000s, most research on chemotherapy safety focused on inpatient care and primarily employed retrospective reviews. With increased cancer treatment in outpatient and ambulatory settings, little is known about the rates of errors, types of harm, and the potential for verification by pharmacists and nurses. To fill this gap, Gandhi et al. (2005) conducted one of the first prospective cohort studies of ambulatory chemotherapy safety at Dana-Farber Cancer Institute. Three adult and pediatric infusion units were examined, with 10,112 medication orders from 1,606 patients (1,380 adults and 226 children). The researchers reported 306 medication errors in 10,112 orders, including 2% of potentially harmful orders. Among these, 82% of adult errors (203 of 249) and 60% of pediatric errors (34 of 57) were potentially adverse drug events (ADEs), with one-third being serious. Pharmacists and nurses in ambulatory oncology identified and rectified 45% of possible ADEs prior to the drugs reaching patients, indicating the significance of professional checks.

The paper has shown that the smallest mistakes may lead to dramatic or potentially fatal outcomes, particularly in pediatric chemotherapy, where dose accuracy is paramount and therapeutic indices are low. On the basis of these results, the authors suggested system-level measures such as the Computerized Provider Order Entry (CPOE) and standard chemotherapy templates, as well as pharmacist review. According to Gandhi and colleagues, outpatient chemotherapy safety, a reduction in unnecessary mishaps, and the maintenance of performance levels can be significantly enhanced by organized electronic programs and multidisciplinary management (Gandhi et al., 2005).

In- and Outpatient Oncology System Surveillance

Past safety education in oncology has focused primarily on individual variations in prescription or administration mistakes, generally addressed retrospectively. Most hospitals use manual checking of orders by pharmacists or nurses with minimal coordination between pharmacies, clinical wards, and quality-assurance teams. Although electronic order entry and standard chemotherapy regimens are used, few institutions have implemented department-wide, proactive systems to track medication errors and severe adverse events in real time.

Markert et al. (2009) developed a dual-surveillance system to address this gap: the PERMIT system, which identifies prescription and administrative chemotherapy errors, and the MERKE system, which documents severe adverse events (SAECTx). A multidisciplinary clinical service center (CSC) comprising oncologists, pharmacists, nurses, and data specialists would confirm all chemotherapy orders prior to administration, which is a conceptual change from a single double check to a system-wide safety approach. The team prospectively studied 22,216 chemotherapy requests from 2,337 patients over two years (January 2005–December 2006).

Of these, 83.5% were error-free, while 17.1% contained deviations: 3.8% chemotherapy-related, 4.5% patient-data errors, and 8.7% incomplete consent forms. Errors were less frequent among outpatients (3.3%) than among inpatients (4.5%), and outpatient errors decreased from 4.0% (2005) to 2.8% (2006) following electronic order refinement. Among the 3,792 detected errors, only three (0.079%) reached patients, corresponding to a 99.9% prevention rate and a patient risk of 0.13% for receiving incorrect chemotherapy. The additional quality-assurance cost was estimated at € 1 per order (approximately € 23,000 per year) (Markert et al., 2009).

This pioneering model demonstrated that multidisciplinary preverification and continuous feedback loops can achieve near-zero transmission of chemotherapy errors at minimal cost, providing a template for institutional learning systems that combine error detection, adverse event monitoring, and process improvement within routine oncology care. Table 1 summarizes the design, scope, and major outcomes of three pivotal chemotherapy safety studies that collectively characterize the spectrum of medication use errors in cancer care, from inpatient to ambulatory and mixed oncology settings.

Table 1. Comparative overview of chemotherapy error studies

Setting/ design	Sample size & scope	Error incidence/ rate	Predominant error types	Key findings and safety interventions	Study (Year)
Prospective observational; inpatient oncology (France)	6,607 chemotherapy prescriptions (~22,138 doses)	449 errors (5.2%); 97% identified before administration; 2.9% reached patients	Prescribing (~ 91%), dose or selection errors	13.4% temporary, 2.6% permanent, 2.6% life-threatening if uncorrected; € 92,900 annual cost; emphasized pharmacist verification and double checks	Ranchon et al. (2011)
Prospective cohort; ambulatory chemotherapy (USA)	1,606 patients; 10,112 orders (8,008 adult + 2,104 pediatric)	306 errors (3%); 2% potentially harmful; 45% corrected before administration	Dose/ calculation errors; potential ADEs (82% adult, 60% pediatric)	One-third serious; advocated CPOE, standardized templates, and pharmacist review	Gandhi et al. (2005)
Prospective 2-year cohort; inpatient and outpatient oncology (Germany)	2,337 patients; 22,216 chemotherapy orders	17.1% any error (3.8% chemo, 4.5% data, 8.7% consent); 0.079% reached patients	Regimen, patient data, documentation	99.9% prevented before administration; dual surveillance and team verification achieved near-zero harm	Markert et al. (2009)

Note: Computerized provider order entry (CPOE)

In all these studies, prescribing and order verification were the most vulnerable stages of chemotherapy. The difficulty of individualizing the dose and selecting a regimen can be noted by the fact that 70–90% of all mistakes occur when a prescription is written or transcribed (Gandhi et al., 2005; Markert et al., 2009; Ranchon et al., 2011).

In inpatient oncology, the error rates were 5%, 3% in ambulatory chemotherapy, and 17% in a mixed inpatient–outpatient cohort *(Gandhi et al., 2005; Markert et al., 2009; Ranchon et al., 2011)*, most of which were administrative. Strong pharmacist and nurse review systems maintained patient errors between 0.08–3%.

The prevention rates reported in all the studies were greater than 97, which implies the importance of multidisciplinary verification. System design, not individual vigilance, ensures chemotherapy safety. This problem is prevented with a structured design, changing handwritten orders to CPOE, introducing real-time verification, and establishing a centralized surveillance center such as Markert's Clinical Service Center.

These findings suggest a systems-integration paradigm involving

1. Electronic prescriptions, standardized dose-verification algorithms,
2. independent nurse and pharmacist verification and
3. Regular check-ups and feedback about negative events.

Oncology systems that are highly reliable are marked by redundancy, resilience, and continuous learning on how to learn near misses, which includes implementing protocols for regular check-ups and feedback of negative events to enhance patient safety. Chemotherapy remains fundamentally the responsibility of humans, even when technical advancements are made. Automation and electronic safety can minimize the risk of error, but they cannot replace the clinical judgment required for subtle decisions made by oncology pharmacists and nurses who interpret laboratory information, organ operations, and treatment regimens. The economic and human cost inputs of over EUR 90,000 per year reported by Ranchon et al. (2011) in avoidable near misses prove that safety investments have paybacks (Ranchon et al., 2011).

In the context of the organization, interdisciplinary communication is the core of prevention. An organized briefing, standardized sets of orders, and active integration of the pharmacist in real time during medical rounds will consistently decrease the number of prescribing discrepancies. Even in low-resource/high-volume centers, simplified visual differentiation plans (e.g., separate packaging, tall-man lettering, color coding, and physical segregation of LASA drugs) are still pragmatic supplements. Clinician well-being is also a vital requirement. In the case of system malfunctions, the so-called second-victim effect (e.g., guilt, anxiety, and loss of confidence) in healthcare workers can take place, and it regularly undermines morale and entails defensive treatment. Building just-culture structures that decouple system responsibility and individual culpability is thus essential to maintaining engagement and endless improvement (Ahuja & Ahuja, 2024; Cohen, 2007a; Cohen et al., 2007; Cohen & Smetzer, 2007; Cohen et al., 2012; Neelakantan et al., 2024; Supapaan et al., 2024; World Health Organization, 2023).

PREVENTING CHEMOTHERAPY ERRORS

Structured systems, standardized processes, interdisciplinary communication, and safety-focused culture across all stages of care are needed to prevent chemotherapy errors. Cancer drugs are high-risk because most are given at or near the maximum tolerated dose, leaving little room for error (Kloth, 2002). Kloth's seminal review revealed that systemic fragmentation, not individual negligence, causes catastrophic chemotherapy errors such as intrathecal vincristine administration, which kills everyone. He advised comprehensive safeguards on the basis of incidents at top U.S. cancer centers:

1. Standardized chemotherapy order templates reduce transcription and dose-calculation errors.
2. Elimination of verbal chemotherapy orders: only written or electronic.
3. Before compounding or administering, the pharmacist and nurse verify every order.
4. Indications for high-alert drugs include “For IV use only—Fatal if given intrathecally.”
5. All oncology staff undergo annual competency testing.

Kloth also advocated system redesign and continuous education to replace a punitive “blame” culture with transparency and learning. The framework shaped national oncology safety guidelines and Joint Commission vincristine sentinel event alerts.

Schulmeister (2006) examined the ongoing threat of LASA medication errors in oncology to complement this system-level view. In her analysis of the U.S. Pharmacopeia (USP) Medication Errors Reporting Program (1996–2001), 15% of all reports were related to name or labeling confusion, with oncology drugs disproportionately represented. The ISMP estimated that name and label confusion causes nearly half of medication errors. Cisplatin/carboplatin, vincristine/vinblastine, paclitaxel/docetaxel, and daunorubicin/idarubicin have caused overdoses, route errors, and fatal mix-ups. Schulmeister suggested practical solutions.

1. Tall-man lettering (CISplatin vs. CARBOplatin).
2. LASA drug storage in separate bins.
3. Protocol bans abbreviations and nicknames.

4. Each chemotherapy dispensing and administration step requires two-person verification.
5. CPOE and barcode scanning reduce transcription and dispensing errors.

The findings revealed that oncology nurses and pharmacists are key frontline interceptors of LASA and compounding errors, especially in high-volume outpatient infusion units (Schulmeister, 2006).

On the basis of these foundations, the American Society of Clinical Oncology (ASCO) and Oncology Nursing Society (ONS) created the Chemotherapy Administration Safety Standards, which were updated in 2016 to include pediatric oncology and oral chemotherapy (Neuss et al., 2017). Two qualified practitioners must independently verify patient identifiers, drug name, dose, route, rate, and cycle for all chemotherapy orders before compounding or infusion. In intrathecal drug facilities, vinca alkaloids must be dispensed in minibags, never syringes. The update promotes full CPOE implementation with built-in decision support, standardized preprinted templates, and auditable verification step documentation.

These studies and standards highlight the shift in oncology from reactive error correction to proactive risk prevention. Kloth's preventive framework, Schulmeister's LASA-mitigation strategies, and ASCO/ONS verification protocols have reduced catastrophic chemotherapy errors. Given the ever-growing complexity of the oncology-therapy environment, institutional safety culture, pharmacist leadership, and interprofessional collaboration should be vigilant in safeguarding patients. The approach required is a systems-based approach to minimize the occurrence of chemotherapy errors by performing standardized verification, LASA mitigation, and technological safeguards (see Figure 2).

Figure 2. Protecting oncology practices by preventing chemotherapy errors

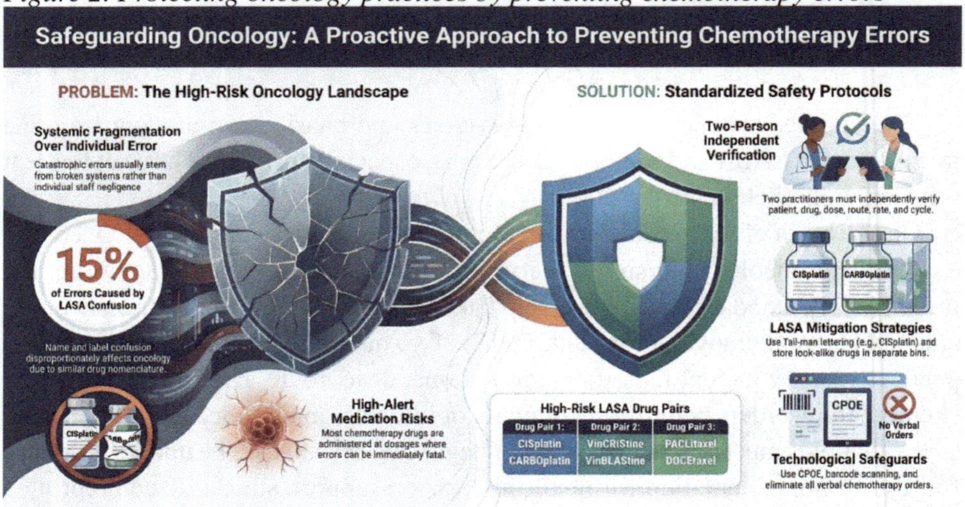

The figure outlines the major oncology medication safety risks, including LASA confusion, high-alert medications, and system fragmentation, as well as prevention strategies such as two-person verification, tall man lettering, separate storage, CPOE, barcode scanning, and the removal of verbal chemotherapy orders.

COMMON LASA PAIRS IN ONCOLOGY PRACTICE

An extensive range of LASA pairs and high-annuity medicines is provided in the realms of oncology. LASA-related errors are especially prone to these agents because of the peculiarities of oncology drugs. They usually possess a small therapeutic index, with a minor dosing error being fatal or ineffective. Prescriptions are given in complex regimens involving numerous cycles, doses, and combinations. They are commonly packed in comparable containers or vials, which could also be confusing at the dispensing or administration stage (Kaushal et al., 2001; Schulmeister, 2006; World Health Organization, 2017). The following LASA pairs are often linked to medication errors and serious safety events. Vials that look alike, names that sound similar, and active ingredient formulations with different dosing regimens are all risks. These risks must be addressed to prevent oncological harm.

Leading LASA Offenders in Oncology

An extensive range of LASA pairs and high-annuity medicines is provided in the realms of oncology. LASA-related errors are especially prone to these agents because of the peculiarities of oncology drugs. They usually possess a small therapeutic index, with a minor dosing error being fatal or ineffective. Prescriptions are provided in complicated regimens with many cycles, doses, and combinations. They are commonly packed in comparable containers or vials, which could also be confusing at the dispensing or administration stage (Kaushal et al., 2001; Schulmeister, 2006; World Health Organization, 2017). Table 2 provides a list of significant high-risk LASA drug pairs used in oncology, with the relationship of each pair to its clinical application, major error mechanisms, and mitigation measures. These two pairs demonstrate that similarity in name, look-alike packaging, regimen differences, or differences in dose can result in severe or disastrous drug errors. VinCRIStine vs. vinblastine, DAUNOrubicin vs. DOXOrubicin, and CARBOplatin vs. CISplatin are classic instances where special care is needed to prevent confusion, which might require tall man type, bar-code checking, standard order sets, and double-checking. Table 2 facilitates oncology practices in the strategy of medication error reduction by matching certain LASA risks with the corresponding preventive measures.

Table 2. Major high-risk LASA drug pairs in oncology and their clinical uses, primary error risks with each pair, and approaches for compensating for all major risk factors

LASA Pair	Clinical use/ route	Primary error risk	Practical mitigation	Reference
vinCRIStine vs vinblastine.	Vinca alkaloids; IV for hematologic/ solid tumors	Wrong route (intrathecal vinca is catastrophic); name similarity contributes to selection risk. Fatalities reported globally; rationale for minibag-only dispensing	Dispense vinca only in minibags; never syringes; Tall man lettering; independent double-check; explicit route warnings.	The Institute for Safe Medication Practices (ISMP) (2023a); The Joint Commission (2023) Grissinger (2016) ISMP News/ECRI (2020)
DAUNOrubicin vs DOXOrubicin	Anthracyclines; IV	Name confusion, wrong drug/dose; both cardiotoxic; regimen efficacy impacted.	Tall man; barcode-assisted verification; standardized order sets with max-dose/Clinical Decision Support (CDS) checks.	Schulmeister (2006); The Institute for Safe Medication Practices (ISMP) (2023a)
CARBOplatin vs CISplatin	Platinum agents; IV	Wrong-drug selection compounded by dose-basis differences (AUC vs mg/m^2); severe toxicity if interchanged. MedMARX reports document transcription errors leading to cisplatin overdose	Tall man; CPOE hard stops confirming agent and dose basis; independent dose check; storage separation.	Hicks et al. (2008); Schulmeister (2006); The Institute for Safe Medication Practices (ISMP) (2023a)
DOCEtaxel vs PACLitaxel	Taxanes; IV	Name similarity and similar indications and wrong-drug selection.	Tall man; barcode scan at preparation/administration; standardized regimen templates with sequencing.	Institute for Safe Medication Practices Canada (2015); Schulmeister (2006)
LEVOleucovorin vs Leucovorin	Rescue with Methotrexate (MTX) and adjunct to 5-FU; IV/PO	Look-alike names; wrong-product selection between leucovorin and levoleucovorin formulations	Tall man (LEVOleucovorin vs leucovorin); configure CPOE to force indication + strength; barcode verification.	The Institute for Safe Medication Practices (ISMP) (2023a)

continued on following page

Table 2. Continued

LASA Pair	Clinical use/ route	Primary error risk	Practical mitigation	Reference
epiRUBicin vs eriBULin	Epirubicin (anthracycline) vs eribulin (microtubule inhibitor); IV	Orthographic similarity leading to wrong-drug selection.	Tall man; storage separation by class; barcode scan; pharmacist double-check.	Institute for Safe Medication Practices Canada (2015)
vinorelbine vs vinBLAStine/ vincristine	Vinca alkaloids; IV	Cluster similarity within class; high-risk selection errors identified in proactive formulary analysis	Tall man across the cluster; vinca minibag-only policy; double-check with read-back of drug name.	Kovacic and Chambers (2011)
soraFENIB vs sunitinib	Oral Tyrosine kinase inhibitors (TKIs)	High orthographic similarity; recurrent LASA signal in oncology reviews	Tall man; patient education with brand/strength images; large auxiliary labels.	Institute for Safe Medication Practices Canada (2015); Kovacic and Chambers (2011)

Antineoplastic LASA Medication Errors: An Investigation Based on MedMARX and the ISMP/FDA/WHO

Drug name confusion, or LASA errors, can be a significant risk factor in oncology, as high-alert medication is often administered. Table 3 provides a summary of LASA drug pairs that have been reported in the MedMARX 2008 database and classified according to the NCC MERP index in terms of severity of reported outcomes (Hicks et al., 2008). Table 4 presents LASA drug pairs commonly used in oncology practice, compiled from ISMP and Schulmeister, highlighting antineoplastic and supportive care agents frequently involved in name-related errors (Schulmeister, 2006; The Institute for Safe Medication Practices (ISMP), 2024a).

Table 3. Selected antineoplastic LASA pairs reported in MedMARX 2008, with NCC MERP categories and pharmacologic classifications

No.	Drug 1	Drug 2	Category (NCC MERP)	Meaning
1	Cisplatin*	Carboplatin*	C–D, E-H	Error reached patient; caused no harm to possible harm.
2	Cyclophosphamide*	Cyclosporine (Immunological agents, immunomodulators)	B, C–D	Error intercepted or reached patient without harm.
3	Doxorubicin*	Daunorubicin*	A, B, C–D	Potential error or intercepted/reached without harm.
4	Fluorouracil (5-FU)*	Fluocinonide	B, C–D, E-H	Error intercepted, reached without harm, or caused harm.
5	Methotrexate*	Minoxidil (Antihypertensive/ dermatologic agent)	E–H	Error reached patient and caused harm.
6	Methotrexate*	Mercaptopurine*	A, B	Potential error or intercepted before reaching patient.
7	Methotrexate*	Methylprednisolone Sodium Succinate (Glucocorticoid, Corticosteroid)	B	Error intercepted before reaching patient.
8	Methotrexate*	Metolazone (Antihypertensive)	A, B, C–D	Potential, intercepted, or reached patient without harm.
9	Methotrexate*	Metronidazole (Antiprotozoal)	C–D	Error reached patient but caused no harm.
10	Paclitaxel*	Docetaxel*	B, C–D	Error intercepted or reached patient without harm.
11	Rituximab*	Infliximab (Monoclonal antibodies; oncology & autoimmune)	B, C-D, E–H	Error intercepted, reached without harm, or caused harm.
12	Tamoxifen*	Temazepam (Benzodiazepine, sedative/hypnotic)	A, C–D	Potential error or reached patient without harm.
13	Tamoxifen*	Tamsolosin (Alpha-1 Adrenergic Blocker)	B, C–D	Error intercepted or reached patient without harm.
14	VinBLAStine*	VinCRIStine*	B	Error intercepted before reaching patient.

(Hicks et al., 2008)

*Marked drugs are antineoplastic agents (chemotherapy/oncology-related).

Table 4. LASA drug pairs are commonly used in cancer patient care, as compiled from ISMP (2024) and Schulmeister (2006). Antineoplastic agents are indicated with an asterisk (*), while nonchemotherapy drugs are annotated with their pharmacologic categories in parentheses

Drug 1	Drug 2	Category	Reference
Adriamycin® (doxorubicin)*	Idamycin® (idarubicin)*	Both antineoplastics	Schulmeister (2006)
Adriamycin® (doxorubicin)*	Aredia® (pamidronate)	Antineoplastic vs Bisphosphonate derivative	Schulmeister (2006)
aldesleukin	oprelvekin	Immunotherapy (cytokine) versus supportive care agent	Schulmeister (2006)
Alkeran® (melphalan)*	Leukeran® (chlorambucil)*	Both antineoplastics	Schulmeister (2006)
asparaginase*	pegaspargase*	Both antineoplastics	Schulmeister (2006)
Adriamycin® (doxorubicin)*	Doxil® (liposomal doxorubicin)*	Both antineoplastics	Schulmeister (2006)
Adriamycin (doxorubicin)*	daunorubicin*	Both antineoplastics	Schulmeister (2006)
Adriamycin (doxorubicin)*	epirubicin*	Both antineoplastics	Schulmeister (2006)
Adriamycin (doxorubicin)*	Droxia (hydroxyurea)	Both antineoplastics	Schulmeister (2006)
BiCNU® (carmustine)*	CeeNU® (lomustine)*	Both antineoplastics	Schulmeister (2006)
CARBOplatin*	CISplatin*	Both antineoplastics	The Institute for Safe Medication Practices (ISMP) (2024a) Schulmeister (2006)
carboplatin*	Paraplatin® (carboplatin)*	Both antineoplastics	Schulmeister (2006)
capecitabine*	gemcitabine*	Both antineoplastics	Schulmeister (2006)
carmustine*	lomustine*	Both antineoplastics	Schulmeister (2006)
cyclophosphamide*	cyclosporine*	Antineoplastic vs Immunosuppressant agent	Schulmeister (2006)
Cytosar® (cytarabine)*	Cytoxan® (cyclophosphamide)*	Both antineoplastics	Schulmeister (2006)
Cytoxan® (cyclophosphamide)*	Cytarabine*	Both antineoplastics	Schulmeister (2006)
DACTINomycin*	DAPTOmycin (antibiotic, lipopeptide)	Antineoplastic vs antibiotic	The Institute for Safe Medication Practices (ISMP) (2024a)
darbepoetin alpha	epoetin alpha	Both hematopoietic agents	Schulmeister (2006)
docetaxel (Taxotere®)*	paclitaxel (Taxol®)*	Both antineoplastics	Schulmeister (2006)

continued on following page

Table 4. Continued

Drug 1	Drug 2	Category	Reference
docetaxel (Taxotere®)*	Paxil® (paroxetine)	Antineoplastic vs Antidepressant	Schulmeister (2006)
DOCEtaxel*	PACLitaxel*	Both antineoplastics	The Institute for Safe Medication Practices (ISMP) (2024a) Schulmeister (2006)
DOXOrubicin*	DAUNOrubicin*	Both antineoplastics; different uses/toxicity	The Institute for Safe Medication Practices (ISMP) (2024a) Schulmeister (2006)
DOXOrubicin*	DOXOrubicin liposomal*	Both antineoplastics (Conventional vs liposomal, major dosing difference)	The Institute for Safe Medication Practices (ISMP) (2024a)
Doxorubicin*	Idarubicin*	Both antineoplastics	Schulmeister (2006)
Doxorubicin*	Doxacillin	Antineoplastics vs antibiotics	Schulmeister (2006)
epiRUBicin*	eriBULin*	Anthracycline vs microtubule inhibitor	The Institute for Safe Medication Practices (ISMP) (2024a)
epirubicin*	daunorubicin*	Both antineoplastics	Schulmeister (2006)
epirubicin*	doxorubicin*	Both antineoplastics	Schulmeister (2006)
epirubicin*	idarubicin*	Both antineoplastics	Schulmeister (2006)
Epogen® (epoetin alpha)	Neupogen® (filgrastim)	Both hematopoietic agents	Schulmeister (2006)
filgrastim	pegfilgrastim	Both hematopoietic agents	Schulmeister (2006)
filgrastim	sargramostim	Both hematopoietic agents	Schulmeister (2006)
fluorouracil*	flucytosine	Antineoplastic agent & antifungal agent	Schulmeister (2006)
fluorouracil*	fluocinonide	Antineoplastic agent & corticosteroid	Schulmeister (2006)
gemcitabine*	capecitabine*	Both antineoplastics	Schulmeister (2006)
IDArubicin*	DOXOrubicin*	Both antineoplastics	The Institute for Safe Medication Practices (ISMP) (2024a)
IDArubicin*	DAUNOrubicin*	Both antineoplastics	The Institute for Safe Medication Practices (ISMP) (2024a)
IDArubicin*	idaruCIZUmab	Antineoplastic vs monoclonal antibody fragment, antidote	The Institute for Safe Medication Practices (ISMP) (2024a)

continued on following page

Table 4. Continued

Drug 1	Drug 2	Category	Reference
Leukeran® (chlorambucil)*	Leukine® (sargramostim, CSF)	Antineoplastic agent vs supportive care (hematopoietic growth factor)	Schulmeister (2006)
Leukeran® (chlorambucil)*	leucovorin (rescue agent)	Antineoplastic vs rescue/ supportive agent	Schulmeister (2006)
Leukeran® (chlorambucil)*	Alkeran®	Both antineoplastic agents	Schulmeister (2006)
lomustine*	carmustine*	Both antineoplastic agents	Schulmeister (2006)
melphalan*	Myleran®*	Both antineoplastic agents	Schulmeister (2006)
methotrexate*	methohexital (barbiturate anesthetic)	Antineoplastic vs Anesthetic	Schulmeister (2006)
mitoMYcin*	mitoXANTRONE*	Both are antineoplastic agents	The Institute for Safe Medication Practices (ISMP) (2024a) Schulmeister (2006)
nelarabine (Arranon®)	Navelbine® (vinorelbine tartrate)	Both antineoplastic agents	Schulmeister (2006)
neratinib*	nilotinib*	Both are oral targeted antineoplastic agents.	The Institute for Safe Medication Practices (ISMP) (2024a)
neratinib*	niraparib*	Both are oral targeted antineoplastic agents.	The Institute for Safe Medication Practices (ISMP) (2024a)
Neumega® (oprelvekin, IL-11)	Neupogen® (filgrastim, G-CSF)	Both supportive care agents	Schulmeister (2006)
Neumega® (oprelvekin, IL-11)	Neulasta® (pegfilgrastim, CSF)	Both supportive care agents	Schulmeister (2006)
Neupogen® (filgrastim, G-CSF)	aldesleukin (IL-2)	Both supportive care agents	Schulmeister (2006)
nilotinib*	niraparib*	Both are oral targeted antineoplastic agents.	The Institute for Safe Medication Practices (ISMP) (2024a)
PACLitaxel*	PACLitaxel protein-bound particles (nab-paclitaxel)*	Same antineoplastic agent with different formulations (not interchangeable)	The Institute for Safe Medication Practices (ISMP) (2024a)
paclitaxel	docetaxel	Both antineoplastic agents	Schulmeister (2006)
paclitaxel	Paxil® (paroxetine)	Antineoplastic agent vs antidepressant (SSRI)	Schulmeister (2006)
paclitaxel	paroxetine	Antineoplastic agent vs antidepressant (SSRI)	Schulmeister (2006)
Paraplatin®	Platinol-AQ®	Both antineoplastic agents	Schulmeister (2006)

continued on following page

Table 4. Continued

Drug 1	Drug 2	Category	Reference
Platinol-AQ®	Paraplatin®	Both antineoplastic agents	Schulmeister (2006)
Proleukin®	Leukine	Immunotherapy vs supportive care agent	Schulmeister (2006)
PAZOPanib*	PONATinib*	Both antineoplastic agents	The Institute for Safe Medication Practices (ISMP) (2024a)
PEMEtrexed*	PRALAtrexate*	Both antineoplastic agents	The Institute for Safe Medication Practices (ISMP) (2024a)
oprelvekin	aldesleukin	Supportive care agent vs immunotherapy	Schulmeister (2006)
romiDEPsin*	romiPLOStim	Antineoplastic vs hematopoietic agent	The Institute for Safe Medication Practices (ISMP) (2024a)
SORAfenib*	SUNItinib*	Both are oral multikinase inhibitors.	The Institute for Safe Medication Practices (ISMP) (2024a)
talquetamab-tgvs*	teclistamab-cqyv*	Both are bispecific T-cell engagers.	The Institute for Safe Medication Practices (ISMP) (2024a)
tamoxifen	Tamiflu® (oseltamivir)	Antineoplastic vs antiviral	Schulmeister (2006)
tamoxifen	tamsulosin	Antineoplastic vs urologic agent	Schulmeister (2006)
Talvey*	Tecvayli*	Both antineoplastics (bispecific T-cell engagers for MM)	The Institute for Safe Medication Practices (ISMP) (2024a)
Taxol® (paclitaxel)	Paxil® (paroxetine)	Antineoplastic agent vs antidepressant (SSRI)	Schulmeister (2006)
Taxol® (paclitaxel)*	Taxotere® (docetaxel)*	Both antineoplastic agents	Schulmeister (2006)
traSTUZumab*	ado-traSTUZumab emtansine*	Both antineoplastic agents	The Institute for Safe Medication Practices (ISMP) (2024a)
vinBLAStine*	vinCRIStine*	Both antineoplastic agents (vinca alkaloids)	The Institute for Safe Medication Practices (ISMP) (2024a) Schulmeister (2006)
vinblastine*	vindesine*	Both antineoplastic agents (vinca alkaloids)	Schulmeister (2006)
vinblastine*	vinorelbine*	Both antineoplastic agents (vinca alkaloids)	Schulmeister (2006)

continued on following page

Table 4. Continued

Drug 1	Drug 2	Category	Reference
vincristine*	vinblastine*	Both antineoplastic agents (vinca alkaloids)	Schulmeister (2006)
vincristine*	vindesine*	Both antineoplastic agents (vinca alkaloids)	Schulmeister (2006)
vincristine*	vinorelbine*	Both antineoplastic agents (vinca alkaloids)	Schulmeister (2006)

(National Library of Medicine, 2025; Schulmeister, 2006; The Institute for Safe Medication Practices (ISMP), 2024a)

LASA ERRORS OF DRUG NAME STEMS

Drug name stems, specific linguistic fragments embedded in the generic (non-proprietary) names of medicines, play a pivotal role in the occurrence of look-alike, sound-alike (LASA) errors in oncology pharmacotherapy. The World Health Organization (WHO) International Nonproprietary Name (INN) system (World Health Organization, 2024) uses stems to indicate the mechanistic class, molecular origin, or pharmacological traits of drugs (for example, the suffix "mAb" denotes monoclonal antibodies) (Bryan et al., 2015; DrugPatentWatch, 2025; Karet, 2019).

The stems are meant to serve as cognitive aids to help healthcare workers categorize and recognize medicines. For example, a clinician who hears the suffix -nib could organizationally relate it to a tyrosine kinase inhibitor (DrugPatentWatch, 2025; Karet, 2019).

These similarities between agents can, however, be confusing. The use of multiple drug names that have common stems or stem clusters, particularly in similar treatment groups, leads to an increase in prescribing, dispensing, and administration errors. The suffixes of names ending with -mab can share similar prefixes, phonetics, or orthographs, which puts the possibility of auditory or visual errors at risk (Bryan et al., 2015).

Mechanisms by which drug names stem from the risk of LASA: This spread of risk is in two main dimensions:

(1) Phonetic similarity—how two names sound like when they are pronounced or heard in a busy clinical setting; and

(2) Orthographic similarity—the appearance of two names printed, typed, or scanned (on a CPOE screen or a medication label). Bryan et al. emphasize the importance of shared linguistic properties in the aspects of wrong-drug substitution events: LASA errors occur because of shared linguistic properties between two

or more names and result in misplaced substitution of a single medicinal product (Bryan et al., 2021a).

Making the patterns visible in groups of stems makes it possible to apply specific mitigation measures such as alerts in prescribing software, specialized educational efforts to health-care staff, and refined labeling practices (e.g., tall-man lettering, differentiation of shelf tags, and distinct packaging).

A lack of awareness of these linguistic features can result in practitioners not foreseeing or detecting possible confusion in prescribing, dispensing, or administering drugs. In this way, systematic LASA error prevention can be based on a structural comprehension of drug-name stem linguistics. An example of the naming scheme, as explicated by the AMA Journal of Ethics, is as follows: "Pharmaceutical names are assigned according to a scheme in which specific syllables in the drug name (called stems) convey information about the chemical structure, action, or indication of the drug." (Karet, 2019).

Finally, it should be mentioned that linguistic factors themselves do not work in isolation: the risk of error due to the similarity in naming stems from linguistic factors is further increased by cognitive load, flaws in organizational design (e.g., high workload, inadequate double-check processes), and system-level flaws. A recent umbrella review of contributory factors to medication errors revealed that latent conditions (such as inadequate staffing or education) combine with active failures in complex systems to increase risk across medication use phases (Naseralallah et al., 2022).

Historical Perspective: From Legacy to Modern Oncology Therapies

Oncology has in turn moved out of classical cytotoxic chemotherapy to highly selective targeted and immune-modulatory therapies in the past five decades. This change is not only apparent in the mechanisms of therapy; the stems of the International Nonproprietary Names (INN) system have also been developed to indicate mechanisms or molecular roots (e.g., -mab (monoclonal antibody), -tinib (tyrosine kinase inhibitor), and -degib (SMO antagonist). The antineoplastic drugs are still named with historical suffixes such as -platina, -mustina, -rubicina, -trexate, and vin- (innovation in therapy is denoted by -rafenib or -tansine), according to the World Health Organization INN list (World Health Organization, 2024).

With the increase in the number of treatment modalities, drug nomenclature has become complicated. This is a scientifically systematic evolution of the language that, however, realized new dangers of LASA confusion between more similar nonproprietary names (Karet, 2019, 2023; Kovacic & Chambers, 2011).

The Legacy of Chemotherapy

Early cytotoxic chemotherapies are still vital for cancer therapy and include vin- (vinca alkaloids, vindesine, vincristine), -rubicin (anthracyclines, doxorubicin, daunorubicin), -mustine, -platin, and -trexate. Numerous LASA mix-ups, including cisplatin-carboplatin and vinblastine-vincristine, have been reported in safety databases and fatal-error reports because of shared orthographic and phonetic elements (Hicks et al., 2008; Schulmeister, 2006; The Institute for Safe Medication Practices (ISMP), 2024b, 2024c). Although still embedded in formularies and electronic order sets, these legacy stems maintain LASA vulnerability decades after their introduction.

Implementing Modern Targeted Therapies

The development of molecularly targeted agents and biologics in the late 1990s, such as monoclonal antibodies, tyrosine kinase inhibitors, fusion proteins and PARP inhibitors, signaled a great shift in cancer therapy. Although these developments were beneficial for making treatment specific, they increased the number of medicines with similar naming patterns and linguistic stems. As a result, the current trend of using targeted and biologic approaches and integrating long-standing cytotoxic drugs into complex portfolios initiated by oncology clinicians can increase the risk of incorrect drug selection, especially in high-tension clinical care (Bryan et al., 2021a; Bryan et al., 2021b; World Health Organization, 2023). The concept of stem clusters offers a beneficial structural format that may be applied to ascertain LASA danger in historical and contemporary oncology medicines containing similar phonetic or orthographic units. A pharmacist can fill prescriptions containing agents with endings -platin and -nib during the same shift, which provides the chances of phonological overlap and near-miss events. Susceptibility is also enhanced by regular changes in the regimen, intricate compounding and verification procedures, and multitasking of the oncology pharmacy processes (Kovacic & Chambers, 2011; Naseralallah et al., 2022). Notably, chemotherapy and targeted anticancer agents are always categorized as high-alert medications, and name confusion errors may have clinical consequences because of their small therapeutic index (Schulmeister, 2006). Since the risk of LASA can be seen as crossing various treatment eras, instead of a single drug-class effort, a long-term, system-wide approach to safety is needed and not a single therapeutic-class-specific intervention.

Persistence of Risk

Oncology medication use analyses have shown that a large number of look-alike and sound-alike drug pairs that are used in treating cancer are not completely reflected in institutional safety lists or other external lists, which suggests that fixed reference tools should not be used to manage LASA risk in oncology. Oncology formularies as well as chemotherapy error reporting have shown that both older cytotoxic agents and newer treatments can share similar naming patterns without being automatically identified, especially when the formularies grow and become diversified with time (Kovacic & Chambers, 2011; Schulmeister, 2006; World Health Organization, 2023).

The data on incident reporting and safety further show that even today, the malpractices related to the wrong-drug errors in question are yet to be removed in regard to long-established chemotherapy agents or the products of oncology by nature. Such mistakes are very common in the process of prescription, dispensing, and preparation when drugs that share similar names, packaging, or even the same therapeutic effect are in the same complex treatment regimen. According to reports of medication-error surveillance systems, antineoplastic drugs continue to be overrepresented in high-severity LASA events and already have one of the thinnest therapeutic indices and the most complex workflows in the oncology department (National Coordinating Council for Medication Error Reporting and Prevention (NCC MERP), 2022; The Institute for Safe Medication Practices (ISMP), 2023b; Weingart et al., 2003).

Vulnerability of the Oncology-Relevant Drug Name Stem and LASA

Drug name stems play a central role in the identification, categorization, and safe use of oncology medicines. Although standard naming systems (especially the International Nonproprietary Names (INN) system) provide pharmacological clarity, the extensive use of common stems among antineoplastic agents has provided systematic susceptibility to look-alike, sound-alike (LASA) medication errors. Physical harm, particularly in cancer, has on numerous occasions been linked to stem-driven confusion, which has been in many instances and has a narrow therapeutic index, a complex dose regimen, and overlapping indications.

The literature on the safety of LASA by peer review has demonstrated an increased risk of LASA where the agents bear the same suffixes (e.g., -platin, -rubicin, and -mab) when used together with other similar prefixes, packaging, or storage sites. The most typical ones are cisplatin-carboplatin substitution errors and interclass confusion with anthracyclines and monoclonal antibodies, with lethal results and very high toxicity. New classes of therapies, including tyrosine kinase inhibitors, PARP inhibitors, and cell- and gene-based therapies, create even greater risks because of dense multisyllabic names with poor discriminatory characteristics (Hicks et al., 2008; Kovacic & Chambers, 2011; Neuss et al., 2017; Schulmeister, 2006).

Table 5 provides a summary of oncology-relevant drug name stems, therapeutic classes, and representative agents, as well as known LASA mechanisms and verified reference examples in published peer-reviewed PubMed-indexed literature, the WHO International Nonproprietary Names Program, and Institute for Safe Medication Practices (ISMP) safety reports.

Table 5. Oncology-relevant drug name stems and LASA risk commentary

Stem	Therapeutic Class/ Mechanism	Representative Examples	LASA Risk Commentary	Reference
–mab	Monoclonal antibodies targeting tumor antigens or immune checkpoints	Rituximab; Trastuzumab; Pertuzumab; Obinutuzumab	High phonetic and orthographic similarity among biologics with overlapping indications	(Kovacic & Chambers, 2011); Schulmeister (2006); (World Health Organization, 2024)
–nib/–tinib	Tyrosine kinase inhibitors (TKIs)	Imatinib; Dasatinib; Nilotinib; Sunitinib; Sorafenib	Short prefixes and identical suffixes increase prescribing and dispensing errors	(Kovacic & Chambers, 2011; Schulmeister, 2006; The Institute for Safe Medication Practices (ISMP), 2024a; World Health Organization, 2024)
–parib	PARP inhibitors (DNA damage response modulators)	Olaparib; Niraparib; Rucaparib; Talazoparib	Limited syllabic variation and similar indications promote substitution errors	The Institute for Safe Medication Practices (ISMP) (2024a); World Health Organization (2024)
–cept	Fusion proteins combining receptor and immunoglobulin components	Aflibercept; Etanercept; Abatacept	Visual and orthographic overlap with other biologics increases misidentification risk	Pottier et al. (2017); World Health Organization (2024)
–platin	Platinum-based DNA-crosslinking cytotoxic agents	Cisplatin; Carboplatin; Oxaliplatin	Well-documented LASA pair with fatal overdose and renal toxicity reports	(Fyhr & Akselsson, 2012; Schulmeister, 2006; The Institute for Safe Medication Practices (ISMP), 2024c)
–rubicin	Anthracycline topoisomerase II inhibitors	Doxorubicin; Daunorubicin; Epirubicin; Idarubicin	Intraclass confusion may result in cumulative cardiotoxicity	(Schulmeister, 2006; The Institute for Safe Medication Practices (ISMP), 2024a)
–mustine	Nitrosourea alkylating agents	Carmustine; Lomustine	Orthographic similarity and limited product range increase compounding errors	(Kovacic & Chambers, 2011; Schulmeister, 2006; World Health Organization, 2024)
–trexate	Antifolate antimetabolites	Methotrexate; Pemetrexed; Pralatrexate	LASA risk amplified by dosing frequency differences and rescue therapy confusion	(Kaushal et al., 2001; The Institute for Safe Medication Practices (ISMP), 2024a)
–leucel/–gene	Cell- and gene-based immunotherapies (e.g., CAR-T therapies)	Tisagenlecleucel; Lisocabtagene maraleucel; Idecabtagene vicleucel	Emerging LASA cluster affecting labeling and chain-of-identity processes	(West Virginia University School of Pharmacy, 2021; World Health Organization, 2024)

The historical evolution of oncology therapeutics has been significantly accompanied by changes in drug-naming conventions, with progressive pharmacologic innovations introducing more complex patterns of linguistic forms that have unwittingly added to the risk of LASA medication errors. Early cytotoxic drugs, such as alkylating agents and antimetabolites, were introduced not only when handwritten prescriptions and few system controls were the norm but also when transcriptional and visual name confusion was a key cause of initial medication errors in chemotherapy (Grissinger et al., 2007; Schulmeister, 2006). With the increase in cancer treatment practices in the second half of the twentieth century, an increasing number of agents with structural and therapeutic similarity, including platinum compounds, vinca alkaloids, and others, were introduced into common clinical practice, which resulted in well-reported wrong-drug errors with serious and even fatal outcomes, especially when the drugs had orthographic similarity or were abbreviated during practice (Hicks et al., 2008; Schulmeister, 2006).

With the subsequent appearance of targeted therapeutics, such as monoclonal antibodies and tyrosine kinase inhibitors, in the early 2000s, the proliferation of comparable nonproprietary names significantly increased, increasing phonemic and visual overlap across the biological platform as well as the small-molecule platform and creating new prospects of LASA errors in very intricate medication-use frameworks. Oncology medication safety research evidence suggests that LASA vulnerability has remained constant for many decades, not because of the characteristics of any particular drug class but because of the dynamic process of changing naming conventions, increasing formularies, and shifting clinical systems within which high-risk medications are prescribed, prepared, and administered (Chotsampancharoen et al., 2016; Cohen, 2007b; Hicks et al., 2008; Kovacic & Chambers, 2011; Neuss et al., 2017).

By showing how oncology drug names originate from different therapeutic eras, Figure 3 illustrates the longitudinal relationship and highlights that LASA risk remains an ongoing safety issue that increases with pharmacologic and linguistic complexity rather than being confined to a specific generation of anticancer agents. This chronology shows how oncology drug names have changed over time alongside significant therapeutic advances and how the naming convention of any period of time spawned unique look-alike, sound-alike (LASA) medication errors (Cohen, 2007b; Kloth, 2002; Lambert et al., 2005; Neuss et al., 2017; Ranchon et al., 2011; Schulmeister, 2006).

- 1950–1970s (Cytotoxic Foundations): -mustine, -trexate, and -rubicin are the earliest classes of chemotherapeutic agents. Inadequate automation and manual orders frequently created transcriptional mix-ups that created the first recorded LASA events (Cohen et al., 2007; Grissinger et al., 2007; Schulmeister, 2006).

- 1980-1990s (Expansion of Alkylating and Antimetabolite Classes): Stems such as "platin" and "bine" were introduced; look-alike vial labels and handwritten abbreviations of the regimen were both common causes of wrong-drug errors (including the notoriously documented cisplatin-carboplatin and vinblastine-vincristine errors) (Grissinger, 2016; Neuss et al., 2017; Schulmeister, 2006; The Joint Commission, 2023).
- From 2000–2010 (Targeted-Therapy Revolution), mAb monoclonal antibodies and -nib kinase inhibitors, emerging during this period, caused a large number of similar-sounding names, which created cross-stem LASA risk across biologic and small-molecule platforms in much more complex medical-use systems (Kovacic & Chambers, 2011; Ocvirk et al., 2013).
- 2015-Present (Immunotherapy and Cell-Based Era): New names such as -leucel, -gene, -parib, and -cept are characterized by unprecedented mechanistic diversity, whereas they come with unintuitive and elongated, multimorphemic names that are difficult to visualize or pronounce. Increasing reliance on complex digital security measures such as computerized prescriber order entry (CPOE) controls and barcode verification is becoming standard for ensuring patient safety (West Virginia University School of Pharmacy, 2021; World Health Organization, 2024)

Figure 3. Oncology drug name stems evolution and the LASA-risk continuum (1950–2025)

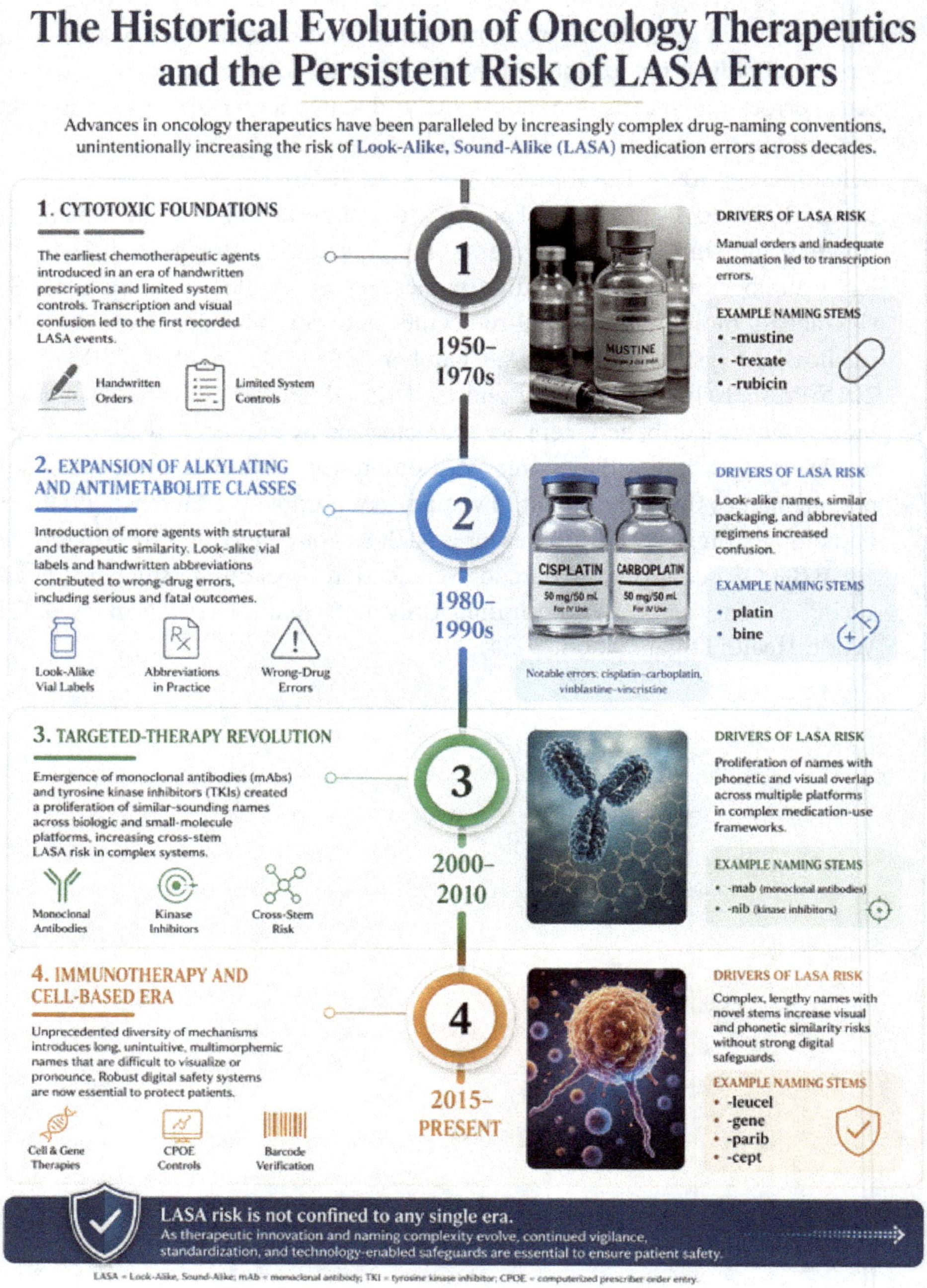

Collectively, these changes can be used to prove that LASA susceptibility is not confined to one or two generations of oncology agents but is a series of decades of pharmacologic development. The illustration highlights the idea that effective LASA error prevention should develop along with the rise of therapeutic and linguistic complexity (Neuss et al., 2017; Poon et al., 2010; Schulmeister, 2006; Schwappach & Wernli, 2010).

CONCLUSION

Oncology medication safety is a constantly evolving and dynamic phenomenon. Although progress in anticancer therapy has led to considerable improvements in patient outcomes, the complexity, toxicity, and narrow therapeutic index of these drugs, especially LASA drugs, remain highly vulnerable to medication error. Decades of evidence prove that LASA risk is long-term but can be prevented. The implementation of a multilayered defense mechanism involving the redesign of a system, digital protection, and human watchfulness is needed to minimize the effects of any threat or possible attack. The problem of safe medication in oncology is a joint concern for clinicians, leaders of health systems, and researchers, who must always be informed of the errors that have caused the problem and constantly change with the new treatments and nomenclature systems to protect patients in high-risk cancer care settings, particularly as these errors can lead to severe adverse effects and compromise patient safety.

REFERENCES

Ahuja, A., & Ahuja, V. (2024). LASA (Look alike sound alike) medicament errors-What a dental personnel needs to know? *Journal of Dental Panaceal*, *6*(3), 113–114. DOI: 10.18231/j.jdp.2024.023

American Society of Health-System Pharmacists (ASHP). (2018). *ASHP Guidelines on Preventing Medication Errors with Chemotherapy and Biotherapy*. Retrieved 14 Oct from https://www.ashp.org/-/media/assets/policy-guidelines/docs/guidelines/preventing-medication-errors-chemotherapy-biotherapy.pdf?utm

Bryan, R., Aronson, J. K., ten Hacken, P., Williams, A., & Jordan, S. (2015). Patient safety in medication nomenclature: Orthographic and semantic properties of International Nonproprietary Names. *PLoS One*, *10*(12), e0145431. DOI: 10.1371/journal.pone.0145431 PMID: 26701761

Bryan, R., Aronson, J. K., Williams, A., & Jordan, S. (2021a). The problem of look-alike, sound-alike name errors: Drivers and solutions. *British Journal of Clinical Pharmacology*, *87*(2), 386–394. DOI: 10.1111/bcp.14285 PMID: 32198938

Bryan, R., Aronson, J. K., Williams, A. J., & Jordan, S. (2021b). A systematic literature review of LASA error interventions. *British Journal of Clinical Pharmacology*, *87*(2), 336–351. DOI: 10.1111/bcp.14644 PMID: 33197079

Chanakit, T., Napaporn, J., Chiempattanakajohn, T., Sangkhawan, S., & Wichakot, S. (2013). The survey of look alike/sound alike (LASA) drugs available in hospitals in Thailand. *African Journal of Pharmacy and Pharmacology*, *7*(6), 227–239. DOI: 10.5897/AJPP11.812

Chotsampancharoen, T., Sripornsawan, P., & Wongchanchailert, M. (2016). Two Fatal Cases of Accidental Intrathecal Vincristine Administration: Learning from Death Events. *Chemotherapy*, *61*(2), 108–110. DOI: 10.1159/000441380 PMID: 26636546

Cohen, M. R. (2007a). Causes of medication errors. In Cohen, M. R. (Ed.), *Medication Errors* (2nd ed., pp. 55–66). The American Pharmacists Association. DOI: 10.21019/9781582120928.ch4

Cohen, M. R. (2007b). Preventing Medication Errors in Cancer Chemotherapy. In *Medication Errors* (2nd ed.). The American Pharmacists Association. DOI: 10.21019/9781582120928.ch16

Cohen, M. R., Domizio, G. D., & Lee, R. E. (2007). The role of drug names in medication errors. In Cohen, M. R. (Ed.), *Medication Errors* (2nd ed., pp. 87–110). The American Pharmacists Association. doi:10.21019/9781582120928.ch6

Cohen, M. R., & Smetzer, J. L. (2007). Preventing dispensing errors. In *Medication Errors* (2nd ed.). The American Pharmacists Association. DOI: 10.21019/9781582120928.ch10

Cohen, M. R., Smetzer, J. L., Westphal, J. E., Comden, S. C., & Horn, D. M. (2012). Risk models to improve safety of dispensing high-alert medications in community pharmacies. *Journal of the American Pharmacists Association, 52*(5), 584–602. DOI: 10.1331/JAPhA.2012.10145 PMID: 23023839

Donaldson, M. S., Corrigan, J. M., & Kohn, L. T. (2000). To err is human: building a safer health system.

DrugPatentWatch. (2025). *A Comprehensive Generic Drug Naming Resource: Decoding the Pharmaceutical Alphabet*. Retrieved 20 Oct from https://www.drugpatentwatch.com/blog/a-comprehensive-generic-drug-naming-resource/

Eiland, L. S., Benner, K., Gumpper, K. F., Heigham, M. K., Meyers, R., Pham, K., & Potts, A. L. (2018). ASHP-PPAG Guidelines for Providing Pediatric Pharmacy Services in Hospitals and Health Systems. *The Journal of Pediatric Pharmacology and Therapeutics, 23*(3), 177–191. DOI: 10.5863/1551-6776-23.3.177 PMID: 29970974

Elmzughi, R. F., Abuhasina, A., & Abdulsalam, O. (2025). Impact of Illegible Handwritten Prescriptions on Dispensing Errors: A Focus on Look-Alike Sound-Alike Medications in Libyan Community Pharmacies. *Journal of Pharmacy and Pharmacology, 7*(3), 73–82. https://doi.org/10.36349/easjpp.2025.v07i03.004

Fyhr, A., & Akselsson, R. (2012). Characteristics of medication errors with parenteral cytotoxic drugs. *European Journal of Cancer Care, 21*(5), 606–613. DOI: 10.1111/j.1365-2354.2012.01331.x PMID: 22335508

Gandhi, T. K., Bartel, S. B., Shulman, L. N., Verrier, D., Burdick, E., Cleary, A., Rothschild, J. M., Leape, L. L., & Bates, D. W. (2005). Medication safety in the ambulatory chemotherapy setting. *Cancer, 104*(11), 2477–2483. DOI: 10.1002/cncr.21442 PMID: 16245353

Grissinger, M. (2016). Death and Neurological Devastation From Intrathecal Vinca Alkaloids. *P&T : a Peer-Reviewed Journal for Formulary Management, 41*(8), 464–525. PMID: 27504060

Grissinger, M., Cohen, H., & Vaida, A. J. (2007). Using rechnology to prevent medication errors. In *Medication Errors* (2nd ed.). The American Pharmacists Association. DOI: 10.21019/9781582120928.ch15

Hicks, R., Becker, S., & Cousins, D. (2008). *MEDMARX data report. A report on the relationship of drug names and medication errors in response to the institute of Medicine's call for action.* Center for the Advancement of Patient Safey, US Pharmacopeia.

Institute for Safe Medication Practices Canada. (2015). *TALLman lettering for look-alike/sound-alike drug names in Canada.* Retrieved 11 Sep from https://www.ismp-canada.org/download/TALLman/TALLman_lettering.pdf

Institute of Medicine Committee on Quality of Health Care in America. (2000). To err is human: building a safer health system. In L. T. Kohn, J. M. Corrigan, & M. S. Donaldson (Eds.). National Academies Press (US). DOI: 10.17226/9728

ISMP News/ECRI. (2020). *Due to ISMP Advocacy, VinCRIStine Labeling and Packaging Changed to Prevent Wrong Route Administration.* Retrieved 5 Sep from https://home.ecri.org/blogs/ismp-news/due-to-ismp-advocacy-vincristine-labeling-and-packaging-changed-to-prevent-wrong-route-administration?

Joint Commission International. (2017). *Quick Safety Issue* 37: *Eliminating vincristine administration events*. Retrieved 5 Sep from https://www.jointcommission.org/en/knowledge-library/newsletters/quick-safety/issue-37?

Karet, G. B. (2019). How do drugs get named? *AMA Journal of Ethics*, *21*(8), E686–E696. DOI: 10.1001/amajethics.2019.686 PMID: 31397664

Karet, G. B. (2023). Linguistic analysis of generic-generic drug name pairs prone to wrong-drug errors for which tall-man lettering is recommended. *Therapeutic Innovation & Regulatory Science*, *57*(4), 751–758. DOI: 10.1007/s43441-023-00526-0 PMID: 37171707

Kaushal, R., Bates, D. W., Landrigan, C., McKenna, K. J., Clapp, M. D., Federico, F., & Goldmann, D. A. (2001). Medication Errors and Adverse Drug Events in Pediatric Inpatients. *Journal of the American Medical Association*, *285*(16), 2114–2120. DOI: 10.1001/jama.285.16.2114 PMID: 11311101

Kloth, D. D. (2002). Prevention of Chemotherapy Medication Errors. *Journal of Pharmacy Practice*, *15*(1), 17–31. DOI: 10.1106/EXK5-5F5M-T5QV-45CW

Kopp, B. J., Erstad, B. L., Allen, M. E., Theodorou, A. A., & Priestley, G. (2006). Medication errors and adverse drug events in an intensive care unit: Direct observation approach for detection. *Critical Care Medicine*, *34*(2), 415–425. DOI: 10.1097/01.CCM.0000198106.54306.D7 PMID: 16424723

Kovacic, L., & Chambers, C. (2011). Look-alike, sound-alike drugs in oncology. *Journal of Oncology Pharmacy Practice*, *17*(2), 104–118. DOI: 10.1177/1078155209354135 PMID: 20118216

Lambert, B. L., Lin, S.-J., & Tan, H. (2005). Designing Safe Drug Names. *Drug Safety*, *28*(6), 495–512. DOI: 10.2165/00002018-200528060-00003 PMID: 15924503

Lustig, A. (2000). Medication error prevention by pharmacists-An Israeli solution. *Pharmacy World & Science*, *22*(1), 21–25. DOI: 10.1023/A:1008774206261 PMID: 10815296

Markert, A., Thierry, V., Kleber, M., Behrens, M., & Engelhardt, M. (2009). Chemotherapy safety and severe adverse events in cancer patients: Strategies to efficiently avoid chemotherapy errors in in- and outpatient treatment. *International Journal of Cancer*, *124*(3), 722–728. DOI: 10.1002/ijc.23991 PMID: 18989899

Nagamotoo, Y., Lai, K., & Cavell, G. (2022). Measuring drug name similarity to prioritize the application of tall-man lettering in a computerized pharmacy dispensing system. *The International Journal of Pharmacy Practice*, *30*(S2), ii35–ii36. DOI: 10.1093/ijpp/riac089.041

Naseralallah, L., Stewart, D., Azfar Ali, R., & Paudyal, V. (2022). An umbrella review of systematic reviews on contributory factors to medication errors in health-care settings. *Expert Opinion on Drug Safety*, *21*(11), 1379–1399. DOI: 10.1080/14740338.2022.2147921 PMID: 36408597

National Coordinating Council for Medication Error Reporting and Prevention (NCC MERP). (2022). *Types of Medication Errors*. Retrieved 11 Oct from https://www.nccmerp.org/types-medication-errors

National Library of Medicine. (2025). *The DailyMed database* Retrieved 17 Sep from https://dailymed.nlm.nih.gov/dailymed/index.cfm

Nchinech, N., Benhasna, O., Achour, S., Elkartouti, A., Bousliman, Y., Lamsaouri, J., & Tadlaoui, Y. (2023). Medication Errors Related to Look Alike and Sound Alike Medications: About a Moroccan City University Hospital and Community Pharmacies Experience. *Sch Acad J Pharm*, *12*(12), 271–277. DOI: 10.36347/sajp.2023.v12i12.003

Neelakantan, M., Sharma, P., & Kulkarni, A. (2024). Look-alike, sound-alike (LASA) drugs in India. *The Lancet Regional Health. Southeast Asia*, *26*, 100425. DOI: 10.1016/j.lansea.2024.100425 PMID: 38798984

Neuss, M. N., Gilmore, T. R., Belderson, K. M., Billett, A. L., Conti-Kalchik, T., Harvey, B. E., Hendricks, C., LeFebvre, K., Mangu, P., McNiff, K., Olsen, M. K., Schulmeister, L., Von Gehr, A., & Polovich, M. (2017). 2016 Updated American Society of Clinical Oncology/Oncology Nursing Society Chemotherapy Administration Safety Standards, Including Standards for Pediatric Oncology. *Oncology Nursing Forum*, *44*(1), 31–43. DOI: 10.1188/17.ONF.31-43 PMID: 28067033

Noble, D. J., & Donaldson, L. J. (2010). The quest to eliminate intrathecal vincristine errors: A 40-year journey. *Quality & Safety in Health Care*, *19*(4), 323–326. DOI: 10.1136/qshc.2008.030874 PMID: 20211962

Ocvirk, J., Heeger, S., McCloud, P., & Hofheinz, R.-D. (2013). A review of the treatment options for skin rash induced by EGFR-targeted therapies: Evidence from randomized clinical trials and a metaanalysis. *Radiology and Oncology*, *47*(2), 166–175. DOI: 10.2478/raon-2013-0014 PMID: 23801914

Poon, E. G., Keohane, C. A., Yoon, C. S., Ditmore, M., Bane, A., Levtzion-Korach, O., Moniz, T., Rothschild, J. M., Kachalia, A. B., Hayes, J., Churchill, W. W., Lipsitz, S., Whittemore, A. D., Bates, D. W., & Gandhi, T. K. (2010). Effect of Bar-Code Technology on the Safety of Medication Administration. *The New England Journal of Medicine*, *362*(18), 1698–1707. DOI: 10.1056/NEJMsa0907115 PMID: 20445181

Pottier, J., Chastang, R., Dumet, C., & Watier, H. (2017). Rethinking the INN system for therapeutic antibodies. *mAbs*, *9*(1), 5–11. DOI: 10.1080/19420862.2016.1255520 PMID: 27808597

Ranchon, F., Salles, G., Späth, H. M., Schwiertz, V., Vantard, N., Parat, S., Broussais, F., You, B., Tartas, S., Souquet, P. J., Dussart, C., Falandry, C., Henin, E., Freyer, G., & Rioufol, C. (2011). Chemotherapeutic errors in hospitalized cancer patients: Attributable damage and extra costs. *BMC Cancer*, *11*(1), 478. DOI: 10.1186/1471-2407-11-478 PMID: 22067636

Reason, J. (2000). Human error: Models and management. *BMJ (Clinical Research Ed.)*, *320*(7237), 768–770. DOI: 10.1136/bmj.320.7237.768 PMID: 10720363

Schulmeister, L. (2006). Look-alike, sound-alike oncology medications. *Clinical Journal of Oncology Nursing*, *10*(1), 35–41. DOI: 10.1188/06.CJON.35-41 PMID: 16482726

Schwappach, D. L., & Wernli, M. (2010). Medication errors in chemotherapy: Incidence, types and involvement of patients in prevention. A review of the literature. *European Journal of Cancer Care*, *19*(3), 285–292. DOI: 10.1111/j.1365-2354.2009.01127.x PMID: 19708929

Supapaan, T. S., Songmuang, A., Napaporn, J., Sangsukwow, P., Boonrod, P., Intarapongsakul, P., Jaturapattarawong, A., & Pitchayajittipong, C. (2024). Look-alike/sound-alike medication errors: An in-depth examination through a hospital case study. *Pharmacy Practice*, *22*(2), 1–13. DOI: 10.18549/PharmPract.2024.2.2959

The Institute for Safe Medication Practices (ISMP). (2023a). *FDA and ISMP lists of look-alike drug names with recommended tall man (mixed case) letters*. Retrieved 16 Apr from https://www.ismp.org/system/files/resources/2023-01/ISMP_Tallman_Letters_012523_MS5087%20%282%29.pdf

The Institute for Safe Medication Practices (ISMP). (2023b). *List of confused drug names*. Retrieved 16 Apr from https://www.ismp.org/recommendations/confused-drug-names-list

The Institute for Safe Medication Practices (ISMP). (2024a). *ISMP List of Confused Drug Names*. Retrieved 07 Sep from https://online.ecri.org/hubfs/ISMP/Resources/ISMP_ConfusedDrugNames.pdf

The Institute for Safe Medication Practices (ISMP). (2024b). *ISMP list of error-prone abbreviations, symbols, and dose designations*. Retrieved 12 April from https://www.ismp.org/recommendations/error-prone-abbreviations-list?check_logged_in=1

The Institute for Safe Medication Practices (ISMP). (2024c). ISMP list of high-alert medications in acute care settings. *ISMP An ECRI Affiliate*, *29*(1), 6.

The Joint Commission. (2023). *Quick Safety Issue* 37: *Eliminating vincristine administration events*. Retrieved 07 Sep from https://www.jointcommission.org/en-us/knowledge-library/newsletters/quick-safety/issue-37

Weingart, S. N., Toth, M., Sands, D. Z., Aronson, M. D., Davis, R. B., & Phillips, R. S. (2003). Physicians' decisions to override computerized drug alerts in primary care. *Archives of Internal Medicine*, *163*(21), 2625–2631. DOI: 10.1001/archinte.163.21.2625 PMID: 14638563

West Virginia University School of Pharmacy. (2021). *Idecabtagene vicleucel (ABECMA®) drug monograph*. Retrieved 29 Dec from https://pharmacy.wvu.edu/media/3385/abecma-monograph.pdf

World Health Organization. (2007). *The importance of pharmacovigilance: safety monitoring of medicinal products*. Retrieved 10 Sep from https://www.who.int/publications/i/item/10665-42493

World Health Organization. (2017). *Medication without harm.* Retrieved 10 Feb from https://www.who.int/initiatives/medication-without-harm

World Health Organization. (2023). *Medication safety for look-alike, sound-alike medicines.* World Health Organization. Retrieved 3 June from https://iris.who.int/bitstream/handle/10665/373495/9789240058897-eng.pdf?sequence=1

World Health Organization. (2024). *Use of stems in the selection of International Nonproprietary Names (INN) for pharmaceutical substances.* World Health Organization. (Original work published 2024)

Wu, A. W. (2000). Medical error: the second victim. *The doctor who makes the mistake needs help too*, 320(7237), 726-727. DOI: 10.1136/bmj.320.7237.726

ABBREVIATIONS

CAR-T: Chimeric Antigen Receptor T-cell Therapy
CDS: Clinical Decision Support
CPOE: Computerized Provider Order Entry
IV: Intravenous
ISMP: Institute for Safe Medication Practices
LASA: Look-Alike, Sound-Alike
MTX: Methotrexate
PO: Oral Administration
TKI: Tyrosine Kinase Inhibitor
WHO: World Health Organization

Chapter 7
Clinical Consequences of Look-Alike, Sound-Alike Medication Errors

ABSTRACT

Look-Alike, Sound-Alike (LASA) medication errors are one of the preventable causes of patient harm on the global level. This chapter discusses the possible LASA mistakes and clinical outcomes, pointing out that it may cause harm both due to improper administration of the drug and due to the lack of treatment of the targeted disorder. It explains a continuum of consequences including treatment failure and mild adverse effects, hospitalization, irreversible harm, and death based upon real-world case scenarios and reports of patient-safety. The most critical impacts are high-alert medicines and drugs of narrow therapeutic index where minor selection or dosing mistakes can easily result into lethal choices. Other psychological and system-level effects not related to direct clinical damage are also emphasized in the chapter.

INTRODUCTION

Medication errors represent among the most frequent sources of avoidable harm in healthcare globally and are omnipresent, costly, and cross-border burdens in all types of clinical settings. One particularly challenging kind of mistake arises from the mix-up of look-alike, sound-alike (LASA) drugs. It is easy to dismiss these as simple typos or careless errors, but they are indicative of deeper, more systemic issues with the way that the systems support our healthcare work. The pair of drug names are so close in their visual and oral appearance that only one mistaken selec-

DOI: 10.4018/979-8-3373-5478-1.ch007

tion can be presented in a decision cascade chain with severe and sometimes fatal effects (World Health Organization, 2023).

In combination with complex modern drug formularies and the fast-paced, high-stress environment in which healthcare providers work, you have the perfect storm for these mistakes. The issue is not just about a "single point of failure" but an intricate concertina of human error, technical shortcomings, and fundamentally defective processes. A LASA mistake may occur at many points and involve various role players, such as a doctor's barely legible handwriting in the prescription, an oversight by the pharmacist during the hasty filling stage, or a nurse's distractive action at the bedside of the patient. Moreover, the puzzle is made more confusing by the lack of uniform packaging, labels that all look alike, and pressure on clinicians to move quickly.

These mistakes have a significant clinical impact on patients, ranging from minor issues that provide no assistance to catastrophic, fatal consequences. By recognizing the harm and obtaining a better picture of how a system can breakdown, we can begin to divert our attention from blaming individuals and toward creating a safer environment for everyone to receive care. The following analysis will deconstruct LASA errors; it goes beyond hearing about an incident to dissect the depth of the associated clinical effects and the systemic flaws that make them causal (Cohen & Smetzer, 2007; Leape, 2007; Leape et al., 1995).

Objectives of the Chapter

The aims of this chapter are as follows:

(1) To introduce LASA medication errors as a systems-level patient-safety problem and explain why they occur across the medication-use process.
(2) To describe the spectrum of LASA-related clinical harm—from treatment failure to severe injury and death—and link severity to the NCC MERP framework.
(3) To illustrate real-world LASA consequences through selected case studies across high-risk drug pairs.
(4) To examine impacts beyond clinical harm, including psychological effects on patients/families and clinicians, and economic/system-level burden.
(5) To define practical prevention roles for patients and caregivers, particularly in transitions of care and outpatient/home medication use.
(6) To explain how reporting and pharmacovigilance systems detect LASA signals and inform risk-reduction actions.

Organization of the Chapter

Chapter 7 starts with an introduction to LASA medication errors as a patient safety problem at the system level. It describes a continuum of clinical harm and shows LASA outcomes to the NCC MERP severity index. The chapter then presents several case studies illustrating the actual consequences of LASA errors, followed by a discussion of their effects beyond clinical harm, including psychological and economic impacts at the system level. The next point of the chapter is the prevention roles of patients and caregivers, and the conclusion point is an explanation of how reporting and pharmacovigilance systems contribute to the risk prevention of LASA and safer practices.

SPECTRUM OF CLINICAL HARM

LASA medication errors have varying clinical significance depending on the drugs involved, patient vulnerability, and the promptness with which the error is detected. LASA-related harm can be conceptualized as a graded spectrum from mild therapeutic failure to catastrophic injury or death (**Figure 1**). All stages of damage manifest different clinical pathways and vulnerabilities in the system, which highlights the importance of risk-stratified prevention measures.

Figure 1. LASA error harm spectrum

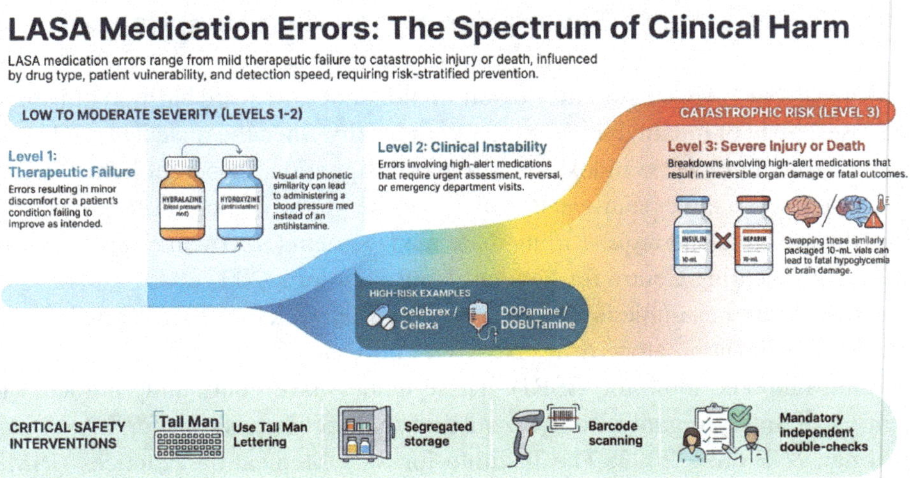

This figure shows conceptual demonstrations of the increasing clinical outcomes of LASA medication errors, including mild (therapeutic failure and minor discomfort), moderate (hospitalization and clinical instability), and severe injury or death with irreversible organ damage.

Level 1: Failure of Treatment and Mild Adverse Effects

On the mild end of the spectrum, there may be a LASA error that results in therapeutic failure, meaning that the patient's condition did not improve to the expected or intended level; minor adverse events that cause slight discomfort but do not cause permanent injury. These errors often occur when a pair of LASA drugs, which are from different drug classes and have names that resemble each other, are confused. A key LASA risk example is hydralazine, an antihypertensive agent, and hydroxyzine, an antihistamine. The resemblance of their names is visually and phonetically misleading, particularly when these drugs appear near one another in dispensing systems and when written in lists (Cohen, 2020; ISMP, 2016; The Institute for Safe Medication Practices (ISMP), 2015, 2023). In one reported case, a patient developed hypotensive symptoms after receiving hydralazine instead of hydroxyzine because of a medication dispensing error, which was later identified during an emergency department visit (The Institute for Safe Medication Practices (ISMP), 2016). These cases reflect instances where harm from LASA is more than just toxicity following the administration of the wrong drug and includes harm from the failure to treat (Abrishami et al., 2024).

Level 2: Moderate to Severe Harm, Including Hospitalization

More severe LASA errors may result in moderate-to-severe harm, requiring urgent assessment or inpatient management, especially when the mistaken medication has a narrow therapeutic index, a high-alert designation, or potent hemodynamic effects. These mistakes can cause patients to be slightly uncomfortable and feel clinically unstable and require immediate management (Hoffman & Proulx, 2003; WHO Collaborating Centre for Patient Safety Solutions, 2007).

A well-known example is the confusion between Celebrex® (celecoxib, a nonsteroidal anti-inflammatory drug, NSAID) and Celexa® (citalopram, a selective serotonin reuptake inhibitor, SSRI). These names have continually attracted the attention of safety organizations because of their predisposition for LASA error (Hoffman & Proulx, 2003; The Institute for Safe Medication Practices (ISMP), 2024). A patient expecting Celebrex®, who is administered Celexa®, could experience uncontrolled pain and, when mixed with other serotonergic agents, a greater risk of serotonin toxicity (Hoffman & Proulx, 2003).

On the other hand, if the prescribed drug is Celexa® and Celebrex® is the drug that was actually handed out, the patient—especially if it is an elderly patient or a patient with comorbidities—may experience known adverse events as a result of being treated with an NSAID, such as renal insufficiency or cardiovascular events (Hoffman & Proulx, 2003; WHO Collaborating Centre for Patient Safety Solutions, 2007). Another high-risk duo in the acute care setting is dopamine (a vasopressor) and dobutamine (mainly an inotrope). They also LASA, and they are often prescribed under time pressures in hemodynamically unstable patients, a situation that increases the likelihood of LASA errors.

The FDA/ISMP tall man lettering separates DOBUTamine and DOPamine in all capital letters because of continuing postmarketing confusion (ISMP, 2016; The Institute for Safe Medication Practices (ISMP), 2024; U.S. Department of Health and Human Services Food and Drug Administration (FDA), 2020). Misadministering either agent in the reverse direction could result in safety risks: giving dobutamine instead of dopamine could worsen hypotension, resulting in insufficient vasoconstriction, while administering dopamine in place of dobutamine could provoke tachyarrhythmias and increase afterload, reducing cardiac output in certain types of shock (Grissinger, 2012; ISMP, 2016; U.S. Department of Health and Human Services Food and Drug Administration (FDA), 2020). These examples represent how LASA errors, even those of Tier-2 severity, can cascade rapidly to emergency department presentations or intensive care unit (ICU) admissions, frequently requiring reversal, observation, and occasionally transfusion or vasopressor support (Hoffman & Proulx, 2003; WHO Collaborating Centre for Patient Safety Solutions, 2007).

Level 3: Severe Injury and Death

The most serious outcomes of LASA incidents include patient harm/death, which is commonly associated with high-alert medications that can result in serious harm or death if used incorrectly. These mistakes are all examples of avoidable yet devastating breakdowns in medication safety. The risk of potentially fatal LASA arises from the use of heparin, an anticoagulant, and insulin, which are hypoglycemic agents, especially since they are packaged in similar 10-mL vials, their dosing units are drawn similarly, and they are frequently stored adjacent to one another in treatment settings. Error reports published in the literature describe several deaths due to neonatal total parenteral nutrition (TPN) solutions in which insulin was added instead of heparin being administered to central line catheters receiving a flush of insulin rather than heparin (Cohen, 2007; Grissinger, 2011).

Consequences included severe hypoglycemia of the sort in which blood glucose in a premature infant fell to 17 mg/dL, seizures, coma, irreparable brain damage and death, and fatal bleeding when heparin was given rather than insulin. Similar cases have also been reported previously. Cohen (1991) described pharmacy admixture errors in which the pharmacists added 200 units and 1,000 units of insulin instead of heparin to TPN solutions with subsequent severe hypoglycemia (Cohen, 1991). In their efforts to minimize this potential for error, the ISMP and state patient safety reporting programs recommend segregated storage and employing prefilled syringes or pen devices; checking doses through barcode scanning; and enforcing mandatory independent doublechecking when preparing IV admixtures or TPN solutions. Some institutions have moved away from adding insulin to TPN and are now providing it as a separate infusion to minimize confusion (Grissinger, 2011).

LASA ERROR CLASSIFICATION ACCORDING TO NCC MERP CATEGORIES

To understand the significance of LASA errors, it is important to correlate these errors with the National Coordinating Council for Medication Error Reporting and Prevention (NCC MERP) Index. This classification separates errors from Category A (error with little potential for harming a patient) to Category I (error that causes a patient's death). Applying LASA events to this framework helps visualize how a LASA event is not just somewhere a mistake goes wrong but is instead a spectrum of harm from close calls to mortality. MedMARX demonstrates the association of LASA errors with the NCC MERP Index of Severity, ranging from near misses to death. These cases highlight the need to report, monitor, and apply responses and interventions according to the severity of the errors (Hicks et al., 2008). **Table 1** shows examples of LASA cases identified from MedMARX 2008 according to NCC MERP levels (A–I). In the case of a paired-drug combination, it can be a single episode of confusion, and it can result in different levels of harm, depending on the effect.

Table 1. Examples of LASA cases associated with medication errors from MedMARX 2008

Category	Definition	MedMARX LASA Examples
A – Potential for error	Circumstances with capacity to cause error, but no error occurred.	*Ampicillin vs. Amoxicillin* *Atropine vs. Apresoline*
B – Error, Did not reach patient	An error occurred but was caught before reaching patient.	*Glyburide and Metformin vs. Glipizide and Metformin* *Haloperidol vs. Hydralazine*
C – Error, No harm	Error reached patient but caused no harm, no intervention needed.	*Granisetron vs. Ondansetron (Category C-D)* *Glutamine vs. Galantamine (Category C-D)*
D – Error, Monitoring needed	Error reached patient; monitoring is required to confirm no harm.	*Apresoline vs. Aldactone (Category C-D)* *Levetiracetam vs. Levofloxacin (Category C-D)*
E – Temporary harm, intervention needed	Error contributed to temporary harm and required treatment.	*Methotrexate vs. Minoxidil (Category E-H)* *Morphine Sulfate vs. Meperidine (Category B, C-D, E-H)*
F – Temporary harm, Hospitalization	Error caused harm requiring initial or prolonged hospitalization.	*Niacin vs. Niacinamide (Category B, E-H)* *Infliximab vs. Rituximab (Category B, C-D, E-H)*
G – Permanent harm	Error caused permanent patient harm.	*Isosorbide Dinitrate vs. Isosorbide Mononitrate (Category A, B, C-D, E-H)* *Lamivudine vs. Efavirenz (Category B, E-H)*
H – Life-sustaining intervention	Error required life-saving intervention.	*Lamotrigine vs. Labetalol (Category A, B, C-D, E-H)* *Lansoprazole vs. Omeprazole (Category A, B, C-D, E-H)*
I – Death	Error caused patient death.	*Phenobarbital vs. Phenytoin Sodium (Category B, C-D, E-H, I)* *Glimepiride vs. Galantamine (Category A, B, C-D, E-H, I)*

(Hicks et al., 2008)

CHOSEN CASE STUDIES WITH DEMONSTRATION OF THE EFFECT OF LASA MEDICATION ERRORS

Even though most LASA risks are now proactively identified by means of name review and safety screening, the postmarketing experience indicates that confusion still occurs in clinical practice. The examples below, which are based on peer-reviewed sources and regulatory safety reports, demonstrate how LASA errors have appeared in real-life scenarios and provide opportunities to enhance medication safety at the system level.

1. Avandia® (rosiglitazone) and Coumadin® (warfarin)

The risk of LASA errors has been described in patient safety surveillance systems in which handwritten orders, verbal orders, and familiarity bias with commonly used drug names have been associated with confusion between the oral antidiabetic agent rosiglitazone (Avandia®) and the oral anticoagulant warfarin (Coumadin®). The clinical outcomes of these mistakes are two-way and could be critical. Note that the unwarranted prescription of warfarin rather than rosiglitazone will lead to unintended anticoagulation without proper tracking, and patients are at risk of major bleeding incidents, such as gastrointestinal or intracranial bleeding.

On the other hand, avoiding warfarin treatment by replacing it with rosiglitazone could put patients at risk of thromboembolism, including stroke or venous thromboembolism. These consequences are heightened by the fact that warfarin has a small therapeutic index and needs frequent follow-ups of the international normalized ratio (INR) level, which are well-known determinants of anticoagulant-related morbidity in clinics (Gaunt, 2007; Holbrook et al., 2012; Institute for Safe Medication Practices (ISMP), 2015; Senior Care Consultant Group (SCCG), 2006).

2. Cerebyx® (Fosphenytoin), Celexa® (Citalopram), and Celebrex® (Celecoxib)

The three-way LASA cluster of Cerebyx® (Fosphenytoin), Celexa® (Citalopram), and Celebrex® (Celecoxib) represents the potential of phonetic and orthographic similarity between therapeutic classes to cause clinically significant medication errors. Misunderstanding of these brand names has been specifically reported in patient safety studies of drug name-related errors, which have found Celebrex®, Celexa®, and Cerebyx® to be classic examples of proprietary names that could be confused, especially when poor handwriting, verbal order, and bias in clinical familiarity were involved (Hoffman & Proulx, 2003; Senior Care Consultant Group (SCCG), 2006).

Clinical outcomes of such errors are determined by the kind of medication that is missed or wrongly given. When celecoxib or citalopram is substituted with fosphenytoin, failure to control seizures or breakthrough seizures may ensue, and the reverse is also true; using fosphenytoin instead of an antidepressant or anti-inflammatory agent will expose patients to unwarranted adverse effects such as central nervous system depression, cardiac conduction abnormalities, or hypotension. Additionally, failing to use an effective analgesic or antidepressant can result in the loss of pain control or worsening mental status. All these effects are in line with the known pharmacologic effects and safety profiles of antiepileptic agents, selective serotonin reuptake inhibitors, and nonsteroidal anti-inflammatory agents (Hoffman & Proulx, 2003; Perucca & Gilliam, 2012).

3. Clonidine and Clonazepam (Klonopin®)

Misinterpretation of clonidine, a centrally acting α2-adrenergic agonist that is administered to treat hypertension and specific neuropsychiatric conditions, and clonazepam (Klonopin®), a benzodiazepine that is used to treat seizure disorders and anxiety, is a clinically important LASA drug. The Joint Commission specifically sets this duo as a problem because the generic name clonidine is easily mixed with the trade name or generic name clonazepam, especially in health care settings where handwritten or oral orders are utilized. In addition to the regulatory issue, first-hand clinical experience of injury that follows clonidine-clonazepam confusion has been reported.

In one published letter to the editor in the Journal of Clinical Psychopharmacology, a patient admitted to the hospital was accidentally exposed to clonazepam instead of clonidine, and his clinical condition showed significant bradycardia, hypotension, and anaerobic behavior, necessitating immediate clinical intervention. Dispensing errors took place during the dispensing phase, and the patient swallowed two doses of the incorrect drug, which shows how LASA types of errors can spread to the stage of repeated dose taking before they are detected.

Clinically, the effects of this pair of LASA are directional in terms of their pharmacologic effects. Accidental intake of clonazepam can result in oversedation, respiratory depression, bradycardia, and hypotension, especially when other drugs that exert central or cardiovascular effects are used. On the other hand, the omission or substitution of clonidine can lead to a loss of blood pressure and even a rebound in hypertension among chronic users in the case of sudden withdrawal. These processes demonstrate the seriousness of the consequences that are presented in a case (Gutierrez et al., 1991). The identified system factors are phonetic similarity, overlapping dosage strength, and proximal storage of medications, all of which are in line with known LASA error mechanisms. As a reaction, the Joint Commission suggests a series of general LASA risk-reduction recommendations to this pair, such as the explicit use of brand and generic names, adequate documentation of medication indication, and the avoidance of verbal orders where possible, as well as wider system-wide provisions that involve computerized prescribing and independent double checks (Senior Care Consultant Group (SCCG), 2006).

4. Cisplatin and Carboplatin

Misidentification of cisplatin and carboplatin is an example of a high-risk look-alike, sound-alike (LASA) oncology medication error that is caused by a combination of high orthographic and phonetic similarity and shared clinical application. These chemotherapeutic agents, which are made of platinum, are not dose interchangeable and vary greatly in terms of different dosing regimens and supportive care needs. Carboplatin doses that are safe often go beyond the maximum safe dose of cisplatin, which presents a severe risk in situations where the name or product is selected incorrectly.

A case report on a landmark case revealed an unimaginable mistake that took place: A woman who was 68 years old was given an enormous dose of cisplatin after being accidentally given carboplatin but without the intensive intravenous hydration needed by cisplatin therapy (Chu et al., 1993). The patient developed extreme systemic toxicity, such as intense emesis, myelosuppression, acute renal failure, and permanent hearing loss. Other toxicities, including seizures, hallucinations, visual loss, and hepatic dysfunction, were present and were explained by the exceptionally high dose. The extraordinarily high concentrations of systemic platinum and plasma platinum were verified to be greater than 2,900 ng/mL and showed lasting cellular effects even 19 days after exposure, which was evidence of the long-term biological action of cisplatin.

Aggressive multimodal intervention is needed for management. Plasmapheresis significantly decreased the levels of circulating platinum and sustained hydration, despite end-stage renal failure, increasing the level of urinary platinum excretion. Treatment with granulocyte–macrophage colony-stimulating factor (GM-CSF) was used to treat severe myelosuppression. Eventually, the patient required renal transplantation from a monozygotic twin and survived, but they were permanently deaf and had no other significant residual deficits. The cisplatin-carboplatin pair represents a significant LASA risk within the system, since cisplatin doses over 100 mg/kg every 3–4 weeks are almost never safe and must prompt immediate warnings. Its LASA consequence guidance points to the fact that name mix-ups in chemotherapy may lead to serious or potentially deadly harm and proposes strong protection, such as maximum-dose warnings in computerized prescribing systems, physical isolation of look-alike agents, and use of the full generic name without abbreviations when the prescription is being made (Chu et al., 1993; Senior Care Consultant Group (SCCG), 2006)

5. Depo-Medrol® (methylprednisolone acetate) and Depo-ProVera® (medroxyprogesterone acetate)

There have been numerous recorded cases of confusion between injectable products with the prefix Depo- and Depo-Medrol® (methylprednisolone acetate) and Depo-ProVera® (medroxyprogesterone acetate). A case narrative published through the Institute of Safe Medication Practices (ISMP) discusses a 44-year-old man who was intraarticularly injected with Depo-ProVera rather than Depo-Medrol because of shoulder pain. The mistake occurred when a drug and its administration were chosen and was triggered by the procedure of storing and binning, which made the two products close to each other and resulted in a lack of verification before administration.

The clinical outcome recorded in this case involved exposure to inappropriate hormones and failure to take planned corticosteroid therapy. In addition to this narrative report, ISMP research based on reports received in The FDA Adverse Event Reporting System (FAERS) and the ISMP Medication Error Reporting Program revealed several similar cases in healthcare, such as reverse mix-ups, which led to contraceptive failure or untimely treatment. The similarity in names, injectable formulations, and storage habits exemplified in this LASA pair highlights the possibility of convergence to overcome traditional safety boundaries (Institute for Safe Medication Practices (ISMP), 2016; U.S. Department of Health and Human Services Food and Drug Administration, 2016).

6. Ephedrine and Epinephrine

Confusion between ephedrine and epinephrine, also known as adrenaline, is a well-known high-risk LASA medication error, particularly in obstetric and perioperative care. Patient safety reports have highlighted that these two medications seem to be similar in terms of name and that their clinical application in the management of hypotension is likely to be combined, particularly in labor and delivery units. The fact that both agents are usually provided in a similar format, i.e., 1 mL amber ampules and vials (**Figure 2**), further exacerbates this risk, thus increasing the chance of selection errors in cases of urgent clinical situations.

Although ephedrine and epinephrine have only superficial similarities, ephedrine and epinephrine have significant differences in terms of their pharmacologic potency and receptor selectivity (Senior Care Consultant Group (SCCG), 2006). Epinephrine is an α- and β-adrenergic agonist, whereas ephedrine stimulates sympathetic effects (both direct and indirect). Therefore, unintended use of epinephrine instead of ephedrine can cause excessive vasoconstriction, extremely high blood pressure, tachyarrhythmia, heart attack, heart ischemia, or pulmonary edema, whereas the use of ephedrine instead of epinephrine may cause an insufficient response to hypotension or anaphylaxis and thereby postpone life-saving treatment. Such negative conditions fit into the known cardiovascular risks of improper dosing of epinephrine and are well supported in the clinical literature (Brown, 2004; Kemp et al., 2008).

Figure 2. Ephedrine and epinephrine (adrenaline) appear similar in appearance

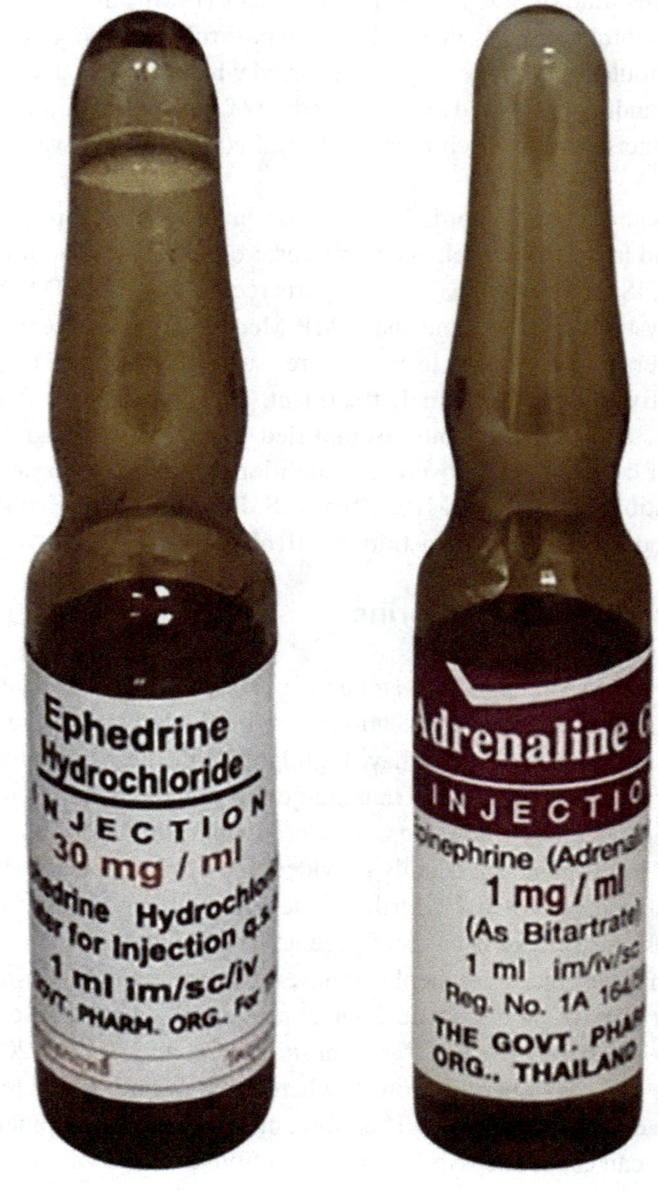

7. Fentany and Sufentanil

Sufentanil and fentanyl are powerful synthetic opioid medications utilized in anesthesia and critical care, but these are not interchangeable. The efficacy of sufentanil is 5–10 times stronger than that of fentanyl; i.e., any mistake in selection or dosing may easily cause opioid toxicity. Pharmacologic research has reported that the respiratory depression caused by sufentanil is dose dependent and progresses to respiratory arrest and that this effect is reversible by naloxone. This process is consistent with the well-known opioid toxicology, whereby activation of μ-opioid receptors inhibits central respiratory drive and is the main factor leading to morbidity and mortality caused by opioids. (Ghelardini et al., 2015; Wang et al., 2022).

Patient safety reports have shown that LASA confusion of fentanyl and sufentanil leads to respiratory arrest, especially when sufentanil is accidentally administered instead of fentanyl and most commonly during fentanyl shortages, when substitution is unaccompanied by a suitable increase or decrease in the dose. The potential occurrence of such errors is further increased when both agents are stored close to each other, particularly in pharmacy or anesthesia supply areas, or when sufentanil is not stored in operating room (OR) or postanesthesia care unit (PACU) settings, where familiarity with its increased potency may be limited. Unintentional substitution may lead to hypoventilation, deep hypoxia, naloxone rescue, prolonged mechanical ventilation, or death; therefore, the importance of the role of strict separation in storing and limited stocking as a prevention measure is paramount (Ghelardini et al., 2015; Huang et al., 2024; Senior Care Consultant Group (SCCG), 2006).

8. Foradil® (formoterol) and Toradol® (ketorolac)

Regulatory documentation from the U.S. Food and Drug Administration (FDA) confirms that medication error reports on confusion of Foradil® (formoterol), a long-acting bronchodilator, and Toradol® (ketorolac), a nonsteroidal anti-inflammatory drug, occurred. These mistakes were detected during proprietary name examination and in postmarketing oversight, which shows that misinterpretation indicates practical medication faults in the real world and not hypothetical danger. Even though there is no description of patient-specific clinical outcomes in the FDA summaries, the errors are clinically significant, as they are omissions of necessary bronchodilator therapy and unintended exposure to NSAIDs. In patients with asthma or those with chronic obstructive pulmonary disease, the inability to take bronchodilators may negatively affect the ability to control symptoms, whereas the use of inappropriate ketorolac can increase the risk of NSAID toxicity, such as gastrointestinal and renal side effects. This illustration highlights the importance of regulatory name review as a medication safety tool, as well as how residual LASA risk may also persist despite a drug being approved on the market (Center for Drug Evaluation and Research (CDER), 2000, 2006).

9. Lamictal® (lamotrigine) and Lamisil® (terbinafine)

Lamictal® (lamotrigine), an antiepileptic, and Lamisil® (terbinafine), an antifungal medication, have been reported as the subject of confirmed medication error reports because of name similarity. Surveillance-enabled analyses of reported errors have revealed examples of dispensing terbinafine rather than lamotrigine, which are due mainly to the orthographic similarity between the proprietary names. Although such reports do not always present patient-specific clinical outcomes, the error is a loss of antiepileptic therapy, which is clinically significant in the management of epilepsy. The literature on epilepsy and regulatory agencies emphasizes that the discontinuation or absence of lamotrigine can lead to breakthrough seizures and clusters of seizures and explains how delays in discovering an error can cause serious harm to chronic neurologic drugs (Hoffman & Proulx, 2003; Sullivan; The Institute for Safe Medication Practices (ISMP) Canada, 2001).

10. Mercaptamine (cysteamine) and Mercaptopurine

Mercaptamine (synonymous with cysteamine) and mercaptopurine are associated with one of the clinically significant LASA drug risks of high orthographic and phonetic similarity with very different indications to use. Mercaptamine is used to treat nephropathic cystinosis, whereas mercaptopurine is a cytotoxic antimetabolite that is mainly used to treat acute leukemia and other malignant or immune-mediated diseases (Medicines and Healthcare products Regulatory Agency (MHRA), 2014; Therapeutic Goods Administration, 2016).

There have been reported real-world injuries that have been caused by this name confusion as prescribed by regulatory safety alerts. One such case involved a 9-month-old child with nephropathic cystinosis who was mistakenly prescribed mercaptopurine rather than mercaptamine in primary care. One month later, the child was admitted to a hospital with pancytopenia due to incorrect therapy, which was taken for approximately one month, which is evidence of the serious negative consequences that may arise in the case of a high-risk LASA substitution. The patient was eventually cured after the discontinuation of the wrong medicine and proper care, but the case highlights how dangerous the risk can be (MHRA, 2010).

Nomenclaturewise, the example of this drug pair is that even minor differences in prefixes (e.g., mercap-) and minimal dissimilarity at the letter level make LASA errors more prone to occur, especially when drugs are prescribed manually, when an order is being typed, and when they are communicating via words. The analysis of the linguistic properties of the International Nonproprietary Names has presented mercaptamine-mercaptopurine as a typical example of LASA susceptibility based on the orthographic similarity in place of pharmacological relatedness, which supports the need to create system-wide protection that cannot be limited to the familiarity of the clinician In reaction to this, regulatory bodies suggest increased vigilance in the prescription of these agents, such as explicit indication documentation, the prevention of using abbreviations, and the introduction of electronic prescribing alerts that distinguish the two names at the order entry point. They are aligned with general patient safety models expected to compel healthcare organizations to actively detect high-risk LASA drug pairs and introduce specific measures to avert accidental interchange and patient injury (Bryan et al., 2015; Bryan et al., 2021a; Medicines and Healthcare products Regulatory Agency (MHRA), 2014; Therapeutic Goods Administration, 2016).

11. Morphine and Hydromorphone

The risk of a high LASA mistake in medication in this case was confusion between morphine and hydromorphone, which are not interchangeable opioid injections. The LASA consequence appendix of the Joint Commission explicitly records that there has been a misconception in some quarters of the clinicians that hydromorphone is the generic counterpart of morphine and that fatal mistakes have occurred when hydromorphone was taken to be morphine, especially when the products were stored together and in similar strength; the LASA consequence appendix has further indicated that such confusion has led to incidences of respiratory arrest that can be explained by the difference in potency.

In addition to this safety signal, a review article summarizing the reports provided by the Pennsylvania Patient Safety Reporting System (PA-PSRS) reports that 32% of the opiate/narcotic look-alike name reports were morphine and hydromorphone and that a portion of the events involving this combination proved to be fatal, with contributing factors of the consistent misconception of generic equivalence and the fact that the two drugs are available in 1, 2, and 4 mg/mL prefilled syringes. Although research on the epidemiologic outcomes does not identify LASA name confusion as the causal pathway, the data from the hospital population prove that patients who were administered hydromorphone had a higher rate of naloxone rescue use (as an adverse event measure) and higher 30-day all-cause readmission rates than patients who received morphine did, which highlights the low harm threshold when hydromorphone is used in inpatient care. A combination of these pieces of evidence makes system-level controls on this LASA-vulnerable opioid pair, such as tall man lettering, physical segregation, uniform concentrations, and mandatory independent checks, a priority (Grissinger, 2008; Gulur et al., 2015; Rahman & Parvin, 2015; Senior Care Consultant Group (SCCG), 2006).

12. Navane® (thiothixene) and Norvasc® (amlodipine)

Drug name confusion at the outpatient level of pharmacy was an example of a well-documented look-alike, sound-alike medication error, where a 71-year-old female patient received the antipsychotic thiothixene (Navane®) instead of the antihypertensive amlodipine (Norvasc®) approximately three months by mistake because of the drug name mismatch (da Silva & Krishnamurthy, 2016). The mistake was not detected immediately, despite frequent contact with healthcare providers, and exposure to unwanted medication continued. In this case, the patient showed progressive physical and neuropsychiatric manifestations, such as tremor, impaired locomotion, bradykinesia, personality change, and mood alteration, which were eventually attributed to drug-induced parkinsonism as a result of taking thiothixene.

This case demonstrates that LASA-associated errors can go unnoticed and may be incorrectly attributed to underlying neurologic or psychiatric diseases; consequently, diagnostic overshadowing and the lack of medication reconciliation can lead to further patient harm. The literature on patient safety often refers to the incident as an example of how systemic weaknesses allow a single LASA mishap to spread through various phases of care (Palasuberniam et al., 2018).

13. Reminyl® (galantamine) and Amaryl® (glimepiride)

One of the most influential LASA cases in U.S. medication safety involved confusion between Reminyl® (galantamine), an acetylcholinesterase inhibitor for Alzheimer's disease, and Amaryl® (glimepiride), a sulfonylurea antidiabetic agent. Shortly after Reminyl entered the U.S. market, a published report reported that at least ten prescriptions intended for Reminyl were incorrectly dispensed as Amaryl, primarily at the pharmacy dispensing stage, because of the orthographic and phonetic similarity between the brand names.

These dispensing errors resulted in patients inadvertently receiving a hypoglycemic agent, leading to severe hypoglycemia and hypoglycemia-related complications, with at least one confirmed fatality; secondary safety reports have cited two deaths associated with this confusion. The seriousness of these outcomes prompted regulatory action, culminating in the U.S. brand name change of galantamine from Reminyl® to Razadyne®, representing a landmark example of postmarketing name change driven by patient safety concerns rather than pharmacologic issues (Center for Drug Evaluation and Research (CDER), 2004; Pharmacy Times, 2005; Reines, 2005; U.S. Department of Health and Human Services Food and Drug Administration, 2015).

14. Seroquel® (Quetiapine) and Serzone® (Nefazodone)

Seroquel® (quetiapine) and Serzone® (Nefazodone) have reported LASA medication errors in patient safety studies. In addition to the similarity of the names, the medicines are offered in the same tablet strengths (100 mg and 200 mg), similar dose ranges and instructions and are applicable in the same psychiatric clinical environment, which increases the danger of mistakes in selection and dispensing. Some of the reported effects include sedation or dizziness when Seroquel® was dispensed in place of Serzone® and decompensation or worsening of mental status when Serzone® was administered in place of Seroquel®.

Furthermore, nefazodone has a high possibility of severe drug interactions, with severe reactions and sometimes fatal effects reported upon the administration of drugs with pharmacologic properties similar to those of nefazodone alongside monoamine oxidase inhibitors. These results emphasize the potential for possible harm that can be caused by the combination of particular characteristics of name similarity, dosing overlap, and shared clinical use and emphasize the necessity of increased precautions in the prescription and dispensing of these agents (Institute for Safe Medication Practices (ISMP) Canada, 2002; Senior Care Consultant Group (SCCG), 2006; The Health and Disability Commissioner, 2003).

15. Taxol® (paclitaxel) and Taxotere® (docetaxel)

Taxol® (paclitaxel) and Taxotere® (docetaxel) are well-known LASA drugs used in oncology practice. These two are among the problematic drug names listed by the Joint Commission related to a risk of severe medication errors, since confusion is possible between paclitaxel and docetaxel, as they are administered differently yet are used in different types of cancer. This risk is further justified by the World Health Organization (WHO), which cites the use of LASA medication names as one of the leading causes of preventable medication errors across the globe. The WHO urges that the resemblance of drug names can cause unintentional replacement and unsuitable doses, particularly with high-alert drugs such as antineoplastic agents, and advises system-level interventions to mitigate confusion (WHO Collaborating Centre for Patient Safety Solutions, 2007). In line with these suggestions, the Joint Commission recommends that computerized prescribing systems should have a maximum-dose warning to alert the staff about the potential name mix-ups when they are entering orders and to avoid storing paclitaxel and docetaxel in close areas in the pharmacy and medication storage areas to reduce the occurrence of LASA-related chemotherapy errors (Schulmeister, 2006; Senior Care Consultant Group (SCCG), 2006).

16. Vinblastine and Vincristine

LASA name confusion of the similarity between vinblastine and vincristine, especially the administration of vincristine intravenously instead of vinblastine as the equivalent dose, has resulted in a number of fatal medication errors. Both agents are dosed differently, although they fall in the same category as the vinca alkaloid group. The maximum dosage of vincristine is typically approximately 1.4 mg/m^2 per week, but the dosage of vinblastine is less predictable, and in most adult patients, the range of the average dosage per week is approximately 5.5–7.4 mg/m^2. Misidentification of these agents in turn puts patients at a substantial risk of overdosing and has cost several people lives.

To reduce this LASA risk, patient safety experts suggest the use of maximum dose warnings in computerized and prescribing systems to help staff recognize a possible name mix-up when entering an order. Other system-level precautions involve not storing vinblastine and vincristine in close physical proximity, ensuring that all personnel involved with chemotherapy handling know the critical difference between these drugs and ensuring that the prescription is performed using the brand name or both the brand and generic names. These drug names should never be abbreviated to minimize the chances of misunderstanding and confusion (ISMP News/ECRI, 2020; Schulmeister, 2006; Senior Care Consultant Group (SCCG), 2006).

17. Zyprexa® (olanzapine) and Zyrtec® (cetirizine)

Zyprexa® (olanzapine) and Zyrtec® (cetirizine) are well-known look-alike/sound-alike (LASA) errors that have the potential to cause clinically significant harm. The Joint Commission includes this duo in the list of problematic drug names and provides a list of frequent confusion cases when patients who should receive Zyprexa receive Zyrtec instead and patients who should receive Zyprexa receive Zyrtec instead. An FDA/Eli Lilly communication, which states that there were prescribing/dispensing substitutions between olanzapine and cetirizine and that these substitutions can cause adverse events and possibly relapse in schizophrenia or bipolar disorder, is summarized. The report identifies contributory factors to similarities in the brand-name prefix "ZY," possible proximal storage, and similarities in dosage strength and once-a-day dosing (NBC News, 2005; The Associated Press, 2005; Waknine, 2005).

This LASA risk is also supported by regulatory documentation in the FDA Drugs@FDA archive, where an FDA approval letter of a supplement of changes being implemented says that Zyprexa bottle labels were changed to help minimize the possibility of medication errors involving Zyprexa and Zyrtec. The fact that this type of mix-up has been observed in reality within the context of actual clinical practice is also evidenced by the fact that a published set of patient-safety cases explicitly mentions one such scenario where a patient was given Zyprexa, rather than Zyrtec, by a pharmacy, as an example of how LASA confusion may spread to patients beyond the hospital oncology environment (Campbell & Sumner, 2005). In line with these sources, system-level controls, including but not limited to the separation of storage locations, not placing adjacent items on the selection screens, explicit written prescriptions (brand and generic), and strengthening of indication verification and patient counseling, should be considered as the priority of the prevention process, which is consistent with the Joint Commission's general recommendations of LASA risk mitigation (Senior Care Consultant Group (SCCG), 2006).

IMPACT OF LASA ERRORS BEYOND CLINICAL HARM

LASA medication errors can cause more than just direct clinical harm. LASA errors have cascading consequences that are not limited to patient injury and include the psychological distress of patients and families, second-victim effects on clinicians, and economic and organizational costs to healthcare systems in the form of resource consumption, incident investigations, and preventive measures, as shown in **Figure 3.**

Figure 3. LASA errors can have simultaneous, layered effects on patients, families, healthcare professionals, and healthcare systems

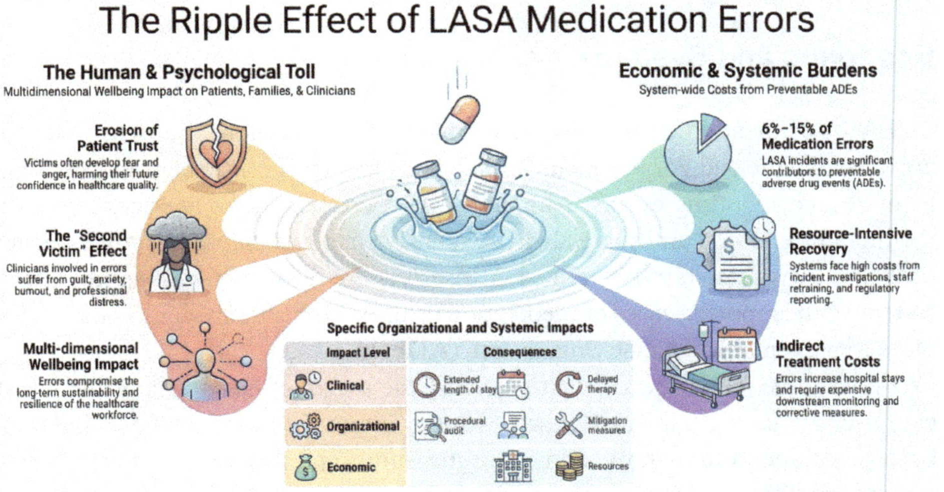

Psychological Impact

Patients and Families

Medication errors and patient safety studies have shown that patients who have been victims of avoidable medical errors often develop emotional distress, fear, and anger and lack trust. Incomplete or poor disclosure also contributes to psychological damage and harms future views on the quality of care and the desire to use healthcare systems (Gallagher et al., 2003; Mazor et al., 2004). Although LASA-specific psychological outcomes are not well studied, these findings may reasonably be extended to LASA events because these events are known to be preventable and have system-based causes.

Clinicians and Other Healthcare Workers

The second victim effect may manifest among clinicians who have been involved in LASA and other medication errors, and it may result in much emotional and professional distress. Empirical studies have revealed strong correlations with guilt, anxiety, sleep disturbance, lower job satisfaction, burnout, and professional reputation concerns. Distress is also reported after notably significant errors as well as near accidents, especially when the support of the organization is perceived as weak (Scott et al., 2009; Waterman et al., 2007). These findings suggest that LASA errors have a multidimensional impact on the well-being of patients, confidence in healthcare systems, and the sustainability and resilience of the healthcare workforce.

Economic and System-Level Impact

LASA medication errors cause economic and organizational burdens since they are an avoidable category of medication errors, and their presence is usually in the form of incorrect drug events. Although LASA cost estimates are not provided in the literature, LASA errors are always expensive and resource-consuming because of their downstream ramifications. LASA errors are responsible for approximately 6–15% of the reported cases of medication errors, making them significant contributors to preventable adverse drug events (ADEs).

Preventable ADEs are known to increase the length of hospital stay and healthcare use, indicating that LASA errors lead to increased treatment costs indirectly because of delays in therapy, corrective measures, and further monitoring. LASA errors at the system level result in additional costs in economic terms, investigations of incidents, retraining of staff, reporting of regulatory results, and mitigation measures, such as barcode medication administration, computerized prescribing, and medication-naming control. Since LASA errors are largely due to changes in system factors that can be managed, e.g., the nomenclature of drugs, labeling, and packaging look-alikes, as well as selection interfaces, their economic effects support the need to implement system-based prevention measures proactively (Bryan et al., 2015; Bryan et al., 2021a; Bryan et al., 2021b; Rodziewicz et al., 2023; World Health Organization, 2023).

THE ROLE OF THE PATIENT AND CAREGIVER IN PREVENTION

Patients and caregivers play a key role in preventing LASA medication errors, especially during changes in care and medication care given outside the health care setting. It has been shown that the lack of medication literacy and a preference to evaluate drugs on the basis of their physical appearance, such as the color of pills, their packaging, or the shape of the blisters, instead of using the medicine names can predispose them to the risk of LASA confusion (World Health Organization, 2023, 2024). Research has indicated that a significant proportion of patients cannot accurately name their drugs and rely on visual cues, which can be misleading in the case of medicine resemblance in terms of their appearance or name. Older adults, patients with polypharmacy, and those with limited health literacy are more susceptible to this type of vulnerability; therefore, caregivers play a vital role in safety (Davis et al., 2006; World Health Organization, 2023).

Involving patients and caregivers in medication safety—by stimulating them to be familiar with the name of the medicine, the cause of use, its strength, and the schedule of administration and asking about sudden changes in appearance by asking questions—has been shown to enhance the detection of errors and prevent unnecessary injuries. Active involvement of patients, such as dispensing and administration verification, is another safety measure of the medication use system. In line with this, patient and caregiver education, shared decision-making, and open communication with healthcare professionals are highlighted as the key measures to prevent LASA medication errors, especially at the community and home-care levels (World Health Organization, 2017, 2023).

Both patients and caregivers play important roles in the prevention of LASA medication errors, as shown in **Figure 4,** because they can identify their typical weaknesses and take part in simple precautions, such as verifying medication labels, asking about sudden changes, and maintaining effective communication with healthcare providers.

Figure 4. Patients and caregivers: their role in the prevention of LASA medication errors, which dwells on the areas of weakness and positive interventions such as verification, inquiring about appearance changes, and open communication with medical practitioners

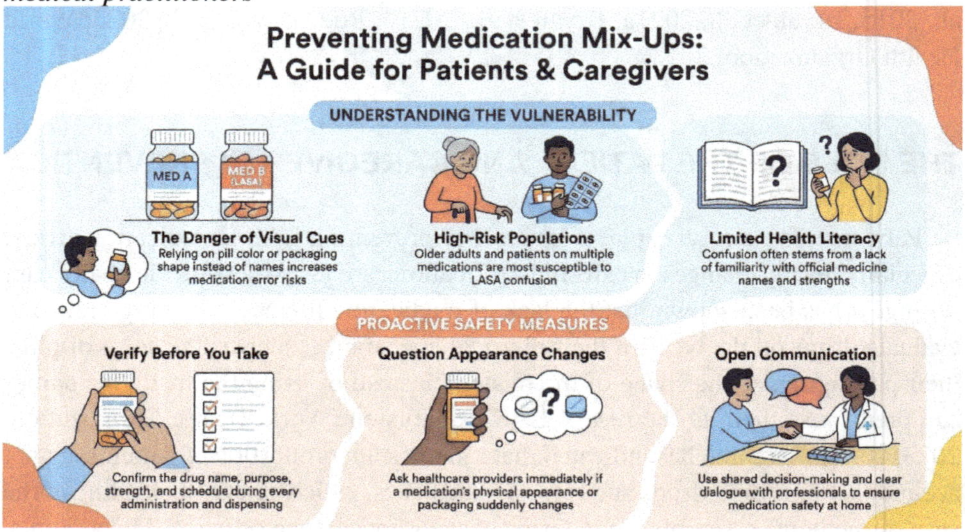

THE ROLE OF REPORTING SYSTEMS IN IDENTIFYING LASA ERRORS

The field of postmarketing pharmacovigilance is based mainly on spontaneous reports on adverse events by health workers, patients, and pharmaceutical companies. These reports form the major data source in signal detection, which can be defined as the identification of new or partially documented safety issues that could be further evaluated and taken into action (Hauben & Aronson, 2009). Medication errors, such as LASA errors, can be included in the data captured in spontaneous reports when the error mechanism or unintended encounter with a drug is outlined (Ostini et al., 2012).

United States: FDA and FAERS

The FDA Adverse Event Reporting System (FAERS) is the database in the United States that is the center of reporting of safety surveillance after the product has been marked. FAERS is a compilation of spontaneous reports submitted by healthcare professionals, consumers, and manufacturers and is typically utilized to detect signals by trend and pattern analysis of reported incidents. FAERS contains reports of adverse events and medication errors, which can be used to identify potential safety signals in situations of incorrect drug administration when there is enough clinical information (Sakaeda et al., 2013). In the context of established pharmacovigilance systems, such signals are indicators of possible relationships instead of being actually definitive; thus, they must be confirmed by means of clinical examination and other sources of information (Hauben & Aronson, 2009). In the cases when such credible risks are detected regarding medication use, the most frequent regulatory actions involve labeling changes, packaging/name differentiation, and specific safety communications, which are in line with a systems approach to preventing name confusion errors reported in the LASA literature (Ostini et al., 2012).

European Union: EMA and EudraVigilance

EudraVigilance assists EU-wide signal management activities in the European Union. According to the EMA, a safety signal is the information that might be induced by a medicine and needs further investigation, and the responsibility to detect and manage the signals lies with the EMA and member states along with marketing authorization holders. The Pharmacovigilance Risk Assessment Committee (PRAC) is the committee of the EMA that tests and observes the safety of human medicines. On this basis, medication errors, such as LASA errors that can be detected in case reports, are within the range of practices of pharmacovigilance signal management and risk-minimization interventions (European Medicines Agency (EMA), 2021a, 2021b; Ostini et al., 2012).

Global Relevance

Since LASA vulnerabilities occur because of linguistic similarity and system-level issues as opposed to national practices, international pharmacovigilance collaboration aids in the timely detection and distribution of safety signals across jurisdictions. An interdisciplinary approach suggests involving solutions throughout the medication-use process (production, dispensing, preparation, and administration) and encompassing them with consumer-oriented initiatives, including education and empowerment to pose questions (Ostini et al., 2012).

Reporting systems such as FAERS and EudraVigilance are important for detecting LASA-related safety signals, as indicated in **Figure 5,** and contribute to regulatory and collaborative actions to mitigate the risks of medication errors.

Figure 5. The role of reporting systems in detecting LASA errors, with a special emphasis on the role of FAERS and EudraVigilance in detecting signals, regulatory response, and international pharmacovigilance cooperation

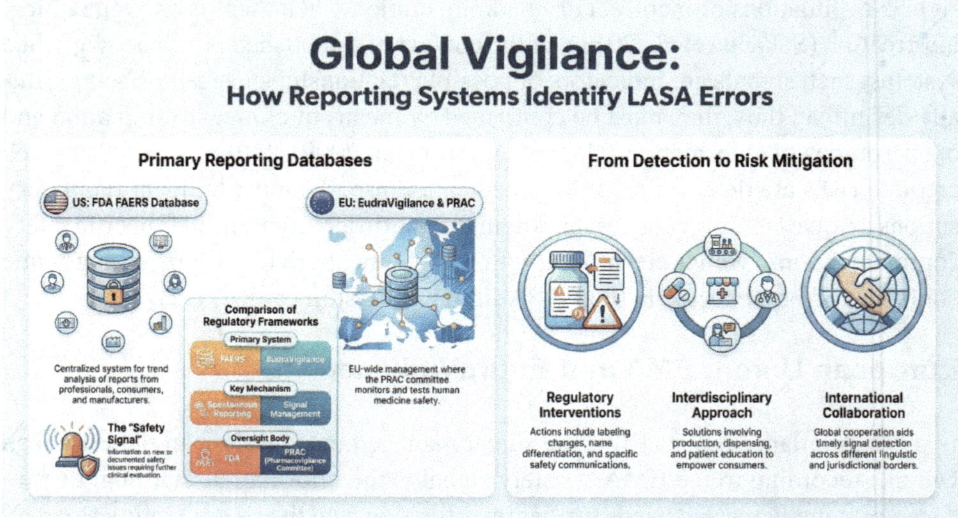

CONCLUSION

Potential errors arising from LASA medications can lead to a wide range of clinical consequences, from treatment failure and mild adverse effects to hospitalization, permanent injury, and death, depending on the drug pair involved, patient vulnerability, and the timeliness of detection. The worst outcomes are always high-alert drugs and drugs with narrow therapeutic indices, in which minor selection or dosing mistakes can quickly result in life-threatening events. Among the reviewed cases, LASA-related errors, such as hemodynamic instability due to the use of vasoactive agents, metabolic or anticoagulation crisis due to the use of high-risk injectables, breakthrough seizures due to anticonvulsant omission, and fatal respiratory depression due to potent opioids, were consistently observed. These trends underscore the relevance of focusing on early interception and high-reliability controls of high-risk classes of drugs with severity frameworks such as the NCC MERP Index, which should help balance prevention and response efforts with the severity of harm these drugs could cause to patients.

REFERENCES

Abrishami, R., Aghili, S. H., Farhang Ranjbar, M., & Lashgari, N.-A. (2024). Assessment of Transcription Errors and their Effects on Medical Approach, Hospitalization Duration, and Financial Costs of Traumatic Patients: How Can We Prevent Them? *Epidemiol Health System J, 11*(3), 121–127. DOI: 10.34172/ehsj.26193

Brown, S. G. A. (2004). Clinical features and severity grading of anaphylaxis. *The Journal of Allergy and Clinical Immunology, 114*(2), 371–376. DOI: 10.1016/j.jaci.2004.04.029 PMID: 15316518

Bryan, R., Aronson, J. K., ten Hacken, P., Williams, A., & Jordan, S. (2015). Patient safety in medication nomenclature: Orthographic and semantic properties of International Nonproprietary Names. *PLoS One, 10*(12), e0145431. DOI: 10.1371/journal.pone.0145431 PMID: 26701761

Bryan, R., Aronson, J. K., Williams, A., & Jordan, S. (2021a). The problem of look-alike, sound-alike name errors: Drivers and solutions. *British Journal of Clinical Pharmacology, 87*(2), 386–394. DOI: 10.1111/bcp.14285 PMID: 32198938

Bryan, R., Aronson, J. K., Williams, A. J., & Jordan, S. (2021b). A systematic literature review of LASA error interventions. *British Journal of Clinical Pharmacology, 87*(2), 336–351. DOI: 10.1111/bcp.14644 PMID: 33197079

Campbell, J., & Sumner, W.II. (2005). OOPS: Test of a structure for recording patient safety events. *AMIA ... Annual Symposium Proceedings - AMIA Symposium. AMIA Symposium, 2005*, 910. PMID: 16779197

Center for Drug Evaluation and Research (CDER). (2000). *Proprietary name review: Foradil aerolizer*. Retrieved 11 Jan from https://www.accessdata.fda.gov/drugsatfda_docs/nda/2001/20831_Foradil_admindocs_P1.pdf

Center for Drug Evaluation and Research (CDER). (2004). *Approval package for: Application number NDA* 21-615 *medical review (s)*. Retrieved 11 Jan from https://www.accessdata.fda.gov/drugsatfda_docs/nda/2004/021615s000_Razadyne_medr.pdf

Center for Drug Evaluation and Research (CDER). (2006). *Proprietary name review(s): Foradil certihaler*. https://www.accessdata.fda.gov/drugsatfda_docs/nda/2006/021592s000_NameR.pdf

Chu, G., Mantin, R., Shen, Y. M., Baskett, G., & Sussman, H. (1993). Massive cisplatin overdose by accidental substitution for carboplatin. Toxicity and management. Cancer, 72(12), 3707-3714. https://doi.org/10.1002/1097-0142

Cohen, M. R. (1991). Insulin overdoses that originated in the pharmacy IV admixture area. Hosp Pharm, 26, 998-999.

Cohen, M. R. (2007). Action needed to prevent dangerous heparin-insulin confusion; sorting things out; staff unaware of fentanyl patch starting doses. *Hospital Pharmacy*, *42*(8), 675–679. DOI: 10.1310/hpj4208-675

Cohen, M. R. (2020). Medication Errors. *Nursing*, *50*(11), 72. https://doi.org/DOI-10.1097/01.NURSE.0000719696.41409.94. DOI: 10.1097/01.NURSE.0000719696.41409.94 PMID: 6907778

Cohen, M. R., & Smetzer, J. L. (2007). Preventing dispensing errors. In *Medication Errors* (2nd ed.). The American Pharmacists Association. DOI: 10.21019/9781582120928.ch10

da Silva, B. A., & Krishnamurthy, M. (2016). The alarming reality of medication error: A patient case and review of Pennsylvania and National data. *Journal of Community Hospital Internal Medicine Perspectives*, *6*(4), 31758. DOI: 10.3402/jchimp.v6.31758 PMID: 27609720

Davis, T. C., Wolf, M. S., Bass, P. F.III, Middlebrooks, M., Kennen, E., Baker, D. W., Bennett, C. L., Durazo-Arvizu, R., Bocchini, A., Savory, S., & Parker, R. M. (2006). Low literacy impairs comprehension of prescription drug warning labels. *Journal of General Internal Medicine*, *21*(8), 847–851. DOI: 10.1111/j.1525-1497.2006.00529.x PMID: 16881945

European Medicines Agency (EMA). (2021a). *Pharmacovigilance Risk Assessment Committee (PRAC)*. Retrieved 16 Jan from https://www.ema.europa.eu/en/committees/pharmacovigilance-risk-assessment-committee-prac

European Medicines Agency (EMA). (2021b). *Signal management*. Retrieved 16 Jan from https://www.ema.europa.eu/en/human-regulatory-overview/post-authorisation/pharmacovigilance-post-authorisation/signal-management

Gallagher, T. H., Waterman, A. D., Ebers, A. G., Fraser, V. J., & Levinson, W. (2003). Patients' and physicians' attitudes regarding the disclosure of medical errors. *Journal of the American Medical Association*, *289*(8), 1001–1007. DOI: 10.1001/jama.289.8.1001 PMID: 12597752

Gaunt, M. (2007). Error Trifecta: Avandia, Coumadin, and Cardura. *Pharmacy Times*, *73*(11), 53.

Ghelardini, C., Di Cesare Mannelli, L., & Bianchi, E. (2015). The pharmacological basis of opioids. *Clinical Cases in Mineral and Bone Metabolism*, *12*(3), 219–221. DOI: 10.11138/ccmbm/2015.12.3.219 PMID: 26811699

Grissinger, M. (2008). Morphine and Hydromorphone: An Omnipresent Risk of Mix-ups. *P&T : a Peer-Reviewed Journal for Formulary Management, 33*(4), 194–247. PMID: 19750160

Grissinger, M. (2011). Action is neeeded to prevent heparin-insulin mixups. *P&T : a Peer-Reviewed Journal for Formulary Management, 36*(4), 177–202. PMID: 21572772

Grissinger, M. (2012). Tall man letters are gaining wide acceptance. *P&T : a Peer-Reviewed Journal for Formulary Management, 37*(3), 132–148. PMID: 22605902

Gulur, P., Koury, K., Arnstein, P., Lee, H., McCarthy, P., Coley, C., & Mort, E. (2015). Morphine versus Hydromorphone: Does Choice of Opioid Influence Outcomes? *Pain Research and Treatment, 482081*, 1–6. Advance online publication. DOI: 10.1155/2015/482081 PMID: 26609431

Gutierrez, M. A., Todd, K., & Nagy, R. M. (1991). On the alert for clonazepam (Klonopin) versus clonidine. *Journal of Clinical Psychopharmacology, 11*(4), 269–270. DOI: 10.1097/00004714-199108000-00018 PMID: 1918426

Hauben, M., & Aronson, J. K. (2009). Defining 'Signal' and its Subtypes in Pharmacovigilance Based on a Systematic Review of Previous Definitions. *Drug Safety, 32*(2), 99–110. DOI: 10.2165/00002018-200932020-00003 PMID: 19236117

Hicks, R., Becker, S., & Cousins, D. (2008). MEDMARX data report. A report on the relationship of drug names and medication errors in response to the institute of Medicine's call for action. Center for the Advancement of Patient Safey, US Pharmacopeia.

Hoffman, J. M., & Proulx, S. M. (2003). Medication errors caused by confusion of drug names. *Drug Safety, 26*(7), 445–452. DOI: 10.2165/00002018-200326070-00001 PMID: 12735783

Holbrook, A., Schulman, S., Witt, D. M., Vandvik, P. O., Fish, J., Kovacs, M. J., . . . Guyatt, G. H. (2012). Evidence-based management of anticoagulant therapy: Antithrombotic Therapy and Prevention of Thrombosis, 9th ed: American College of Chest Physicians Evidence-Based Clinical Practice Guidelines. *Chest*, 141(2 Suppl), e152S-e184S. DOI: 10.1378/chest.11-2295

Huang, D., Luo, Z., Song, X., & Zou, K. (2024). Global research on sufentanil use in anesthesiology from 2003 to 2023: a bibliometric analysis [Systematic Review]. *Frontiers in Pharmacology, Volume* 15 - 2024. DOI: 10.3389/fphar.2024.1412726

Institute for Safe Medication Practices (ISMP). (2015). *Community/ambulatory care IMSP Medication Safety Allert! Health alert! Avandia, not Coumadin*. Retrieved 16 Jan from https://www.ismp.org/sites/default/files/attachments/2018-03/community201512.pdf

Institute for Safe Medication Practices (ISMP). (2016). *ISMP Medication Safety Alert! Do not let "Depo-" medications be a depot for mistakes*. Retrieved 11 Jan from https://www.ismp.org/sites/default/files/attachments/2018-03/20160324.pdf

Institute for Safe Medication Practices (ISMP) Canada. (2002). Confusion Between SEROQUEL® and SERZONE-5HT2® Reported in Canada. *ISMP Canada Safety Bulletin*, *2*(10), 1–2.

ISMP. (2016). *FDA and ISMP lists of look-alike drug names with recommended tall man letters*. Retrieved 5 Sep from https://www.ismp.org/sites/default/files/attachments/2017-11/tallmanletters.pdf?

ISMP News/ECRI. (2020). *Due to ISMP Advocacy, VinCRIStine Labeling and Packaging Changed to Prevent Wrong Route Administration*. Retrieved 5 Sep from https://home.ecri.org/blogs/ismp-news/due-to-ismp-advocacy-vincristine-labeling-and-packaging-changed-to-prevent-wrong-route-administration?

Kemp, S. F., Lockey, R. F., & Simons, F. E. (2008). Epinephrine: The drug of choice for anaphylaxis. A statement of the World Allergy Organization. *Allergy*, *63*(8), 1061–1070. DOI: 10.1111/j.1398-9995.2008.01733.x PMID: 18691308

Leape, L. L. (2007). Chapter 1. Systems Analysis and Redesign: The Foundation of Medical Error Prevention. In *Medication Errors, 2nd Edition*. The American Pharmacists Association. https://doi.org/doi:10.21019/9781582120928.ch1

Leape, L. L., Bates, D. W., Cullen, D. J., Cooper, J., Demonaco, H. J., Gallivan, T., & Edmondson, A. (1995). Systems Analysis of Adverse Drug Events. *Journal of the American Medical Association*, *274*(1), 35–43. DOI: 10.1001/jama.1995.03530010049034 PMID: 7791256

Mazor, K. M., Simon, S. R., Yood, R. A., Martinson, B. C., Gunter, M. J., Reed, G. W., & Gurwitz, J. H. (2004). Health plan members' views about disclosure of medical errors. *Annals of Internal Medicine*, *140*(6), 409–418. DOI: 10.7326/0003-4819-140-6-200403160-00006 PMID: 15023706

Medicines and Healthcare products Regulatory Agency (MHRA). (2014). *Mercaptamine and mercaptopurine: confusion between drug names*. Retrieved 15 June from https://www.gov.uk/drug-safety-update/mercaptamine-and-mercaptopurine-confusion-between-drug-names

News, N. B. C. (2005). *Zyprexa, Zyrtec similarities causing confusion*. Retrieved 15 Apr from https://www.nbcnews.com/health/health-news/zyprexa-zyrtec-similarities-causing-confusion-flna1c9439578

Ostini, R., Roughead, E. E., Kirkpatrick, C. M., Monteith, G. R., & Tett, S. E. (2012). Quality use of medicines—Medication safety issues in naming; look-alike, sound-alike medicine names. *The International Journal of Pharmacy Practice*, *20*(6), 349–357. DOI: 10.1111/j.2042-7174.2012.00210.x PMID: 23134093

Palasuberniam, P., Chin, S., Thangiah, V., & Dsouza, U. J. A. (2018). Medication Errors: A Review of Classifications. *Borneo Journal of Medical Sciences*, *12*(3), 11–18. DOI: 10.51200/bjms.v12i3.1173

Perucca, P., & Gilliam, F. G. (2012). Adverse effects of antiepileptic drugs. *The Lancet. Neurology*, *11*(9), 792–802. DOI: 10.1016/S1474-4422(12)70153-9 PMID: 22832500

Pharmacy Times. (2005). *Reminyl Is Now Razadyne*. Retrieved 11 Jan from https://www.pharmacytimes.com/view/2005-08-9769

Rahman, Z., & Parvin, R. (2015). Medication errors associated with look-alike/sound-alike drugs: A brief review. *J Enam Med Col*, *5*(2), 110–117. DOI: 10.3329/jemc.v5i2.23385

Reines, S. A. (2005). Look-alike, sound-alike drug errors with Reminyl and Amaryl. *American Journal of Health-System Pharmacy*, *62*(1), 35–36. DOI: 10.1093/ajhp/62.1.35 PMID: 15658069

Rodziewicz, T. L., Houseman, B., & Hipskind, J. E. (2023). *Medical error reduction and prevention*. StatPearls Publishing.

Sakaeda, T., Tamon, A., Kadoyama, K., & Okuno, Y. (2013). Data Mining of the Public Version of the FDA Adverse Event Reporting System [Review]. *International Journal of Medical Sciences*, *10*(7), 796–803. DOI: 10.7150/ijms.6048 PMID: 23794943

Schulmeister, L. (2006). Look-alike, sound-alike oncology medications. *Clinical Journal of Oncology Nursing*, *10*(1), 35–41. DOI: 10.1188/06.CJON.35-41 PMID: 16482726

Scott, S. D., Hirschinger, L. E., Cox, K. R., McCoig, M., Brandt, J., & Hall, L. W. (2009). The natural history of recovery for the healthcare provider "second victim" after adverse patient events. *Quality & Safety in Health Care*, *18*(5), 325–330. DOI: 10.1136/qshc.2009.032870 PMID: 19812092

Senior Care Consultant Group (SCCG). (2006). *Appendix* 17: *sound alike/look alike medications*. Retrieved 22 May from http://mysccg.com/generalDocuments/Look%20and%20Sound%20Alike%20Meds.pdf

Sullivan, P. (2003, March 4). New US labeling to eliminate drug conFUSION. *Canadian Medical Association Journal, 168*(5), 598. PMID: 12615765

The Associated Press. (2005). *Zyprexa, Zyrtec similarities causing confusion*. Retrieved 8 Feb from https://www.nbcnews.com/health/health-news/zyprexa-zyrtec-similarities-causing-confusion-flna1c9439578

The Health and Disability Commissioner. (2003). *Antidepressant nefazodone (Serzone) dispensed instead of prescribed antipsychotic quetiapine (Seroquel)*. Retrieved 16 Jan from https://www.hdc.org.nz/media/exujf0qh/01hdc11914pharmacists.pdf

The Institute for Safe Medication Practices (ISMP). (2015). *ISMP's list of confused drug names*. Retrieved 16 Apr from https://www.ismp.org/sites/default/files/attachments/2017-11/confuseddrugnames%2802.2015%29.pdf?

The Institute for Safe Medication Practices (ISMP). (2016). Hydralazine, hydroxyzine confused again. *America's Pharmacist*.

The Institute for Safe Medication Practices (ISMP). (2023). *List of confused drug names*. Retrieved 16 Apr from https://www.ismp.org/recommendations/confused-drug-names-list

The Institute for Safe Medication Practices (ISMP). (2024). *ISMP List of Confused Drug Names*. Retrieved 07 Sep from https://online.ecri.org/hubfs/ISMP/Resources/ISMP_ConfusedDrugNames.pdf

The Institute for Safe Medication Practices (ISMP) Canada. (2001). Multiple reports of confusion between lamotrigine (LAMICTAL®) and products with 'sound alike'/'look alike' name. *ISMP Canada Safety Bulletin*, 1(3).

Therapeutic Goods Administration. (2016). *Mercaptamine (cysteamine) and mercaptopurine*. Retrieved 13 Jan from https://www.tga.gov.au/safety/safety-monitoring-and-information/safety-alerts/mercaptamine-cysteamine-and-mercaptopurine

U.S. Department of Health and Human Services Food and Drug Administration. (2015). *Galantamine hydrobromide (marketed as Razadyne, formerly Reminyl) Information*. Retrieved 11 Jan from https://www.fda.gov/drugs/postmarket-drug-safety-information-patients-and-providers/galantamine-hydrobromide-marketed-razadyne-formerly-reminyl-information

U.S. Department of Health and Human Services Food and Drug Administration. (2016). *October - December* 2016 *Report | Potential Signals of Serious Risks/New Safety Information Identified by the FDA Adverse Event Reporting System (FAERS)*. Retrieved 11 Jan from https://www.fda.gov/drugs/fdas-adverse-event-reporting-system-faers/october-december-2016-report-potential-signals-serious-risksnew-safety-information-identified-fda

U.S. Department of Health and Human Services Food and Drug Administration (FDA). (2020). *FDA name differentiation project*. Retrieved 06 Aug from https://www.fda.gov/drugs/medication-errors-related-cder-regulated-drug-products/fda-name-differentiation-project

Waknine, Y. (2005). *Zyprexa and Zyrtec substitution errors may lead to adverse events, relapse of schizophrenia or bipolar disorder*. Retrieved 14 Jan from https://www.medscape.com/viewarticle/499062?form=fpf

Wang, W., He, Q., Wang, M., Kang, Y., Ji, P., Zhu, S.,…Sun, X. (2022). Associations of Fentanyl, Sufentanil, and Remifentanil With Length of Stay and Mortality Among Mechanically Ventilated Patients: A Registry-Based Cohort Study [Original Research]. *Frontiers in Pharmacology, Volume* 13 - 2022. DOI: 10.3389/fphar.2022.858531

Waterman, A. D., Garbutt, J., Hazel, E., Dunagan, W. C., Levinson, W., Fraser, V. J., & Gallagher, T. H. (2007). The emotional impact of medical errors on practicing physicians in the United States and Canada. *Joint Commission Journal on Quality and Patient Safety*, *33*(8), 467–476. DOI: 10.1016/S1553-7250(07)33050-X PMID: 17724943

WHO Collaborating Centre for Patient Safety Solutions. (2007). *Look-alike, sound-alike medication names*. Retrieved 9 August from https://cdn.who.int/media/docs/default-source/patient-safety/patient-safety-solutions/ps-solution1-look-alike-sound-alike-medication-names.pdf?sfvrsn=d4fb860b_8

World Health Organization. (2017). *Medication without harm*. Retrieved 10 Feb from https://www.who.int/initiatives/medication-without-harm

World Health Organization. (2023). *Medication safety for look-alike, sound-alike medicines*. World Health Organization. Retrieved 3 June from https://iris.who.int/bitstream/handle/10665/373495/9789240058897-eng.pdf?sequence=1

World Health Organization. (2024). *Medication safety: WHO webinar on the Global Patient Safety Challenge Medication Without Harm*. Retrieved 24 July from https://cdn.who.int/media/docs/default-source/integrated-health-services-%28ihs%29/psf/medication-without-harm/medication-safety-who-webinar-7march2024.pdf

ABBREVIATIONS

ADE: Adverse Drug Events
FAERS: The FDA Adverse Event Reporting System
ICU: Intensive Care Unit
INR: International Normalized Ratio
ISMP: Institute for Safe Medication Practices
LASA: Look-Alike, Sound-Alike
NCC MERP: National Coordinating Council for Medication Error Reporting and Prevention
NSAID: Non-Steroidal Anti-Inflammatory Drug
OR: Operating Room
PACU: Postanesthesia Care Unit
PA-PSRS: Pennsylvania Patient Safety Reporting System
TPN: Total Parenteral Nutrition
WHO: World Health Organization

Chapter 8
Look-Alike, Sound-Alike in Dietary Supplements

ABSTRACT

Look-alike, sound-alike (LASA) errors are a patient safety issue that is not well understood yet is becoming increasingly important. A combination of high rates of supplement use, a high rate of concomitant use with prescription drugs, and insufficient pre-market screening of supplement names and packaging provides circumstances that are favorable to confusion based on name and appearance. When compared to pharmaceuticals, dietary supplements are regularly placed on the market without a systematic LASA review, which means that the products with names, indications, or even graphic designs similar to prescription drugs could find their place in the market. This chapter analyzes the regulatory loopholes, marketing-based LASA processes, and practical case studies, such as herbal packaging similarities in hospitals. It highlights the necessity of applying the dietary supplements to medication safety systems by increasing their regulation, the participation of pharmacists, and patient education.

INTRODUCTION

Medication errors cause extreme patient safety risks in any healthcare environment, and look-alike/sound-alike (LASA) medication names have become among the most challenging and persistent contributors to preventable adverse drug events (Cohen, 2007; Cohen et al., 2007; Marovino et al., 2022; Supapaan et al., 2024). Notably, one of the typical causes of drug mistakes that may result in patient harm or even death is the presence of confusing drug names (Rahman & Parvin, 2015). LASA drugs are drugs that can be mixed because of their orthographic (look-alike) and phonetic (sound-alike) features and can lead to mistakes in prescribing, dispensing, administering, monitoring, transcribing, or documenting (Muchu, 2024). This

DOI: 10.4018/979-8-3373-5478-1.ch008

issue is not limited to the conventional line of pharmaceutical products but also to dietary supplements, which makes the regulatory boundaries, therapeutic claims, and nomenclature overlap in an especially convoluted landscape. More than 50% of adults in the U.S. are dietary supplement users, and the National Health and Nutrition Examination Survey (NHANES) 1999–2000 records that 52% of American adults had used at least one dietary supplement within the past month (Radimer et al., 2004). The prevalence of this broadly applied use has risen significantly over the past few decades, with more recent data from NHANES 2009–2010 still indicating high rates of supplement use in all categories (Chen et al., 2019).

This high prevalence of supplement usage exists in a regulatory framework that is essentially dissimilar to that used in prescription drugs and thus presents the possibility of confusion when supplement names mirror those of pharmaceutical products. Recent reports of certain dietary supplement products whose names are intentionally similar to prescription drugs have shown the deliberate nature of most supplement-drug LASA risks (Kelling, 2017). In contrast to LASA errors, which are usually caused by accidental similarities, there is some evidence that there are certain manufacturers of nutritional supplements who particularly construct the names of their products in a manner that resembles the already existing prescription drugs. As shown in Figure 1, LASA risk is also caused by orthographic and phonetic similarities in drug names, as well as by weak points throughout the medication-use process and the overlap between prescription drugs and dietary supplements across different regulatory systems.

Figure 1. Overview of LASA risk, representing how orthographic and phonetic similarity, major medication-use vulnerabilities, and overlap between prescription drugs and dietary supplements contribute to patient safety risk

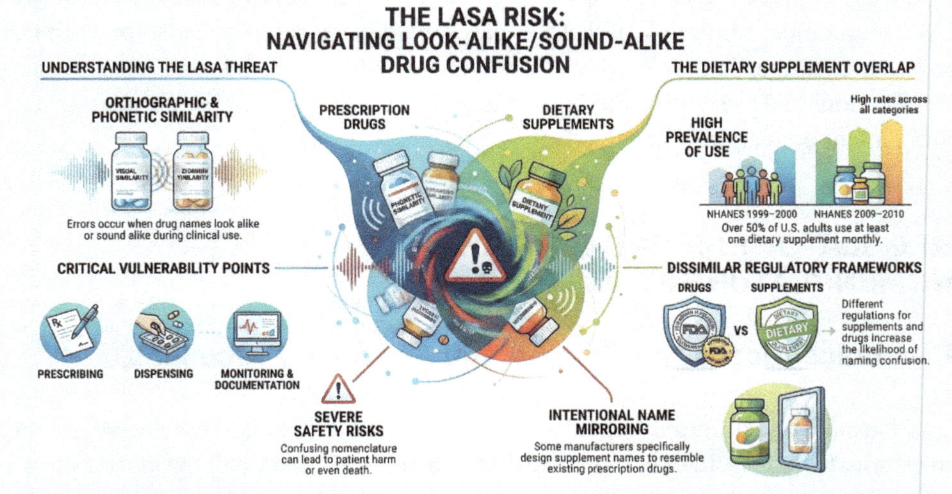

Objectives of the Chapter

The aims of this chapter are as follows:

(1) To describe LASA errors and briefly review the history of medication safety concerns.
(2) To compare pharmaceutical and dietary supplement regulatory frameworks, with emphasis on naming and labeling controls.
(3) To identify key LASA risk mechanisms related to dietary supplements, including name, indication, and packaging similarity.
(4) To present representative case examples of dietary supplement–related LASA errors from international and Thai settings.
(5) To outline prevention strategies that integrate regulation, pharmacy practice, and patient education.

Organization of the Chapter

Chapter 8 begins by providing an overview of LASA errors, as well as a historical outlook on medication safety. Afterward, it undergoes a review of pharmaceutical drug naming and approval procedures and then an examination of dietary supplement regulation with a focus on regulatory lapses in name, labeling, and premarket regulation. The chapter then argues about the international differences in the regulations of dietary supplements and how they contribute to the risk of LASA. It is followed by documented examples of LASA cases in dietary supplements, prescription supplements, and herbal products. The chapter ends by discussing patient safety implications and prevention methods in terms of regulatory authorities, pharmacists, and patient education.

REGULATORY FRAMEWORK AND NOMENCLATURE STANDARDS

Pharmaceutical Drug Naming and Approval Processes

Pharmaceutical drug approval and naming involve stakeholders and regulatory measures to reduce LASA risk. The FDA in the U.S. evaluates proposed proprietary (brand) names for confusion with existing products using a wide range of criteria. Health Canada searches for similar proprietary and nonproprietary names, orthographic or phonetic computer analyses, verbal and handwritten prescription testing studies, literature reviews of medication errors, or systematic evaluations of the proposed name, considering contributing factors (i.e., dosage form or route of administration) and the propensity for drug confusion when manufacturers submit a drug product. Laboratory-based memory and perception tests can predict error rates related to drug name confusion in a pharmacy chain, with the best models explaining 37–45% of the dispensing error rate (Cheung & Goodwin, 2013; Schroeder et al., 2017).

Drug nomenclature is internationally coordinated by the World Health Organization (INN) program, which gives pharmaceutical substances generic names. The INN system uses standardized stems to denote the pharmacological class (e.g., "-olol" in beta-blockers, "-pril" in ACE inhibitors, and "-statin" in HMG-CoA reductase inhibitors) and makes it easier to recognize therapeutic types. Nonetheless, the methodical application of common stems ironically may increase the risk of LASA among drug classes because several drugs are named in a similar manner. A study of 7,987 International Nonproprietary Names revealed that the WHO guidelines of using stems to serve meaning and the goal of minimizing similarities in nomenclature created a conflict between WHO guidelines and the intention to minimize similarities and the tendency to use a stem shared by two INNs to create a higher level of orthographic similarity (less than 5 Levenshtein edit distances), thus increasing the risk of confusion (Bryan et al., 2015).

Postmarketing surveillance systems such as adverse event reporting systems, medication error databases maintained by organizations such as the Institute of Safe Medication Practices (ISMP), and voluntary reporting by professionals identify LASA pairs that have escaped preapproval detection (Karet, 2023). The List of Confused Drug Names is actively updated and implemented in the ISMP and serves as a source of information for healthcare organizations conducting error prevention programs, and lists are made available through authorized channels, which can be referred to by healthcare facilities to implement the precautions since they use the same drugs. The list is, however, only the documented cases that may not represent all the clinically significant pairs of LASA, particularly new medications or products that apply to fewer patients. The LASA category presents a variety of options based on different brands in each country (Dhande et al., 2021).

Dietary Supplement Regulation Under DSHEA

The Dietary Supplement Health and Education Act (DSHEA) of 1994 is the regulatory framework that governs the field of dietary supplements in the United States and defines dietary supplements as products that are expected to be added to the diet and that include vitamins, minerals, herbs, amino acids, or any dietary substances (Bekker et al., 2023). The dietary supplements in the United States are mostly marketed without prior safety or efficacy approval by the premarket mechanisms under the Dietary Supplement Health and Education Act of 1994 (DSHEA). Rather, supplements are assumed to be safe unless the U.S. Food and Drug Administration (FDA) concludes that after the product is marketed, it poses a serious or unreasonable risk to the health of the population. This level of regulation is in contrast to that applied to pharmaceutical substances, where manufacturers must prove their safety and efficacy before being approved (Avigan et al., 2016). In line with this scenario, dietary supplements do not need to be taken through standardized premarket dosages, pharmacokinetics, or systematic evaluations of adverse effects and then sold to consumers (Avigan et al., 2016; Dwyer et al., 2018). A review of regulatory systems has suggested that compared with pharmaceutical products, the premarket regulation of some areas of dietary supplement labeling and marketing takes place less under this model.

One of the main regulatory aspects of DSHEA is product claim classification. Dietary supplements affect the structure/function of the body, but supplements cannot cause disease; i.e., supplements affect the structure or function of the body, thus suggesting a cure, prevention, diagnosis, or treatment of a disease (Bekker et al., 2023; Dwyer et al., 2018; U.S. Food and Drug Administration, 2011). In such a regulatory framework, dietary supplements are not obligated to prove safety and efficacy before they are sold, unlike pharmaceutical products that are subject to official premarket testing (Avigan et al., 2016; Dwyer et al., 2018). Regulatory issues related to pharmaceutical and dietary supplements have some implications for LASA. The brand names of pharmaceuticals are also subjected to the FDA review process, which aims to minimize medication-name confusion, including the inspection of orthographic and phonetic resemblance.

Conversely, the name of a dietary supplement product does not undergo proactive screening of LASA before the product comes to the market, which means that the name of the supplement, similar to the prescription drug name, can be introduced to the market. Alprazium®, Glucocil®, and Mitadone® are among the products that have also been found to be dietary supplements whose names sound like those of the already established prescription drugs. The products were reported in a category of LASA dietary supplements that are commercially sold, especially via online retailers, and that can take up a top spot in search results when consumers query the name of prescription drugs. In addition to the similarity of names, these supplements are frequently sold for health-related purposes, which overlap with the therapeutic uses of the prescription drugs that they look similar to, which can also add to the problem of sorting supervised pharmaceutical products and uncontrolled dietary supplements (Kelling, 2017).

This type of naming has been singled out as a possible cause of confusion for consumers. In other cases, the consumers might buy these products on the assumption that they are identical to or that they are suitable replacements for prescription drugs, especially in situations where the names of the products and their marketed application are similar to prescription drugs. This is demonstrated in the following examples of how the naming of dietary supplements can confuse the boundary between regulated pharmaceuticals and dietary supplements, particularly in the face of a lack of proactive screening of LASA potential before a dietary supplement receives its name (Kelling, 2017).

Regulatory measures against misleading dietary supplement products, such as warning letters, product seizures, and injunction, are normally taken after the product has been introduced to the market, with the identification of safety, adulteration, or misbranding (Cohen, 2009). The information gathered after marketing also revealed that dietary supplements are linked to adverse events, such as hepatotoxicity and other severe clinical events (Avigan et al., 2016). Observational research and surveillance systems have reported that adverse events related to dietary supplements can lead to hospitalization or emergency department admission, especially for some categories of products (Bent et al., 2003; Geller et al., 2015). Ongoing difficulties in adverse-event monitoring and reporting of dietary supplements have been reported in the literature (Dwyer et al., 2018). These observations highlight the need to continue paying attention to LASA considerations in regulatory policy, pharmacy practice, and patient education (Dwyer et al., 2018; Kelling, 2017).

INTERNATIONAL REGULATORY VARIATIONS AND GLOBAL DIETARY SUPPLEMENT REGISTRATION AND LASA CHALLENGES

Global inconsistency in the regulation and registration of dietary supplements is a valuable contextual obstacle in the prevention of look-alike/sound-alike (LASA) errors. Unlike pharmaceutical products, which are regulated using more or less harmonized principles and are backed by internationally accepted naming codes such as International Nonproprietary Names (INNs) of the World Health Organization, dietary supplements are regulated by different legal frameworks in different countries. These frameworks vary considerably in terms of product classification, premarket requirements, and postmarketing oversight, leading to uneven regulatory environments across the globe (Dwyer et al., 2018).

Dietary supplements in the U.S. fall under the Dietary Supplement Health and Education Act of 1994 (DSHEA). The Dietary Supplement Health and Education Act of 1994, 21 U.S.C. SS 321[ff], defines a dietary supplement as a dietary intake supplement, a product comprising a dietary ingredient (e.g., vitamin, mineral, herb or other botanical, amino acid, or some other substance) or a group of dietary ingredients (e.g., calcium, iron, vitamins), designed to be added to a diet. In this statutory definition, herbal products are specifically covered when they are being sold as dietary supplements as opposed to for medical purposes. In the United States, dietary supplements are not preapproved as safe or effective and are assumed to be safe unless postmarketing studies can prove that a product poses a serious or unreasonable risk to the health of the population (Avigan et al., 2016; Gardiner et al., 2008).

The regulatory status of herbal and botanical products is, however, significantly different internationally. Analysis of world regulatory standards reveals that these products can be regulated as dietary supplements, foods, or medicinal products on the basis of the country's legislation, intended purpose, and historical background (Dwyer et al., 2018). Herbal products are also classified as a subgroup of dietary supplements or food and have relatively lenient premarket regulations (in some jurisdictions) or as a subgroup of herbal or traditional medicines and are regulated as pharmaceutical (Vlietinck et al., 2009). In the European Union (EU), e.g., herbal products can be regulated as food supplements or as traditional herbal medicinal products on the basis of their presentation, claims, and intended use. The Traditional Herbal Medicinal Products Directive (2004/24/EC) created a distinct regulatory route for traditional herbal medicinal products, where they may receive registration on the basis of documented traditional use instead of using the evidence of randomized clinical trials. The route involves demonstration of a period of at least 30 years of traditional use, of which at least 15 years are in the EU (Vlietinck et al., 2009). Products listed under this directive are deemed to be regulated like medicines as opposed to dietary supplements, and similar herbal components may be marketed as dietary supplements in the United States under DSHEA or foods in other jurisdictions (Dwyer et al., 2018).

The World Health Organization (WHO) has recognized this international regulatory variation and has stressed that traditional and herbal medicines are integrated into national regulatory frameworks in various forms across nations. According to the WHO, herbal products can be classified as medicines, dietary supplements, or traditional products in accordance with national legal frameworks, which subsequently determines registration, safety monitoring, and postmarketing surveillance requirements (World Health Organization, 2004). The WHO guidance on these matters, however, does not achieve a globally harmonized nomenclature or registration system for dietary supplements or herbal products to which pharmaceutical substances have an equivalent, the INN system.

This disjointed regulatory environment can pose a challenge to an LASA way of trying to systematically avoid name-based confusion. The brand names of pharmaceuticals are expected to undergo systematic regulatory assessment procedures aimed at decreasing the risk of confusion because of orthographic or phonetic inequalities. In contrast, similar proactive name screening systems for dietary supplements do not exist or are inconsistently implemented across jurisdictions. Consequently, a legally marketable dietary supplement product in one country may be under the name of a prescription drug, whereas an equivalent name would be rebuffed in a name-approval procedure in a pharmaceutical company (Kelling, 2017).

Currently, no published global study is known that precisely quantifies the LASA risks that are due to differences in dietary supplement registration or naming practices between different countries. Regulatory heterogeneity, safety monitoring restrictions, and adverse event reporting of dietary supplements and herbal products are the major themes of the literature but do not necessarily empirically correlate variability in international registration with LASA error rates (Dwyer et al., 2018; Kelling, 2017). As a result, the existing information on the risk of LASA associated with global dietary supplements is indirect.

Overall, the global diversity in the regulation and registration of dietary supplements adds to the fragmented international environment where the practices of naming, labeling, and safety regulation vary considerably across borders. Despite the fact that these differences are arguably applicable to LASA risk, evidence is abundant, and additional studies are necessary to directly test how cross-border regulatory heterogeneity can affect name-based confusion in relation to dietary supplements. There is a high possibility that this gap needs to be addressed through coordinated international studies, an improved system of the pharmacovigilance of dietary supplements, and increased pharmacist involvement in the detection and management of LASA risks in ever-globalizing product markets.

A significant disparity in the rigor of the regulatory process of pharmaceuticals and dietary supplements, especially with respect to premarket approval, proactive screening of LASA names, and postmarket enforcement, is shown in Figure 2, which establishes a significant gap in safeguarding against name confusion.

Figure 2. A comparison of regulatory gaps between pharmaceutical and dietary supplements reveals differences in premarket approval, LASA name screening, naming standards, and postmarket oversight

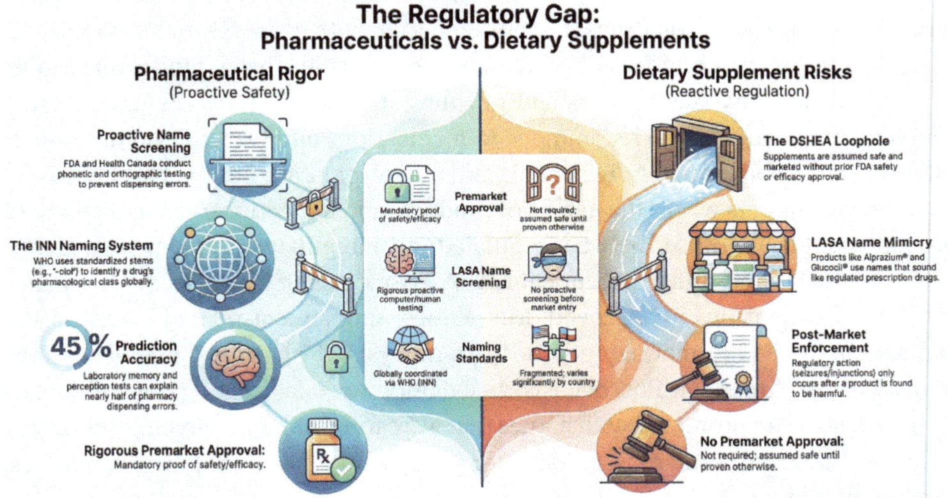

DIETARY SUPPLEMENT-RELATED LASA ERRORS

LASA medication errors were historically studied as prescriptions and over-the-counter pharmaceutical drugs. The pharmacy practices and the literature on the health of the population have suggested otherwise; however, evidence indicates that dietary supplements represent an extra and poorly understood aspect of this patient safety concern. This growth of the dietary supplement market, coupled with the lack of premarket regulation of supplement naming and labeling, has left confusion between dietary supplements and prescription drugs that may arise during the process of selecting products and self-administering them to patients (Dwyer et al., 2018; Kelling, 2017).

The consumption of dietary supplements is very high in the United States. According to nationally representative data provided by the NHANES, more than 50% of the U.S. adult population reports taking some dietary supplements, with prevalence estimates between approximately 52% and more than 70%, depending on age group, cycle of survey, and population factors (Bailey et al., 2013; Gahche et al., 2011). Analyses of surveys also show that a large portion of consumers consider dietary supplements safe and helpful, even though no consideration of the safety and efficacy of these products is given before the market (Bailey et al., 2013; Dwyer et al., 2018). Combined with the high frequency of using dietary supplements in combination with prescription drugs, the possible topicality of LASA risk is increased. Observational research and narrative reviews have revealed that a significant number of adults, especially older adults and people with chronic illnesses, take dietary supplements in addition to recommended medications and that they do not inform medical staff about them (Avigan et al., 2016; Dwyer et al., 2018). This confusion forms environments where the names of products and indications/visual displays of products could be confused between regulated and unregulated supplement products.

In contrast to most pharmaceutical LASA errors, which tend to occur by chance because of similarities in approved drug names, supplement-related LASA issues can also be related to marketing issues. An analysis of pharmacy practices in the Journal of the American Pharmacists Association revealed that a range of dietary supplements were promoted with names that were too similar to known prescription drugs and covered numerous therapeutic groups, such as anxiolytics, hypnotics, stimulants, opioids, and antidiabetic agents (Kelling, 2017). These products were heavily featured in search results whenever prescription drugs were searched online, and these products were promoted as health-related when they tended to overlap with the prescription medications that they imitate.

Confusion between dietary supplements and prescription drugs has been identified as a potential cause of consumer confusion, especially among people with low health literacy. According to the statistics of the U.S. National Assessment of Adult Literacy, a small percentage of adults possess basic or below-basic health literacy, which could hamper their skills in reading product labels and distinguishing between supplements and prescription drugs (Kutner et al., 2006). Kelling (2017) reported that consumers can replace LASA dietary supplements with prescribed medication or accidentally buy a supplement and believe that it is a prescribed drug.

In terms of safety surveillance, adverse events related to dietary supplements have been well documented but underreported. A mixed study on adverse events associated with supplements revealed that some serious events (such as hospitalization) were experienced when a group of users took some type of product, especially those advertised as weight loss supplements and performance-enhancing products (Bent et al., 2003). Follow-up studies of emergency department data in the United States estimated that tens of thousands of emergency department visits are due to dietary supplements each year, with older adults and children being disproportionately impacted (Geller et al., 2015). It has also been noted that the pharmacovigilance systems in the field of dietary supplements have weaknesses: inadequate product identification and slowness to respond to these products (Avigan et al., 2016; Dwyer et al., 2018).

These surveillance restrictions apply to LASA risk. Adverse events due to confusion or substitution of dietary supplements with prescription drugs may not be considered medication errors, may be seen as a consequence of the disease, or may not be communicated using formal safety monitoring systems. The fact that no standardized methods of naming and international product identifiers of dietary supplements exist also makes identifying name-related safety signals more difficult. Systemic LASA risks associated with dietary supplements present a challenge to medication safety models, which are largely based on regulated pharmaceuticals. The use of dietary supplements is often not captured in a standardized way during medication reconciliation procedures, electronic health records, and clinical decision-support tools, which is why the risks associated with LASA related to supplements are not adequately addressed by the tools that are effective in the case of prescription medications (Dwyer et al., 2018).

Overall, the LASA errors related to dietary supplements are clinically significant when the medication safety risk is extended. The high prevalence of supplement use, the common and concurrent use of prescription drugs, inadequate regulatory measures on the naming of supplements, and inadequate pharmacovigilance all provide an environment where name-based confusion can take place. The inclusion of dietary supplements within the larger LASA risk environment is critical for the formulation of prevention initiatives that incorporate pharmacy practices, regulatory supervision, and patient education.

Combined with the above-described epidemiologic situation and regulatory deficiencies, the given factors precondition a definite reason to discuss LASA errors related to dietary supplements using real-life examples. The lack of premarket regulation of the naming and marketing of supplements, high levels of concomitant use with prescription medications, and limited indication-based and visual confusion make the possibility of name-based, indication-based, and visual confusion potentially transform into patient harm. Notably, in addition to phonetic or orthographic similarity, the aspect of semantic similarity, or similarity of the implied therapeutic meaning of a product name or the intended clinical use depicted by a product name or marketing language, is critical in supplement-related LASA risk. Semantic information in product names (e.g., glucose control, anxiety relief, increased attention, or management of withdrawal) can result in patients assuming clinical similarity to prescription drugs, even if there are marked regulatory differences (Dwyer et al., 2018; Kelling, 2017).

To overcome the theoretical risk and provide an example of how these mechanisms can be used in real-life situations, the following subsections provide documented cases of LASA confusion concerning prescription medicines and dietary supplements. These are the cases of opioids, antidiabetic agents, anxiolytics, antidepressants, stimulants, and hypnotics, and the overlap of phonetic and semantic similarity, deceptive therapeutic messages, and consumer self-selection with regulatory restrictions that the U.S. Food and Drug Administration, the World Health Organization, and the Institute for Safe Medication Practices have found in relation to dietary supplements, which places dietary supplements as a clinically relevant extension of the larger LASA medication-safety issue(Bent et al., 2003; Kelling, 2017; National Institutes of Health; U.S. Food and Drug Administration, 2011; World Health Organization, 2017a).

Methadone (Dolophine®) and Mitadone® (U4Life, LLC)

Methadone (Dolophine®) is a prescription opioid drug that is administered in tightly controlled clinical practice for the treatment of opioid use disorder and opioid pain. Mitadone®, developed by U4Life, LLC, is a branded product that is advertised as a dietary supplement that is an anti-opioid aid. In the LASA approach, the pharmacy practice literature has identified Mitadone® as a dietary supplement composed of nondrug ingredients such as vitamins, minerals, and botanical substances, whose name closely resembles the prescription opioid methadone, thereby creating a risk of medication name confusion (Center for Food Safety and Applied Nutrition, 2018; Kelling, 2017; U.S. Food and Drug Administration, 2016). This similarity is a manifestation of phonetic likeness that can cause consumers to have more problems when they distinctly differentiate between a controlled prescription drug and an unregulated supplement product, especially when it is presented out of the clinical context.

In addition to the similarity of names, regulatory issues about Mitadone® could be discussed in terms of a warning letter provided by the U.S. Food and Drug Administration (FDA) in January 2018. The FDA in this letter said that Mitadone® was being sold with claims that it was used to treat or mitigate opioid dependence and withdrawal. The FDA concluded that these claims were more than those allowed for dietary supplements and that the product was deemed misbranded and an unapproved new drug under the Federal Food, Drug, and Cosmetic Act (U.S. Food and Drug Administration, 2016, 2018).

The communication of the FDA noted that the products, which are positioned as opioid dependent or withdrawn, have to be approved by the FDA to be safe and effective. The agency was also worried that such products might influence the health of the population negatively if they cause them to postpone or forego evidence-based medical care. The warning letter required the manufacturer to implement appropriate remedial measures, but there is no publicly available record of any further enforcement actions taken after the initial warning. Collectively, the Mitadone® case indicates that the phonetic similarity of names, coupled with overlapping treatment messages, could be a source of LASA-related issues in the dietary supplement market. Although the pharmacy literature takes naming similarity as a possible cause of confusion (Kelling, 2017), the FDA warning letter also shows that such products can lead to regulatory and safety problems after marketing. This case highlights why dietary supplements should be included in wider LASA risk discourses, especially where the product names are similar to those of prescription drugs that are administered in high-risk treatment fields (Center for Food Safety and Applied Nutrition, 2018).

Metformin (Glucophage®) and Glucocil®

One example of a dietary supplement for LASA risk, which is well documented, is the confusion of metformin (Glucophage®) with a first-line pharmacologic intervention for type 2 diabetes mellitus and Glucocil® with a dietary supplement promoted as supporting blood sugar. In contrast to Glucocil®, which is not authorized to diagnose, treat, cure, or prevent diabetes, metformin is an approved prescription drug whose indications, dose, contraindications, and long-term clinical outcome evidence are well known and established (ClinicalTrials.gov, 2024; U.S. Food and Drug Administration, 2016).

Glucocil® is an example of a common LASA dietary supplement, the name of which and its active use are very similar to those of metformin. It could pose a significant risk of patients being confused, especially in online shopping, where dietary supplements may stand side by side with prescription drugs in search results (Kelling, 2017). Glucocil® is a multi-ingredient dietary supplement that contains vitamins D3, B1, B6, and B12; chromium picolinate; fish oil/omega-3 fatty acids; and a proprietary blood glucose management blend that includes *Phellodendron chinense* bark extract, alpha-lipoic acid, *Morus alba* leaf extract, *Gymnema sylvestre* leaf extract, *Cissus quadrangularis* leaf extract, banaba extract (*Lagerstroemia speciosa* leaf), Insulina (*Cissus sicyoides* leaf), and cinnamon (*Cinnamomum cassia* bark) (National Institutes of Health, 2026a).

Name and indication mimicry is the main force behind the LASA mechanism here since the similarity between "gluco-" and "glucemic" control can be considered a strong indicator, which can create a certain impression of therapeutic similarity to patients, particularly those who are less health literate (Kelling, 2017). This process is in line with the World Health Organization Medication Without Harm program, which labels drug name confusion, improper substitution, and patient misconception as the situations that lead to preventable medication-related harm in all healthcare systems (World Health Organization, 2017a, 2017b). In this view, dietary supplements such as LASA products expand medication safety risks into the real-world context of the patient and the environment of traditional prescribing and dispensing.

Regulatory bodies have consistently reiterated that dietary supplements that promise the treatment of diabetes are being sold illegally and could cause health fraud. The FDA has issued alert messages to consumers that products being marketed as substitutes for prescription antidiabetic drugs are unlawful and may be hazardous and clearly state that no dietary supplement has been given green light in the treatment of diabetes (U.S. Food and Drug Administration, 2016). The dietary supplement labeling instructions also serve to further explain that a product can be regarded as a misbranded product provided that its names, labeling, or marketing information suggest treatment of a disease, even without specific therapeutic labeling. Glucocil® ingredient disclosure, as recorded in the National Institutes of Health Dietary Supplement Label Database, confirms that Glucocil® is a dietary supplement of vitamins, minerals, and botanical substances and not an approved pharmacologic agent and does not prove clinical equivalence to metformin (ClinicalTrials.gov, 2024; National Institutes of Health; U.S. Food and Drug Administration, 2016).

Considering medication safety, this LASA combination also reflects the ideas suggested by the Institute of Safe Medication Practices (ISMP), which has consistently recognized drug name confusion and misleading product nomenclature as the continuing reasons for the errors in medication. ISMP instructions also underscore the fact that the names appear similar and are pronounced in a similar way, and their intended meaning may be inappropriate product use where patients on their own choose products without the oversight of professionals. Although ISMP recommendations have typically been applied to prescription and over-the-counter medications, the case of metformin (Glucophage®) and Glucocil® shows that the risk mechanisms can also be applied to dietary supplements that are visually or semantically similar to prescription drugs (Kelling, 2017; The Institute for Safe Medication Practices (ISMP), 2019).

Although clinical studies examining nonpharmacologic or adjunctive glycemic control strategies remain ongoing, with some registered clinical trials comparing supplement-based interventions, these studies have no effect on the regulatory difference between antidiabetic drugs approved by the FDA and dietary supplements and are not justifiable to replace current antidiabetic treatment in routine clinical care (ClinicalTrials.gov, 2024). In terms of patient safety, there is a significant risk of misconfusion between Glucophage® and Glucocil®, including the incorrect discontinuation of effective antidiabetic therapy, late treatment escalation, and avoidable onset of complications caused by diabetes. In line with the WHO and ISMP recommendations, active monitoring of dietary supplement use, clear patient education about regulatory status, and any misleading claims or adverse event reporting using FDA reporting mechanisms are critical approaches to reducing harm related to dietary supplementation with LASA products (ClinicalTrials.gov, 2024; U.S. Food and Drug Administration, 2016).

Alprazolam (Xanax®) and Alprazium®

Alprazolam (Xanax®), a benzodiazepine prescribed to treat anxiety and panic attacks. It is a prescription central nervous system depressant with relatively well-known pharmacologic effects, safety issues, and regulatory restrictions. Alprazium®, a dietary supplement used to treat anxiety and mood, is still a regulated dietary supplement and has no approval to diagnose, treat, cure, or prevent anxiety disorders. Kelling (2017) reported that Alprazium® is an LASA dietary supplement where the name shares both phonetic and orthographic similarity with alprazolam, which heightens the chances of confusion as patients select supplemental products during self-selection, especially in cases of online shopping where the supplement products are placed next to the prescription drug information. The fact that this is similar to alprazolam can cause patients to wrongly believe that Alprazium® is an equivalent to alprazolam that is natural and safer and, as a consequence, may lead to inappropriate substitution, untreated anxiety, or a lack of evidence-based pharmacotherapy (Kelling, 2017).

Alprazolam (Xanax®) and Zanivan®

Alprazolam (Xanax®) and Zanivan® pose a LASA risk in dietary supplements. Another occurrence of LASA mishaps in dietary supplements is the association of alprazolam (Xanax®), a benzodiazepine prescribed to manage anxiety and panic disorders, with Zanivan®, a dietary supplement sold to manage stress and emotional balance. The pharmacologic effects, safety issues, and regulatory oversight of alprazolam have been well characterized, whereas Zanivan® is regulated as a dietary supplement and is not indicated for the diagnosis, treatment, cure, or prevention of anxiety-related illnesses. One specific LASA dietary supplement, Zanivan®, shares the phonetic similarity of alprazolam, and therefore, the likelihood of confusion is enhanced, especially in consumer-driven purchasing markets where a patient transacts on their devices/means by looking up the name of a medication and choosing a dietary supplement bearing its name. Patients can be mistaken because of such similarity; Zanivan® is perceived as a more natural and safer choice than alprazolam is, which increases the chances of inappropriate substitution, untreated anxiety symptoms, or delays in accessing evidence-based pharmacologic therapy (Kelling, 2017).

Bupropion (Zyban®) and Zypan®

Bupropion (Zyban®) is a prescription antidepressant that is also used for smoking cessation, and it has established indications, dosages, contraindications, and safety concerns. Zypan® is a nutritional supplement that is sold to assist in digestive support, and it has not been approved to diagnose, treat, cure, or prevent depression or nicotine dependence. The fact that there are both Zyban® (a brand name) and Zypan® (a dietary supplement name) is a LASA risk, which is primarily due to phonetic resemblance and could contribute to patient confusion in consumer-driven purchasing scenarios. The drug most frequently purchased, Zypan®, which is not indicated as a smoking cessation or mood medication, may be erroneously chosen by individuals who happen across the name because of a lack of understanding of its indication and who do not have depression or tobacco dependence. This confusion can lead to incorrect substitution, delay in the onset of evidence-based therapy, or continuation of untreated symptoms, which highlights patient safety issues related to dietary supplementation with LASA products (Kelling, 2017).

Dextroamphetamine/Amphetamine (Adderall®) and Adderplex®

It is a prescription central nervous system stimulant (dextroamphetamine/amphetamine (Adderall®)) used to treat attention-deficit/hyperactivity disorder and narcolepsy with known efficacy, dose specifications, contraindications, and side effects, which include the risk of abuse and cardiovascular and psychiatric events. Adderplex® is a dietary supplement that is sold to support focus and attention and is not approved to diagnose, treat, cure, or prevent neuropsychiatric disorders. The resemblance of the brand names Adderall® and Adderplex® is an LASA risk based essentially on phonetic similarity that can result in patient confusion in consumer-directed purchasing settings. Patients who are looking to have a stimulant prescription to address problems in either focus or concentration can easily pick Adderplex(r) by mistake because of its nondrug status and unproven ability to treat Attention-Deficit/Hyperactivity Disorder (ADHD). This confusion can result in a wrong substitution, late introduction of evidence-based therapy, or the continuation of untreated symptoms, highlighting the dangers to patient safety in terms of dietary supplementation with LASA products (Kelling, 2017).

Eszopiclone (Lunesta®) and Luna®

Eszopiclone (Lunesta®) is a prescription sedative-hypnotic that is used to treat insomnia, and its use has proven to be effective. Dosage, contraindications, and safety issues are linked to central nervous system depression and impaired psychomotor functions the next day. Luna® is a diet supplement that is being sold on the value of sleep quality and relaxation and is not intended to be used to diagnose, cure, treat, or prevent sleep disorders. The resemblance of the Lunesta® and Luna® names constitutes a LASA risk motivated by phonetic and orthographic closeness, which can be the cause of confusion among patients in consumer-driven purchasing settings. The National Institutes of Health Dietary Supplement Label Database lists products sold under the Luna® brand name as being based on nondrug ingredients commonly found in sleep-support products, including botanical extracts and nutraceutical components such as valerian root, melatonin, chamomile, and lemon balm that may change across manufacturers and eras (National Institutes of Health, 2026b). Patients who want pharmacologic insomnia treatment might thus fall into the trap of wrongfully making an uninformed choice of the wrong medication by the name Luna® and end up receiving the wrong replacement, continuing with sleeping disturbances, or may end up receiving evidence-based therapy late. This LASA combination is a perfect example of patient safety issues related to dietary supplements whose names are similar to those of prescription sedative-hypnotic drugs (Kelling, 2017).

Dietary supplements resembling prescription drug names have the potential to produce clinically significant LASA risks, as shown in Figure 3, by fostering confusion, inappropriate self-selection, and delaying the administration of evidence-based treatment.

Figure 3. Confusion of dietary supplementation-related LASA is an example of how the name of the supplement can sound like a prescription drug and cause inappropriate substitution, delayed treatment, and harm to patients

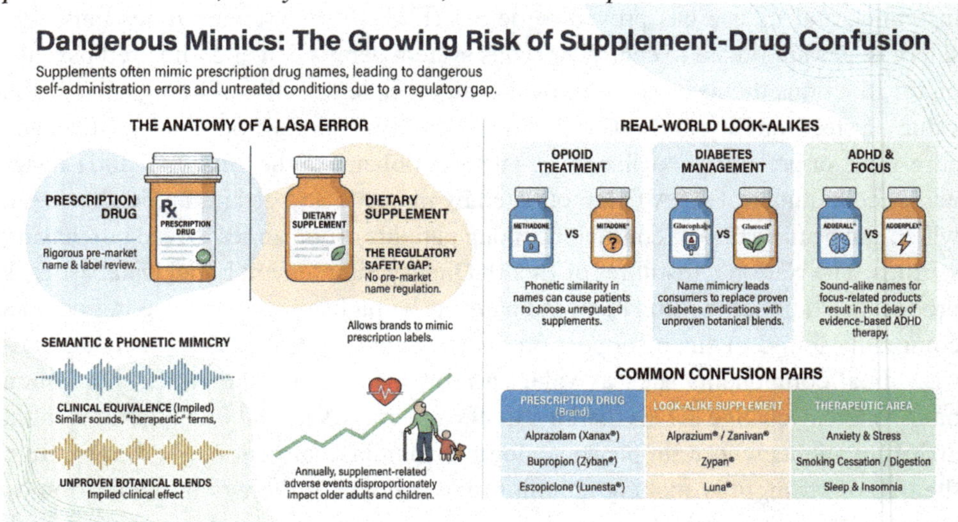

PRESCRIPTION DRUG (Brand)	LOOK-ALIKE SUPPLEMENT	THERAPEUTIC AREA
Alprazolam (Xanax®)	Alprazium® / Zanivan®	Anxiety & Stress
Bupropion (Zyban®)	Zypan®	Smoking Cessation / Digestion
Eszopiclone (Lunesta®)	Luna®	Sleep & Insomnia

In addition, LASA risk has been documented in herbal dietary supplements in hospitals in Thailand, where similarity in names is not the only issue to be confused by; similar packaging and visual presentation of the product, as seen in Figure 4, also contribute. An in-hospital medication safety report reported a case in which herbal products were dispensed in pharmaceutical-like packages with dissimilar colors, types of capsules, and label designs, which heightened the chances of selection and administration mistakes by the patients and their caregivers. Another example is that Thaowan Priang, or Jewel Vine (*Derris scandens*), and Fah Talai Jone (*Andrographis paniculata*), Bitter Cucumber (*Momordica charantia),* and Senna *(Senna alexandrina)* were sold in almost the same green blister packs, although their therapeutic indications were different. This visual similarity can cause misunderstandings of regulatory equivalence and therapeutic interchangeability, which further increase the LASA risk beyond name-based confusion to packaging-related look-like effects in the Thai healthcare environment (Bueng Kan Hospital, 2021).

Figure 4. Examples of look-alike packaging of herbal dietary supplements in a hospital setting in Thailand. Drug pair (A) Thaowan Priang (Jewel Vine; Derris scandens) and Fah Talai Jone (Andrographis paniculata), whereas drug pair (B) Bitter Cucumber (Momordica charantia) and Senna (Senna alexandrina). Even though they have different indications for therapy, both pairs are given almost identical green blister packs, which demonstrates packaging-related visual similarity

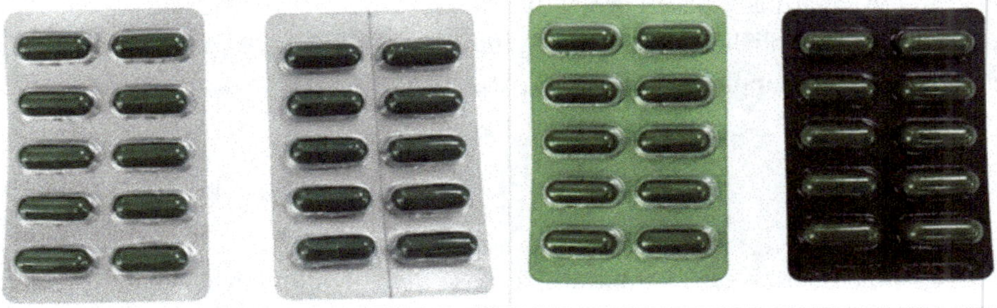

A) Thaowan Priang (Jewel Vine; *Derris scandens*) and Fah Talai Jone (*Andrographis paniculata*)

(B) Bitter Cucumber (*Momordica charantia*) and Senna (*Senna alexandrina*)

PREVENTION STRATEGIES THAT INCLUDE REGULATION, PHARMACY PRACTICE, AND PATIENT EDUCATION

To prevent dietary supplement-related look-alike and sound-alike (LASA) errors, a multilevel approach should be used. Regulatory measures include enhancing the control of the naming, labeling, and packaging of dietary supplements, especially in the area of misleading disease-related claims and the presentation of products, which can create the impression of therapeutic equivalence to prescription drugs (Avigan et al., 2016; Radimer et al., 2004; U.S. Food and Drug Administration, 2011). In contrast to pharmaceuticals, dietary supplements do not undergo proactive premarket screening of LASA names, which enables goods with potentially confusing names or appearances to be on the market (Kelling, 2017).

Systematic medication reconciliation, which explicitly records dietary supplement intake; the detection of LASA-prone products during dispensing and counseling; and the reporting of suspected LASA-related incidents using established medication safety systems, are regarded as pharmacy practice interventions (Institute for Safe Medication Practices, 2019). These practices correspond to international medication safety principles that focus on avoiding name- and appearance-based confusion (World Health Organization, 2017a).

Incorrect beliefs about the safety and regulatory status of dietary supplements should be considered when patients are educated. In counseling, it should be stressed that FDA-approved medicines and dietary supplements differ when the first is used over the second and that the risks of their inappropriate substitution are quite significant, and healthcare professionals should notify healthcare professionals about supplement consumption (Dwyer et al., 2018; Kelling, 2017). Combining regulatory intervention, pharmacy-based protective measures, and patient-centered education as part of the established patient safety models can decrease preventable injuries related to dietary supplement-related LASA risks.

CONCLUSION

LASA medication errors continue to pose a challenging and avoidable patient safety risk to all healthcare systems. Although LASA risks have been historically discussed in the context of prescription and over-the-counter drugs, this chapter proves that dietary supplements present a neglected but rapidly growing aspect of LASA-related harm. The high prevalence of supplement use, common concomitant use of prescription drugs, insufficient regulation of supplement names and packaging, and limitations in pharmacovigilance systems create an environment where confusion based on name and appearance can occur.

This risk is compounded by the regulatory difference between pharmaceuticals, which undergo strict premarket screening of names prior to market launch and postmarketing surveillance, and dietary supplements, which are frequently marketed without proactive LASA evaluation. The evidence reviewed in this chapter demonstrates that certain names and other presentation features of the supplements closely resemble existing prescription drugs, with some being deliberately intended to do so, and this creates uncertainty regarding the distinction between controlled therapies and uncontrolled products. Additionally, the hospital-based examples provided in Thailand demonstrate that the risk of LASA is not limited to the nomenclature but also to look-alike packaging and even similarity in visual representation, even among herbal-based products with various therapeutic indications.

The interventions needed to resolve dietary supplement-related LASA errors are more comprehensive medication safety programs involving a combination of pharmacy practices, relevant regulatory policies, and patient education. The strategies required include active medication reconciliation that incorporates supplements, better regulatory oversight of naming and packaging procedures, better reporting of adverse events, and patient-centered counseling. The identification of dietary supplements as components of the LASA risk environment is important for expanding overall prevention programs and enhancing global patient safety.

REFERENCES

Avigan, M. I., Mozersky, R. P., & Seeff, L. B. (2016). Scientific and Regulatory Perspectives in Herbal and Dietary Supplement Associated Hepatotoxicity in the United States. *International Journal of Molecular Sciences*, *17*(3), 331. DOI: 10.3390/ijms17030331 PMID: 26950122

Bailey, R. L., Gahche, J. J., Miller, P. E., Thomas, P. R., & Dwyer, J. T. (2013). Why US adults use dietary supplements. *JAMA Internal Medicine*, *173*(5), 355–361. DOI: 10.1001/jamainternmed.2013.2299 PMID: 23381623

Bekker, J. L., Flores, A., & Sinha, M. S. (2023). Re-regulating dietary supplements. *Journal of Food Law & Policy, 19*(2), 1–22. https://doi.org/10.54119/jflp.eqso5002

Bent, S., Tiedt, T. N., Odden, M. C., & Shlipak, M. G. (2003). The relative safety of ephedra compared with other herbal products. *Annals of Internal Medicine*, *138*(6), 468–471. DOI: 10.7326/0003-4819-138-6-200303180-00010 PMID: 12639079

Bryan, R., Aronson, J. K., ten Hacken, P., Williams, A., & Jordan, S. (2015). Patient safety in medication nomenclature: Orthographic and semantic properties of International Nonproprietary Names. *PLoS One*, *10*(12), e0145431. DOI: 10.1371/journal.pone.0145431 PMID: 26701761

Bueng Kan Hospital. (2021). *Look Alike Sound Alike Drug*. Retrieved 17 Jan from https://bkh.moph.go.th/bkhweb/uploads/media/202303310725123_4.LASA_update-_2566.pdf#page=6.00

Center for Food Safety and Applied Nutrition. U. S. F. a. D. A. (2018). *U4Life LLC dba Mitadone*. Retrieved 18 Jan from https://www.fda.gov/inspections-compliance-enforcement-and-criminal-investigations/warning-letters/u4life-llc-dba-mitadone-542731-01112018

Chen, F., Du, M., Blumberg, J. B., Ho Chui, K. K., Ruan, M., Rogers, G., & Zhang, F. F. (2019). Association Among Dietary Supplement Use, Nutrient Intake, and Mortality Among U.S. Adults: A Cohort Study. *Annals of Internal Medicine*, *170*(9), 604–613. DOI: 10.7326/M18-2478 PMID: 30959527

Cheung, R. Y., & Goodwin, S. H. (2013). What's in a drug name? *Canadian Pharmacists Journal/Revue des Pharmaciens du Canada*, 146(1), 8-9. DOI: 10.1177/1715163512472651

ClinicalTrials.gov. (2024). *A study to assess effect of Glucocil® on metabolic health in individuals with prediabetes and type 2 diabetes mellitus (ClinicalTrials.gov Identifier: NCT*06496893). *U.S. National Library of Medicine.* Retrieved 18 Jan from https://www.clinicaltrials.gov/study/NCT06496893#study-plan

Cohen, M. R. (2007). Causes of medication errors. In Cohen, M. R. (Ed.), *Medication Errors* (2nd ed., pp. 55–66). The American Pharmacists Association. DOI: 10.21019/9781582120928.ch4

Cohen, M. R., Domizio, G. D., & Lee, R. E. (2007). The role of drug names in medication errors. In Cohen, M. R. (Ed.), *Medication Errors* (2nd ed., pp. 87–110). The American Pharmacists Association. https://doi.org/doi:10.21019/9781582120928.ch6

Cohen, P. A. (2009). American Roulette — Contaminated Dietary Supplements. *The New England Journal of Medicine*, *361*(16), 1523–1525. DOI: 10.1056/NEJMp0904768 PMID: 19812394

Dhande, P. P., Mule, A. V., & Chaudhari, A. P. (2021). Retrospective analysis of look-alike and sound-alike drug incidents in a tertiary care hospital. *Indian Journal of Pharmacy Practice*, *14*(2), 115. DOI: 10.5530/ijopp.14.2.21

Dwyer, J. T., Coates, P. M., & Smith, M. J. (2018). Dietary Supplements: Regulatory Challenges and Research Resources. *Nutrients*, *10*(1), 41. Advance online publication. DOI: 10.3390/nu10010041 PMID: 29300341

Gahche, J., Bailey, R., Burt, V., Hughes, J., Yetley, E., Dwyer, J., & Sempos, C. (2011). Dietary supplement use among U.S. adults has increased since NHANES III (1988-1994). *NCHS Data Brief*, (61), 1–8. PMID: 21592424

Gardiner, P., Sarma, D. N., Low Dog, T., Barrett, M. L., Chavez, M. L., Ko, R., & Giancaspro, G. I. (2008). The state of dietary supplement adverse event reporting in the United States. *Pharmacoepidemiology and Drug Safety*, *17*(10), 962–970. DOI: 10.1002/pds.1627 PMID: 18613260

Geller, A. I., Shehab, N., Weidle, N. J., Lovegrove, M. C., Wolpert, B. J., Timbo, B. B., Mozersky, R. P., & Budnitz, D. S. (2015). Emergency Department Visits for Adverse Events Related to Dietary Supplements. *The New England Journal of Medicine*, *373*(16), 1531–1540. DOI: 10.1056/NEJMsa1504267 PMID: 26465986

Karet, G. B. (2023). Linguistic analysis of generic-generic drug name pairs prone to wrong-drug errors for which tall-man lettering is recommended. *Therapeutic Innovation & Regulatory Science*, *57*(4), 751–758. DOI: 10.1007/s43441-023-00526-0 PMID: 37171707

Kelling, S. E. (2017). Look-alike/sound-alike dietary supplements. *Journal of the American Pharmacists Association*, *57*(3), 300–301. DOI: 10.1016/j.japh.2017.03.001 PMID: 28411012

Kutner, M., Greenberg, E., & Baer, J. (2006). *A First Look at the Literacy of America's Adults in the 21st Century. NCES 2006-470*. National Center for Education Statistics.

Marovino, E., Morgillo, A., Mancino, N., Di Feo, V., & Genito, E. (2022). Therapeutic error: Types and prevention strategies and focus about" Look Alike/Sound Alike" and" High Risk" drugs. *Journal of Pharmaceutical Research International*, *34*(48A), 9–16. DOI: 10.9734/jpri/2022/v34i48A36409

Muchu, P. (2024). Look Alike Sound Alike Drugs in Adults. *International Journal of Health Care and Biological Sciences*, *5*(1), 18–23. DOI: 10.46795/ijhcbs.v5i1.609

National Institutes of Health. (2026a). *Dietary Supplement Label Database: Glucocil® product label*. Retrieved 18 Jan from https://dsld.od.nih.gov/label/301431

National Institutes of Health. (2026b). *Dietary Supplement Label Database: Luna Gentle Sleep Aid*. Retrieved 18 Jan from https://dsld.od.nih.gov/label/255959

Radimer, K., Bindewald, B., Hughes, J., Ervin, B., Swanson, C., & Picciano, M. F. (2004). Dietary Supplement Use by US Adults: Data from the National Health and Nutrition Examination Survey, 1999–2000. *American Journal of Epidemiology*, *160*(4), 339–349. DOI: 10.1093/aje/kwh207 PMID: 15286019

Rahman, Z., & Parvin, R. (2015). Medication errors associated with look-alike/sound-alike drugs: A brief review. *J Enam Med Col*, *5*(2), 110–117. DOI: 10.3329/jemc.v5i2.23385

Schroeder, S. R., Salomon, M. M., Galanter, W. L., Schiff, G. D., Vaida, A. J., Gaunt, M. J., Bryson, M. L., Rash, C., Falck, S., & Lambert, B. L. (2017). Cognitive tests predict real-world errors: The relationship between drug name confusion rates in laboratory-based memory and perception tests and corresponding error rates in large pharmacy chains. *BMJ Quality &amp. Safety (Basel, Switzerland)*, *26*(5), 395–407. DOI: 10.1136/bmjqs-2015-005099 PMID: 27193033

Supapaan, T. S., Napaporn, J., Ruthirakanok, R., Srichathum, S., Songmuang, A., & Pitchayajittipong, C. (2024). Look-alike sound-alike (LASA) medication errors in Thai hospitals. *Pharmacy Practice*, *22*(1), 2886.

The Institute for Safe Medication Practices (ISMP). (2019). *ISMP list of confused drug names*. Retrieved 11 Oct from https://www.ismp.org/recommendations/confused-drug-names-list

U.S. Food and Drug Administration. (2011). *Guidance for Industry: Substantiation for Dietary Supplement Claims Made Under Section* 403(*r*) (6) *of the Federal Food, Drug, and Cosmetic Act*. Retrieved 17 Jan from https://www.fda.gov/regulatory-information/search-fda-guidance-documents/guidance-industry-substantiation-dietary-supplement-claims-made-under-section-403r-6-federal-food

U.S. Food and Drug Administration. (2016). *Questions and Answers: FDA alerts companies to stop the illegal sale of products claiming to treat diabetes*. https://www.fda.gov/consumers/health-fraud-scams/questions-and-answers-fda-alerts-companies-stop-illegal-sale-products-claiming-treat-diabetes

U.S. Food and Drug Administration. (2018). *Illegally sold opioid cessation products*. Retrieved 18 Jan from https://www.fda.gov/consumers/health-fraud-scams/illegally-sold-opioid-cessation-products#:~:text=U4Life%2C%20LLC%20dba%20Mitadone%20%C2%B7%20Mitadone%20Anti%2DOpiate,Product%20name%20linked%20to%20Flickr%20image%20when

Vlietinck, A., Pieters, L., & Apers, S. (2009). Legal requirements for the quality of herbal substances and herbal preparations for the manufacturing of herbal medicinal products in the European union. *Planta Medica*, *75*(7), 683–688. DOI: 10.1055/s-0029-1185307 PMID: 19204891

World Health Organization. (2004). *WHO guidelines on safety monitoring of herbal medicines in pharmacovigilance systems*. Retrieved 18 Jan from https://www.who.int/publications/i/item/9241592214

World Health Organization. (2017a). *Guidance on the use of International Non-proprietary Names (INNs) for pharmaceutical substances*. Retrieved 16 June from https://cdn.who.int/media/docs/default-source/international-nonproprietary-names-(inn)/who-pharm-s-nom-1570.pdf

World Health Organization. (2017b). *Medication without harm*. Retrieved 10 Feb from https://www.who.int/initiatives/medication-without-harm

ABBREVIATIONS

DSHEA: Dietary Supplement Health and Education Act
FDA: U.S. Food and Drug Administration
INN: International Nonproprietary Names
ISMP: Institute for Safe Medication Practices
LASA: Look-Alike, Sound-Alike
NHANES: National Health and Nutrition Examination Survey

U.S.: United States
WHO: World Health Organization

Chapter 9
Oral Liquid Medications and LASA Errors

ABSTRACT

Oral liquid drugs are necessary for both pediatric and geriatric populations and dysphagic patients but are unique to look-alike and sound-alike (LASA) medication mistakes. The chapter summarizes international and Thai data on the epidemiology of LASA errors with oral liquids and identifies the risk mechanisms of similarity between the packaging, consistency in labelling, different concentrations, and the necessity of measuring doses and administration by the caregiver. National data on Thailand indicate that oral liquid LASA pairs comprise 3.39 percent of all LASA pairs reported, with the similarity of packaging as the predominant mechanism. Examples of generic-name oral liquid LASA pairs are used to provide case studies and analyze vulnerabilities in prescribing and administration and focus on system-level issues to allow safer utilization.

INTRODUCTION

Oral liquid drugs contribute significantly to drug therapy for children and geriatric and dysphagic patients since they allow the individualization of doses and provide easy administration when oral direct dosage forms cannot be used. Nevertheless, oral fluids are invariably linked with frequent susceptibilities in drug-taking procedures, especially in the measurement and administration of drugs in outpatient and home-care facilities, where the precision of dosing relies on the skill of the caregiver and the dosing device applied (Yin et al., 2014; Yin et al., 2010). These susceptibilities are compounded further in look-alike, sound-alike (LASA) situations, including similar names of drugs, labeling, or even the presence of more than one strength, where errors in selection and administration can exist at various stages of prescribing, dispensing, and caregiver administration. On the international scale, the

DOI: 10.4018/979-8-3373-5478-1.ch009

Medication Without Harm program by the World Health Organization highlights medication safety as a system-level goal in any healthcare environment, which also implies that one will need to focus on the preventable error processes that continue re-emerging in actual practice (World Health Organization, 2017, 2021). The data from Thailand also indicate that the risks of LASA medications remain despite the already developed safety measures, and the similarity of the names and pronunciation is often the cause, which is why it is necessary to implement more intensive control by the system of risk factors (Supapaan T et al., 2024; Supapaan TS, Kamnuek J, et al., 2024; Supapaan TS, Songmuang A, et al., 2024; Supapaan, Napaporn, et al., 2024; Supapaan, Songmuang, et al., 2024).

Objectives of the Chapter

The aims of this chapter are as follows:

(1) To briefly outline LASA issues and the history of medication errors.
(2) To summarize the epidemiology of LASA errors associated with oral liquid medications.
(3) To report Thai case reports and recorded LASA error incidences.
(4) To investigate human factors throughout the medication-use process that lead to LASA risk.
(5) To determine the weaknesses of prescribing and dosing expressions in oral liquids.
(6) To examine measurement tools and administration errors that are related to the use of oral liquids.
(7) To assess the determinants of LASA risk, such as labeling, packaging, and health literacy.
(8) To identify risk-reduction measures for compounded oral liquid medications.

Organization of the Chapter

Chapter 9 starts by providing an overview of look-alike, sound-alike (LASA) medication errors and a historical overview of medication safety, particularly oral liquid formulations. It subsequently analyzes the epidemiology of LASA errors in oral liquids and combines international evidence with Thai evidence at the national level to explain prevalence trends and major risk mechanisms. The chapter then provides case studies of the Thai LASA to depict the life consequences and the vulnerability of the system. The chapter subsequently evaluates human factors in the medication-use process, such as prescribing, dispensing, administering, and monitoring. Vulnerabilities have to do with dose expression, measurement equipment, labeling, packaging, and health literacy. Dedicated sections clarify how these aspects increase the risks of LASA in oral liquids. This chapter presents reduction strategies for compounded and commercial oral liquid preparations on the basis of evidence; it also includes system-level strategies to minimize avoidable harm.

EPIDEMIOLOGY OF LASA ERRORS IN ORAL LIQUIDS

LASA errors are a clinically important and consistent subgroup of reported medication errors in all parts of the world. Confusion due to similar drug names or appearances has been found to explain a significant portion of medication errors (range of 6–15% based on study design) in medication-error surveillance systems, narrative reviews, and large retrospective studies, with much greater variation in provisional beliefs based on study design, operationalization, clinical setting, and reporting culture (Bryan et al., 2021a; Bryan et al., 2021b; Hoffman & Proulx, 2003; World Health Organization, 2017). LASA errors occur because of orthographic (similarity of look-alikes) and phonetic (similarity of sounds) similarities and are often exacerbated by similarities in the package form, the dosage form, its strength, or the indication, which increase the risk of wrong-drug or wrong-strength selection (Allard et al., 2002; Bryan et al., 2021a; Bryan et al., 2021b; Cohen MR et al., 2021).

LASA confusion has been extensively recognized as a frequent cause of wrong-drug and wrong-strength errors throughout the medication-use process through medication-error surveillance. Initial findings regarding U.S. reports of medication errors revealed LASA mechanisms as a factor that frequently contributes to wrong-drug events, and oral liquid formulations were frequently the focus of problems since product choice decisions may be based heavily on visual cues as well as the coexistence of multiple strengths and formulations within the same therapeutic class (Cohen & Davis, 1992). Later, extensive retrospective studies of reporting systems, such as the United States Pharmacopeia (USP) Medication Error Reporting Program (MEDMARX®), a voluntary medication error reporting system (Hicks et al., 2006; Santell et al., 2003), verified that LASA errors are found throughout the use of medications and that dispensing was repeatedly found to be a significant point of failure. Wrong products were repeatedly selected among liquid drugs of similar packaging, labeling, or concentration. Although most of the events were intercepted prior to patient exposure, a consistent group of events occurred among patients, which proved the unavoidable risk when system defenses were weak (Chumchit et al., 2015; Hicks et al., 2008).

The use of oral liquid preparations is a unique and clinically relevant subcategory of LASA error epidemiology. In addition to similarity in name and packaging, oral liquids also add the additional complication of dose administration and caregiver administration, which increases the chances that an initial selection error will become a dose administration error at the point of use. Medication-safety efforts are focused on liquid medication that must be administered by a caregiver; these efforts focus on the fact that this type of error is a frequent location of error, especially in outpatient and home-care environments where formal safety measures are constrained (World Health Organization, 2017, 2023). Even minor deviations in an administered volume can lead to a clinically significant underdose or overdose, particularly in children and in those drugs with a small therapeutic index (Yin et al., 2014; Yin et al., 2010).

Medication errors associated with the administration of oral liquids that involve LASA are not limited to pediatric practice. Adult populations and evidence-based studies conducted in different countries that involve multiple countries indicate that oral liquid preparations are frequently involved in various healthcare settings. European, Asian, and Australian published analyses and reviews have reported LASA with cough and cold syrup, gastrointestinal liquid preparations, antihistamines, and iron preparations in adults and mixed populations. In these studies, the visual attributes of the product, including the shape of the container, color, and layout of the label, always have a more profound effect on product choice than the phonetic similarity of the drug names to each other does. In situations that involve a high workload, frequent interruptions, and the use of visual memory during the dispensing process, similarity in the type of packaging and the appearance of the containers becomes among the most influential factors leading to wrong-product selection even in cases where the medications are therapeutically unrelated (Bryan et al., 2021a; Bryan et al., 2021b; Hoffman & Proulx, 2003).

Pediatric-oriented studies, however, indicate that oral liquid preparations are overrepresented among reported medication errors compared with solid-dose preparations. Pediatric-based systematic reviews and observational studies repeatedly indicate that liquids are found in wrong-drug and wrong-dose reports, and LASA confusion is often mentioned as a causative factor. Even though the rate of interception across hospital settings is quite high, most of the reported incidences fall into the National Coordinating Council for Medication Error Reporting and Prevention (NCC MERP) categories, implying that an error after discharge, during caregiver administration, is more likely to reach the patient, which shows a change in the risk factor from controlled institutional settings to home environments (Yin et al., 2014).

Extemporaneous compounding activities increase the LASA risks of oral liquids. In the case of the nonavailability of age-commercial liquid preparation formulations, inconsistency in concentrations, containers, and labeling results in latent vulnerability of the system. In Thailand, cross-sectional studies continuously reflect LASA involving the use of pediatric antipyretics, antibiotics, gastrointestinal agents, and traditional mixtures, which are more representative of structural and process-related weaknesses than a specific error (Supapaan, Napaporn, et al., 2024).

Among the national Thai LASA dataset of 2,510 pairs of drugs in all dosage forms, 85 pairs (3.39%) were found to have liquid dose forms. Even though oral liquids reflect a smaller percentage of LASA pairs than tablets/capsules do (66.69%) and injectable preparations do (17.01%), their epidemiologic significance is not because of their absolute frequency but because of their similarity and downward risk mechanisms. The type of similarity analysis of LASA shows that similarity in oral liquid LASA errors is mostly packaging similarity-based. The percentage of liquid dosage forms contributed 6.87 to the total number of all the pairs of packaging-related LASA, and only 2.68% were related to name or pronunciation similarity. Conversely, none of the LASA pairs that had liquid dosage forms were ascribed to the similarity of the appearance of tablets/capsules, emphasizing that the LASA risk profile of oral liquids is essentially different from that of solid dosage forms (Supapaan, Napaporn, et al., 2024).

This trend cuts across the structural properties of liquid drugs. Commercially prepared oral liquids (as well as extemporaneously prepared liquids) are usually dispensed in standardized containers (such as amber bottles) with only minor visual distinctions related to shape, color, or label arrangement. As a result, the label design and appearance of containers, but not the orthography of drug names, are primary signals during dispensing. When there is pressure to work and interruption, the probability of selecting the wrong product increases with the use of these visual cues.

With respect to safety, the relatively small percentage of liquid LASA pairs cannot be regarded as having low clinical importance. The mechanisms underlying the risk amplification of oral liquids include volume measurement, administration by caregivers, and frequent use by children. Consequently, one oral LASA selection error is more likely to persist in causing a dosing error at the administration point, especially in an outpatient and home-care environment.

Altogether, oral liquid LASA errors are a qualitatively different subgroup of LASA risk, where packaging-related similarity and augmented downstream toxicity occur. These results support the importance of dosage-form-specific prevention strategies such as standardized labeling, container differentiation, and storage segregation in lieu of similar LASA controls on all preparations.

Across regions and populations, the literature converges on four verified conclusions. First, oral liquid medications are consistently represented among reported LASA events. Although they constitute a smaller proportion of LASA pairs than tablets/capsules and injectable preparations do, oral liquids exhibit distinct and recurrent risk mechanisms related to packaging similarity, labeling uniformity, and the need for dose measurement. Second, dispensing and caregiver administration emerge as critical risk points, reflecting a heavy reliance on visual cues during product selection in pharmacy workflows and the downstream amplification of errors during home administration. Third, while most reported oral liquid LASA events are intercepted—with many classified in early medication error categories—their repeated identification across multiple datasets indicates persistent system-level vulnerabilities rather than isolated human error. Finally, pediatric liquid formulations requiring volume measurement represent a particularly high-risk subgroup, although adult oral liquids, including cough, gastrointestinal, antihistamine, and iron preparations, are also frequently used. Collectively, the patterns summarized in Table 1 support the prioritization of system-level interventions—such as standardized labeling, packaging differentiation, storage segregation, and clear dosing communication—over reliance on individual vigilance alone.

Table 1. Reported prevalence and patterns of oral liquid LASA errors

Study Type	Oral Liquid Involvement	Dominant LASA Mechanisms	Error Stage Most Reported	Severity Pattern	Setting/ Data Source
Narrative analysis of medication-error reports	Oral liquids frequently cited in LASA wrong-drug events	Similar names; similar packaging; multiple strengths	Dispensing	Many intercepted; some reached patients	U.S. national reports Cohen and Smetzer (2018)
Retrospective database analysis	Liquids recurrent among LASA cases	Packaging similarity; strength confusion	Dispensing	Predominantly NCC MERP B, C–D	MedMARx database (U.S.) Hicks et al. (2008)
Cross-sectional national analysis	85 liquid LASA pairs (3.39% of 2,510)	Similar packaging; similar names; multiple strengths	Dispensing	Mostly NCC MERP B–C	Thailand (multihospital) Supapaan, Napaporn, et al. (2024)

THAI REPORTS OF THE LASA ERROR CASE STUDIES

Case reports in the real world are important for critically understanding how LASA medication errors can be seen in noncontrollable institutional environments and how seemingly minor system vulnerabilities can culminate in severe patient injury. A few well-publicized cases in Thailand show that the errors of LASA are not limited to the mix-up of two oral drugs; there are also mix-ups between internal and externally used products as well as, in the worst-case scenario, between pharmaceutical agents and nonmedicinal chemicals when packaging, labeling, or storage procedures have not been differentiated adequately. These incidents highlight the heightened risk of similarity in the appearance of containers, time constraints during dispensing, and lack of verification, especially when the medication is dispensed to be used at home and administered by the caregiver.

The cases described below are based on adult, pediatric, and infant populations as reported in Thai media and hospital releases and demonstrate near-miss cases of severe toxicity, necessitating intensive care. Together, they demonstrate common system-wide failure points, such as the proximity of internal and external products to storage, excessive dependability on container looks, and the lack of protective measures against high-risk pediatric drugs.

Case 1: Shampoo Administration in the Place of Cough Syrup (Near Miss in an Elderly Adult)

The case of a 66-year-old woman with asthma and a cardiac operation history who came to a hospital to receive treatment for a cough is presented. Owing to a mistake in dispensing, she was given a bottle of shampoo instead of oral cough syrup as prescribed (Figure 1). At home, she tried to take the medication but was notified right away about the bitter and foamy taste and realized that the product was shampoo, and she spit it out and did not swallow it. There was no severe clinical harm, and it was defined as a near miss. In turn, the hospital responded by physically segregating internal- and external-use products and administrators, with an apology to the patient at her home, formally admitted to system failure (Kapook, 2023).

Figure 1. Example of the visual similarity between two bottles involved in a LASA error: a tar-based shampoo for external use and an oral cough syrup

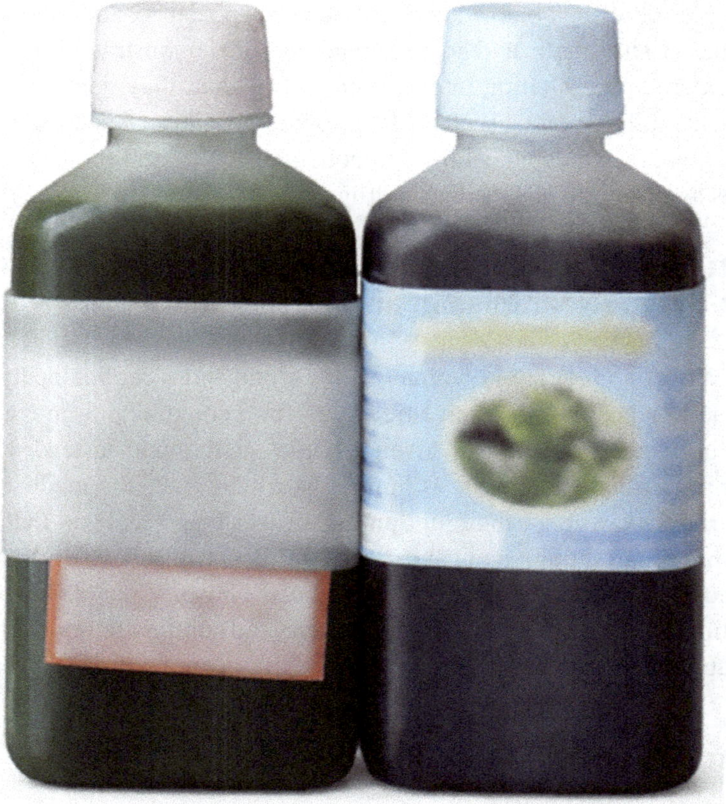

Case 2: Topical Anti-itch Lotion and Cough Syrup Dispensed (Adults and Infants)

In a case of cough management in an adult outpatient, a woman who came to seek treatment was given a topical anti-pruritic lotion rather than an oral cough syrup. She tried to swallow the product as she was told, but very soon she understood that it was not an oral drug and avoided being exposed to it. The case resulted in media attention to the problem with pharmacy checks (Thairath, 2018). Another even more seriously related case involved a 1-month-old girl who had been prescribed cough syrup. The intended oral formulation was applied topically and was administered to the infant by her mother, who was given a topical lotion against it.

The baby suffered vomiting and diarrhea and had to be hospitalized in the intensive care unit, where he was under observation and supportive care. The case revealed the increased sensitivity of infants to LASA errors and the exaggerated effects of nonprofessional administration by the caregiver (Sanook, 2022).

Case 3: Trichloroacetic Acid Given out of Chloral Hydrate (Severe Pediatric LASA Error)

A 1-year-old patient with head trauma underwent procedural sedation for diagnostic imaging, and the use of chloral hydrate, which is a pediatric sedative, was prescribed. Because of a LASA dispensing error, trichloroacetic acid (TCA), which is a caustic dermatologic agent, was given instead. After ingestion, the child experienced mucosal irritation and initial signs of esophageal and gastric damage, necessitating hospitalization, parenteral nutrition, close observation, and long-term follow-up. Despite the fact that no life-threatening burns or perforations were observed, the risk of these events was high. The hospital terminated the personnel in question, provided thorough assistance to the family, and released a public statement of apology. The given case is the worst extreme of the LASA error scale, as the visual similarity of containers and names may result in life-threatening injuries in children (Figure 2) (Khaosod, 2023; Thairath., 2023).

Figure 2. Example of the visual similarity of two bottles involved in a LASA error: Chloral hydrate (pediatric sedative) and Trichloroacetic acid (TCA) (caustic dermatologic agent)

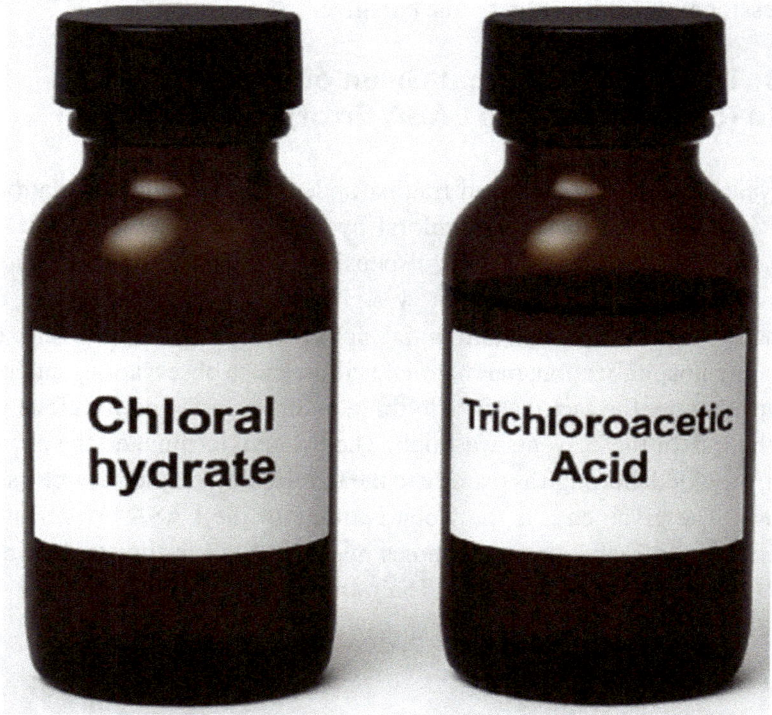

Oral liquid medications are especially susceptible to LASA errors since these medications frequently have similar formulation attributes, package designs, and labeling patterns and, at the same time, demand that dosages be measured precisely during dispensing and administration. According to the evidence provided in the international literature on medication safety, liquid preparations, particularly those used in the field of pediatric and outpatient services, are overrepresented in LASA error reports because of the similarity of drug names, concentrations, and container looks and because of the use of visual clues during high-workload dispensing. Such risks increase further when several strength- or therapy-unrelated drugs are sold in the same bottle or dispensed as an extemporaneously prepared mixture (Supapaan et al., 2023; Supapaan, Napaporn, et al., 2024).

The results of a Thai multihospital-based study provide a quantitative background for this risk. Among the 2,510 identified LASA pairs of drugs (in different levels of hospitals), 85 (3.39%) consisted of oral liquid preparations. Oral liquids represented a lower percentage of all reported LASA pairs than tablets/capsules and injectable medications did but, by virtue of repeated occurrence, indicated system-level susceptibility, especially in regard to the proximity of storage and nonstandardized labeling and inadequate visual differentiation of products with similar names or similar appearances. Notably, the majority of the reported oral liquid LASA incidents fell under the early medication error categories (NCC MERP Categories B-C), meaning that the event often went unnoticed or was exposed without harm, but it also indicates that the risk will persist in the case of safeguards being breached or the medication being given in nonhospital settings (Supapaan, Napaporn, et al., 2024).

Table 2 further shows examples of LASA oral liquid preparation pairs that are found in this subset (N = 85 pairs) and are listed in order of frequency. As shown in the table, the most frequently affected pairs are similar drug names, similar packaging, or both and often include items in multiple concentrations or that use traditional mixtures (e.g., Mixtura carminativa, Mixtura tussis). These cases represent how even such seemingly low-risk oral liquid drugs can become repeat causes of medication errors when there are limitations in system design, labeling practices, and human-factor pressures that come into conflict.

Table 2. Examples of LASA liquid preparations reported in Thailand

Drug names	Drug names	Frequency of pairs	Percentage	Types of LASA pairs	Error Category
1. Milk of magnesia	Alum milk	11	11.47	Similar name, Similar packaging	A, B, C
2. Ferrous fumarate drop	Simethicone drop	6	7.89	Similar name, Similar packaging	B, C
3. Paracetamol 120 mg/5 ml	Paracetamol 250 mg/5 ml	5	6.58	Similar name, Similar packaging	A, B
4. Amoxicillin 125 mg/5 ml	Amoxicillin 250 mg/5 ml	4	4.71	Similar name, Similar packaging	B
5. Amoxicillin	Dicloxacillin	2	2.35	Similar packaging	B
6. M. carminative*	M. tussis**	2	2.35	Similar name, Similar packaging	B
7. *Phyllanthus emblica* extract (Amla) cough syrup	M. tussis	1	1.18	Similar name, Similar packaging	B
8. Hydroxyzine	Dicyclomine	1	1.18	Similar packaging	B, C

continued on following page

Table 2. Continued

Drug names	Drug names	Frequency of pairs	Percentage	Types of LASA pairs	Error Category
9. Dimenhydrinate	Domperidone	1	1.18	Similar packaging	B, C
10. Dicyclomine	Brompheniramine + Phenylephrine	1	1.18	Similar packaging	B, C
11. Hyoscine	Paracetamol	1	1.18	Similar name	B
12. Chlorpheniramine maleate	Glyceryl guaiacolate (Guaifenesin)	1	1.18	Similar packaging	B

(Supapaan, Napaporn, et al., 2024)

Note: *M. carminative = Carminative mixture (Mixtura carminativa); **M. tussis = Cough mixture (Mixtura tussis)

Additional investigations of LASA processes within Thai hospital records revealed that the most common confusion with oral liquid products was represented by similar drug names and similar packaging. The standardization of labeling protocols and the extensive use of amber glass or plastic bottles were some factors that diminished visual product distinction; therefore, the chances of selecting the wrong drug increased. The majority of reported LASA incidences of oral liquids were categorized as Category B errors, which are incidences that did not reach the patient and therefore showed that there were successful interception mechanisms. Nevertheless, the continued occurrence of such close calls indicates high-level system vulnerability and not individual errors (Supapaan TS, Kamnuek J, et al., 2024; Supapaan TS, Songmuang A, et al., 2024; Supapaan, Napaporn, et al., 2024).

These findings are reflected in international pediatric literature outside of an institutional context. Caregiver-administered medication studies have also demonstrated that oral liquid preparations are some of the most commonly involved dosage forms in medication errors in the home, especially in cases where caregivers possess low health literacy or apply nonstandard dosing tools (Yin et al., 2014; Yin et al., 2010). Owing to the absence of formal reporting systems for the majority of LASA errors, the actual epidemiologic burden of LASA-related harm in relation to oral liquid medications is probably underreported in hospital-based surveillance data (Cohen, 2007; Cohen et al., 2007; Hoffman & Proulx, 2003; World Health Organization, 2023).

HUMAN FACTORS AND THE MEDICATION-USE PROCESS

LASA errors, where oral liquid medicines are confused with similar-sounding words, are now conceptualized as multifactorial phenomena that emerge from human performance–task requirement–tool–environment interactions. These mistakes do not necessarily indicate isolated individual lapses but can occur in any phase of the medication-use process—prescribing, transcription, dispensing, administration, and monitoring—and the risk is likely to accumulate as medications are transferred among different handoffs (Agency for Healthcare Research and Quality (AHRQ)-Patient Safety Network (PSNET), 2024; Tariq et al., 2021; World Health Organization, 2017, 2023).

Oral liquid medications should receive special consideration through a human-factor prism since they necessitate repetitive oral-to-oral doses, concentrations, and volume translations, which are frequently conducted by various parties in various care environments. Prescribers, pharmacists, nurses, caregivers, and patients may interact with the medication at various stages; they often face time pressure and not all the contextual information needed. Similarities in drug names or packaging may also cause more mental load and the risk of making mistakes when there are variable concentrations and dosing devices, which occur along with LASA similarities (Bryan et al., 2015; Bryan et al., 2021a; Bryan et al., 2021b; Hoffman & Proulx, 2003).

Prescribing Stage

Prescription in oral liquid therapy can be a very initial stage in which ambiguity may be brought in. Orders containing doses expressed in milligrams but do not specify the volume (milliliter, mL) or the concentration of the product should be interpreted downstream by pharmacists or caregivers. Such reliance on interpretation can lead to the possibility of unintended selection of products or strength, especially when there are several concentrations or formulations of the same oral liquid (The Institute for Safe Medication Practices (ISMP), 2011; World Health Organization, 2017).

Such issues are exacerbated in pediatric and geriatric practice when off-label or unlicensed use of oral liquids is the norm because of the paucity of commercially available age-specific preparations. Scientific research into the use of medications in pediatrics has revealed that off-label prescription often requires changes in dose, formulation, or route of administration, which contributes to the complexity and vulnerability of LASA errors during the prescribing phase (Bellis et al., 2013; Pandolfini & Bonati, 2005). The use of oral liquid prescriptions in Thai hospitals is often associated with extemporaneous compounding, which only increases the significance of clarity and standardization at the prescription point (Supapaan TS, Songmuang A, et al., 2024; Supapaan, Napaporn, et al., 2024).

Dispensing Stage

Environmental and cognitive conditions influence LASA errors at the dispensing stage, as they are workload, interruption, time pressure, and storage configuration. Commercially produced and extemporaneously prepared oral liquid medications are usually stored in similar amber bottles with uniform label designs, which can inhibit the visual distinction of products. Visual clues or location memory can be used by pharmacy staff because LASA medicines are stored near each other and are prone to selection errors when high volumes of these medicines are dispensing (Cohen, 1992; Hoffman and Proulx, 2003; Bryan et al., 2015).

Thai Hospital's experience suggests that oral liquid preparations constitute a large share of extemporaneously formulated medicines, but there is still a significant difference between hospitals regarding the method of preparation, labeling standards, and storage procedures (Supapapaan et al., 2023). This variability is capable of introducing latent system vulnerabilities, especially when compounded liquids of similar names or indications are dispensed as a normal outpatient workflow stressor.

Administration Stage

Administration is among the most important areas of weakness related to LASA mistakes of oral liquid medications where the dosage needs to be calculated by hand at the point of administration. In contrast to solid dosage forms, oral liquid drugs are dependent not only on the proper and correct interpretation of instructions but also on the proper choice and application of dosing devices. Experiments have always revealed that dosing mistakes are more likely to occur when dosing cups are used than when dosing by means of oral syringes and that both underdosing and overdosing are common. Notably, errors in administration have been identified at different levels of caregiver education and language proficiency, which implies that task complexity and the characteristics of the device rather than the individual characteristics of the caregivers should be considered the factors that influence errors in administration (Shiffman et al., 2011; Yin et al., 2014; Yin et al., 2010).

The contribution of task complexity to administration errors is further confirmed by recent extensive observational studies. A prospective evaluation of pediatric inpatients revealed that oral drugs that need solvents or diluents were linked to significantly elevated error rates compared with oral drugs that did not necessitate any preparation, which emphasizes the cumulative hazard posed by extra preparation measures (Westbrook et al., 2024). Even though this study was performed in a general context of medication administration errors, the results of this study apply directly to the risk of oral liquid LASA, especially in pediatric settings where the manipulation of dosage is widespread. The study of human factors also revealed that dosing units that are not standard, including teaspoons (tsp) and tablespoons (tbsp), are more likely to cause clinically significant dosing discrepancies. The combination of LASA confusion with the lack of clarity in labeling, similarity in packaging, or the use of an incorrect dosing device can lead to an even greater risk, particularly in the conditions of home-care patients, in which formal verification procedures are restricted (The Institute for Safe Medication Practices (ISMP), 2011; World Health Organization, 2017).

System-Wide System Monitoring and Learning

The monitoring stage is important for the detection and reduction of LASA-related harm. Early indicators of upstream errors may be detected by near-miss reports, inquiries made by caregivers, and unanticipated therapeutic reactions. Nevertheless, the instances of medication errors in oral liquids, especially in regard to community and home-based environments, are often underreported, restricting organizational learning and making the actual scale of LASA-related risk dim (Hoffman & Proulx, 2003; World Health Organization, 2017). It is necessary to build greater reporting mechanisms and feedback loops to facilitate continuous improvement and system-level learning. Taken together, such evidence suggests a systems-based approach to LASA medication error prevention, i.e., one that prioritizes effective prescribing habits, standardized compounding and labeling, proper dose-delivery devices, and effective monitoring systems coupled with education and professional training.

Errors in LASA with oral liquid drugs are increasingly being viewed as system-wide, multifactorial phenomena that occur because of the interaction between human performance, task demands, tools, and the care environment and not as a result of individual performance failures. The risk of LASA confusion increases at consecutive levels of the medication-use process—prescribing, dispensing, and administration—and the medication safety results are defined in Figure 3. In every stage, the cognitive load, time constraints, interference, and dependence on visual stimuli may increase the likelihood of making a mistake, especially when oral liquid preparations need to be interpreted regularly by drug name, concentration, volume, and dosing apparatus. This cumulative risk pathway highlights the importance of including vulnerabilities in any one stage to propagate to the other step as well as why successful LASA prevention should target the entire medication-use system and not individual steps (Agency for Healthcare Research and Quality (AHRQ)-Patient Safety Network (PSNET), 2024; Tariq et al., 2021; World Health Organization, 2017, 2023).

Figure 3. Human factors throughout the medication-use process that have led to LASA errors in oral liquid drugs

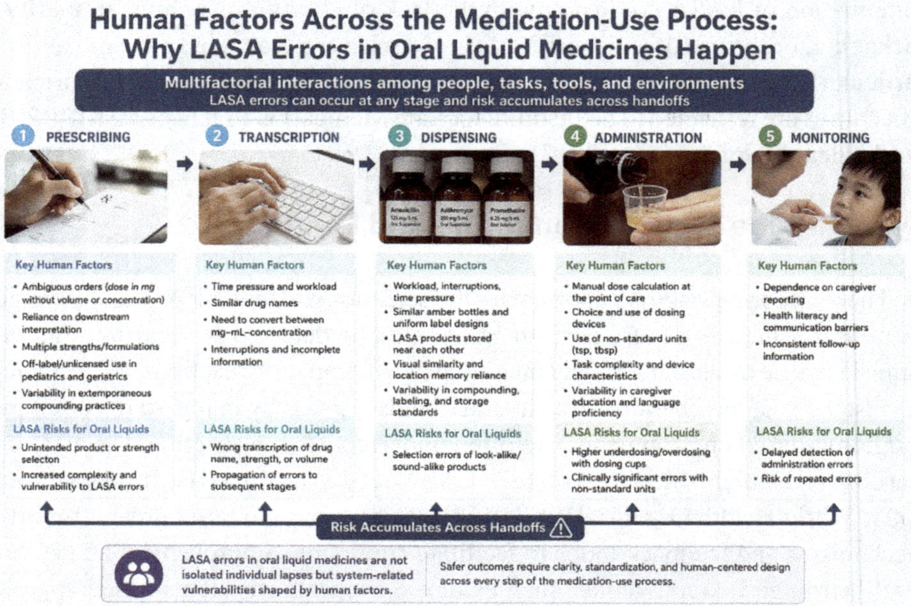

DOSING EXPRESSION AND PRESCRIBING VULNERABILITIES

The first and strongest point of control of LASA errors with oral liquid drugs is prescribing. Pediatric literature on medication safety invariably indicates that a high number of medication errors occur during the prescription phase and later spread to subsequent dispensing and administration phases unless they are intercepted during the error-prone phases (Payne et al., 2007; Rinke et al., 2007). Decisions to prescribe in the pediatric context are particularly important since the choice made can frequently be the basis of the following actions and prescribers' assumptions about formulation and concentration.

One of the most well-known prescribing weaknesses is an expression of doses in terms of mass only (such as milligrams) without providing a particular volume (mL) or product concentration. When oral liquid therapy is used, there is a problem of ambiguity, as several concentrations of the same medication might be sold commercially or compounded in the same healthcare system. It has been stressed by the World Health Organization that partial dose expression leads to the risk of misguided choice of product/strength and can lead to a clinically significant deviation in dosing when the prescription is adhered to (Institute for Safe Medication Practices (ISMP), 2016; NCPDP, 2021; World Health Organization, 2017).

This matter is directly connected with LASA risk mechanisms. Ambiguity in dose expression wipes out an important verification anchor where there is similarity in the drug names, labeling, or packaging to distinguish between a look-alike product or strength. In these cases, assumptions based on the idea of what are considered normal concentrations may be used, which puts the pharmacists and caregivers at risk of choosing a look-alike formulation and exposing them to the wrong dose (Institute for Safe Medication Practices (ISMP), 2016; World Health Organization, 2017).

Reported Cases of Prescribing Errors and LASA Applicability

The cases of mistreatment caused by vague prescribing recorded by the community analyzed by the Institute of Safe Medication Practices are an example of how harm can be. A common example is seen in a newborn infant where the prescription was ten times that of levetiracetam oral solution when the prescription was typed only in volume (mL) rather than in body weight and concentration. Since the drug was in high-strength preparation, the mistake was not realized at the time of dispensing and persisted for more than a few weeks at home (Institute for Safe Medication Practices, 2016). Even though this incident was not related to the wrong drug choice, the process is similar to LASA pathways since it illustrates how the absence of explicit links between dose and concentration allows severe mistakes to pass through various safety checks.

The same pattern has also been reported with oral flecainide suspensions, with the prescribers adjusting the doses by varying the volume injected but maintaining a constant concentration. In instances whereby the infants were refilled in other pharmacies that dispensed higher-strength formulations, they were overdosed several times, leading to cardiotoxic conditions. These examples demonstrate the interactions between the variability of formulation, care transitions, and missing prescribing information, which are quite similar to amplification mechanisms in LASA (Institute for Safe Medication Practices (ISMP), 2016).

Complexity in Prescriptions and Changes in Formulations in Pediatrics

Compared with adults, the complexity of the prescribing stage has greater effects on pediatric patients since weight-based dosing is a standard practice and many medicines have commercially available pediatric-specific preparations. Consequently, the prescription of oral liquid drugs for pediatric use often involves the calculation of doses, dilution, and interpretation by pharmaceutical personnel and caregivers before administration. Reviews and systematic studies in hospitals consistently report that such prescriptions based on calculations led to additional cognitive work in downstream processes, and there is a high probability of causing the propagation of errors along the medication-use pathway (Gonzales, 2010; Payne et al., 2007). According to evidence provided by pediatric medication safety research, problems in the prescribing stage play a significant role in the occurrence of future dispensing and administration errors.

In a prospective study of medication errors in children, Payne et al. reported that prescription was a primary source of medication error in children and that the work of calculating and interpreting the dose was recurrent (Payne et al., 2007). On the same note, a systematic review emphasized that pediatric prescriptions frequently have intermediate stages of transformation, including milligram doses to volumes, increasing the risk of misinterpretation, especially when nonstandardized or incomplete instructions are received (Gonzales, 2010). This is complicated by the variability of the formulations. Numerous oral liquid drugs are sold at various concentrations, and such preparations may vary among manufacturers, hospitals, or pharmacies. There is a greater likelihood of confusion when there is similarity, both visual and phonetic, between product labels and brand names. Pediatric medication error studies have demonstrated that the presence of multiple strengths of a single oral liquid medication is a repeated factor in wrong-dose and wrong-product incidences, particularly when the instructions about the prescriptions fail to directly connect dose, concentration, and volume (Miller et al., 2007; World Health Organization, 2017).

The use of oral liquid drugs off-label and without a license is also a common practice in the pediatric setting and adds further confusion in the prescribing process. A large prospective cohort study revealed that off-label and unlicensed medicines were more prone to adverse drug events among children, and dosing and formulation variables explained a significant number of such occurrences instead of inappropriate clinical decision-making (Bellis et al., 2013). Under these conditions, prescribers can use extemporaneous prepared liquids or nonstandard concentrations, which further compounds the requirement of accurate dosage expression. These prescribing features have especially consequential effects on LASA. Ambiguous prescriptions, e.g., prescriptions that contain only a mass dose (mg) or a volume (mL), allow numerous interpretation options. When used together with names of look-alike or sound-alike medication or with similar packaging at different concentrations, the likelihood of picking an incorrect product or strength increases. A mass-only order could be accompanied by the wrong concentration, and a volume-only order could be used on a stronger formulation, which would subsequently result in clinically significant under- or overdosing even if it seems that the prescription was fulfilled.

The full and standardized dose expression is thus a key LASA risk-reduction measure of oral liquid drugs as described by international safety guidelines. Prescriptions are always recommended to contain the name of the medication, its concentration, total mass dose in milliliters, patient mass weight where necessary, and the use of metric units only, and household measures are discouraged (NCPDP, 2021; World Health Organization, 2017). These actions are aimed at minimizing later interpretation downstream and restricting the relationship between ambiguity in prescribing and LASA conditions. Taken together, the results of pediatric systematic reviews with evidence, national error-reporting databases, and ISMP case studies suggest that dose expression practices, formulation variability, and calculation needs are the leading contributing factors to the vulnerability of oral liquid prescription due to its use in pediatric therapy. These problems are system-related design features and not the performance of some prescribers. Enhancing prescribing criteria, including clear concentration and volume, metric-only dosing, and increasing patient weight, is important for the prevention of LASA-related harm in the use of oral liquid medicine among children.

MEASUREMENT DEVICES AND ADMINISTRATION ERRORS

Medication errors in the use of oral liquids are often linked to drug administration since the dose must be measured at the point of administration (hospital, outpatient, or home). In contrast to solid dosage forms, oral liquids have the user convert instructions to a volume, select a suitable measuring instrument, and dose oneself with the required amount at every administration, which means that the patient can err despite correct prescriptions and dispensing processes. This is congruent with medication-safety frameworks, which narrate errors to occur throughout the medication-use process and highlight vulnerabilities in system design and processes, instead of problems rooted only in individual performance (Agency for Healthcare Research and Quality (AHRQ)-Patient Safety Network (PSNET), 2024).

The Choice of Device is Important, as Different Devices are More Accurate and Easier to Use

Dosing cups are linked to greater variations in the dosage that was planned relative to oral syringes, especially when small quantities are measured (a frequent circumstance in pediatrics). In an experimental experiment comparing oral liquid measuring devices, dosing cups were more variable than oral syringes were, which confirms that cup-based measurements have the potential to increase the risk of under- or overmeasurement in practice.

Pediatric studies that are caregiver centered further confirm the notion that device type has a significant effect on the elements of dosing. According to a study on parents using liquid medication, dosing errors were prevalent, and the probability of errors varied by instrument, indicating that even postcounseling, errors may occur and that device design/usability is a key factor in determining performance at the administration level (Agency for Healthcare Research and Quality (AHRQ)-Patient Safety Network (PSNET), 2024; Sobhani et al., 2008).

Nonmetric Units Introduce Unnecessary Ambiguity (Teaspoon/Tablespoon)

One of the largest, most reported causes of error at the administration stage is the propagation of nonmetric units (teaspoon and tablespoon) in the labels and instructions. These words may be misunderstood, and abbreviations are not used consistently, increasing the cognitive load of caregivers and increasing the likelihood of misunderstanding when the markings on dosing tools are not aligned with written instructions.

The difference in teaspoon-tablespoon volume is clinically significant because 1 tablespoon (15 mL) has 3 times the amount of 1 teaspoon (5 mL); thus, misuse of the two can result in a threefold difference in administered volume. This is one of the risks, which is why policy and standards documents strongly emphasize the need to eliminate teaspoon/tablespoon instructions about oral liquids and shift them to one, nonambiguous unit (mL) (Commitee on Drugs, 2015).

The Evidence-Based System Controls are Metric-Only Dosing (Ml) and Syringe Distribution

According to the American Academy of Pediatrics policy statement, dosing of orally administered liquid medications must be in milliliters (mL), and it states that teaspoon and tablespoon dosing is no longer to be used; it also strongly recommends the use of accurate devices (preferably syringes with metric markings) instead of household spoons and dispensing specific devices with the medication.

Simultaneously, the National Council for Prescription Drug Programs (NCPDP) Professional Pharmacy Services Work Group (WG10) recommendations support the idea that a household unit should have standardized designations of oral liquid dosing and that misunderstanding in terms of which direction to execute leads to clinically significant results, which makes the idea of system-level standardization, i.e., mL-based expressions and consistent device labeling, a viable mitigation measure (NCPDP, 2021).

Oral Liquid LASA Risk Implications

These weaknesses during the administration phase are compounded by LASA risks in oral liquid products. The possibility of an incorrect dosage increases further when a misselected product is administered because of additional confusion arising from unit expressions (i.e., teaspoon vs. tablespoon) or the use of incorrect measuring devices (i.e., dosing cups or improperly used household spoons) after an already incorrectly chosen product has been given. The ISMP has documented instances where pharmacy labels have converted metric doses into household measurements, potentially leading to serious overdoses.

As an illustration, an amoxicillin/clavulanate oral suspension (Augmentin ES-600) connection of 5 mL to a pediatric patient was wrongly labeled as 5 teaspoons (5-fold dosing error), which was detected only when the caregiver crosschecked the dosage in an electronic patient portal (Cohen & Smetzer, 2018). Such unit-based ambiguities are further enhanced in the case of LASA, where upstream drug misidentification has already taken place, increasing the chances of injury at the administration point. Therefore, not only are the best practices, standardization of dosing devices (use of oral syringes), only metric units (mL-only), and common communication between prescribing, dispensing, and patient education scalable system-level measures, but they can also be used to prevent downstream harm when LASA conditions are present (Cohen & Smetzer, 2018; Commitee on Drugs, 2015). As shown in Figure 4, administration-stage errors in oral liquid medications may be worsened by inappropriate measuring devices, ambiguous units, and LASA-related confusion.

Figure 4. Measurement devices and administration errors associated with oral liquid medications

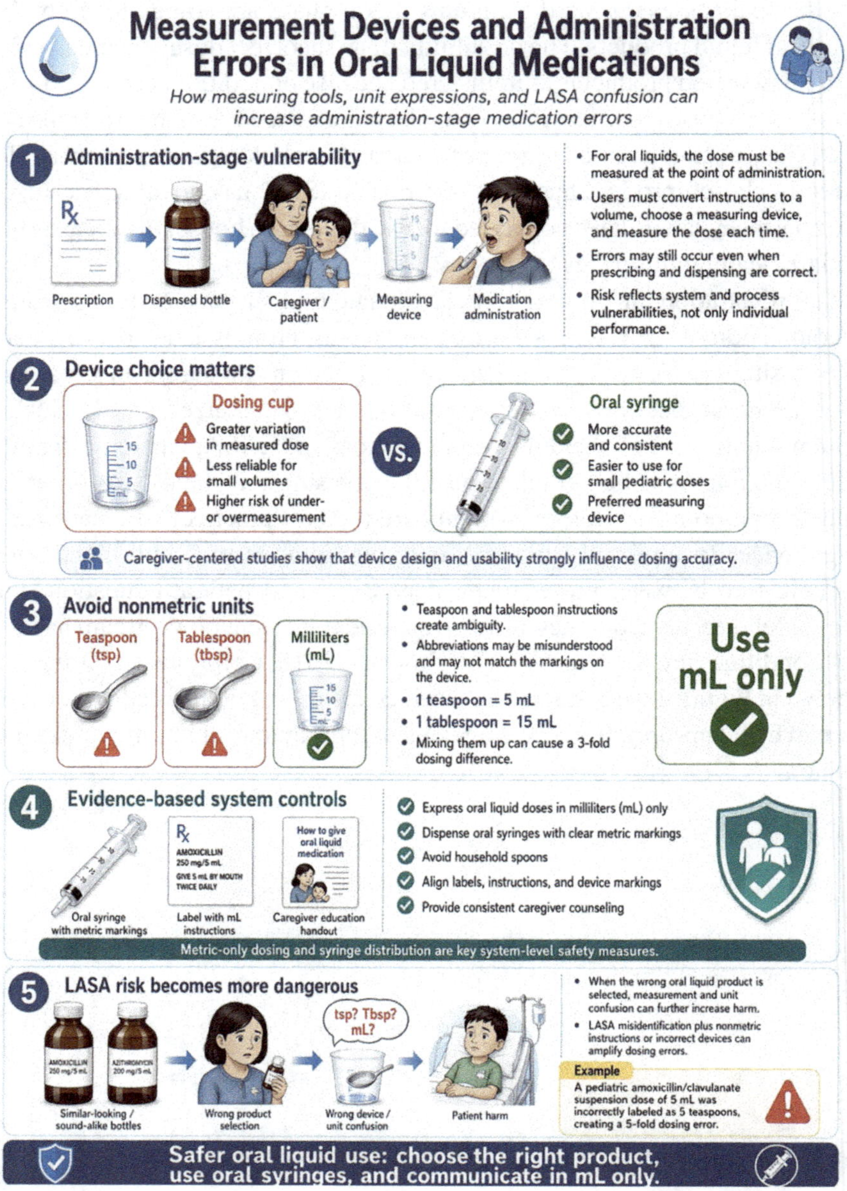

The figure shows how oral liquid medication errors may occur during administration because of inaccurate device selection, nonmetric units, and LASA-related product confusion and emphasizes metric-only dosing and oral syringe use as key safety measures.

LABELING, PACKAGING, AND HEALTH LITERACY

The practices of labeling and packaging play a leading role in influencing the risk of look-alike, sound-alike (LASA) mistakes with oral liquid drugs. Poor readability of labels, which is seen in small font, overcrowded designs, poor contrast, and poor consistency in the positioning of important information, has been consistently linked to the misinterpretation of drug strength, concentration, and dosing regimens by both medical practitioners and caregivers. Oral liquid preparations magnify these weaknesses where the accuracy of dosage given lies not only in the right choice of product but also in the accurate deciphering of instructions given in terms of volumes (The Institute for Safe Medication Practices (ISMP), 2011, 2023; World Health Organization, 2017).

In LASA, brand or generic name similarity often comes along with almost identical label designs, color schemes and bottle shapes. This visual homogeneity decreases the likelihood of users detecting a wrong-drug error, especially in situations of time pressure or cognitive load. Reports submitted to the Institute for Safe Medication Practices (ISMP) indicate that medication errors associated with liquid formulas are commonly related to confusion and label-related malfunctions but not to one cause (Cohen & Smetzer, 2018; The Institute for Safe Medication Practices (ISMP), 2023). The lack of concentration prominently and standardized to display (e.g., in mg/mL) makes the risk even higher that even with the right product dispensed, caregivers might still administer the wrong dosage.

Health literacy is not a significant protective-moderating factor in the process. LHPs with low literacy or numeracy levels are particularly susceptible to ambiguous labels, nonmetric dose phrases and discrepant instructions at various phases of prescription, dispensing, and administration. Nonetheless, experimental and observational research has shown that medication dosing errors are common even when the caregiver is literate, if the labels are poorly developed or if the dosing calculators are used incorrectly. Parents with adequate reading ability continued to make important dosing errors in a series of controlled studies when the instructions were given in household measures or when the layout of the labels obscured important information, indicating that failure of the design of the system is more critical than an individual's ability to determine safety (Agency for Healthcare Research and Quality (AHRQ), 2017; Yin et al., 2014).

In the Thai hospital setting, these risks are indirectly proven by evidence. Surveys of the national population and studies conducted in hospitals indicate that a significant percentage of LASA errors with oral liquid medications are prevented at the stage of reaching patients, with the majority of them being identified at the dispensing and checking steps in institutional procedures. Nevertheless, this labeling standard, package features, and other features of the formulation remain the same when the drugs are given for home use, where there is no direct professional control or real-time verification. This shift to unregulated home conditions is a critical escalation factor that may cause harm to patients, especially in pediatric and geriatric groups who depend on carers to administer medication (Pitchayajittipong et al., 2025; Pitchayajittipong et al., 2021; Supapaan et al., 2023; Supapaan TS, Songmuang A, et al., 2024; Supapaan, Napaporn, et al., 2024). Oral liquid preparations that are prepared and administered extemporely have added safety issues and are commonly used in pediatric care to offer age-specific dosing in the event of nonavailability of commercial preparations. The existing body of systematic evidence suggests that these compounded liquids are often not equal with respect to stability, dose consistency, and vehicle formulation, making accurate dosing difficult and increasing the risks of adverse effects in the case of improper labeling and packaging. A pediatric oral extemporaneous compounds practice survey, the first global survey, also indicated great differences in formulation practices throughout the WHO regions, which suggests a lack of standardized methods that could decrease the risk of errors in either clinical or domestic practice (Fadda et al., 2024; Yuliani et al., 2023). Even with well-informed caregivers, oral liquid medication errors can be increased by weaknesses in labeling and packaging design in both institutional and home-use contexts, as illustrated in Figure 5.

Figure 5. Naming, packaging, and health literacy as factors in oral liquid medication errors. The figure demonstrates that dosing errors can be augmented by look-alike packaging, unclear labels, confusion over concentrations, and home use circumstances and that system design can play a greater role in safety than individual health literacy

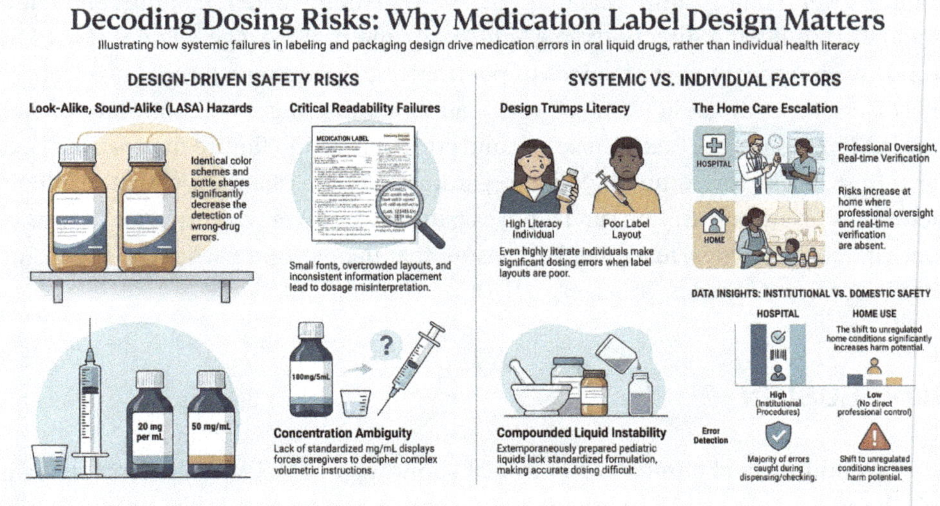

RISK MITIGATION STRAGEGIES FOR COMPOUNDED ORAL LIQUIDS

The results of the ISMP medication error analyses demonstrate that the risk mitigation process related to compounded oral liquids must focus on standardization as well as process controls to avoid both LASA and dosing errors. As compounding may be needed, the recommended approaches are to make use of standardized concentrations and recipes (master formulations), an adequate vehicle/excipient system, and a reduction in variability in the preparation procedures. In the study of tacrolimus errors by ISMP, compounding issues related to 10-fold overdoses/underdoses were identified in the case of using the wrong capsule strength and clinically significant variability in the case of using the incorrect suspending agent; consequently, ISMP advised the standardization of the compounding concentrations and recipes and clearly and extensively described how to prepare them (Cohen & Smetzer, 2018). Since many adverse events take place downstream during administration (commonly in the domestic environment), labeling and dosing-device development are fundamental safety measures. Recommendations to use standardized dosing of oral liquid medicines include the use of metric units (mL-only) on packages and equipment, not household units (e.g., teaspoons and tablespoons), and the use of dosing devices that match the dose. In the case of prescription oral liquids, oral syringes are usually favored at 10 mL, and equipment should not introduce several unit systems that may cause caregiver misunderstandings and faults (standardized dosing directions; e.g., mL-only and oral-syringe choice) (NCPDP, 2021). With respect to the practices of pharmacies, these sources encourage central pharmacists' positions in terms of verification, counseling, and continuity of safe use. ISMP emphasizes that counseling and communication failure may cause direct harm (e.g., a lack of communication regarding strength changes, which results in incorrect self-administration) and advises patient/caregiver education and a type of confirmation known as teach-back to ensure that the use of a particular dispensing item is correct (Cohen & Smetzer, 2018).

CONCLUSION

The common and clinically significant subgroup of LASA medication errors is oral liquid medications. Even though oral liquids constitute a lower proportion of LASA pairs than tablets/capsules and injectable preparations do, their risk profiles are qualitatively different and are frequently more complicated. The similarity of packaging and labeling, the presence of different dosages, the necessity of dose administration, and administration by caregivers create numerous error propagation possibilities throughout the medication-use process.

The results summarized in this chapter indicate that LASA errors associated with oral liquids occur mainly at the dispensing point and are highly dependent on human-factor circumstances such as workload, interruptions, dependence on visual cues, and storage arrangement. Although many reported incidents are prevented prior to inflicting any damage, the fact that they have been repeatedly detected in international data and in national surveillance within the Thai context indicates that there are still systematic vulnerabilities of the system, not just specific failures by individuals. Weight-based dosing, off-label or extemporaneous, and reliance on caregivers make pediatric patients especially susceptible, but even adult liquid preparations of drugs, including cough, gastrointestinal, antihistamine, and iron preparations, are commonly used.

The data concerning Thai hospitals offer a rather useful country outlook, revealing that oral liquid LASA pairs constitute 3.39% of the total reported LASA pairs and that packaging similarity is the predominant mechanism. These results are consistent with the global evidence, and they highlight the fact that the absolute frequency is insufficient to assess the clinical relevance of oral liquid LASA errors, since they have increased dose-harm potential in outpatient and home care settings.

This means that system-level interventions are necessary to prevent LASA errors in oral liquid medications. They are standardized and distinctively differentiated labeling, segregation of packaging and storage, use of metric-based expressions of dosing, the delivery of a fitting measuring apparatus, uniform principles of compounding, and intensive training of the caregiver by teaching-back protocols. To identify near misses and prevent them, the increased use of surveillance, reporting, and organizational learning is also needed. All these steps contribute to the transition process from individual vigilance-based interventions to resilient system design, which is necessary to minimize avoidable damage related to oral liquid LASA medication errors.

REFERENCES

Agency for Healthcare Research and Quality (AHRQ). (2017). *Guide to patient and family engagement in hospital quality and safety*. Retrieved 23 Jan from https://www.ahrq.gov/patient-safety/patients-families/engagingfamilies/guide.html

Agency for Healthcare Research and Quality (AHRQ)-Patient Safety Network (PS-NET). (2024). *Medication errors and adverse drug events*. Retrieved 22 Jan from https://psnet.ahrq.gov/primer/medication-errors-and-adverse-drug-events

Allard, J., Carthey, J., Cope, J., Pitt, M., & Woodward, S. (2002). Medication errors: Causes, prevention and reduction. *British Journal of Haematology*, *116*(2), 255–265. DOI: 10.1046/j.1365-2141.2002.03272.x

Bellis, J. R., Kirkham, J. J., Thiesen, S., Conroy, E. J., Bracken, L. E., Mannix, H. L., Bird, K. A., Duncan, J. C., Peak, M., Turner, M. A., Smyth, R. L., Nunn, A. J., & Pirmohamed, M. (2013). Adverse drug reactions and off-label and unlicensed medicines in children: A nested case–control study of inpatients in a pediatric hospital. *BMC Medicine*, *11*(1), 238. DOI: 10.1186/1741-7015-11-238

Bryan, R., Aronson, J. K., ten Hacken, P., Williams, A., & Jordan, S. (2015). Patient safety in medication nomenclature: Orthographic and semantic properties of International Nonproprietary Names. *PLoS One*, *10*(12), e0145431. DOI: 10.1371/journal.pone.0145431

Bryan, R., Aronson, J. K., Williams, A., & Jordan, S. (2021a). The problem of look-alike, sound-alike name errors: Drivers and solutions. *British Journal of Clinical Pharmacology*, *87*(2), 386–394. DOI: 10.1111/bcp.14285

Bryan, R., Aronson, J. K., Williams, A. J., & Jordan, S. (2021b). A systematic literature review of LASA error interventions. *British Journal of Clinical Pharmacology*, *87*(2), 336–351. DOI: 10.1111/bcp.14644

Chumchit, C., Amrumpai, Y., & Treesak, C. (2015). Recognition on medication safety and look-alike/sound-alike medication problems in Thai public hospitals. *Silpakorn U Science & Tech J*, *9*(2), 40–51.

Cohen, M. R. (2007). Causes of medication errors. In Cohen, M. R. (Ed.), *Medication Errors* (2nd ed., pp. 55–66). The American Pharmacists Association. DOI: 10.21019/9781582120928.ch4

Cohen, M. R., & Davis, N. M. (1992). Dispensing the Wrong Medication. *American Pharmacy*, *32*(5), 32. DOI: 10.1016/S0160-3450(15)31197-1

Cohen, M. R., Domizio, G. D., & Lee, R. E. (2007). The role of drug names in medication errors. In Cohen, M. R. (Ed.), *Medication Errors* (2nd ed., pp. 87–110). The American Pharmacists Association. https://doi.org/doi:10.21019/9781582120928.ch6

Cohen, M. R., Harris, D., Zanoletty, A., & Linvill-Neal, D. (2021). *The inside track on drug naming safety standards*. Retrieved 15 June from https://www.ismp.org/sites/default/files/attachments/2021-07/The%20Inside%20Track%20on%20Drug%20Naming%20Standards-%20Handouts.pdf

Cohen, M. R., & Smetzer, J. L. (2018). Multifactorial Causes of Tacrolimus Errors: Confusion With Strength/Formulation, Look-Alike Names, Preparation Errors, and More Ensuring Safety of Recipes for Drug Compounding Please, no more teaspoon dosing. *Hospital Pharmacy, 53*(3), 142–145. DOI: 10.1177/0018578718769757

Fadda, H. M., Weiler, H., Carvalho, M., Lee, Y. Z., Dassouki, H., AbuBlan, R., & Li, Z. (2024). Pediatric oral extemporaneous preparations and practices: International Pharmaceutical Federation (FIP) global study. *European Journal of Pharmaceutics and Biopharmaceutics : Official Journal of Arbeitsgemeinschaft für Pharmazeutische Verfahrenstechnik e.V, 204*, 114483. DOI: 10.1016/j.ejpb.2024.114483

Gonzales, K. (2010). Medication Administration Errors and the Pediatric Population: A Systematic Search of the Literature. *Journal of Pediatric Nursing, 25*(6), 555–565. DOI: 10.1016/j.pedn.2010.04.002

Hicks, R., Becker, S., & Cousins, D. (2008). *MEDMARX data report. A report on the relationship of drug names and medication errors in response to the institute of Medicine's call for action*. Center for the Advancement of Patient Safey, US Pharmacopeia.

Hicks, R. W., Becker, S. C., & Cousins, D. D. (2006). Harmful medication errors in children: A 5-year analysis of data from the USP's MEDMARX program. *Journal of Pediatric Nursing, 21*(4), 290–298. DOI: 10.1016/j.pedn.2006.02.002

Hoffman, J. M., & Proulx, S. M. (2003). Medication errors caused by confusion of drug names. *Drug Safety, 26*(7), 445–452. DOI: 10.2165/00002018-200326070-00001

Institute for Safe Medication Practices (ISMP). (2016). Prescribing and dispensing errors with oral solutions. *ISMP Medication Safety Alert! Community. Ambulatory Care, 15*(5), 1–6.

Kapook. (2023). *Shampoo dispensed instead of cough syrup; 66-year-old patient spit it out after tasting*. Retrieved 23 Jan from https://hilight.kapook.com/view/233483

Khaosod. (2023). *Hospital error: TCA acid dispensed instead of chloral hydrate in pediatric case*. Retrieved 23 Jan from https://www.khaosod.co.th/breaking-news/news_8000990

Miller, M. R., Robinson, K. A., Lubomski, L. H., Rinke, M. L., & Pronovost, P. J. (2007). Medication errors in pediatric care: A systematic review of epidemiology and an evaluation of evidence supporting reduction strategy recommendations. *Quality & Safety in Health Care*, *16*(2), 116–126. DOI: 10.1136/qshc.2006.019950

NCPDP. (2021). NCPDP recommendations for standardizing dosing in metric units (mL) on prescription container labels of oral liquid medications, version 2.0. *American Journal of Health-System Pharmacy*, *78*(7), 578–605. DOI: 10.1093/ajhp/zxab023

Pandolfini, C., & Bonati, M. (2005). A literature review on off-label drug use in children. *European Journal of Pediatrics*, *164*(9), 552–558. DOI: 10.1007/s00431-005-1698-8

Payne, C. H., Smith, C. R., Newkirk, L. E., & Hicks, R. W. (2007). Pediatric medication errors in the postanesthesia care unit: Analysis of MEDMARX data. *AORN Journal*, *85*(4), 731–740. DOI: 10.1016/S0001-2092(07)60147-1

Pitchayajittipong, C., Purachaka, S., Kruaysungnoen, A., Fangseekam, N., Noisri, A., Songmuang, T., & Prachuabaree, L. (2025). Extemporaneous compounding practices: Case study in Thai Hospitals. *Pharmacy Practice*, *23*(1), 1–16. DOI: 10.18549/PharmPract.2025.1.3134

Pitchayajittipong, C., Sriboon, S., Kulmee, S., Prachuabaree, L., Srisawai, K., Wattanawong, W., Sripa, S., Anderson, C., & Supapaan, T. (2021). An overview of pharmaceutical production in Thai hospitals. *Hospital Pharmacy*, *56*(4), 265–275. DOI: 10.1177/0018578719890090

Rinke, M. L., Shore, A. D., Morlock, L., Hicks, R. W., & Miller, M. R. (2007). Characteristics of pediatric chemotherapy medication errors in a national error reporting database. *Cancer*, *110*(1), 186–195. DOI: 10.1002/cncr.22742

Sanook. (2022). *Mother shocked: Infant fed lotion instead of cough syrup, admitted to ICU*. Retrieved 23 Jan from https://www.sanook.com/news/8700410/

Santell, J. P., Hicks, R. W., McMeekin, J., & Cousins, D. D. (2003). Medication errors: Experience of the United States Pharmacopeia (USP) MEDMARX reporting system. *Journal of Clinical Pharmacology*, *43*(7), 760–767. DOI: 10.1177/0091270003254831

Shiffman, S., Gerlach, K. K., Sembower, M. A., & Rohay, J. M. (2011). Consumer understanding of prescription drug information: An illustration using an antidepressant medication. *The Annals of Pharmacotherapy*, *45*(4), 452–458. DOI: 10.1345/aph.1P477

Sobhani, P., Christopherson, J., Ambrose, P. J., & Corelli, R. L. (2008). Accuracy of Oral Liquid Measuring Devices: Comparison of Dosing Cup and Oral Dosing Syringe. *The Annals of Pharmacotherapy*, *42*(1), 46–52. DOI: 10.1345/aph.1K420

Supapaan, T., Jamlongpeng, C., Yangyuen, N., Srisawai, K., Prachuabaree, L., Wattanawong, W., & Pitchayajittipong, C. (2023). Enhancing extemporaneous preparations in Thai Hospitals: Exploring variation, common formulations, and challenges and needs related to extemporaneous preparations. *Pharmacy Practice*, *21*(4), 1–12. DOI: 10.18549/PharmPract.2023.4.2892

Supapaan, T., Pitchayajittipong, C., Sonrasawan, K., Chittawee, C., & Napaporn, J. (2024). Development of the database for look-alike, sound-alike drugs in Thailand. *Thai J Pharm Pract*, *16*(1), 112–125.

Supapaan, T. S., Kamnuek, J., Khakaew, C., Jungsuwadee, T., Songmuang, A., Saksit, S., & Napaporn, J. (2024). Assessment of look-Alike, Sound-Alike similarities among brand names of tablets and capsules: A cross-sectional survey in Thailand. *Pharmacy Practice*, *22*(3), 2955. DOI: 10.18549/PharmPract.2024.3.2955

Supapaan, T. S., Napaporn, J., Ruthirakanok, R., Srichathum, S., Songmuang, A., & Pitchayajittipong, C. (2024). Look-alike sound-alike (LASA) medication errors in Thai hospitals. *Pharmacy Practice*, *22*(1), 2886.

Supapaan, T. S., Songmuang, A., Napaporn, J., Sangsukwow, P., Boonrod, P., Intarapongsakul, P., Jaturapattarawong, A., & Pitchayajittipong, C. (2024). Look-alike/sound-alike medication errors: An in-depth examination through a hospital case study. *Pharmacy Practice*, *22*(2), 2959. DOI: 10.18549/PharmPract.2024.2.2959

Supapaan, T. S., Songmuang, A., Napaporn, J., Sangsukwow, P., Boonrod, P., Intarapongsakul, P., Jaturapattarawong, A., & Pitchayajittipong, C. (2024). Look-alike/sound-alike medication errors: An in-depth examination through a hospital case study. *Pharmacy Practice*, *22*(2), 1–13. DOI: 10.18549/PharmPract.2024.2.2959

Tariq, R. A., Vashisht, R., Sinha, A., & Scherbak, Y. (2021). Medication dispensing errors and prevention. In *StatPearls*. StatPearls Publishing.

Thairath. (2018). *Hospital dispensed anti-itch lotion instead of cough syrup*. Retrieved 23 Jan from https://www.thairath.co.th/news/society/1206147

Thairath. (2023). *Hospital dispensed TCA (trichloroacetic acid) instead of chloral hydrate to 1-year-old; staff suspended*. Retrieved 23 Jan from https://www.thairath.co.th/news/society/2746607

The Institute for Safe Medication Practices (ISMP). (2011). *ISMP list of high-alert medications in community/ambulatory healthcare*. Retrieved 20 March from https://www.ismp.org/sites/default/files/attachments/2017-11/highAlert-community.pdf

The Institute for Safe Medication Practices (ISMP). (2023). *List of confused drug names*. Retrieved 16 Apr from https://www.ismp.org/recommendations/confused-drug-names-list

Westbrook, J. I., Li, L., Woods, A., Badgery-Parker, T., Mumford, V., Merchant, A., Fitzpatrick, E., & Raban, M. Z. (2024). Risk Factors Associated with Medication Administration Errors in Children: A Prospective Direct Observational Study of Pediatric Inpatients. *Drug Safety*, *47*(6), 545–556. DOI: 10.1007/s40264-024-01408-6

World Health Organization. (2017). *Medication without harm*. Retrieved 10 Feb from https://www.who.int/initiatives/medication-without-harm

World Health Organization. (2021). Global patient safety action plan 2021–2030: Towards eliminating avoidable harm in health care. Retrieved 10 Feb from https://iris.who.int/handle/10665/343477.

World Health Organization. (2023). *Medication safety for look-alike, sound-alike medicines*. World Health Organization. Retrieved 3 June from https://iris.who.int/bitstream/handle/10665/373495/9789240058897-eng.pdf?sequence=1

Yin, H. S., Dreyer, B. P., Moreira, H. A., van Schaick, L., Rodriguez, L., Boettger, S., & Mendelsohn, A. L. (2014). Liquid medication dosing errors in children: Role of provider counseling strategies. *Academic Pediatrics*, *14*(3), 262–270. DOI: 10.1016/j.acap.2014.01.003

Yin, H. S., Mendelsohn, A. L., Wolf, M. S., Parker, R. M., Fierman, A., van Schaick, L., Bazan, I. S., Kline, M. D., & Dreyer, B. P. (2010). Parents' medication administration errors: Role of dosing instruments and health literacy. *Archives of Pediatrics & Adolescent Medicine*, *164*(2), 181–186. DOI: 10.1001/archpediatrics.2009.269

Yuliani, S. H., Putri, D. C. A., Virginia, D. M., Gani, M. R., & Riswanto, F. D. O. (2023). Prevalence, risk, and challenges of extemporaneous preparation for pediatric patients in developing nations: A review. *Pharmaceutics*, *15*(3), 840. DOI: 10.3390/pharmaceutics15030840

ABBREVIATIONS

AHRQ: Agency for Healthcare Research and Quality

PSNET: Patient Safety Network

MEDMARX®: United States Pharmacopeia (USP) Medication Error Reporting Program

NCC MERP: National Coordinating Council for Medication Error Reporting and Prevention

NCPDP: National Council for Prescription Drug Programs

WG10: NCPDP Professional Pharmacy Services Work Group

tsp: teaspoons

tbsp: tablespoons

ISMP: Institute for Safe Medication Practices

LASA: Look-Alike, Sound-Alike

WHO: World Health Organization

Chapter 10 Monograph of Look-Alike, Sound-Alike (LASA) Drugs Reported in Thailand (Oral Liquid Preparations)

ABSTRACT

LASA medication errors continue to present a patient-safety threat that is preventable in hospitals whose formularies are complex, especially when dealing with oral liquid formulations in pediatrics and geriatrics. The chapter presents a standardized, component-based LASA drug monograph that aims to transform incidents of LASA reported by the hospital into viable risk-management recommendations. Based on evidence in a national survey of Thailand, the chapter uses oral liquid LASA examples and combines drug identification, mechanisms of similarity, NCC MERP error severity, and safety resources into one framework. The monograph facilitates uniform interpretation, prioritization, and prevention of LASA-related medication errors.

INTRODUCTION

Look-alike, sound-alike (LASA) medication errors continue to be a significant and avoidable patient safety issue, especially in hospital environments where medication formularies are both heterogeneous and intricate. The lack of a standardized and systematic format for reporting LASA drug pairs and interpreting them has impeded the transformation of reported incidents into risk-management strategies despite the growing awareness of the risks of LASA. The reporting practices, mit-

DOI: 10.4018/979-8-3373-5478-1.ch010

igation approaches, and list of hospital LASA are quite different, and determining the risks at the institutions and prioritizing the preventive measures are difficult. This inconsistency indicates the need to create a unified LASA drug monograph that incorporates drug identification, drug similarity mechanisms, real-life events, and the extent of errors in a single organized structure to achieve consistent interpretation and decision-making.

The prevalence of LASA drugs among medication errors in hospital settings is quite high, especially in hospitals with large and complex formularies. The drug lists used in hospitals in Thailand are heterogeneous, with each institution having a LASA drug list and its strategies to prevent and mitigate LASA errors. It was thus a cross-sectional study with a national scope to investigate the prevalence of LASA drug lists in hospitals, types of LASA drug pairs reported, and categories of medication errors reported in Thai hospitals (Supapaan et al., 2024). A sample of 500 government hospitals was sampled from 1309 hospitals across the country using structured questionnaires that were mailed between April and June 2021. One hundred eighty-eight hospitals (response rate of 25.6%), consisting of tertiary, secondary, large primary, small primary and private hospitals, participated. All of these hospitals had 2,510 LASA drug pairs, with the most frequent being tablet and capsule formulations (66.69%), followed by injectable preparations (17.01%) and oral liquid dosage forms (3.39%). These results indicate that LASA risks are still widespread in various dosage forms and at different levels of hospitals in normal clinical practice in Thailand (Supapaan et al., 2024).

Although tablets and capsules represented the most common dosage forms, oral liquid preparations were a common and emerging clinical form of LASA. Oral liquid preparations are mostly applied in pediatrics, geriatrics, and patients with impaired swallowing. Oral liquid medicines can be available in many brands, strengths, and concentrations and might be labeled similarly or even packaged the same, which means that there might be a chance of confusion in the process of prescribing, dispensing, administering, and patient use. Among them, magnesium hydroxide and aluminum milk-based preparations were mentioned as the most common pairs of oral liquid antacids for LASA, which demonstrates the susceptibility of liquid antacid preparations to name and appearance confusion. In all dosage forms, the most prevalent LASA mechanisms included similar drug names or pronunciations, followed by similar packaging names.

Most of the reported medication errors were identified as NCC MERP Category B, which consisted of errors that occurred but no longer reached the patient. This chapter is in reaction to these findings, and it presents a standardized LASA drug monograph that is designed to facilitate systematic LASA risk management in hospitals. The monograph provides fundamental data, such as the list of LASA drug pairs, the type of similarity (name-based and appearance-based), the kind of medication error that is defined by the NCC MERP structure, and the types of hospitals that report such incidents in a logical way. The main goal of this method is to improve patient safety by guaranteeing that patients are provided with the right, suitable, and safe drugs, as well as allowing healthcare specialists to consider high-risk LASA partners and implement proportionate and evidence-based prevention measures.

In addition to clinical use, the monograph is designed to serve as a system-level tool for preventing medication errors. The data in this chapter can be utilized by various stakeholders, such as regulatory bodies, drug manufacturers, healthcare organizations, and policy-making organizations, and can also be used as a source of information by healthcare workers and healthcare students in Thailand, who may research and develop medication safety programs concerning LASA drugs in Thailand (Supapaan et al., 2024).

In line with this, this chapter has two objectives. First, it explains the format and contents of the standardized LASA pair monograph, which outlines the role of each element to assist in identifying systematic risk and comparing and prioritizing risks. Second, it provides illustrative examples of oral liquid LASA drug pairs on the basis of hospital-reported research data, showing how national evidence can be operationalized to promote medication safety practices, education, and subsequent actions that will help to harmonize LASA management strategies in Thailand.

A panel of subject-matter experts informed and consulted on the classification framework of the LASA significance level development. The authors express their gratitude for the assistance of Assoc. Prof. Dr. Thida Ningsanont, Assoc. Prof. Wibul Wongpoowarak, and Assoc. Prof. Dr. Payom Wongpoowarak, whose professional opinions helped develop the criteria for defining the levels of significance of LASA. The authors also deeply appreciate the fact that pharmacists at hospitals in Thailand participated in the survey, provided LASA drug pair data, and provided constructive recommendations, all of which were critical in the development of this monograph.

Objectives of the Chapter

The aims of this chapter are as follows:

(1) To clarify the scope to be covered, the intended use and nonregulatory nature of the LASA drug monograph were determined by the use of disclaimers.
(2) To recognize methodological and data-related flaws that are inherent to hospital-reported LASA incidence records and retrospective analyses.
(3) To provide direction to readers on the standardized use and interpretation of LASA drug monography for systematic risk assessment and comparison.
(4) To promote clear and accountable use of LASA evidence in medication safety practices, education and research.

Organization of the Chapter

Chapter 10 begins by presenting an overview of LASA medication errors and their connection to patient safety, with a particular emphasis on oral liquid preparations. The structure and methodology of the LASA drug monograph are then introduced in the chapter, and detailed presentations of hospital-reported LASA oral liquid drug pairs in Thailand are given. Both monographs combine medication identification, the nature of the incidents, the severity of the errors, and global safety sources. The chapter ends by identifying the practical implications of medication safety practices, education, and future research.

DISCLAIMER AND LIMITATION

In this section, the range, purpose, and limitations involved in using the standardized LASA drug monograph in this chapter are clarified. Since the monograph is created on the basis of retrospective survey data covered by hospitals, it is necessary to provide explicit disclaimers and limitations to facilitate adequate interpretation and utilization of the findings.

Disclaimer

This monograph is intended solely for educational, research, and quality improvement purposes. It does not constitute legal, regulatory, or clinical decision-making guidance. The classifications and recommendations presented may not be universally applicable and should not replace institutional policies, professional judgment, or official regulatory requirements issued by national or international authorities.

Limitations

The data used in this monograph are based on voluntary, self-reported hospital LASA data and therefore are prone to underreporting, reporting bias, and variability in institutional practices of error classification. Therefore, the LASA drug pairs outlined below are not a full national inventory of LASA risks in Thailand, and the actual incidence of medication errors is underreported.

Moreover, the reported LASA incidents might be a manifestation of heterogeneous contributing factors, such as illegible handwriting, verbal miscommunication, similarity of brands, or similarities in packaging, which cannot always be fully decomposed with the help of retrospective survey data. Despite these limitations, hospital-reported LASA events continue to form a source of hard-to-obtain safety intelligence in the real world and are very popular in medication safety studies across the globe (National Coordinating Council for Medication Error Reporting and Prevention (NCC MERP), 2022; World Health Organization, 2023)

HOW TO USE DRUG MONOGRAPH

The entries of this chapter under the LASA monographs provide an organized and standardized report of the reported LASA oral liquid drug pairs in Thailand. This format allows systematic risk evaluation and interhospital comparison and the translation of LASA evidence into feasible medication safety interventions.

All LASA drug pairs are evaluated with the same predetermined components to ensure consistency and transparency. These sections combine drug identification, real-life incident data, the severity of the error, and international medication safety tools so that the reader can distinguish between the hypothetical LASA risk and the actual hospital-reported incidents. The fundamental elements of the LASA pair monograph are summarized in Table 1, and the nine important elements (Components 1 through 9) are presented in Figure 1. They provide complementary textual and visual information on the arrangement of these elements in the monograph system.

Table 1. An overview of the components of the LASA pair monograph and their respective purposes

No.	Component	Description and Rationale
1	Drug names of LASA pairs	- This report provides the essence of each LASA pair, including generic names, brand names, and marketed strengths, as part of the LASA survey conducted in Thailand (Supapaan et al., 2024). - Registered dosage by the Thai Food and Drug Administration (Thai FDA) - Lexi-Drugs (UpToDate Lexidrug) is used in classifying pharmacologic categories. - When they are available, drug identification characteristics (e.g., color, formulation, labeling characteristics, etc.) are provided to aid in proper differentiation of what may be similar in practice.
2	LASA incidents and safety alerts	- Compiles reported LASA events and institutional safety notifications related to the pair of drugs. This element separates the confirmed and real-world medication-use issues and hypothetical or theoretical LASA risks.
	2.1 Type of LASA pair reported	- Indicates whether the confusion is mostly caused by similarities in the name (spelling or pronunciation) or appearance (primary or secondary packaging). This differentiation is crucial to the choice of preventive measures.
	2.2 Number of hospitals reporting incidents	- Shows the number of hospitals that have reported LASA incidents with the drug pair, which is the extent of actual incidence and the greater the external validity of the risk signal.

continued on following page

Table 1. Continued

No.	Component	Description and Rationale
3	Significant level of LASA errors	- Cluster individual LASA drug pairs based on the most severe medication error reports using a standardized error-severity framework. The level indicates both the possible clinical implications and need to intervene and helps prioritize high-risk LSA pairs.
4	Medication error (ME) category	- Provides the list of the particular categories of medication errors reported in the LASA drug pair, according to the hospital error-reporting systems, in line with the NCC MERP classification. This section explains whether mistakes were caught prior to reaching the patient or causing exposure or injury to the patient.
5	Suggested tall man lettering	- Follows the recommendations of the Institute for Safe Medication Practices (ISMP) and the Australian Commission on Safety and Quality in Health Care (ACSQHC) on safe medication practices when there is a report. The availability or unavailability of tall man lettering assists in the identification of similarity of names as a major cause of LASA risk.
6	High-alert medication status	- Shows whether one or both medications are high-alert medications that need extra precautions during prescribing, dispensing, and administration. These are categorized as per established lists in Siriraj Hospital and ISMP, and especially the pediatric and oral liquids, which need to be carefully dosed.
7	LASA issues identified in Lexi-Drugs	- Reports on LASA-related warnings and risk information in the Lexi-Drugs database put them into perspective by listing known confusion risks with each individual drug with other drugs beyond the two LASA drugs being evaluated.
8	Inclusion in other safety databases	- Determines the presence of the LASA drug pair in the international medication-safety databases, e.g., the MedMARx Data Report 2008 of the United States Pharmacopeia. Inclusion implies that the LASA risk should be known better in healthcare systems.
9	Conclusion	- Synthesizes the key LASA risks identified for the drug pair, highlights dominant confusion mechanisms (name-based, appearance-based, or both), and emphasizes the assigned severity level and clinical relevance.

Figure 1. Components of the LASA pair monograph and their purpose

1. ALUMINIUM HYDROXIDE+MAGNESIUM HYDROXIDE+SIMETHICONE - MILK OF MAGNESIA

$Al(OH)_3$ compressed gel 960 mg+ $Mg(OH)_2$ 330 mg, simethicone 60 mg/15 mL – Magnesium hydroxide 8 g/100 mL

<table>
<tr><th></th><th></th><th colspan="8">Drug 1</th><th colspan="3">Drug 2</th></tr>
<tr><td rowspan="3">1</td><td>Generic name and strength (Chanakit et al., 2013; Supapaan et al., 2024)</td><td colspan="8">$Al(OH)_3$ compressed gel 960 mg+ $Mg(OH)_2$ 330 mg, simethicone 60 mg/15 mL (BOWA GEL®)</td><td colspan="3">Magnesium hydroxide 8 g/100 mL (MILK OF MAGNESIA®)</td></tr>
<tr><td>Dosage form (Thailand Food and Drug Administration, 2025)</td><td colspan="8">Oral liquids, suspension</td><td colspan="3">Oral liquids, suspension</td></tr>
<tr><td>Pharmacologic category (Lexi-Drugs., 2025)</td><td colspan="8">Antacid; antiflatulent (Aluminium [Aluminum] Hydroxide, 2025)</td><td colspan="3">Antacid; laxative; magnesium salt (Magnesium Hydroxide, 2025)</td></tr>
<tr><td rowspan="5">2</td><td colspan="12">LASA incidents and safety alerts</td></tr>
<tr><td colspan="9">Type of LASA pairs reported</td><td colspan="3"></td></tr>
<tr><td colspan="9">Similar name (spelling/ pronunciation)</td><td colspan="3">No</td></tr>
<tr><td colspan="9">Similar appearance (primary/ secondary packaging)</td><td colspan="3">Yes</td></tr>
<tr><td colspan="9">Number of hospitals that reported the LASA incidents</td><td colspan="3">1</td></tr>
<tr><td>3</td><td>Significant level of LASA errors</td><td colspan="11">3</td></tr>
<tr><td rowspan="2">4</td><td rowspan="2">Medication error (ME) category</td><td>A</td><td>B</td><td>C</td><td>D</td><td>E</td><td>F</td><td>G</td><td>H</td><td>I</td><td>No ME report, but listed in LASA hospital records</td><td>Number of hospitals reporting the issue</td></tr>
<tr><td>-</td><td>1</td><td>-</td><td>-</td><td>-</td><td>-</td><td>-</td><td>-</td><td>-</td><td>-</td><td>1</td></tr>
<tr><td rowspan="3">5</td><td colspan="12">Suggested Tallman lettering</td></tr>
<tr><td>ISMP (The Institute for Safe Medication Practices (ISMP), 2023)</td><td colspan="8">Not found in the list</td><td colspan="3">Not found in the list</td></tr>
<tr><td>ACSQHC 2024 (Australian Commission on Safety and Quality in Health Care (ACSQHC), 2024)</td><td colspan="8">Not found in the list</td><td colspan="3">Not found in the list</td></tr>
<tr><td>6</td><td>High-alert medication (HAM) status (The Institute for Safe Medication Practices (ISMP), 2011)</td><td colspan="8">N/A</td><td colspan="3">N/A</td></tr>
<tr><td>7</td><td>LASA issues from Lexi-Drugs (Lexi-Drugs., 2025)</td><td colspan="8">Aluminium [Aluminum] Hydroxide, Magnesium Hydroxide, and Simeticone [Simethicone](Aluminium [Aluminum] Hydroxide, 2025)
-According to Lexi-Drugs, LASA medication errors primarily arise from brand names that appear or sound similar.</td><td colspan="3">N/A (Magnesium Hydroxide, 2025)</td></tr>
<tr><td rowspan="3">8</td><td colspan="12">Listed as LASA in other safety databases</td></tr>
<tr><td>MedMarx (Hicks et al., 2008)</td><td colspan="8">Not found in the list</td><td colspan="3">Not found in the list</td></tr>
<tr><td>Other reports</td><td colspan="8">N/A</td><td colspan="3">N/A</td></tr>
<tr><td>9</td><td>Conclusion</td><td colspan="11">The $Al(OH)_3$ compressed gel combined with $Mg(OH)_2$, simethicone suspensions, and magnesium hydroxide suspensions presents a LASA risk due to their similar appearance, as evidenced by one reported hospital medication error. A significance level of 3 has been assigned to this drug pair due to a reported medication error classified as Category B.</td></tr>
<tr><td></td><td colspan="12">Abbreviations: LASA = Look-alike, sound-alike; ISMP = The Institute for Safe Medication Practices; ACSQHC = Australian Commission on Safety and Quality in Health Care; MedMarx = The United States Pharmacopeia (USP) MedMarx Reporting System 2008; N/A: No available reports.</td></tr>
</table>

The figure illustrates key monograph components, including (1) drug names of LASA pairs; (2) LASA incidence and safety alerts, including (2.1) type of LASA pair reported; (2.2) number of hospitals reporting incidents; (3) significant level of LASA errors; (4) medication error (ME) category; (5) suggested tall man lettering; (6) high-alert medication status; (7) LASA issues identified in Lexi-Drugs; (8) inclusion in other safety databases; and (9) conclusion.

PURPOSE OF THE MONOGRAPH STRUCTURE

By applying a standardized, component-based structure, the LASA drug monograph is designed to support healthcare professionals in the systematic identification, interpretation, and mitigation of LASA-related risks. Specifically, the monograph enables users to do the following:

- Rapidly identify high-risk oral liquid LASA drug pairs requiring heightened attention;
- Understand the underlying mechanisms, frequency, and severity of reported LASA medication errors; and
- Targeted, evidence-based prevention strategies that are proportionate to the identified risk profile are selected.

In addition to its routine clinical application, this systematic methodology is also used in pharmacy education, institutional quality improvement, and future national efforts to standardize LASA reporting, analysis, and risk-reduction plans in Thailand.

EXPLANATION OF COMPONENTS IN THE LASA PAIR MONOGRAPH

All LASA pairs are monographs that have standardized components that together identify drug identity, mechanism of error, real-life evidence, and clinical significance.

Component 1. Names of LASA Pair Drugs

This element provides essential identification information for each LASA drug pair, including the following:

- Brand names and generic names,
- Marketed dosage forms and strengths, and
- Pharmacologic categories, by Lexi Drugs (UpToDate Lexidrug), where available.

Drug identification characteristics (color, formulation qualities, or physical properties) are also reported when available. The combination of these elements aids in the proper differentiation of potentially confusing medicines because of similar names, labels, or physical appearances.

Component 2. LASA Incidents and Safety Alerts

It is a summary of recorded LASA incidents and safety warnings related to each drug pair, based mostly on the records of medication errors reported by hospitals. This information is based on real clinical experience and not on theoretical risks but is the evidentiary basis of further classification.

Component 2.1 Classification of LASA Drug Types

The LASA drug pairs are categorized on the basis of the major mechanism of confusion, which is determined by reported cases.

2.1.1 Name-Based LASA

Name-based LASA errors are caused by spelling, pronunciation, or both similarities that cause confusion during prescribing, dispensing, or administration. This type consists of the following:

1. **Similar spelling:** Drugs with a very similar spelling in written form, including those where the major difference is a difference in drug strength.
2. **Same sound:** Verbal miscommunication: The pronunciation of similar drug names is more likely to occur among healthcare workers.
3. **Similarity of spelling and pronunciation:** Drug names that are similar when written and spoken increase risk at more than one stage of the medication-use process.

2.1.2 Appearance-Based LASA

Appearance-based LASA errors are caused by resemblances in drug formulation or packaging and can cause selection errors when the drug is stored, dispensed, or administered. The similarity of packaging can be divided into two levels:

1. **Primary packaging:** The medication is stored in a direct container and is in direct contact with the drug (e.g., tablets, capsules, vials, ampules, bottles, sachets, prefilled syringes, or intravenous containers).
2. **Secondary packaging:** External wrapping that holds one or more primary packages (e.g., cartons, boxes, injection trays, or shipping containers). Drug or packaging images are incorporated into the monograph, where specific brand names and strengths are known and image data are provided. In the case of nonavailability of images, it is marked as not available (N/A).

Component 2.2 Number of Hospitals with LASA Incidents Reported

This aspect reflects how many healthcare facilities have been reported to have experienced the LASA incident, and this aspect can be used to differentiate between actual real-life occurrences and isolated/hypothetical risks. The greater the number of reporting hospitals is, the greater the vulnerability to the system and the urgency of preventive measures.

Component 3. Severity Level of LASA Errors

The severity level of each drug pair as per the most severe reported medication-error outcome is assigned to each LASA drug pair on the basis of a standardized error-severity framework. This grouping is not only based on the possible clinical effect but also on the urgency of the risk-reduction action and the priority of LASA pairs to receive specific interventions.

3.1 Level of Significance of LASA Errors

There are four levels of significance for LASA drug pairs, including critical risk (level 1) and low risk (level 4), as summarized in Table 2. All levels are associated with certain types of medication errors and provide a visual cue to indicate urgency and necessary measures. An increase in the level of significance means that the potential harm to patients is high, and system-level protection is needed.

3.2 Characterization of the Level of Significance of LASA Errors

1. Significance Level 1 (Critical)
   LASA drug pairs were related to medication errors, which fall into the category of I, which refers to errors that led to patient death or irreversible severe harm.
2. Significance Level 2 (High)
   LASA drug pairs related to mistakes falling under Categories E-H, where the mistake was transmitted to the patient and resulted in temporary or permanent harm, necessitated action, or extended stay in the hospital.
3. Significant Level 3 (Moderate)
   LASA drug pairs, which were related to errors that fell into Categories A to D, such as near misses or errors that did not harm the patient but were detected.
4. Significance Level 4 (Low)

LASA drug pairs that have not been reported to cause medication errors but are included in institutional LASA databases on the basis of perceived risk or similarity as identified.

Table 2. LASA significance levels

	Significant level of LASA errors	Risk Severity Description	Suggested management
🔴 1	Level 1 (Critical)	Errors classified under Category I	Emergency warning
🟠 2	Level 2 (High)	Errors classified under Categories E–H	High-priority alert
🟡 3	Level 3 (Moderate)	Errors classified under Categories A–D	Review and monitoring required
🟢 4	Level 4 (Low)	No reported errors; suspected LASA risk	Caution—routine surveillance

If a LASA drug pair is associated with multiple error categories, it is classified according to the highest level of severity observed. For example:

- A drug pair with reported errors in Categories A and E is classified as Level 2 (High).
- A drug pair with reported errors in Categories B, D, and I is classified as Level 1 (critical).

This conservative, severity-based approach ensures that LASA risks are not underestimated and that preventive strategies are aligned with the worst credible clinical outcome.

Component 4. Medication Error (ME) Category

This element is a listing of the particular medication error types related to the LASA drug pair on the basis of hospital error reports. This classification helps to define whether errors were detected prior to reaching a patient or led to exposure or harm.

The medication error classification in this monograph is based on the system developed by the National Coordinating Council on Medication Error Reporting and Prevention (NCC MERP) in the United States. This is a common classification for evaluating the seriousness of medication errors and their effect on patient safety. The types of mistakes range from those that may go unnoticed to those that can result in severe injuries or fatalities. Table 3 shows the NCC MERP classification.

Table 3. NCC MERP Medication Error Classification System (National Coordinating Council for Medication Error Reporting and Prevention (NCC MERP), 2022)

Error Category	Description
1. Category A	Circumstances or events that have the potential to cause an error but do not actually result in one.
2. Category B	An error occurred but did not reach the patient.
3. Category C	An error reached the patient but did not cause harm.
4. Category D	An error reached the patient and required monitoring or intervention to prevent harm.
5. Category E	An error caused temporary harm and required intervention.
6. Category F	An error resulted in hospitalization or prolonged the patient's hospital stay.
7. Category G	An error led to permanent harm.
8. Category H	An error resulted in a life-threatening event, such as anaphylaxis or cardiac arrest, requiring emergency intervention.
9. Category I	An error resulted in patient death.

It is a categorization system that offers a standard method to assess LASA drug-related errors and their outcomes. By determining errors on the basis of their severity, healthcare providers can use specific measures to minimize risks and enhance medication safety.

Component 5. Recommended Tall Man Lettering

The Institute of Safe Medication Practices (ISMP) and the Australian Commission on Safety and Quality in Health Care (ACSQHC) provide recommendations on tall man lettering, which are reported where available. Tall man lettering is a factor used to identify whether the similarity of names is a main cause of the LASA risk to the two drugs.

Component 6. High-Alert Medication Status

This section highlights high-alert medication, which requires extra precautions to be taken when it is prescribed, dispensed, and administered. The identification of high-alert status involves accepted lists of drugs at Siriraj Hospital and ISMP and is specifically pertinent to pediatric and oral liquid preparations, which demand accurate dosing.

Component 7. The Lexi-Drugs identified Lexi-Drugs issues

This element provides a summary of LASA-related warnings and risk evaluations that are reported in the Lexi-Drugs database. It also evaluates the risks of known drug confusion and considers interactions with other drugs beyond the tested LASA pair.

Component 8. Inclusion in Other Safety Databases

This part determines the presence of the LASA drug pair in international medication safety databases, e.g., in the MedMARx Data Report 2008 (United States Pharmacopeia LASA drug reports) or other database safety reports. The use of these databases implies the need for further acknowledgment of LASA risk in healthcare systems.

Component 9. Conclusion

The conclusion summarizes the main LASA risks determined within the monograph; identifies the most prevalent mechanisms of confusion (name, appearance, or both); and highlights the clinical importance and severity level of the LASA drug pair.

EXAMPLES OF LASA ORAL LIQUID REPORTS IN THAILAND

1. Aluminium Hydroxide+Magnesium Hydroxide+Simethicone - Milk Of Magnesia

Table 4. $Al(OH)_3$ compressed gel (960 mg/15 mL) + $Mg(OH)_2$ (330 mg/15 mL), simethicone (60 mg/15 mL) – magnesium hydroxide (8 g/100 mL)

	Drug 1	**Drug 2**
Generic name and strength (Chanakit et al., 2013; Supapaan et al., 2024)	$Al(OH)_3$ compressed gel 960 mg+ $Mg(OH)_2$ 330 mg, simethicone 60 mg/15 mL (BOWA GEL®)	Magnesium hydroxide 8 g/100 mL (MILK OF MAGNESIA®)
Dosage form (Thailand Food and Drug Administration, 2025) (see Figure 2)	Oral liquids, suspension	Oral liquids, suspension
Pharmacologic category (Lexi-Drugs., 2025)	Antacid; antiflatulent (Aluminium [Aluminum] Hydroxide, 2025)	Antacid; laxative; magnesium salt (Magnesium Hydroxide, 2025)
LASA incidents and safety alerts		
Type of LASA pairs reported		
⚠ Similar name (spelling/pronunciation)		No
⚠ Similar appearance (primary/secondary packaging)		⚠ Yes
Number of hospitals that reported the LASA incidents		1
Significant level of LASA errors	3	

Medication error (ME) category	A	B	C	D	E	F	G	H	I	No ME report, but listed in LASA hospital records	Number of hospitals reporting the issue
	-	1	-	-	-	-	-	-	-	-	1

Suggested Tallman lettering		
ISMP (The Institute for Safe Medication Practices (ISMP), 2023)	Not found in the list	Not found in the list
ACSQHC 2024 (Australian Commission on Safety and Quality in Health Care (ACSQHC), 2024)	Not found in the list	Not found in the list
High-alert medication (HAM) status (The Institute for Safe Medication Practices (ISMP), 2011)	N/A	N/A
⚠ **LASA issues from Lexi-Drugs** (Lexi-Drugs., 2025)	⚠ *Aluminium [Aluminum] Hydroxide, Magnesium Hydroxide, and Simeticone [Simethicone](Aluminium [Aluminum] Hydroxide, 2025)* -Lexi-Drugs states that the main cause of LASA medication errors is similarities in the brand names that look or sound alike.	*N/A (Magnesium Hydroxide, 2025)*
Listed as LASA in other safety databases		
MedMarx (Hicks et al., 2008)	Not found in the list	Not found in the list
Other reports	N/A	N/A
Conclusion	The $Al(OH)_3$ compressed gel combined with $Mg(OH)_2$, simethicone suspensions, and magnesium hydroxide suspensions presents a LASA risk due to their similar appearance, as evidenced by one reported hospital medication error. A significance level of 3 has been assigned to this drug pair due to a reported medication error classified as Category B.	

Abbreviations: LASA = Look-alike, sound-alike; ISMP = The Institute for Safe Medication Practices; ACSQHC = Australian Commission on Safety and Quality in Health Care; MedMarx = The United States Pharmacopeia (USP) MedMarx Reporting System 2008; N/A: No available reports.

Figure 2. LASA pair monograph example for aluminum hydroxide–magnesium hydroxide–simethicone suspension (BOWA GEL®) and magnesium hydroxide suspension (MILK OF MAGNESIA®)

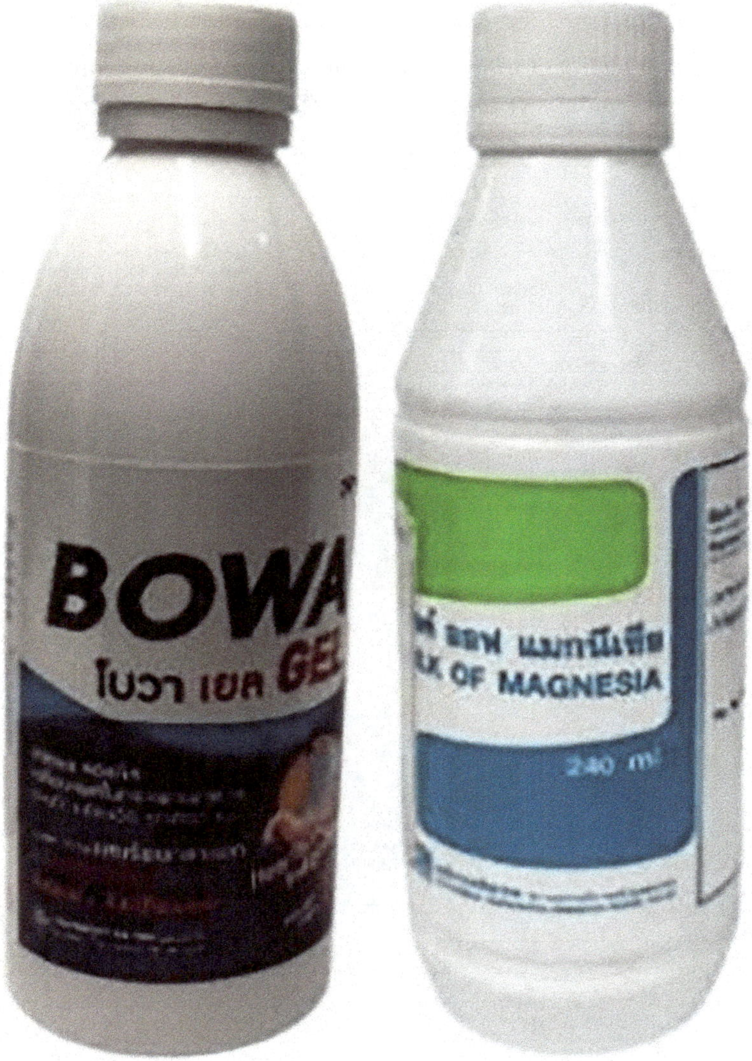

2. Ambroxol Hydrochloride – Diphenhydramine Hydrochloride+Ammonium Chloride+Sodium Citrate

Table 5. Ambroxol hydrochloride (30 mg/5 mL) – diphenhydramine hydrochloride (12.5 mg/5 mL) + ammonium chloride (125 mg/5 mL) + sodium citrate (50 mg/5 mL)

	Drug 1	Drug 2
Generic name and strength (Chanakit et al., 2013; Supapaan et al., 2024)	Ambroxol hydrochloride 30 mg/5 mL (MUCONOR SYRUP®)	Diphenhydramine hydrochloride 12.5 mg + ammonium chloride 125 mg + sodium citrate 50 mg/5 mL (COTUSSIN SYRUP®)
Dosage form (Thailand Food and Drug Administration, 2025)	Oral liquids, syrup	Oral liquids, syrup
Pharmacologic category (Lexi-Drugs., 2025)	Mucolytic agent (Ambroxol, 2025)	Ethanolamine derivative; Expectorant; Histamine H_1 Antagonist; Histamine H_1 Antagonist, First Generation (Diphenhydramine, 2025)
LASA incidents and safety alerts		
Type of LASA pairs reported		
Similar name (spelling/pronunciation)		N/A
Similar appearance (primary/secondary packaging)		Yes
Number of hospitals that reported the LASA incidents		1
Significant level of LASA errors	3	

Medication error (ME) category	A	B	C	D	E	F	G	H	I	No ME report, but listed in LASA hospital records	Number of hospitals reporting the issue
	1	1	-	-	-	-	-	-	-	-	2

	Drug 1	Drug 2
Suggested Tallman lettering		
ISMP (The Institute for Safe Medication Practices (ISMP), 2023)	Not found in the list	diphenhydrAMINE
ACSQHC 2024 (Australian Commission on Safety and Quality in Health Care (ACSQHC), 2024)	Not found in the list	Not found in the list
High-alert medication (HAM) status (The Institute for Safe Medication Practices (ISMP), 2011)	N/A	Yes -Diphenhydramine (oral), a first-generation antihistamine, is considered potentially inappropriate for adults ≥65 according to the Beers Criteria due to its strong anticholinergic effects, which increase the risk of confusion, dry mouth, constipation, and toxicity. Combined use with other anticholinergic drugs further raises the risk of falls, delirium, and dementia, highlighting the need to consider total anticholinergic burden (Diphenhydramine, 2025; The 2023 American Geriatrics Society Beers Criteria® Update Expert Panel, 2023).
LASA issues from Lexi-Drugs (Lexi-Drugs., 2025)	*Ambroxol (Ambroxol, 2025)* -Ambroxol may be mistaken for ambroxol acefyllinate. Its brand names have been reported as being confused with those of other generic drugs.	N/A
Listed as LASA in other safety databases		
MedMarx (Hicks et al., 2008)	Not found in the list	Not found in the list
Other reports	N/A	N/A
Conclusion	Ambroxol hydrochloride and the combination of diphenhydramine hydrochloride with ammonium chloride and sodium citrate present a LASA risk primarily due to their similar appearance in oral liquid/syrup forms. Diphenhydramine is also identified as a high-alert medication in older adults according to the Beers Criteria, due to its strong anticholinergic effects and associated risks such as confusion, constipation, and increased fall risk.	

Abbreviations: LASA = Look-alike, sound-alike; ISMP = The Institute for Safe Medication Practices; ACSQHC = Australian Commission on Safety and Quality in Health Care; MedMarx = The United States Pharmacopeia (USP) MedMarx Reporting System 2008; N/A: No available reports.

3. Amoxicillin Trihydrate – Amoxicillin/Clavulanate

Table 6. Amoxicillin trihydrate (125 mg/5 mL) – Amoxicillin/clavulanate (457 mg/5 mL)

<table>
<tr><th></th><th colspan="8">Drug 1</th><th colspan="3">Drug 2</th></tr>
<tr><td>Generic name and strength (Chanakit et al., 2013; Supapaan et al., 2024)</td><td colspan="8">Amoxicillin trihydrate 125 mg/5 mL (S-MOX 125 DRY SYRUP®)</td><td colspan="3">Amoxycillin trihydrate 400 mg + potassium clavulanate 57 mg (457 mg/5 mL) (CLAVICO 457®)</td></tr>
<tr><td>Dosage form (Thailand Food and Drug Administration, 2025)</td><td colspan="8">Oral liquids, powder for oral suspension</td><td colspan="3">Oral liquids, powder for oral suspension</td></tr>
<tr><td>Pharmacologic category (Lexi-Drugs., 2025)</td><td colspan="8">Antibiotic, penicillin (Amoxicillin and Clavulanate, 2025)</td><td colspan="3">Antibiotic, penicillin (Amoxicillin and Clavulanate, 2025)</td></tr>
<tr><td colspan="12">LASA incidents and safety alerts</td></tr>
<tr><td colspan="9">Type of LASA pairs reported</td><td colspan="3"></td></tr>
<tr><td colspan="9">Similar name (spelling/pronunciation)</td><td colspan="3">Yes</td></tr>
<tr><td colspan="9">Similar appearance (primary/secondary packaging)</td><td colspan="3">N/A</td></tr>
<tr><td colspan="9">Number of hospitals that reported the LASA incidents</td><td colspan="3">1</td></tr>
<tr><td>Significant level of LASA errors</td><td colspan="11">3</td></tr>
<tr><td rowspan="2">Medication error (ME) category</td><td>A</td><td>B</td><td>C</td><td>D</td><td>E</td><td>F</td><td>G</td><td>H</td><td>I</td><td>No ME report, but listed in LASA hospital records</td><td>Number of hospitals reporting the issue</td></tr>
<tr><td>-</td><td>1</td><td>-</td><td>-</td><td>-</td><td>-</td><td>-</td><td>-</td><td>-</td><td>-</td><td>1</td></tr>
<tr><td colspan="12">Suggested Tallman lettering</td></tr>
<tr><td>ISMP (The Institute for Safe Medication Practices (ISMP), 2023)</td><td colspan="8">Not found in the list</td><td colspan="3">Not found in the list</td></tr>
<tr><td>ACSQHC 2024 (Australian Commission on Safety and Quality in Health Care (ACSQHC), 2024)</td><td colspan="8">Not found in the list</td><td colspan="3">Not found in the list</td></tr>
<tr><td>High-alert medication (HAM) status
(The Institute for Safe Medication Practices (ISMP), 2011)</td><td colspan="8">Yes
-The ISMP classifies this pediatric liquid medication as a high-alert medication due to the risk of errors in community settings, especially those that require measurement (The Institute for Safe Medication Practices (ISMP), 2011).</td><td colspan="3">Yes
-The ISMP classifies this pediatric liquid medication as a high-alert medication due to the risk of errors in community settings, especially those that require measurement (The Institute for Safe Medication Practices (ISMP), 2011).</td></tr>
<tr><td>LASA issues from Lexi-Drugs (Lexi-Drugs., 2025)</td><td colspan="8">Amoxicillin (Amoxicillin, 2025)
-Amoxicillin is sometimes confused with amoxapine or Augmentin, and Amoxil is similarly confused with amoxapine.</td><td colspan="3">Amoxicillin and Clavulanate (Amoxicillin and Clavulanate, 2025)
-There is potential for confusion between some brand names and amoxicillin.</td></tr>
<tr><td colspan="12">Listed as LASA in other safety databases</td></tr>
<tr><td>MedMarx (Hicks et al., 2008)</td><td colspan="11">Despite MedMarx not directly reporting the amoxicillin trihydrate-amoxicillin/clavulanate pair, incidents of LASA have been reported using amoxicillin-amoxapine (ME Category B), amoxicillin-ampicillin (ME Categories A, B, C-D), and amoxicillin-Augmentin (ME Categories A, B, C-D, E-H). These reports highlight the significant LASA vulnerability associated with amoxicillin-related names and explain why it is essential to verify specific product choices and strengths, particularly for oral liquid formulations.</td></tr>
<tr><td>Other reports</td><td colspan="8">N/A</td><td colspan="3">N/A</td></tr>
<tr><td>Conclusion</td><td colspan="11">These two drugs have similar names and are both developed as pediatric oral suspension which adds to the possible confusion. The reported LASA incidents, their classification as high-alert medications, and their inclusion in Lexi-Drugs underscore the critical need for enhanced safety strategies, such as distinct labeling and improved prescriber awareness.</td></tr>
<tr><td colspan="12">Abbreviations: LASA = Look-alike, sound-alike; ISMP = The Institute for Safe Medication Practices; ACSQHC = Australian Commission on Safety and Quality in Health Care; MedMarx = The United States Pharmacopeia (USP) MedMarx Reporting System 2008; N/A: No available reports.</td></tr>
</table>

4. Amoxicillin+clavulanic acid – Amoxicillin+clavulanic acid

Table 7. Amoxicillin trihydrate 400 mg + potassium clavulanate 57 mg (457 mg/5 mL) – Amoxicillin trihydrate 600 mg + potassium clavulanate 42.9 (642.9 mg/5 mL)

	Drug 1	Drug 2
Generic name and strength (Chanakit et al., 2013; Supapaan et al., 2024)	Amoxycillin trihydrate 400 mg + potassium clavulanate 57 mg (457 mg/5 mL) (AUGMENTIN (457 MG/5 ML)®)	Amoxycillin trihydrate 600 mg + potassium clavulanate 42.9 (642.9 mg/5 mL) (AUGMENTIN ES®)
Dosage form (Thailand Food and Drug Administration, 2025)	Oral liquids, powder for oral suspension	Oral liquids, powder for oral suspension
Pharmacologic category (Lexi-Drugs., 2025)	Antibiotic, Penicillin (Amoxicillin and Clavulanate, 2025)	Antibiotic, Penicillin (Amoxicillin and Clavulanate, 2025)
LASA incidents and safety alerts		
Type of LASA pairs reported		
⚠️ Similar name (spelling/pronunciation)		⚠️ Yes
⚠️ Similar appearance (primary/secondary packaging)		N/A
Number of hospitals that reported the LASA incidents		1
Significant level of LASA errors	4	

Medication error (ME) category	A	B	C	D	E	F	G	H	I	No ME report, but listed in LASA hospital records	Number of hospitals reporting the issue
	-	-	-	-	-	-	-	-	-	1	1

	Drug 1	Drug 2
Suggested Tallman lettering		
🔍 ISMP (The Institute for Safe Medication Practices (ISMP), 2023)	Not found in the list	Not found in the list
🔍 ACSQHC 2024 (Australian Commission on Safety and Quality in Health Care (ACSQHC), 2024)	Not found in the list	Not found in the list
🚨 **High-alert medication (HAM) status** (The Institute for Safe Medication Practices (ISMP), 2011)	🚨 Yes -The ISMP classifies this pediatric liquid medication as a high-alert medication due to the risk of errors in community settings, especially those that require measurement (The Institute for Safe Medication Practices (ISMP), 2011).	🚨 Yes -The ISMP classifies this pediatric liquid medication as a high-alert medication due to the risk of errors in community settings, especially those that require measurement (The Institute for Safe Medication Practices (ISMP), 2011).
⚠️ **LASA issues from Lexi-Drugs** (Lexi-Drugs., 2025)	⚠️ *Amoxicillin and Clavulanate(Amoxicillin and Clavulanate, 2025)* -There is potential for confusion between some brand names and amoxicillin.	⚠️ *Amoxicillin and Clavulanate (Amoxicillin and Clavulanate, 2025)* -There is potential for confusion between some brand names and amoxicillin.
Listed as LASA in other safety databases		
MedMarx (Hicks et al., 2008)	Despite MedMarx not directly reporting the Amoxycillin trihydrate + potassium clavulanate pair, incidents of LASA have been reported using amoxicillin-amoxapine (ME Category B), amoxicillin-ampicillin (ME Categories A, B, C-D), and amoxicillin-Augmentin (ME Categories A, B, C-D, E-H). These reports highlight the significant LASA vulnerability associated with amoxicillin-related names and explain why it is essential to verify specific product choices and strengths, particularly for oral liquid formulations.	
Other reports	N/A	N/A
Conclusion	The amoxicillin/clavulanate compound preparations of 457 mg/5 mL and 642.9 mg/5 mL oral suspensions present a LASA risk since the names are similar. This pair of drugs was reported in LASA hospital records, though there were no officially reported medication errors. Both formulations are pediatric liquid medications that require accurate measurement, which contributes to their classification as high-alert medications by the ISMP, particularly in community settings. Lexi-Drugs also notes the potential for confusion between amoxicillin and certain brand names.	

Abbreviations: LASA = Look-alike, sound-alike; ISMP = The Institute for Safe Medication Practices; ACSQHC = Australian Commission on Safety and Quality in Health Care; MedMarx = The United States Pharmacopeia (USP) MedMarx Reporting System 2008; N/A: No available reports.

5. Cefaclor – Cefaclor

Table 8. Cefaclor monohydrate (125 mg/5 mL) – Cefaclor monohydrate (250 mg/5 mL)

	Drug 1	Drug 2
Generic name and strength (Chanakit et al., 2013; Supapaan et al., 2024)	Cefaclor monohydrate 125 mg/5 mL (DISTACLOR 125 MG/5 ML®)	Cefaclor monohydrate 250 mg/5 mL (DISTACLOR 250 MG/5 ML®)
Dosage form (Thailand Food and Drug Administration, 2025)	Oral liquids, dry syrup	Oral liquids, dry syrup
Pharmacologic category (Lexi-Drugs., 2025)	Antibiotic, Cephalosporin (Second Generation) (Cefaclor, 2025)	Antibiotic, Cephalosporin (Second Generation) (Cefaclor, 2025)
LASA incidents and safety alerts		
Type of LASA pairs reported		
Similar name (spelling/pronunciation)		Yes
Similar appearance (primary/secondary packaging)		N/A
Number of hospitals that reported the LASA incidents		1
Significant level of LASA errors	4	

Medication error (ME) category	A	B	C	D	E	F	G	H	I	No ME report, but listed in LASA hospital records	Number of hospitals reporting the issue
	-	-	-	-	-	-	-	-	-	1	1

	Drug 1	Drug 2
Suggested Tallman lettering		
ISMP (The Institute for Safe Medication Practices (ISMP), 2023)	Not found in the list	Not found in the list
ACSQHC 2024 (Australian Commission on Safety and Quality in Health Care (ACSQHC), 2024)	Not found in the list	Not found in the list
High-alert medication (HAM) status (The Institute for Safe Medication Practices (ISMP), 2011)	-The ISMP classifies this pediatric liquid medication as a high-alert medication due to the risk of errors in community settings, especially those that require measurement (The Institute for Safe Medication Practices (ISMP), 2011).	-The ISMP classifies this pediatric liquid medication as a high-alert medication due to the risk of errors in community settings, especially those that require measurement (The Institute for Safe Medication Practices (ISMP), 2011).
LASA issues from Lexi-Drugs (Lexi-Drugs., 2025)	*Cefaclor (Cefaclor, 2025)* -Cefaclor and cephalexin have the potential to be confused due to name similarity.	*Cefaclor (Cefaclor, 2025)* -Cefaclor and cephalexin have the potential to be confused due to name similarity.
Listed as LASA in other safety databases		
MedMarx (Hicks et al., 2008)	Even though the cefaclor-cefaclor strength versions were not found as LASA pairs in the MedMarx database, LASA events with cefaclor-cefadroxil (ME category C-D) are reported by MedMarx. This conclusion suggests that cefaclor-containing products are open to name-based errors, which supports the importance of subjecting drug name and intelligence validation and strength testing to dispensing oral liquid cephalosporins.	
Other reports	N/A	N/A
Conclusion	Cefaclor monohydrate oral suspension 125 mg/5 mL and 250 mg/5 mL (similar drug names but not identical concentrations) represent a LASA risk, with one of the hospitals reporting the situation and no case of patient-harm medication errors reported. Defined specification of strengths, standard labeling, and caution of overdose are some of the measures that can be taken to prevent mistakes in pediatric dosing.	

Abbreviations: LASA = Look-alike, sound-alike; ISMP = The Institute for Safe Medication Practices; ACSQHC = Australian Commission on Safety and Quality in Health Care; MedMarx = The United States Pharmacopeia (USP) MedMarx Reporting System 2008; N/A: No available reports.

6. Cefixime Trihydrate – Cetirizine Dihydrochloride

Table 9. Cefixime trihydrate (100 mg/5 mL) and cetirizine dihydrochloride (5 mg/5 mL)

	Drug 1	Drug 2
Generic name and strength (Chanakit et al., 2013; Supapaan et al., 2024)	Cefixime trihydrate 100 mg/5 mL (CEFSPAN®)	Cetirizine dihydrochloride 5 mg/5 mL (STARTEC SYRUP®)
Dosage form (Thailand Food and Drug Administration, 2025) (see Figure 3)	Oral liquids, dry syrup	Oral liquids, syrup
Pharmacologic category (Lexi-Drugs., 2025)	Antibiotic, cephalosporin (third generation) (Cefixime, 2026)	Histamine H_1 antagonist; histamine H_1 antagonist, second generation; piperazine derivative (Cetirizine (systemic), 2026)
LASA incidents and safety alerts		
Type of LASA pairs reported		
Similar name (spelling/pronunciation)		Yes
Similar appearance (primary/secondary packaging)		N/A
Number of hospitals that reported the LASA incidents		1
Significant level of LASA errors	3	

Medication error (ME) category	A	B	C	D	E	F	G	H	I	No ME report, but listed in LASA hospital records	Number of hospitals reporting the issue
	-	1	-	-	-	-	-	-	-	-	1

Suggested Tallman lettering		
ISMP (The Institute for Safe Medication Practices (ISMP), 2023)	Not found in the list	Not found in the list
ACSQHC 2024 (Australian Commission on Safety and Quality in Health Care (ACSQHC), 2024)	Not found in the list	Not found in the list
High-alert medication (HAM) status (The Institute for Safe Medication Practices (ISMP), 2011)	Yes -The ISMP classifies this pediatric liquid medication as a high-alert medication due to the risk of errors in community settings, especially those that require measurement (The Institute for Safe Medication Practices (ISMP), 2011).	Yes -The ISMP classifies this pediatric liquid medication as a high-alert medication due to the risk of errors in community settings, especially those that require measurement (The Institute for Safe Medication Practices (ISMP), 2011).
LASA issues from Lexi-Drugs (Lexi-Drugs., 2025)	Cefixime is similar to cefepime.	Cetirizine may be mistaken for sertraline or stavudine. ZyrTEC may be mistaken for Lipitor, Serax, Xanax, Zantac, Zerit, Zocor, ZyPREXA, or ZyrTEC-D.
Listed as LASA in other safety databases		
MedMarx (Hicks et al., 2008)	Cefixime trihydrate-cetirizine dihydrochlorate was not listed as a LASA pair in the MedMarx database, but was a cefixime-cefepime LASA pair with a ME category B. This fact proves that cefixime is prone to name-based errors, and the safe use of drugs with their names requires the attention to medication-names checks in the process of prescriptions and dispensation.	Not found in the list
Other reports	N/A	N/A
Conclusion	Cefixime trihydrate and cetirizine dihydrochloride show a LASA risk because of the similarity in the pronunciation (e.g., ..span vs ..star) and use of the name as a pediatric oral liquid, where one hospital reported the problem as a ME of type B. Wrong-drug errors need to be avoided by clear indication-based prescribing and close dispensing.	

Abbreviations: LASA = Look-alike, sound-alike; ISMP = The Institute for Safe Medication Practices; ACSQHC = Australian Commission on Safety and Quality in Health Care; MedMarx = The United States Pharmacopeia (USP) MedMarx Reporting System 2008; N/A: No available reports.

Figure 3. LASA pair monograph example for cefixime trihydrate (CEFSPAN®) and cetirizine dihydrochloride (STARTEC SYRUP®)

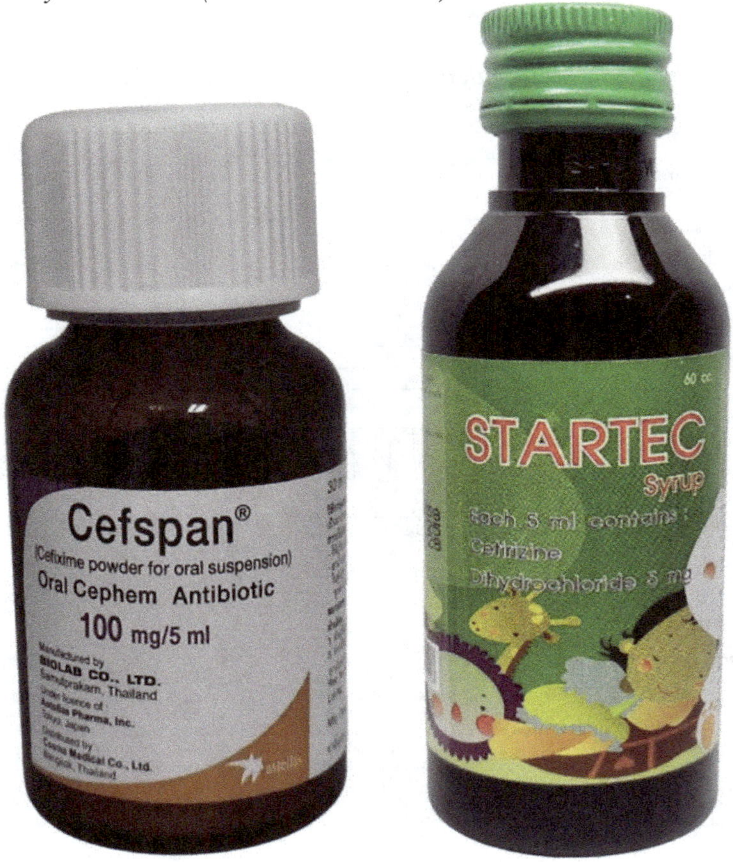

7. Chlorpheniramine Maleate – Hydroxyzine Hydrochloride

Table 10. Chlorpheniramine maleate (2 mg/5 mL)–Hydroxyzine hydrochloride (10 mg/5 mL)

	Drug 1	Drug 2
Generic name and strength (Chanakit et al., 2013; Supapaan et al., 2024)	Chlorpheniramine maleate 2 mg/5 mL (CHLOPHEN SYRUP®)	Hydroxyzine hydrochloride 10 mg/5 mL (R - RAX SYRUP®)
Dosage form (Thailand Food and Drug Administration, 2025)	Oral liquids, syrup	Oral liquids, syrup
Pharmacologic category (Lexi-Drugs., 2025)	Alkylamine derivative; histamine H_1 antagonist; first generation (Chlorphenamine [Chlorpheniramine], 2025)	Antiemetic; histamine H_1 Antagonist; first generation; piperazine derivative (HydrOXYzine, 2025)
LASA incidents and safety alerts		
Type of LASA pairs reported		
Similar name (spelling/pronunciation)		N/A
Similar appearance (primary/secondary packaging)		Yes
Number of hospitals that reported the LASA incidents		1
Significant level of LASA errors	4	
Medication error (ME) category	A: - ; B: - ; C: - ; D: - ; E: - ; F: - ; G: - ; H: - ; I: -	No ME report, but listed in LASA hospital records: 1; Number of hospitals reporting the issue: 1
Suggested Tallman lettering		
ISMP (The Institute for Safe Medication Practices (ISMP), 2023)	Not found in the list	hydrOXYzine
ACSQHC 2024 (Australian Commission on Safety and Quality in Health Care (ACSQHC), 2024)	Not found in the list	Not found in the list
High-alert medication (HAM) status (The Institute for Safe Medication Practices (ISMP), 2011)	Yes -The ISMP classifies this pediatric liquid medication as a high-alert medication due to the risk of errors in community settings, especially those that require measurement (Chlorphenamine [Chlorpheniramine], 2025; The Institute for Safe Medication Practices (ISMP), 2011).	Yes -The ISMP classifies this pediatric liquid medication as a high-alert medication due to the risk of errors in community settings, especially those that require measurement (The Institute for Safe Medication Practices (ISMP), 2011).
LASA issues from Lexi-Drugs (Lexi-Drugs., 2025)	*Chlorphenamine [Chlorpheniramine](Chlorphenamine [Chlorpheniramine], 2025)* -According to Lexi-Drugs, reported LASA incidents include brand name confusion.	*HydrOXYzine* (HydrOXYzine, 2025) -The medication hydrOXYzine is at risk of being confused with hydrALAZINE, hydroCHLOROthiazide, HYDROmorphone, and hydroxyurea. Similarities in brand names may also contribute to confusion.
Listed as LASA in other safety databases		
MedMarx (Hicks et al., 2008)	Chlorpheniramine maleate-hydroxyzine hydrochloride was not listed as an LASA pair in the MedMarx database; however, MedMarx included LASA incidences of chlorpheniramine-cholestyramine (ME Category B) and chlorpheniramine-cyproheptadine (ME Categories B and C-D). These results suggest that chlorpheniramine is recurrently implicated in LASA incidences and therefore necessitate the need to be extra alert in dispensing chlorpheniramine-containing oral liquid preparations.	Not found in the list
Other reports	N/A	N/A
Conclusion	Chlorpheniramine maleate and hydroxyzine hydrochloride present a LASA risk primarily due to the similar appearance of syrup formulations, with one hospital reporting the issue and no patient-harm medication errors documented.	

Abbreviations: LASA = Look-alike, sound-alike; ISMP = The Institute for Safe Medication Practices; ACSQHC = Australian Commission on Safety and Quality in Health Care; MedMarx = The United States Pharmacopeia (USP) MedMarx Reporting System 2008; N/A: No available reports.

8. Chlorpheniramine Maleate - Guaifenesin

Table 11. Chlorpheniramine maleate (2 mg/5 mL)–Guaifenesin (100 mg/5 mL)

<table>
<tr><td></td><td colspan="8">Drug 1</td><td colspan="3">Drug 2</td></tr>
<tr><td>Generic name and strength (Chanakit et al., 2013; Supapaan et al., 2024)</td><td colspan="8">Chlorpheniramine maleate 2 mg/5 mL (CHLORPHENIRAMINE MALEATE SYRUP®)</td><td colspan="3">Guaifenesin 100 mg/5 mL (FENESIN®)</td></tr>
<tr><td>Dosage form (Thailand Food and Drug Administration, 2025) (see Figure 4)</td><td colspan="8">Oral liquids, syrup</td><td colspan="3">Oral liquids, syrup</td></tr>
<tr><td>Pharmacologic category (Lexi-Drugs., 2025)</td><td colspan="8">Alkylamine derivative; histamine H_1 antagonist; first generation (Chlorphenamine [Chlorpheniramine], 2025)</td><td colspan="3">Expectorant (GuaiFENesin, 2025)</td></tr>
<tr><td colspan="12">LASA incidents and safety alerts</td></tr>
<tr><td colspan="9">Type of LASA pairs reported</td><td colspan="3"></td></tr>
<tr><td colspan="9">Similar name (spelling/pronunciation)</td><td colspan="3">No</td></tr>
<tr><td colspan="9">Similar appearance (primary/secondary packaging)</td><td colspan="3">Yes</td></tr>
<tr><td colspan="9">Number of hospitals that reported the LASA incidents</td><td colspan="3">3</td></tr>
<tr><td>Significant level of LASA errors</td><td colspan="11">3</td></tr>
<tr><td rowspan="2">Medication error (ME) category</td><td>A</td><td>B</td><td>C</td><td>D</td><td>E</td><td>F</td><td>G</td><td>H</td><td>I</td><td>No ME report, but listed in LASA hospital records</td><td>Number of hospitals reporting the issue</td></tr>
<tr><td>-</td><td>1</td><td>-</td><td>-</td><td>-</td><td>-</td><td>-</td><td>-</td><td>-</td><td>-</td><td>1</td></tr>
<tr><td colspan="12">Suggested Tallman lettering</td></tr>
<tr><td>ISMP (The Institute for Safe Medication Practices (ISMP), 2023)</td><td colspan="8">Not found in the list</td><td colspan="3">guaiFENesin</td></tr>
<tr><td>ACSQHC 2024 (Australian Commission on Safety and Quality in Health Care (ACSQHC), 2024)</td><td colspan="8">Not found in the list</td><td colspan="3">Not found in the list</td></tr>
<tr><td>High-alert medication (HAM) status (The Institute for Safe Medication Practices (ISMP), 2011)</td><td colspan="8">Yes
-The ISMP classifies this pediatric liquid medication as a high-alert medication due to the risk of errors in community settings, especially those that require measurement (Chlorphenamine [Chlorpheniramine], 2025; The Institute for Safe Medication Practices (ISMP), 2011).</td><td colspan="3">Yes
-This medication may be considered an ISMP high-alert drug in community settings due to its formulation as a pediatric liquid that requires precise measurement (The Institute for Safe Medication Practices (ISMP), 2011).</td></tr>
<tr><td>LASA issues from Lexi-Drugs (Lexi-Drugs., 2025)</td><td colspan="8">Chlorphenamine [Chlorpheniramine](Chlorphenamine [Chlorpheniramine], 2025)
-According to Lexi-Drugs, reported LASA incidents include brand name confusion.</td><td colspan="3">GuaiFENesin (GuaiFENesin, 2025)
-According to Lexi-Drugs, reported LASA incidents include confusion between generic names, such as, guaiFENesin and guanFACINE, as well as brand name confusion.</td></tr>
<tr><td colspan="12">Listed as LASA in other safety databases</td></tr>
<tr><td>MedMarx (Hicks et al., 2008)</td><td colspan="8">-The chlorpheniramine maleate-hydroxyzine hydrochloride was not listed as an LASA pair in the MedMarx database; however, MedMarx included LASA incidences of chlorpheniramine-cholestyramine (ME Category B) and chlorpheniramine-cyproheptadine (ME Categories B and C-D).
-These results suggest that chlorpheniramine is recurrently implicated in LASA incidences and therefore necessitates the need to be extra alert in dispensing chlorpheniramine-containing oral liquid preparations.</td><td colspan="3">-Even though chlorpheniramine maleate-hydroxyzine hydrochloride was not found as a LASA pair in the MedMarx database, MedMarx records LASA events with guaifenesin-gabapentin (ME Categories B, C-D, and E-H) and guaifenesin-gatifloxacin (ME Categories B and C-D).
-These results highlight the fact that the similarities of sound-alike (similar pronunciation) names among commonly used oral drugs are still among the common causes of LASA errors, which supports the importance of drug name checking when prescribing to patients and dispensing.</td></tr>
<tr><td>Other reports</td><td colspan="8">N/A</td><td colspan="3">N/A</td></tr>
<tr><td>Conclusion</td><td colspan="11">Chlorpheniramine maleate and guaifenesin present a LASA risk primarily due to their similar appearance in oral liquid/syrup forms. One medication error, classified as category B, has been reported, resulting in a significance level of 3 for this drug pair.</td></tr>
<tr><td colspan="12">Abbreviations: LASA = Look-alike, sound-alike; ISMP = The Institute for Safe Medication Practices; ACSQHC = Australian Commission on Safety and Quality in Health Care; MedMarx = The United States Pharmacopeia (USP) MedMarx Reporting System 2008; N/A: No available reports.</td></tr>
</table>

Figure 4. LASA pair monograph example for Chlorpheniramine maleate (CHLORPHENIRAMINE MALEATE SYRUP®) and Guaifenesin (FENESIN®)

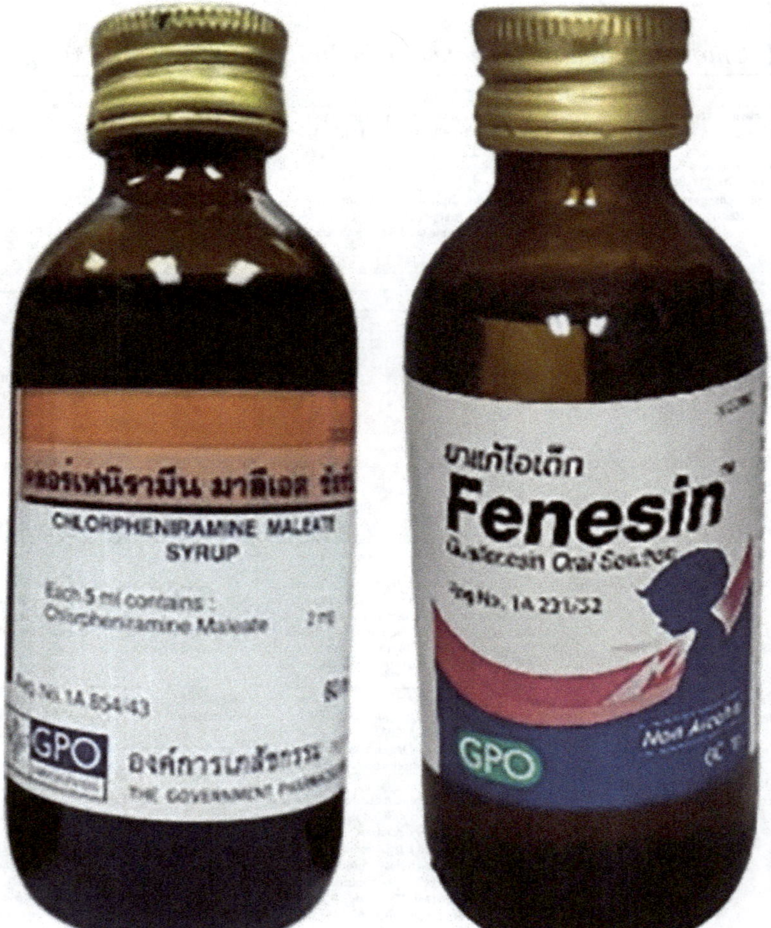

9. Dicyclomine Hydrochloride+Simethicone – Phenylephrine + Brompheniramine

Table 12. Dicyclomine hydrochloride (5 mg/5 mL) + simethicone (50 mg/5 mL) – Phenylephrine (5 mg/5 mL) + brompheniramine (2 mg/5 mL)

<table>
<tr><th></th><th colspan="8">Drug 1</th><th colspan="3">Drug 2</th></tr>
<tr><td>Generic name and strength (Chanakit et al., 2013; Supapaan et al., 2024)</td><td colspan="8">Dicyclomine hydrochloride 5 mg + simethicone 50 mg/5 mL (BERCLOMINE SYRUP®)</td><td colspan="3">Phenylephrine 5 mg + brompheniramine 2 mg/5 mL (NASOTAPP®)</td></tr>
<tr><td>Dosage form (Thailand Food and Drug Administration, 2025) (see Figure 5)</td><td colspan="8">Oral liquids, syrup</td><td colspan="3">Oral liquids, syrup</td></tr>
<tr><td>Pharmacologic category (Lexi-Drugs., 2025)</td><td colspan="8">Anticholinergic Agent; Antiflatulent (Dicycloverine [Dicyclomine] and Simeticone [Simethicone], 2025)</td><td colspan="3">Antihistamine/Decongestant Combination (Brompheniramine and Phenylephrine, 2025)</td></tr>
<tr><td colspan="12">LASA incidents and safety alerts</td></tr>
<tr><td colspan="9">Type of LASA pairs reported</td><td colspan="3"></td></tr>
<tr><td colspan="9">Similar name (spelling/pronunciation)</td><td colspan="3">N/A</td></tr>
<tr><td colspan="9">Similar appearance (primary/secondary packaging)</td><td colspan="3">Yes</td></tr>
<tr><td colspan="9">Number of hospitals that reported the LASA incidents</td><td colspan="3">1</td></tr>
<tr><td>Significant level of LASA errors</td><td colspan="11">3</td></tr>
<tr><td rowspan="2">Medication error (ME) category</td><td>A</td><td>B</td><td>C</td><td>D</td><td>E</td><td>F</td><td>G</td><td>H</td><td>I</td><td>No ME report, but listed in LASA hospital records</td><td>Number of hospitals reporting the issue</td></tr>
<tr><td>-</td><td>1</td><td>1</td><td>-</td><td>-</td><td>-</td><td>-</td><td>-</td><td>-</td><td>-</td><td>2</td></tr>
<tr><td colspan="12">Suggested Tallman lettering</td></tr>
<tr><td>(The Institute for Safe Medication Practices (ISMP), 2023)</td><td colspan="8">Not found in the list</td><td colspan="3">Not found in the list</td></tr>
<tr><td>(Australian Commission on Safety and Quality in Health Care (ACSQHC), 2024)</td><td colspan="8">Not found in the list</td><td colspan="3">Not found in the list</td></tr>
<tr><td>-alert medication (HAM) status (The Institute for Safe Medication Practices (ISMP), 2011)</td><td colspan="8">-The ISMP classifies this pediatric liquid medication as a high-alert medication due to the risk of errors in community settings, especially those that require measurement (The Institute for Safe Medication Practices (ISMP), 2011).</td><td colspan="3">-The ISMP classifies this pediatric liquid medication as a high-alert medication due to the risk of errors in community settings, especially those that require measurement (Brompheniramine and Phenylephrine, 2025; The Institute for Safe Medication Practices (ISMP), 2011).</td></tr>
<tr><td>LASA issues from Lexi-Drugs (Lexi-Drugs., 2025)</td><td colspan="8">N/A</td><td colspan="3">Amoxicillin and Clavulanate(Amoxicillin and Clavulanate, 2025)
-There is potential for confusion between some brand names and amoxicillin.</td></tr>
<tr><td colspan="12">Listed as LASA in other safety databases</td></tr>
<tr><td>MedMarx (Hicks et al., 2008)</td><td colspan="8">The dicyclomine hydrochloride + simethicone-phenylephrine+ brompheniramine pair was not found as a LASA pair in the MedMarx database. Nevertheless, LASA incidents reported by MedMarx include LASA with dicyclomine -declomycin (ME Category B), dicyclomine-demeclocycline (ME Category B), dicyclomine-doxycycline (ME Categories A, B, C-D), and dicyclomine-diphenhydramine (ME Categories A, B, C-D, E-H), meaning that dicyclomine is often involved in name-based medication errors and should get a particular attention during the prescribing and dispensing process</td><td colspan="3">Not found in the list</td></tr>
<tr><td>Other reports</td><td colspan="8">N/A</td><td colspan="3">N/A</td></tr>
<tr><td>Conclusion</td><td colspan="11">The combination of dicyclomine hydrochloride with simethicone, and phenylephrine with brompheniramine, presents a LASA risk due to the similar appearance of their packaging. Two hospitals reported medication errors categorized as B and C. Both products are pediatric oral liquids that require measurement, contributing to their classification as high-alert medications by the ISMP, particularly in community settings.</td></tr>
<tr><td colspan="12">Abbreviations: LASA = Look-alike, sound-alike; ISMP = The Institute for Safe Medication Practices; ACSQHC = Australian Commission on Safety and Quality in Health Care; MedMARx = The United States Pharmacopeia (USP) MedMarx Reporting System 2008; N/A: No available reports.</td></tr>
</table>

Figure 5. LASA pair monograph example for dicyclomine hydrochloride + simethicone (BERCLOMINE SYRUP®) - phenylephrine + brompheniramine (NASOTAPP®)

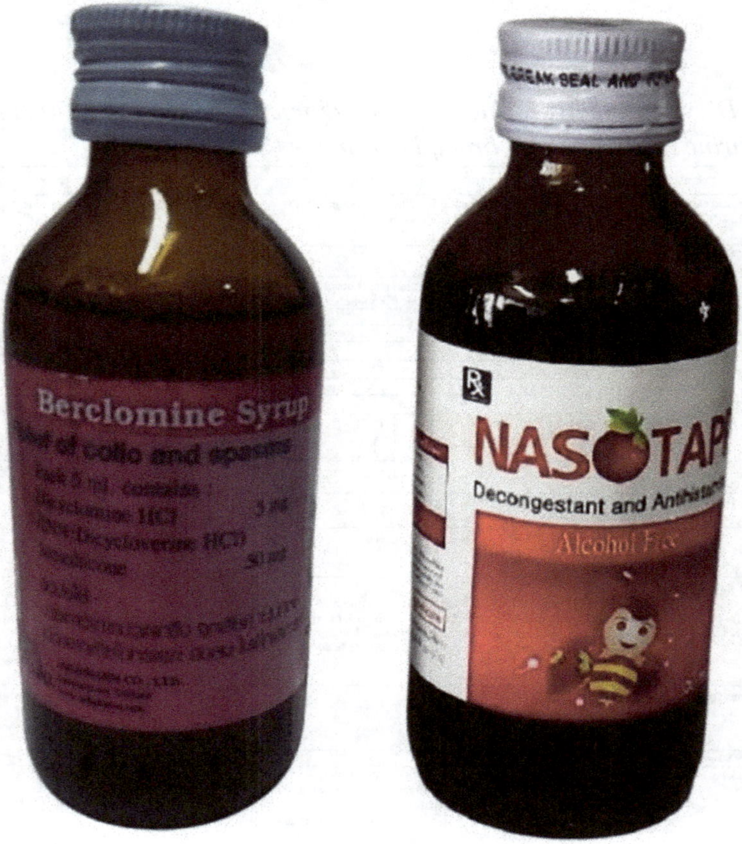

10. Domperidone – Phenylephrine + Brompheniramine

Table 13. Domperidone (5 mg/5 mL)–Phenylephrine (5 mg/5 mL)+brompheniramine (2 mg/5 mL)

<table>
<tr><th></th><th colspan="8">Drug 1</th><th colspan="3">Drug 2</th></tr>
<tr><td>Generic name and strength (Chanakit et al., 2013; Supapaan et al., 2024)</td><td colspan="8">Domperidone 5 mg/5 mL (DOMPERIDONE®)</td><td colspan="3">Phenylephrine 5 mg/5 mL + brompheniramine 2 mg/5 mL (NASOTAPP®)</td></tr>
<tr><td>Dosage form (Thailand Food and Drug Administration, 2025)</td><td colspan="8">Oral liquids, suspension</td><td colspan="3">Oral liquids, syrup</td></tr>
<tr><td>Pharmacologic category (Lexi-Drugs., 2025)</td><td colspan="8">Dopamine antagonist; gastrointestinal agent, prokinetic (Domperidone, 2025)</td><td colspan="3">Antihistamine/decongestant combination (Brompheniramine and Phenylephrine, 2025)</td></tr>
<tr><td colspan="12">LASA incidents and safety alerts</td></tr>
<tr><td colspan="9">Type of LASA pairs reported</td><td colspan="3"></td></tr>
<tr><td colspan="9">Similar name (spelling/pronunciation)</td><td colspan="3">Yes</td></tr>
<tr><td colspan="9">Similar appearance (primary/secondary packaging)</td><td colspan="3">N/A</td></tr>
<tr><td colspan="9">Number of hospitals that reported the LASA incidents</td><td colspan="3">1</td></tr>
<tr><td>Significant level of LASA errors</td><td colspan="11">3</td></tr>
<tr><td rowspan="2">Medication error (ME) category</td><td>A</td><td>B</td><td>C</td><td>D</td><td>E</td><td>F</td><td>G</td><td>H</td><td>I</td><td>No ME report, but listed in LASA hospital records</td><td>Number of hospitals reporting the issue</td></tr>
<tr><td>-</td><td>1</td><td>1</td><td>-</td><td>-</td><td>-</td><td>-</td><td>-</td><td>-</td><td>-</td><td>2</td></tr>
<tr><td colspan="12">Suggested Tallman lettering</td></tr>
<tr><td>ISMP (The Institute for Safe Medication Practices (ISMP), 2023)</td><td colspan="8">Not found in the list</td><td colspan="3">Not found in the list</td></tr>
<tr><td>ACSQHC 2024 (Australian Commission on Safety and Quality in Health Care (ACSQHC), 2024)</td><td colspan="8">Not found in the list</td><td colspan="3">Not found in the list</td></tr>
<tr><td>High-alert medication (HAM) status (The Institute for Safe Medication Practices (ISMP), 2011)</td><td colspan="8">Yes
-The ISMP classifies this pediatric liquid medication as a high-alert medication due to the risk of errors in community settings, especially those that require measurement (The Institute for Safe Medication Practices (ISMP), 2011).</td><td colspan="3">Yes
-The ISMP classifies this pediatric liquid medication as a high-alert medication due to the risk of errors in community settings, especially those that require measurement (The Institute for Safe Medication Practices (ISMP), 2011).</td></tr>
<tr><td>LASA issues from Lexi-Drugs (Lexi-Drugs., 2025)</td><td colspan="8">Domperidone (Domperidone, 2025)
-Iloperidone and paliperidone are sometimes mistaken for domperidone.</td><td colspan="3">N/A</td></tr>
<tr><td colspan="12">Listed as LASA in other safety databases</td></tr>
<tr><td>MedMarx (Hicks et al., 2008)</td><td colspan="8">Not found in the list</td><td colspan="3">Not found in the list</td></tr>
<tr><td>Other reports</td><td colspan="8">N/A</td><td colspan="3">N/A</td></tr>
<tr><td>Conclusion</td><td colspan="11">Domperidone and phenylephrine with brompheniramine present a LASA risk due to the similarity in their names (spelling/pronunciation, e.g., dom-brom). Both products are pediatric oral liquids that require measurement, contributing to their classification as high-alert medications by the ISMP, particularly in community settings.</td></tr>
<tr><td colspan="12">Abbreviations: LASA = Look-alike, sound-alike; ISMP = The Institute for Safe Medication Practices; ACSQHC = Australian Commission on Safety and Quality in Health Care; MedMarx = The United States Pharmacopeia (USP) MedMarx Reporting System 2008; N/A: No available reports.</td></tr>
</table>

11. Hydroxyzine Hydrochloride – Dicyclomine Hydrochloride+Simethicone

Table 14. Hydroxyzine hydrochloride (10 mg/5 mL) – Dicyclomine hydrochloride (5 mg/5 mL) + simethicone (50 mg/5 mL)

	Drug 1	Drug 2
Generic name and strength (Chanakit et al., 2013; Supapaan et al., 2024)	Hydroxyzine hydrochloride 10 mg/5 mL (TARAXIN SYRUP®)	Dicyclomine hydrochloride 5 mg/5 mL + simethicone 50 mg/5 mL (BERCLOMINE SYRUP®)
Dosage form (Thailand Food and Drug Administration, 2025)	Oral liquids, syrup	Oral liquids, syrup
Pharmacologic category (Lexi-Drugs., 2025)	Antianxiety agent; antiemetic; antihistamine; sedative (HydrOXYzine, 2025)	Anticholinergic agent; antiflatulent (Dicycloverine [Dicyclomine] and Simeticone [Simethicone], 2025)
LASA incidents and safety alerts		
Type of LASA pairs reported		
Similar name (spelling/pronunciation)		N/A
Similar appearance (primary/secondary packaging)		Yes
Number of hospitals that reported the LASA incidents		1
Significant level of LASA errors	3	

Medication error (ME) category	A	B	C	D	E	F	G	H	I	No ME report, but listed in LASA hospital records	Number of hospitals reporting the issue
	-	1	1	-	-	-	-	-	-	-	2

	Drug 1	Drug 2
Suggested Tallman lettering		
ISMP(The Institute for Safe Medication Practices (ISMP), 2023)	hydrOXYzine	Not found in the list
ACSQHC 2024(Australian Commission on Safety and Quality in Health Care (ACSQHC), 2024)	Not found in the list	Not found in the list
High-alert medication (HAM) status (The Institute for Safe Medication Practices (ISMP), 2011)	-The ISMP classifies this pediatric liquid medication as a high-alert medication due to the risk of errors in community settings, especially those that require measurement (The Institute for Safe Medication Practices (ISMP), 2011).	-The ISMP classifies this pediatric liquid medication as a high-alert medication due to the risk of errors in community settings, especially those that require measurement (The Institute for Safe Medication Practices (ISMP), 2011).
LASA issues from Lexi-Drugs (Lexi-Drugs., 2025)	*Hydroxyzine* (HydrOXYzine, 2025) -The medication hydrOXYzine is at risk of being confused with hydrALAZINE, hydroCHLOROthiazide, HYDROmorphone, and hydroxyurea. Similarities in brand names may also contribute to confusion.	N/A
Listed as LASA in other safety databases		
MedMarx (Hicks et al., 2008)	The hydroxyzine-dicyclomine pair in the MedMarx database was not found as a LASA pair, but there are various LASA incidents in which hydroxyzine-containing products are involved. Particularly, hydroxyzine hydrochloride has been mixed up with meclizine and hydrocortisone sodium succinate (ME Categories B and C-D), hydroxyzine pamoate with hydrocortisone sodium succinate (ME Categories B and C-D), and hydroxyzine and hydralazine (ME Category C-D). These results demonstrate that hydroxyzine preparations are always potentially confounded with other drugs containing a word in their name, and it is necessary to verify drug names closely during prescriptions and dispensing.	The dicyclomine hydrochloride + simethicone-phenylephrine+ brompheniramine pair was not found as a LASA pair in the MedMarx database. Nevertheless, LASA incidents reported by MedMarx include LASA with Declomycin-Declomycin (ME Category B), dicyclomine-demeclocycline (ME Category B), dicyclomine-doxycycline (ME Categories A, B, C-D), and dicyclomine-diphenhydramine (ME Categories A, B, C-D, E-H), meaning that dicyclomine is often involved in name-based medication errors and should get a particular attention during the prescribing and dispensing process
Other reports	N/A	N/A
Conclusion	The combination of dicyclomine hydrochloride with simethicone and phenylephrine with brompheniramine presents a LASA risk due to the similar appearance of their packaging. Two hospitals reported medication errors categorized as A and B. Both products are pediatric oral liquids that require measurement, contributing to their classification as high-alert medications by the ISMP, particularly in community settings.	

Abbreviations: LASA = Look-alike, sound-alike; ISMP = The Institute for Safe Medication Practices; ACSQHC = Australian Commission on Safety and Quality in Health Care; MedMARx = The United States Pharmacopeia (USP) MedMarx Reporting System 2008; N/A: No available reports.

12. HYOSCINE BUTYLBROMIDE – DOMPERIDONE

Table 15. Hyoscine butylbromide (5 mg/5 mL) - Domperidone (5 mg/5 mL)

<table>
<tr><th></th><th colspan="8">Drug 1</th><th colspan="3">Drug 2</th></tr>
<tr><td>Generic name and strength (Chanakit et al., 2013; Supapaan et al., 2024)</td><td colspan="8">Hyoscine butylbromide 5 mg/5 mL (HYOSCINE STAR SYRUP®)</td><td colspan="3">Domperidone 5 mg/5 mL (MORIDON SUSPENSION®)</td></tr>
<tr><td>Dosage form (Thailand Food and Drug Administration, 2025) (see Figure 6)</td><td colspan="8">Oral liquids, syrup</td><td colspan="3">Oral liquids, suspension</td></tr>
<tr><td>Pharmacologic category (Lexi-Drugs., 2025)</td><td colspan="8">Anticholinergic agent (Scopolamine (hyoscine), 2026)</td><td colspan="3">Dopamine antagonist; gastrointestinal agent, prokinetic (Domperidone, 2025)</td></tr>
<tr><td colspan="12">LASA incidents and safety alerts</td></tr>
<tr><td colspan="9">Type of LASA pairs reported</td><td colspan="3"></td></tr>
<tr><td colspan="9">Similar name (spelling/pronunciation)</td><td colspan="3">Yes</td></tr>
<tr><td colspan="9">Similar appearance (primary/secondary packaging)</td><td colspan="3">N/A</td></tr>
<tr><td colspan="9">Number of hospitals that reported the LASA incidents</td><td colspan="3">1</td></tr>
<tr><td>Significant level of LASA errors</td><td colspan="11">3</td></tr>
<tr><td rowspan="2">Medication error (ME) category</td><td>A</td><td>B</td><td>C</td><td>D</td><td>E</td><td>F</td><td>G</td><td>H</td><td>I</td><td>No ME report, but listed in LASA hospital records</td><td>Number of hospitals reporting the issue</td></tr>
<tr><td>-</td><td>1</td><td>-</td><td>-</td><td>-</td><td>-</td><td>-</td><td>-</td><td>-</td><td>-</td><td>1</td></tr>
<tr><td colspan="12">Suggested Tallman lettering</td></tr>
<tr><td>ISMP (The Institute for Safe Medication Practices (ISMP), 2023)</td><td colspan="8">Not found in the list</td><td colspan="3">Not found in the list</td></tr>
<tr><td>ACSQHC 2024 (Australian Commission on Safety and Quality in Health Care (ACSQHC), 2024)</td><td colspan="8">Not found in the list</td><td colspan="3">Not found in the list</td></tr>
<tr><td>High-alert medication (HAM) status (The Institute for Safe Medication Practices (ISMP), 2011)</td><td colspan="8">Not found in the list</td><td colspan="3">Yes
-The ISMP classifies this pediatric liquid medication as a high-alert medication due to the risk of errors in community settings, especially those that require measurement (The Institute for Safe Medication Practices (ISMP), 2011).</td></tr>
<tr><td>LASA issues from Lexi-Drugs (Lexi-Drugs., 2025)</td><td colspan="8">N/A</td><td colspan="3">Domperidone (Domperidone, 2025)
-Iloperidone and paliperidone are sometimes mistaken for domperidone.</td></tr>
<tr><td colspan="12">Listed as LASA in other safety databases</td></tr>
<tr><td>MedMarx (Hicks et al., 2008)</td><td colspan="8">Not found in the list</td><td colspan="3">Not found in the list</td></tr>
<tr><td>Other reports</td><td colspan="8">N/A</td><td colspan="3">N/A</td></tr>
<tr><td>Conclusion</td><td colspan="11">Hyoscine butylbromide and domperidone show a LASA risk because they are similarly pronounced and because they can be used as pediatric oral liquids, with a single hospital reporting the problem and an ME Category B classification. It is important to prescribe domperidone by clear indication and closely dispense it, especially due to the high alert nature of the substance in liquid formulations of domperidone among the pediatric population.</td></tr>
<tr><td colspan="12">Abbreviations: LASA = Look-alike, sound-alike; ISMP = The Institute for Safe Medication Practices; ACSQHC = Australian Commission on Safety and Quality in Health Care; MedMarx = The United States Pharmacopeia (USP) MedMarx Reporting System 2008; N/A: No available reports.</td></tr>
</table>

Figure 6. LASA pair monograph example for hyoscine butylbromide (HYOSCINE STAR SYRUP®)- domperidone (MORIDON SUSPENSION®)

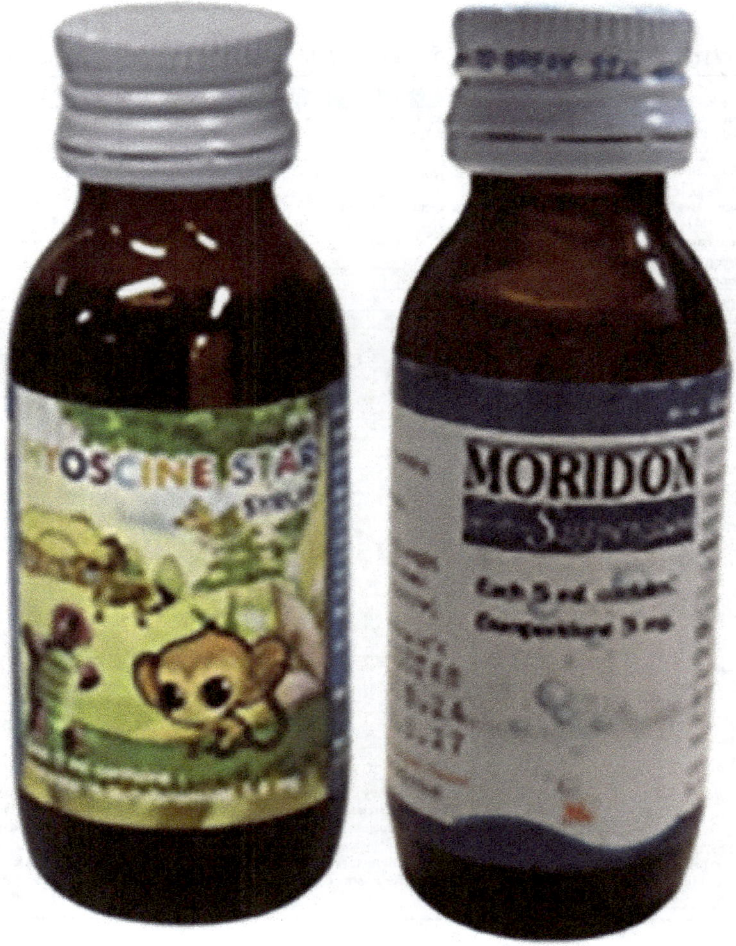

13. Ibuprofen – Sulfamethoxazole/Trimethoprim

Table 16. Ibuprofen (100 mg/5 mL) – Sulfamethoxazole (200 mg/5 mL) + trimethoprim (40 mg/5 mL)

<table>
<tr><th></th><th colspan="10">Drug 1</th><th colspan="2">Drug 2</th></tr>
<tr><td>Generic name and strength (Chanakit et al., 2013; Supapaan et al., 2024)</td><td colspan="10">Ibuprofen 100 mg/5 mL (BUNOFEN®)</td><td colspan="2">Sulfamethoxazole 200 mg/5 ml + trimethoprim 40 mg/5 mL (SULTRIM ORAL SUSPENSION®)</td></tr>
<tr><td>Dosage form (Thailand Food and Drug Administration, 2025)</td><td colspan="10">Oral liquids, suspension</td><td colspan="2">Oral liquids, suspension</td></tr>
<tr><td>Pharmacologic category (Lexi-Drugs., 2025)</td><td colspan="10">Analgesic, nonopioid; nonsteroidal anti-inflammatory drug (NSAID) (Ibuprofen, 2025)</td><td colspan="2">Antibiotic, miscellaneous; antibiotic, sulfonamide derivative (Co-Trimoxazole [Sulfamethoxazole and Trimethoprim], 2025)</td></tr>
<tr><td colspan="13">LASA incidents and safety alerts</td></tr>
<tr><td colspan="11">Type of LASA pairs reported</td><td colspan="2"></td></tr>
<tr><td colspan="11">Similar name (spelling/pronunciation)</td><td colspan="2">N/A</td></tr>
<tr><td colspan="11">Similar appearance (primary/secondary packaging)</td><td colspan="2">Yes</td></tr>
<tr><td colspan="11">Number of hospitals that reported the LASA incidents</td><td colspan="2">1</td></tr>
<tr><td>Significant level of LASA errors</td><td colspan="12">3</td></tr>
<tr><td rowspan="2">Medication error (ME) category</td><td>A</td><td>B</td><td>C</td><td>D</td><td>E</td><td>F</td><td>G</td><td>H</td><td>I</td><td colspan="2">No ME report, but listed in LASA hospital records</td><td>Number of hospitals reporting the issue</td></tr>
<tr><td>-</td><td>1</td><td>-</td><td>-</td><td>-</td><td>-</td><td>-</td><td>-</td><td>-</td><td colspan="2">-</td><td>1</td></tr>
<tr><td colspan="13">Suggested Tallman lettering</td></tr>
<tr><td>ISMP (The Institute for Safe Medication Practices (ISMP), 2023)</td><td colspan="10">Not found in the list</td><td colspan="2">Not found in the list</td></tr>
<tr><td>ACSQHC 2024 (Australian Commission on Safety and Quality in Health Care (ACSQHC), 2024)</td><td colspan="10">Not found in the list</td><td colspan="2">Not found in the list</td></tr>
<tr><td>High-alert medication (HAM) status (The Institute for Safe Medication Practices (ISMP), 2011)</td><td colspan="10">Yes
-The ISMP classifies this pediatric liquid medication as a high-alert medication due to the risk of errors in community settings, especially those that require measurement (Ibuprofen, 2025; The Institute for Safe Medication Practices (ISMP), 2011).</td><td colspan="2">Yes
-The ISMP classifies this pediatric liquid medication as a high-alert medication due to the risk of errors in community settings, especially those that require measurement (The Institute for Safe Medication Practices (ISMP), 2011).
-Sulfonamides are included on the Key Potentially Inappropriate Drugs in Pediatrics (KIDs) list and should be avoided in neonates due to the risk of kernicterus (Co-Trimoxazole [Sulfamethoxazole and Trimethoprim], 2025).</td></tr>
<tr><td>LASA issues from Lexi-Drugs (Lexi-Drugs., 2025)</td><td colspan="10">Ibuprofen (Ibuprofen, 2025)
-According to Lexi-Drugs, reported LASA incidents include brand name confusion.</td><td colspan="2">Co-Trimoxazole [Sulfamethoxazole and Trimethoprim](Co-Trimoxazole [Sulfamethoxazole and Trimethoprim], 2025)
-Co-trimoxazole may be mistaken for clotrimazole, and their brand names have also been reported as a source of confusion with other brand names.</td></tr>
<tr><td colspan="13">Listed as LASA in other safety databases</td></tr>
<tr><td>MedMarx (Hicks et al., 2008)</td><td colspan="10">Not found in the list</td><td colspan="2">Not found in the list</td></tr>
<tr><td>Other reports</td><td colspan="10">N/A</td><td colspan="2">N/A</td></tr>
<tr><td>Conclusion</td><td colspan="12">Ibuprofen and sulfamethoxazole with trimethoprim present a LASA risk primarily due to their similar appearance in oral liquid forms. Both medications are classified by ISMP as high-alert drugs in community settings due to the risks associated with pediatric liquid formulations requiring precise measurement. Additionally, sulfamethoxazole is listed on the KIDs list and should be avoided in neonates due to the risk of kernicterus.</td></tr>
<tr><td colspan="13">Abbreviations: LASA = Look-alike, sound-alike; ISMP = The Institute for Safe Medication Practices; ACSQHC = Australian Commission on Safety and Quality in Health Care; MedMarx = The United States Pharmacopeia (USP) MedMarx Reporting System 2008; N/A: No available reports.</td></tr>
</table>

14. Paracetamol – Simethicone

Table 17. Paracetamol (500 mg/5 mL) - simethicone (40 mg/0.6 mL)

<table>
<tr><td></td><td colspan="8">Drug 1</td><td colspan="3">Drug 2</td></tr>
<tr><td>Generic name and strength (Chanakit et al., 2013; Supapaan et al., 2024)</td><td colspan="8">Paracetamol 500 mg/5 mL
(SARA INFANT DROPS®)</td><td colspan="3">Simethicone 40 mg/0.6 mL
(VIN DROPS®)</td></tr>
<tr><td>Dosage form (Thailand Food and Drug Administration, 2025)</td><td colspan="8">Oral liquids, syrup</td><td colspan="3">Oral liquids, suspension</td></tr>
<tr><td>Pharmacologic category (Lexi-Drugs., 2025)</td><td colspan="8">Analgesic, nonopioid (Paracetamol [Acetaminophen], 2025)</td><td colspan="3">Antiflatulent (Simeticone [Simethicone], 2025)</td></tr>
<tr><td colspan="12">LASA incidents and safety alerts</td></tr>
<tr><td colspan="9">Type of LASA pairs reported</td><td colspan="3"></td></tr>
<tr><td colspan="9">Similar name (spelling/pronunciation)</td><td colspan="3">No</td></tr>
<tr><td colspan="9">Similar appearance (primary/secondary packaging)</td><td colspan="3">Yes</td></tr>
<tr><td colspan="9">Number of hospitals that reported the LASA incidents</td><td colspan="3">1</td></tr>
<tr><td>Significant level of LASA errors</td><td colspan="11">3</td></tr>
<tr><td rowspan="2">Medication error (ME) category</td><td>A</td><td>B</td><td>C</td><td>D</td><td>E</td><td>F</td><td>G</td><td>H</td><td>I</td><td>No ME report, but listed in LASA hospital records</td><td>Number of hospitals reporting the issue</td></tr>
<tr><td>-</td><td>1</td><td>-</td><td>-</td><td>-</td><td>-</td><td>-</td><td>-</td><td>-</td><td>-</td><td>1</td></tr>
<tr><td colspan="12">Suggested Tallman lettering</td></tr>
<tr><td>ISMP (The Institute for Safe Medication Practices (ISMP), 2023)</td><td colspan="8">Not found in the list</td><td colspan="3">Not found in the list</td></tr>
<tr><td>ACSQHC 2024 (Australian Commission on Safety and Quality in Health Care (ACSQHC), 2024)</td><td colspan="8">Not found in the list</td><td colspan="3">Not found in the list</td></tr>
<tr><td>High-alert medication (HAM) status (The Institute for Safe Medication Practices (ISMP), 2011)</td><td colspan="8">Yes
-The ISMP classifies this pediatric liquid medication as a high-alert medication due to the risk of errors in community settings, especially those that require measurement (Paracetamol [Acetaminophen], 2025; The Institute for Safe Medication Practices (ISMP), 2011).</td><td colspan="3">Yes
This medication may be considered an ISMP high-alert drug in community settings due to its formulation as a pediatric liquid that requires precise measurement (The Institute for Safe Medication Practices (ISMP), 2011).</td></tr>
<tr><td>LASA issues from Lexi-Drugs (Lexi-Drugs., 2025)</td><td colspan="8">Paracetamol [Acetaminophen](Paracetamol [Acetaminophen], 2025)
-Acetaminophen may be confused with acetazolamide. Additionally, brand names may cause confusion with other brands or generic names.</td><td colspan="3">Simeticone [Simethicone](Simeticone [Simethicone], 2025)
-Simethicone is at risk of being confused with cimetidine due to name similarity.</td></tr>
<tr><td colspan="12">Listed as LASA in other safety databases</td></tr>
<tr><td>MedMarx (Hicks et al., 2008)</td><td colspan="8">Not found in the list</td><td colspan="3">The paracetamol-simethicone combination was not listed as a LASA combination in the MedMarx database; nevertheless, MedMarx records LASA events with acetaminophen-acetazolamide and recorded Medication Error (ME) Categories B and C-D. Since paracetamol is acetaminophen in the United States, these data points to the possibility of name confusion relating to the presence of paracetamol/acetaminophen, meaning that drug names must be carefully checked when prescribing and dispensing.</td></tr>
<tr><td>Other reports</td><td colspan="8">N/A</td><td colspan="3">N/A</td></tr>
<tr><td>Conclusion</td><td colspan="11">Paracetamol 500 mg/5 mL (drops) and simethicone 40 mg/0.6 mL (drops) present a LASA risk due to their similar appearance, with one reported hospital medication error. A significance level of 3 has been assigned to this drug pair due to a reported medication error classified as Category B.</td></tr>
<tr><td colspan="12">Abbreviations: LASA = Look-alike, sound-alike; ISMP = The Institute for Safe Medication Practices; ACSQHC = Australian Commission on Safety and Quality in Health Care; MedMarx = The United States Pharmacopeia (USP) MedMarx Reporting System 2008; N/A: No available reports.</td></tr>
</table>

15. Simethicone – Ferrous Fumarate

Table 18. Simethicone (40 mg/0.6 mL)–Ferrous fumarate (45 mg/0.6 mL)

<table>
<tr><td></td><td colspan="8">Drug 1</td><td colspan="3">Drug 2</td></tr>
<tr><td>Generic name and strength
(Bueng Kan Hospital, 2021; Chanakit et al., 2013; Supapaan et al., 2024)</td><td colspan="8">Simethicone 40 mg/0.6 mL
(GAS - MED SUSPENSION®)</td><td colspan="3">Ferrous fumarate 45 mg/0.6 mL
(FERDEK DROPS®)</td></tr>
<tr><td>Dosage form (Thailand Food and Drug Administration, 2025) (see Figure 7)</td><td colspan="8">Oral liquids, suspension</td><td colspan="3">Oral liquids, syrup</td></tr>
<tr><td>Pharmacologic category
(Lexi-Drugs., 2025)</td><td colspan="8">Antiflatulent (Simeticone [Simethicone], 2025)</td><td colspan="3">Iron preparations (Ferrous Fumarate, 2025)</td></tr>
<tr><td colspan="12">LASA incidents and safety alerts</td></tr>
<tr><td colspan="9">Type of LASA pairs reported</td><td colspan="3"></td></tr>
<tr><td colspan="9">Similar name (spelling/pronunciation)</td><td colspan="3">Yes</td></tr>
<tr><td colspan="9">Similar appearance (primary/secondary packaging)</td><td colspan="3">Yes</td></tr>
<tr><td colspan="9">Number of hospitals that reported the LASA incidents</td><td colspan="3">2</td></tr>
<tr><td>Significant level of LASA errors</td><td colspan="11">3</td></tr>
<tr><td rowspan="2">Medication error (ME) category</td><td>A</td><td>B</td><td>C</td><td>D</td><td>E</td><td>F</td><td>G</td><td>H</td><td>I</td><td>No ME report, but listed in LASA hospital records</td><td>Number of hospitals reporting the issue</td></tr>
<tr><td>-</td><td>1</td><td>-</td><td>-</td><td>-</td><td>-</td><td>-</td><td>-</td><td>-</td><td>-</td><td>1</td></tr>
<tr><td colspan="12">Suggested Tallman lettering</td></tr>
<tr><td>ISMP(The Institute for Safe Medication Practices (ISMP), 2023)</td><td colspan="8">Not found in the list</td><td colspan="3">Not found in the list</td></tr>
<tr><td>ACSQHC 2024(Australian Commission on Safety and Quality in Health Care (ACSQHC), 2024)</td><td colspan="8">Not found in the list</td><td colspan="3">Not found in the list</td></tr>
<tr><td>High-alert medication (HAM) status
(The Institute for Safe Medication Practices (ISMP), 2011)</td><td colspan="8">Yes
-The ISMP classifies this pediatric liquid medication as a high-alert medication due to the risk of errors in community settings, especially those that require measurement (The Institute for Safe Medication Practices (ISMP), 2011).</td><td colspan="3">Yes
-The ISMP classifies this pediatric liquid medication as a high-alert medication due to the risk of errors in community settings, especially those that require measurement (The Institute for Safe Medication Practices (ISMP), 2011).</td></tr>
<tr><td>LASA issues from Lexi-Drugs
(Lexi-Drugs., 2025)</td><td colspan="8">Simeticone [Simethicone] (Simeticone [Simethicone], 2025)
-Simethicone is at risk of being confused with cimetidine due to name similarity.</td><td colspan="3">N/A(Ferrous Fumarate, 2025)</td></tr>
<tr><td colspan="12">Listed as LASA in other safety databases</td></tr>
<tr><td>MedMarx (Hicks et al., 2008)</td><td colspan="8">Not found in the list</td><td colspan="3">Not found in the list</td></tr>
<tr><td>Other reports</td><td colspan="8">N/A</td><td colspan="3">N/A</td></tr>
<tr><td>Conclusion</td><td colspan="11">-Simethicone drops and ferrous fumarate drops present a LASA risk due to similar names and packaging in oral liquid form. Two hospitals have reported LASA incidents involving this pair, including one medication error classified as Category B.</td></tr>
<tr><td colspan="12">Abbreviations: LASA = Look-alike, sound-alike; ISMP = The Institute for Safe Medication Practices; ACSQHC = Australian Commission on Safety and Quality in Health Care; MedMarx = The United States Pharmacopeia (USP) MedMarx Reporting System 2008; N/A: No available reports.</td></tr>
</table>

Figure 7. LASA pair monograph example for simethicone (GAS - MED SUSPENSION®)-ferrous fumarate (FERDEK DROPS®)

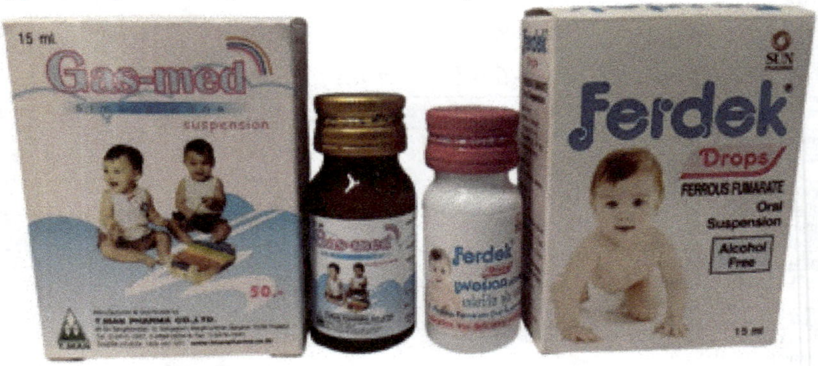

CONCLUSION

This chapter outlines the first ever recorded systematic monograph of LASA drug pairs in liquid form in Thai hospitals, and the national survey data were integrated into internationally recognized medication safety models. The findings suggest that the similarities in terms of the appearance and concentrations of variables in oral liquid preparations and high-alert medication properties are the most common causes of LASA risks of these two variables, particularly in pediatric and community settings. There is no national system of LASA reporting, so this monograph offers a valid tool that hospitals may implement to identify, prioritize, and respond to the risks associated with LASA. Future research should focus on incorporating national data, harmonizing labeling standards, and improving human factor-informed interventions to reduce the harm that can be avoided with LASA medications in Thailand.

REFERENCES

Aluminium [Aluminum] Hydroxide, M. H., and Simeticone [Simethicone], (2025). *Lexi-Drugs Multinational. UpToDate Lexidrug. UpToDate Inc.* Retrieved 19 March from https://online.lexi.com

Ambroxol. (2025). *Lexi-Drugs Multinational. UpToDate Lexidrug. UpToDate Inc.* Retrieved 19 March from https://online.lexi.com

Amoxicillin. (2025). *Lexi-Drugs Multinational. UpToDate Lexidrug. UpToDate Inc.* Retrieved 23 May from https://online.lexi.com

Amoxicillin and Clavulanate. (2025). *Lexi-Drugs Multinational. UpToDate Lexidrug. UpToDate Inc.* Retrieved 19 March from https://online.lexi.com

Australian Commission on Safety and Quality in Health Care (ACSQHC). (2024). *National mixed-case lettering list.* ACSQHC. Retrieved 18 March from https://www.safetyandquality.gov.au/sites/default/files/2024-04/national_mixed-case_lettering_list.pdf

Brompheniramine and Phenylephrine. (2025). *Lexi-Drugs Multinational. UpToDate Lexidrug. UpToDate Inc.* Retrieved 19 March from https://online.lexi.com

Bueng Kan Hospital. (2021). *Look Alike Sound Alike Drug*. Retrieved 17 Jan from https://bkh.moph.go.th/bkhweb/uploads/media/202303310725123_4.LASA_update-_2566.pdf#page=6.00

Cefaclor. (2025). *Lexi-Drugs Multinational. UpToDate Lexidrug. UpToDate Inc.* Retrieved 19 March from https://online.lexi.com

Cefixime. (2026). *Lexi-Drugs Multinational. UpToDate Lexidrug. UpToDate Inc.* Retrieved 25 Jan from https://online.lexi.com

Cetirizine (systemic). (2026). *Lexi-Drugs Multinational. UpToDate Lexidrug. UpToDate Inc.* Retrieved 25 Jan from https://online.lexi.com

Chanakit, T., Napaporn, J., Chiempattanakajohn, T., Sangkhawan, S., & Wichakot, S. (2013). The survey of look alike/sound alike (LASA) drugs available in hospitals in Thailand. *African Journal of Pharmacy and Pharmacology*, *7*(6), 227–239. DOI: 10.5897/AJPP11.812

Chlorphenamine [Chlorpheniramine]. (2025). *Lexi-Drugs Multinational. UpToDate Lexidrug. UpToDate Inc.* Retrieved 19 March from https://online.lexi.com

Co-Trimoxazole [Sulfamethoxazole and Trimethoprim]. (2025). *Lexi-Drugs Multinational. UpToDate Lexidrug. UpToDate Inc*. Retrieved 19 March from https://online.lexi.com

Dicycloverine [Dicyclomine] and Simeticone [Simethicone]. (2025). *Lexi-Drugs Multinational. UpToDate Lexidrug. UpToDate Inc*. Retrieved 19 March from https://online.lexi.com

Diphenhydramine, A. C., and Sodium Citrate, (2025). *Lexi-Drugs Multinational. UpToDate Lexidrug. UpToDate Inc*. Retrieved 19 March from https://online.lexi.com

Domperidone. (2025). *Lexi-Drugs Multinational. UpToDate Lexidrug. UpToDate Inc*. Retrieved 19 March from https://online.lexi.com

Ferrous Fumarate. (2025). *Lexi-Drugs Multinational. UpToDate Lexidrug. UpToDate Inc*. Retrieved 19 March from https://online.lexi.com

GuaiFENesin. (2025). *Lexi-Drugs Multinational. UpToDate Lexidrug. UpToDate Inc*. Retrieved 19 March from https://online.lexi.com

Hicks, R., Becker, S., & Cousins, D. (2008). *MEDMARX data report. A report on the relationship of drug names and medication errors in response to the institute of Medicine's call for action*. Center for the Advancement of Patient Safey, US Pharmacopeia.

HydrOXYzine. (2025). *Lexi-Drugs Multinational. UpToDate Lexidrug. UpToDate Inc*. Retrieved 19 March from https://online.lexi.com

Ibuprofen. (2025). *Lexi-Drugs Multinational. UpToDate Lexidrug. UpToDate Inc*. Retrieved 19 March from https://online.lexi.com

Lexi-Drugs. (2025). *UpToDate Lexidrug. UpToDate Inc*. Retrieved 19 March from https://online.lexi.com

Magnesium Hydroxide. (2025). *Lexi-Drugs Multinational. UpToDate Lexidrug. UpToDate Inc*. Retrieved 19 March from https://online.lexi.com

National Coordinating Council for Medication Error Reporting and Prevention (NCC MERP). (2022). *Types of Medication Errors*. Retrieved 11 Oct from https://www.nccmerp.org/types-medication-errors

Paracetamol [Acetaminophen]. (2025). *Lexi-Drugs Multinational. UpToDate Lexidrug. UpToDate Inc*. Retrieved 19 March from https://online.lexi.com

Scopolamine (hyoscine). (2026). *Lexi-Drugs Multinational. UpToDate Lexidrug. UpToDate Inc*. Retrieved 25 Jan from https://online.lexi.com

Simeticone [Simethicone]. (2025). *Lexi-Drugs Multinational. UpToDate Lexidrug. UpToDate Inc.* Retrieved 19 March from https://online.lexi.com

Supapaan, T. S., Napaporn, J., Ruthirakanok, R., Srichathum, S., Songmuang, A., & Pitchayajittipong, C. (2024). Look-alike sound-alike (LASA) medication errors in Thai hospitals. *Pharmacy Practice*, *22*(1), 2886.

Thailand Food and Drug Administration. (2025). Public pharmaceutical regulatory information: Details of medicinal product.

The 2023 American Geriatrics Society Beers Criteria® Update Expert Panel. (2023). American Geriatrics Society 2023 updated AGS Beers Criteria® for potentially inappropriate medication use in older adults. *Journal of the American Geriatrics Society*, *71*(7), 2052–2081. DOI: 10.1111/jgs.18372

The Institute for Safe Medication Practices (ISMP). (2011). *ISMP list of high-alert medications in community/ambulatory healthcare*. Retrieved 20 March from https://www.ismp.org/sites/default/files/attachments/2017-11/highAlert-community.pdf

The Institute for Safe Medication Practices (ISMP). (2023). *List of confused drug names*. Retrieved 16 Apr from https://www.ismp.org/recommendations/confused-drug-names-list

World Health Organization. (2023). *Medication safety for look-alike, sound-alike medicines*. World Health Organization. Retrieved 3 June from https://iris.who.int/bitstream/handle/10665/373495/9789240058897-eng.pdf?sequence=1

ABBREVIATIONS

AHRQ: Agency for Healthcare Research and Quality
ISMP: Institute for Safe Medication Practices
KIDs: Key Potentially Inappropriate Drugs in Pediatrics
LASA: Look-Alike, Sound-Alike
MedMarx: United States Pharmacopeia (USP) MedMarx Reporting System
mL: milliliter
WHO: World Health Organization

Chapter 11
Look-Alike, Sound-Alike Medication Errors in Vaccines

ABSTRACT

The case of look-alike, sound-alike (LASA) errors in vaccines is a patient safety issue of high impact that applies to immunization systems. Specific attention is given to the risks of LASA associated with vaccines, based on the evidence given by surveillance databases, epidemiological studies, and reported outbreak investigations. The similarity in the name, labeling, packaging, formulations, and storing of vaccines are explored to be the contributing factors to mistakes in wrong-vaccine choice, preparation, and administration, especially in the pediatric, neonatal, and high-throughput vaccination. There are clinical and civic health implications that include poor immunological control and serious negative outcomes and loss of confidence by the population. Prevention strategies that involve manufacturers, healthcare organizations, clinicians, and patients are combined with proven methods to help ensure safer vaccine delivery and strong immunization programs.

INTRODUCTION

Vaccination is among the greatest success stories of the contemporary world. It has saved millions of lives each year and has helped to control and exterminate many different types of viruses and bacteria (Talbird et al., 2022; Whitney et al., 2014). Nevertheless, the problem of safe vaccine administration has become more complicated because of the increasing complexity of immunization timetables, the development of disease threats that can be prevented by vaccination, and the rapid emergence of new vaccines. One such issue is the problem of Look-Alike Sound-

DOI: 10.4018/979-8-3373-5478-1.ch011

Alike (LASA) medication errors in vaccination areas, which has become a hot issue of patient safety with potentially catastrophic outcomes. LASA mistakes are made when pharmaceutical products of similar name, appearance, or package are incorrectly exchanged, with the result being the prescription of a wrong medication or vaccine formulation (Bryan et al., 2021; Emmerton & Rizk, 2012).

These mistakes may occur in several forms in the case of vaccines: they may be confused with other medication types; given an incorrect formulation, their use mixed with other vaccines and other medications or multicomponent vaccines can be confused. The outcomes of these errors include insufficient immunological protection, a need for revaccinate, more severe adverse events, and, in some rare cases, death (Alj et al., 2024; Qureshi et al., 2019). The extent of the decrease in vaccine administration is large and increasing. In the last twenty years, the number of diseases that can be prevented by vaccines has almost doubled, which is associated with the possibility of making vaccine mistakes (Condon & Hayney, 2016; Hibbs et al., 2015). Between 2000 and 2013, the United States obtained 20,585 reports of errors through the Vaccine Adverse Event Reporting System (VAERS), of which 25% of the errors were associated with adverse health events and 8% were described as serious (Hibbs et al., 2015).

The information presented in the summaries of surveillance data published by the Institute for Safe Medication Practices (ISMP) 2022–2023 Biannual Vaccine Error Reports demonstrates that most of the reported errors in medication administration remain the wrong choice of a specific vaccine, most often stipulated by the similarity of the product names, abbreviations, appearance of the vials, and packaging (Institute for Safe Medication Practices (ISMP), 2024). Importantly, most of these mistakes were passed on to the patient, indicating the low efficiency of downstream safety barriers after an incorrect vaccine is chosen. These findings are supported by peer-reviewed studies. A review of the reports to the Vaccine Adverse Event Reporting System (VAERS) in the United States revealed that the majority of errors in vaccination were related to the administration of an inappropriate product, incorrect formulation, or the wrong vaccine altogether, and the pediatric population was disproportionately affected by vaccination errors (Hibbs et al., 2015).

These systematic reviews also support that the most serious burden of immunization errors is observed among children in the underfive age group, as it is defined not only by the complexity of the pediatric schedule but also by the increased vulnerability to LASA (Barboza et al., 2020; Tavares et al., 2024). Redundant human factors and product design are important factors that contribute to LASA-related vaccine errors. Vaccines manufactured by the same manufacturer usually have similar labeling designs, color schemes, vials, and caps, which are more likely to produce confirmation bias when they are chosen. Settings such as outpatient clinics, mass immunization campaigns, and community pharmacies increase these risks because of time pressure, multitasking, and poor use of barcode verification systems (Condon & Hayney, 2016). These states are similar to traditional human-factor error pathways that are outlined in medication safety science. This situation is especially dangerous with combination and multicomponent vaccines that must be properly reconstituted before introduction. The analysis of errors reported for vaccines has demonstrated that two-component vaccines, including Pentacel®, Menveo®, and ActHIB®, are overrepresented in error databases, usually because either one component is omitted or the wrong diluent is used (Samad et al., 2021). Poor distinction of components and a lack of clear labeling have been cited as the main causes.

The COVID-19 epidemic significantly increased the fear of mistakes in the administration of vaccines. The magnitude and urgency of global vaccination campaigns, such as never before, along with the concomitant rapid introduction of several new vaccine platforms with different protocols, became conducive to higher error rates. The point prevalence of vaccine administration errors in Jordan during the COVID-19 pandemic was 2.4%, which is significantly greater than that before the pandemic (Abdel-Qader et al., 2025). This growth highlights the susceptibility of vaccination systems to pressure and the urgency of efficient error prevention measures.

Although many LASA-related vaccine errors do not cause irreversible damage, some cases are infrequent but serious enough to depict their potential clinical implications. Serious adverse events have been reported in case series of the accidental administration of high-dose or improper Bacillus Calmette-Guerin (BCG) formulations to neonates, including extensive lesions on the skin, coagulation anomalies, and intracranial hemorrhage, which require prolonged chemoprophylaxis and follow-up (Qureshi et al., 2019). These incidences highlight the medical and societal morality of LASA vaccine mistakes, especially in tuberculosis-affected areas. Notably, LASA vaccine errors need to be viewed as system failures as opposed to personal failures. The contributing factors are the practices in regulatory naming, the design of the packaging and labeling, the structure of storage, workflow pressure, and training loopholes. These weaknesses require a concerted effort to respond at the regulatory, organizational, and frontline practice levels.

Objectives of the Chapter

The aims of this chapter are as follows:

(1) To determine the prevalence of errors during vaccine administration due to LASA.
(2) To divide significant groups of LASA vaccine errors and risk mechanisms.
(3) To investigate vulnerable populations and an illustrative case study of LASA vaccine errors.

(4) To assess clinical, population health, regulation, and health system implications and prevention measures.

Organization of the Chapter

Chapter 11 starts with an overview of the epidemiology of vaccine administration errors and prevalence and then a systematic classification of the categories of LASA vaccine errors. The following sections look at the special considerations of vulnerable populations and discuss representative case studies to provide a picture of the failure pathways at the system level. Clinical outcomes and severity, pharmaceutical and regulatory sentiments, and contributors to LASA vaccine mistakes at the healthcare system level are discussed subsequently in the chapter. The last sections conclude on the influence of patient and population health and summarize evidence-based and system-based prevention measures to help mitigate safer immunization behaviors.

PREVALENCE OF VACCINE ADMINISTRATION ERRORS

Estimates of Global Prevalence

The actual rate of vaccine administration errors, especially those that are caused by LASA vulnerabilities, is conceptually difficult because of the varying structures of immunization safety surveillance systems, sensitivity, reporting requirements, and definitions of errors across countries and medical environments. Most of the existing data are passive reporting systems, which are known to considerably overestimate the true burden of medication and vaccination errors because of underreporting, fear of being blamed, inconsistent safety culture, and missing documentation. Consequently, the published prevalence estimates can be taken as indicators of low risks and not as risk measurements.

These limitations notwithstanding, systematic reviews and population-based surveillance studies are valuable for understanding the magnitude and distribution of immunization errors in relation to adverse events. Evidence synthesized by a global systematic review and meta-analysis to assess errors that led to events that were supposedly caused by vaccination has a pooled prevalence of 0.044 errors per 10,000 doses administered (95% CI: 0.026–0.075), which was based on 11 studies published between 2010 and 2021. Notably, a large degree of heterogeneity was found among the studies ($I^2 = 99\%$), which may be attributed to variations in the population, surveillance processes, and conditions of healthcare delivery. Age-stratified analysis revealed that the prevalence was significantly greater in children younger than five years (0.334 per 10,000 doses), and the lowest prevalence was among elderly people because of increased susceptibility to complex pediatric immunization schedules and contact with products (Tavares et al., 2024).

Data on national surveillance also reveal the rates of immunization errors depending on the type of vaccines and clinical setting. Surveillance of immunization errors based on the Brazilian online reporting system revealed that the total incidence of error was 4.05 per 100,000 doses of immunization, and routine vaccinations contributed 3.70 per 100,000 doses. Conversely, immunobiological serums had error rates that were a thousand times higher (547.70 per 100,000 doses), reflecting the disproportion of the risk of products not identical in terms of indication, dosing, and presentation. Among the common immunizations, the incidence rates were highest for the human rabies vaccine (24.93 per 100,000 doses), the human papillomavirus vaccine (10.12 per 100,000 doses), and the measles-mumps-rubella (triple viral) vaccine (8.74 per 100,000 doses). These findings suggest that vaccines that need special handling, age-related administration, or nonroutine administration may be especially vulnerable to LASA-related errors in selection and administration (Barboza et al., 2020).

Subnational estimates provide further indications of high levels of geographic heterogeneity in error reporting on immunization. In the Brazilian state of Minas Gerais, 3,866 notifications of immunization errors associated with 57,289,277 doses of vaccines injected between 2015 and 2019 were recorded in surveillance data. The incidence rates differed significantly across health macroregions, with the highest incidence rates in Vale do Aço (26.5 per 100,000 doses) and Triângulo do Norte (22.6 per 100,000 doses) and the lowest incidence rates in Noroeste (1.6 per 100,000 doses) and Nordeste (1.8 per 100,000 doses). It is not possible that such variation represents genuine differences in clinical competence in isolation and is much more likely to be a reflection of differences in reporting practices, safety culture maturity, and local surveillance engagement ((Donnini et al., 2022).

Together, these results highlight that the reported prevalence rates are just a small proportion of immunization errors that occur in practice. With respect to medication safety LASA, the interplay between time-sensitive schedules of complex vaccines, the lookalike phenomenon, age-related dosage, and high-volume settings of immunization predetermines the presence of a set of circumstances when selection and injection errors might take place yet will go undetected. Intensifying the standardized reporting mechanisms, encouraging nonpunitive safety cultures, and including LASA-oriented preventive measures are thus necessary to increase the quality of prevalence estimates and reduce preventable vaccine-related damage.

Impact of the COVID-19 Pandemic on Error Rates

Pandemic vaccination, in contrast to regular immunization activities, involves the concomitant management of many closely related vaccine products with a certain amount of extreme time constraints, increasing vulnerabilities to similarity of names, package similarity, conventions of labeling, and storage propinquity. Both national safety surveillance and direct observational research evidence indicate that the factors related to LASA dominated with respect to vaccine errors during the COVID-19 era.

As 1,987 reports of vaccine errors submitted to the ISMP National Vaccine Errors Reporting Program (VERP) (2022) demonstrate, there was an overrepresentation of COVID-19 vaccines among reported vaccine errors, with 44.3% (n=880) of all reported errors (2022–2023). This disproportion cannot be explained only by a certain level of vaccination but is due to the complexity of the COVID-19 vaccine portfolio, which involves the participation of several manufacturers, formulations, age-specific routes, and changing booster requirements (Institute for Safe Medication Practices (ISMP), 2024).

Wrong-vaccine errors, the most common category of errors, were also particularly salient when LASA mechanisms were used (25.2%, n = 501). Among these wrong-vaccine reports, 79.6% (n = 399) were specifically associated with the resemblances between the names of the vaccines, abbreviations, labeling, packaging, or storage conditions. The most prevalent products in this LASA-associated subset were COVID-19 vaccines (Institute for Safe Medication Practices (ISMP), 2024).

Confusion between monovalent and bivalent COVID-19 preparations and between pediatric and adult presentations, which differed only slightly in terms of labeling or cap color, are examples documented by the ISMP. The increase in these LASA weaknesses also increased when the products were placed near each other when there was a high-volume clinic and when visual discrimination became less effective in times of stress.

The similarities in terms of LASA were also crucial factors in the errors of the expired vaccine and age of administration during the pandemic. The proportion of errors related to expired vaccines included 19.8% (n = 393) of the Institute for Safe Medication Practices National Vaccine Errors Reporting Program (ISMP VERP) reports and 71.0% (n = 279) of the reports concerning COVID-19 vaccines. Most of these occurred as a result of mixing the manufacturer's expiration dates and beyond-use dates, which were exacerbated by the presence of visually similar vials with dissimilar stability regulations (Institute for Safe Medication Practices (ISMP), 2024).

Similarly, the error associated with age was the greatest, with 9.8% (n = 194) of all the reports in which COVID-19 vaccines were included in 34.5% (n = 67) of the cases. These errors were common because of look-alike labeling in age-dependent formulations, with pediatric and adult products having a common brand, similar sizes of the vial, and almost identical label designs. The accelerated change in the age eligibility criteria during the course of the pandemic enhanced the dependency on partial visual cues, which is a risk factor for LASA (Institute for Safe Medication Practices (ISMP), 2024).

Independent evidence of the LASA signal in surveillance data is provided by findings from a prospective covert observational study carried out during the COVID-19 mass vaccination campaign in Jordan. Among the 8,743 doses administered, 209 vaccine administration errors were discovered, with a point prevalence of 2.4. Notably, 20.1% (42/209) of the individual mistakes seen were related to incorrect vaccination products, which in itself is related to LASA mechanisms (Abdel-Qader et al., 2025).

The results also revealed that the occurrence of error was significantly linked to peak hours of vaccination, which is a proxy of workload intensity (adjusted odds ratio 2.18; 95% CI 1.58–3.86; $p = 0.002$). In such circumstances, health workers were more inclined to use quick eye-to-cone recognition at the expense of a thorough check, thus exposing themselves to LASA-induced confusion (Abdel-Qader et al., 2025).

Contributing-factors analysis indicated that the most frequent experience of committed errors belonged to the category of factors related to healthcare providers (54.9%), with heavy workload (16.1%), distractions (12.0%), and knowledge gaps (14.8%). These conditions are known to be synergistic with LASA risks, particularly in operations involving the handling of several similar products simultaneously (Abdel-Qader et al., 2025).

Taken together, these results indicate that the COVID-19 pandemic not only increased the number of administered vaccines but also radically changed the error space by exacerbating LASA weaknesses. Concurrent overlap of different similar COVID-19 vaccine products, constant updates in instructions, and high-throughput delivery conditions decreased the trustworthiness of customary human-based security, such as label reading and memory verification. The convergence of national surveillance data and first-hand observation data supports the idea that LASA systems played a crucial role, rather than a secondary role, in pandemic-era vaccine mistakes. This has dire consequences for future pandemic preparedness with upstream interventions that focus on LASA, such as better distinction of names and labeling of vaccines and physical separation of similar products and the decision support provided by a system that depends less on visual discrimination (Abdel-Qader et al., 2025; Institute for Safe Medication Practices (ISMP), 2024).

United States Surveillance Data

Vaccines represent a unique and high-risk subset of injectable LASA medication errors, as immunization programs tend to have many products with overlapping antigens, age-specific indications, combination products, and similar naming/labeling conventions, all of which are carried out in high-throughput outpatient practice workflows. In national surveillance from the U.S., Hibbs and colleagues used VAERS reports (2000–2013) and reported 20,585 vaccination errors, with 21,843 individual errors. An inappropriate schedule was the most frequent error group (27%), followed by storage and dispensing errors (23%), which included expired vaccines (n=2,746). Wrong vaccines accounted for 3,372 errors (15%) and included classic errors between vaccines with similar antigens, such as varicella vs herpes zoster, DTaP vs Tdap, and pneumococcal conjugates vs pneumococcal polysaccharide vaccines. Importantly, 25% of the error reports (n=5,204) contained an adverse health event; 92% of these were judged as nonserious, and therefore, only a small minority of the error reports associated with an adverse health event were judged as serious (Hibbs et al., 2015).

The up-to-date surveillance metrics from the ISMP National Vaccine Errors Reporting Program (ISMP VERP) provide extensive knowledge about the epidemiology and etiology of wrong-vaccine errors in real-life clinical practice. An examination of 1,987 reports of vaccine errors submitted to the ISMP VERP from 2022–2023 revealed that incorrect vaccine selection accounted for 25.2% of all reported errors and was the most frequently reported error type. Among these erroneous vaccine mistakes, packaging, name, abbreviation, and storage contributed to 79.6% of all errors, indicating that LASA factors constitute the most prevalent error in wrong-vaccine administration (ISMP 2022). The list of the factors related to incorrect vaccine errors provides a clear pattern: similar labels on the vaccine containers or packaging were involved in 22.2% of incorrect vaccine errors, similar brand names were involved in 21.8% of errors, and the products placed near one another played a role in 20.6% of mistakes (**Table 1**).

Among all the reports of vaccine errors reported to the ISMP National Vaccine Errors Reporting Program (VERP) from 2022–2023 (n = 1,987), wrong-vaccine selection was the most common type of report (25.2% of all the reports, n = 501). The results of the analysis of Appendix C indicated that three main contributing factors prevailed in this category: similar vaccine container labels or packaging (22.2, n = 111), similar brand names (21.8, n = 109), and products that are nearby each other (20.6, n = 103). Notably, COVID-19 mRNA vaccines (COV-mRNAs) were involved in all three contributing factors, which included 55.9% (n = 62) of the mistakes that involved similar container labeling, 60.6% (n = 66) of the mistakes involving similar brand names, and 24.3% (n = 25) of the incidences of proximal storage. Other frequently used vaccines also included measles-mumps-rubella-varicella (MMRV) in terms of similarities in container labels (7.2, n = 8) and hepatitis B vaccine (HepB) in terms of similarities in brand names (5.5, n = 6) and storage locations (10.7, n = 11). These results highlight the fact that the mistakes associated with incorrect vaccines are fueled more by visual and organizational factors than by just individual cognitive failures and that COVID-19 vaccines account for a disproportionate portion of LASA-related susceptibilities. The similarity of packaging, naming, and storage patterns leads to high-risk conditions in the area of selection errors, and upstream preventive measures for physical segregation, stronger label differentiation, and algorithm-aided LASA screening before the implementation of the products are necessary (Institute for Safe Medication Practices [ISMP], 2024).

Such data are perfectly consistent with the known mechanisms that were found using published detailed case series and cluster studies. The overwhelming proportion of the contribution factors related to storage highlights the idea that, even though packaging differentiation and naming conventions are significant factors contributing to the risk of making errors, the physical design of medication storage spaces significantly affects the likelihood of making an error (Institute for Safe Medication Practices (ISMP), 2024).

Table 1. Distribution of LASA-related contributing factors in wrong-vaccine selection events by vaccine type (%). All vaccine reports (N = 1,987)

Vaccine (n, % of all reports)	Similar brand names (%)	Similar container labels/package (%)	Similar generic names (%)	Similar vaccine abbreviations (%)	Similar packaging (%)	Total LASA error (%)	Other error (%)	% of All vaccine reports
mRNA COVID-19 (n=863, 43.4%)	7.6	7.2	2.3	1.6	0.1	18.8	81.2	43.4
IIV4 (n=95, 4.8%)	4.2	2.1	1.1	–	–	7.4	92.6	4.8
HepA (n=85, 4.3%)	1.2	2.4	2.4	2.4	–	8.4	91.6	4.3
HepB (n=83, 4.2%)	7.2	10.8	2.4	6.0	–	26.4	73.6	4.2
MMRV (n=71, 3.6%)	5.6	11.3	5.6	12.7	1.4	36.6	63.4	3.6
Tdap (n=65, 3.3%)	7.7	9.2	3.1	18.5	–	38.5	61.5	3.3
DTaP-IPV (n=60, 3.0%)	6.7	3.3	3.3	5.0	–	18.3	81.7	3.0

continued on following page

Table 1. Continued

Vaccine (n, % of all reports)	Similar brand names (%)	Similar container labels/package (%)	Similar generic names (%)	Similar vaccine abbreviations (%)	Similar packaging (%)	Total LASA error (%)	Other error (%)	% of All vaccine reports
DTaP (n=48, 2.4%)	4.2	10.4	4.2	16.7	–	35.5	64.5	2.4
MMR (n=48, 2.4%)	2.1	4.2	–	6.3	2.1	14.7	85.3	2.4
MenACWY-CRM (n=41, 2.1%)	2.4	–	2.4	4.9	7.3	17.0	83.0	2.1
RZV/Shingrix (n=40, 2.0%)	–	5.0	–	–	–	5.0	95.0	2.0
DTaP-IPV/Hib (n=37, 1.9%)	2.7	2.7	2.7	5.4	–	13.5	86.5	1.9
DTaP-HepB-IPV (n=24, 1.2%)	4.2	20.8	8.3	12.5	–	45.8	54.2	1.2
PPSV23 (n=14, 0.7%)	21.4	7.1	7.1	7.1	–	42.7	57.3	0.7
RSV vaccine (n=12, 0.6%)	8.3	8.3	16.7	16.7	–	50.0	50.0	0.6

(Institute for Safe Medication Practices (ISMP), 2024)

Note: Percentages indicate the proportion of wrong-vaccine selection reports for each vaccine type in which the specified LASA-related contributing factor was identified. Multiple factors could be selected per event. The total LASA error (%) represents the cumulative LASA contribution per vaccine. Other error (%) = 100 – Total LASA. % of All Vaccine Reports = (n/1,987) × 100.

Abbreviations: mRNA = messenger ribonucleic acid; CoV-mRNA = mRNA coronavirus disease 2019; IIV4 = quadrivalent inactivated influenza vaccine; HepA = hepatitis A vaccine; HepB = hepatitis B vaccine; MMR = measles, mumps, and rubella vaccine; MMRV = measles, mumps, rubella, and varicella vaccine; Tdap = tetanus toxoid, reduced diphtheria toxoid, and acellular pertussis vaccine; DTaP = diphtheria and tetanus toxoids and acellular pertussis vaccine; DTaP-IPV = diphtheria and tetanus toxoids and acellular pertussis vaccine and inactivated poliovirus vaccine; DTaP-IPV/Hib = diphtheria and tetanus toxoids and acellular pertussis vaccine, inactivated poliovirus vaccine, and Haemophilus influenzae type b vaccine; DTaP-HepB-IPV = diphtheria and tetanus toxoids and acellular pertussis vaccine, hepatitis B vaccine, and inactivated poliovirus vaccine; MenACWY-CRM = meningococcal serogroups A, C, W, and Y conjugate vaccine (CRM19

Beyond aggregate reporting, vaccine-related errors may accumulate in high-severity "wrong product" clusters, especially when confusion of vaccines (or vaccine-like products) with other injectables occurs in neonatal and perinatal workflows. A well-known cluster related to the accidental use of rocuronium instead of the hepatitis B vaccine in 6 newborns, a catastrophic LASA/storage/packaging-related mix-up that demonstrates how high-alert medications can enter the immunization processes when segregation and verification are poor (Alj et al., 2024).

Severe immunization errors were reported in a pediatric population that occurred because of confusion between the look-alike neonatal BCG vaccine and intravesical

ONCO-BCG, a high-potency preparation for bladder cancer therapy. In a case series from a tertiary care hospital in Karachi, 26 babies were accidentally immunized with high-dose ONCO-BCG (80-fold higher potency than standard neonatal BCG) in the standard immunization schedule. Clinically significant adverse events were observed, including local injection-site lesions in 16/26 (61.5%), coagulation derangement in 3/26 (11.5%), and intracranial hemorrhage in 1/26 (3.8%). All infants received chemoprophylaxis and supportive care without mortality or disseminated tuberculosis and achieved recovery at follow-up (Qureshi et al., 2019). A subsequent detailed case report of the same incident confirmed that the error was caused by failures in the LASA-related system, such as similar packaging and labeling, the use of pharmacy dispensing errors, and poor cross-checking before administration. The wrong formulation of BCG reached neonates (Jamil et al., 2025). Together, these reports show that errors in vaccine-related LASA can result in serious harm even when the administered product is still a "vaccine" but is not identical to the vaccine formulation, by indication or by dose, especially the need for treating vaccines—especially live attenuated products such as BCG—as high-alert injectable medications in neonatal immunization systems.

There is observational evidence during mass vaccination of the operational drivers of these events. In a prospective point prevalence study during the COVID-19 pandemic in Jordan, the percentage of vaccination errors was 2.4% (209 errors/8,743 doses), and the most common types of errors were timing/interval (33.0%), dosing (28.7%), and incorrect vaccine products (20.1%). Receiving vaccination during peak hours strongly increased the likelihood of error (aOR 2.18; 95% CI 1.58–3.86), which is quantitatively related to the relationship between vaccination throughput/ pressure and preventable error risk, which are conditions that also increase LASA vulnerability (Abdel-Qader et al., 2025).

One of the key constraints in determining the actual prevalence of vaccine administration error may be significant underreporting. It is estimated that half to two-thirds of vaccine errors are not reported annually (Shastay, 2016a). The obstacles to reporting include the fear of being punished, the absence of a clear definition of the concept of an error, and the scarcity of time and resources (Barboza et al., 2020; Donnini et al., 2022). Even though passive surveillance systems are useful, they can be underreported because they are not mandatory (Tavares et al., 2024). Such underreporting can undermine the introduction of preventive measures and can lead to the development of a false belief about the rarity of errors (Barboza et al., 2020; Donnini et al., 2022). The actual scope of LASA-specific vaccine errors is, in turn, difficult to establish; many surveillance systems fail to systematically differentiate LASA errors from other erroneous vaccine errors. However, research that has investigated contributory factors has indicated that LASA issues are substantial, with other comparable packaging, names, and abbreviations contributing to 79.6% of incorrect vaccine errors in recent ISMP VERP statistics (Institute for Safe Medication Practices (ISMP), 2024).

CATEGORIES OF LASA VACCINE ERRORS

LASA vaccine errors can also be divided into several common patterns, each of which is provoked by specific system, product, and human factors and must be prevented through a specific approach.

Vaccine-to-Vaccine Confusion

Similar Vaccine Names and Brand Confusion

The phonetic and visual resemblance of the vaccine names is known to be a major cause of LASA-related selection error, especially in high-throughput settings where clinicians depend on quick visual search or partial name matching. In the United Kingdom, Lang et al. (2014) reported that the administration of an incorrect vaccine caused 33.3% (n = 52) of all reported immunization mistakes to the Vaccine Advice for Clinicians Service. Interestingly, a quarter of these false-vaccine episodes touched on products whose names started with the same first letter as the desired vaccine; hence, the effect of initial-letter recognition on the choice of products (Lang et al., 2014).

Clusters of confusion were seen to be distinct. Five cases were used for which the initial letters were P, such as Pediacel® (TDaP/IPV/Hib), Prevenar® (PCV13), and Pneumovax® (PPV), and the results revealed that the mistakes were not limited to only vaccines against the same disease. In a dramatic case, the Pediacel® infant combination vaccine was given to a patient aged over 65 years who was given Pneumovax®. Other mistakes involved confusion of similarly named vaccines that contained tetanus, such as Repevax® (Tdap-IPV) and Revaxis® (Td-IPV), which included four reports.

The combination of meningococcal and *Haemophilus influenzae* type b (Hib) vaccines is also featured in the list of errors. Thirteen (25%) of these reports were linked to the Hib/MenC vaccine Menitorix®, accidentally injected instead of the desired vaccine, or not given when necessary. In 10 of these 13 cases, Menitorix® was mistakenly mixed with meningococcal C vaccines (Menjugate®, Meningitec®, or NeisVac®), all of which had initials of M. Another seven reports included the wrong selection of the tetanus-containing vaccine, which included all tetanus formulations that were in existence during that period (Lang et al., 2014).

These results can explain how predictable selection mistakes may occur when such common initial letters, brand prefixes, label aesthetics, and so forth are used with unrelated classes of vaccines. The same risks are reported in other facilities, where vaccines such as Pediacel®, Prevenar®, Pneumovax®, Pentacel®, and Pediarix® have been shown to cause confusion to staff, particularly when the prefixes are used near each other and when there is a time constraint (Condon & Hayney, 2016).

Wrong-vaccine mix-ups remain a common immunization error and are often associated with similar brand names, look-alike packaging, and vaccines intended for the same pediatric age group (Institute for Safe Medication Practices (ISMP), 2024). An example of a vaccine error is the mixture of Hexaxim® (DTaP–IPV–HepB–Hib) and Pentaxim® (DTaP–IPV–Hib) (Supapaan et al., 2024) (**Figure 1**). The consequences may include omission of the hepatitis B component or administration of an unintended antigen, particularly in busy vaccination clinics where multiple vaccines are prepared simultaneously.

Figure 1. Representative Hexaxim® and Pentaxim® labels depict similarities in labeling

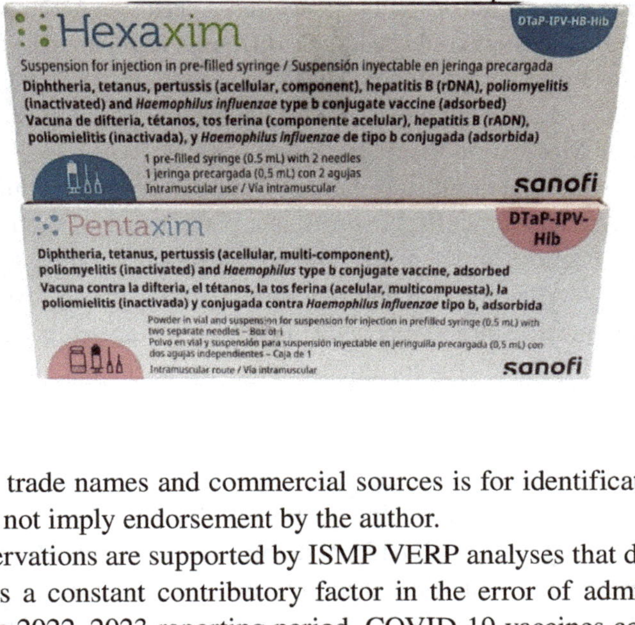

The use of trade names and commercial sources is for identification purposes only and does not imply endorsement by the author.

These observations are supported by ISMP VERP analyses that define naming conventions as a constant contributory factor in the error of administering the vaccine. In the 2022–2023 reporting period, COVID-19 vaccines contributed approximately 17.2% of naming-related events, mainly because of confusion among similar branded formulations (e.g., monovalent and bivalent boosters and pediatric formulations versus adult formulations). They often rely on the color of the vials or the appearance of the boxes instead of verifying the complete label, which is especially dangerous when a specific manufacturer uses the same branding for all of the presentations (Institute for Safe Medication Practices (ISMP), 2024).

Notably, these mistakes are not just due to individual failures; rather, they are predictable human–system interactions. Clinicians put in places where pattern recognition is favored over intelligent verification when similar-sounding vaccines are stored next to each other, when they are packaged differently, or when they are abbreviated differently across electronic systems. In turn, both the ISMP and Condon and Hayney note that effective mitigation should emphasize the upstream redesign of systems, including physical separation of similarly named vaccines, auxiliary labeling with clear signs of age, standard electronic nomenclature, and barcode verification, as opposed to staff vigilance (Condon & Hayney, 2016; Institute for Safe Medication Practices (ISMP), 2024).

Age-Dependent Formulation Errors

Another group of vaccine–vaccine confusion is especially high risk when there are age-specific formulations of the same antigen. Traditional methods involve a case of confusion between pediatric diphtheria-tetanus-acellular pertussis (DTaP) and adolescent/adult tetanus-diphtheria-acellular pertussis (Tdap). Although the indicators of these products could be largely different, CDC-approved abbreviations are separated by a thin line, and they are easy to ignore during handwriting or oral communication or during the hasty look at the screen (Condon & Hayney, 2016; Institute for Safe Medication Practices (ISMP), 2024).

Malpractices that belong to this category include applying adult formulations to children or children to adults, ensuring that patients are of the right age before taking their medication, and choosing the wrong products when working under a high workload. Condon and Hayney reported that age-related formulation errors were among the most common mechanisms of vaccine errors, which is due to the increasing number of available formulations as well as the unequal verification of the age and vaccination history of patients. The results of the ISMP VERP also show that these errors are even extended with several age-specific products that are not clearly differentiated or labeled, which highlights the importance of age-range indicators in storage bins and vaccine containers (ISMP, 2023).

Confusion during the COVID-19 pandemic worsened with the introduction of numerous symptomatic pediatric and adult formulations with short fuses, the visual appearance of which was similar, and with changing recommendations. COVID-19 vaccines represented the most frequent naming-convention error in 2022–2023, with 17.2% of mistakes (n = 86) due to confusion between pediatric and adult doses and monovalent versus bivalent boosters (Institute for Safe Medication Practices (ISMP), 2024).

Proximity to Storage and Pressure on Workflow

The accuracy of vaccine selection is strongly affected by the physical storage scheme and workflow scheme. In the case in which various vaccines are kept in close-performing conditions, especially those that have similar names or signs, the risk of accidental mix-ups increases significantly. Proximate storage was found by Condon and Hayney to be a common cause of wrong-vaccine error, particularly in fridges with various pediatric preparations and combination products. In these settings, the process of checking on products is usually substituted by rushing to obtain the required items during the busiest clinic periods.

These findings are reflected in ISMP VERP reports, which indicate that vaccine-to-vaccine errors are quite common in high-throughput settings with multitasking and interruptions, as well as low use of barcode verification. A high volume of patients in a short period of time, along with the lack of total separation of similar products, leads to a situation in which the staff can operate under the illusion of visual inspection instead of complete label checks (Institute for Safe Medication Practices (ISMP), 2024). These workflow strains are compounded by mass vaccination efforts, where temporary staffing, unknown products, and tightened timelines further diminish safety margins.

When added together, these subtypes paint the picture that vaccine-to-vaccine confusion can hardly be attributed to the actions of individual mistakes that are isolated. Rather, it represents foreseeable vulnerabilities within the system, such as ambiguous naming, lack of product differentiation, proximity storage, and production pressures that should be approached upstream in design and organization between the production and functional units to avoid future occurrences.

Confusion Between Vaccines and Medication

One of the most dangerous types of LASA errors is vaccine-to-medication mix-ups since they often feature high-alert drugs that can inflict immediate and serious damage once used accidentally. These events put patients who are, in most cases, infants or children at risk of the immediate lethal impact of potent pharmacologic agents, unlike the cases of vaccine-to-vaccine errors that lead to inadequate immunization.

Neuromuscular Blocking Drugs

Morocco is a tragic case in which six newborns accidentally received rocuronium in place of the hepatitis B vaccination in routine immunization. A neuromuscular blocking agent called rocuronium led to acute respiratory paralysis, and a baby died even after emergency treatment in this case (Alj et al., 2024). Research on this incident was able to establish several contributory factors, such as the storing of vaccines and injectable drugs in close areas, look-alikes, and the lack of systematic checks before administration. This case is an example of how one error in the process of selecting a product in the context of a neonatal setting may lead to disastrous outcomes.

Insulin Mix-Ups

The same vaccine–medication combinations have been reported in the United States. A retrospective survey of reports reported to the Vaccine Adverse Event Reporting System (VAERS) and the FDA Adverse Event Reporting System (FAERS) between January 2005 and April 2015 revealed 22 cases of inadvertent administration of insulin, rather than the trivalent inactivated influenza vaccine (IIV3) intended, in error. Of these, seven cases were considered highly suggestive, and fifteen were considered suggestive of insulin-influenza vaccine mix-ups.

In 2014, there was a school-based vaccination clinic comprising five highly suggestive cases in one cluster of incidents. Five adult staff members experienced symptoms that were typical of acute hypoglycemia soon after the vaccination in the cluster event. Two patients were in a severe state of hypoglycemia, which implied emergency care and treatment at the hospital; one patient was evaluated at a level of 23 mg/dL of blood sugar and loss of awareness, and another patient had convulsions and had to be given a glucose solution on the way to the emergency room. A multi-dose vial of IIV3 was kept in the same refrigerator where there was a 10 mL vial of Humalog U-100 insulin. The products were not separated into separate and clearly labeled containers or bins. The authors concluded that the factors that could have contributed to the incident included improper storage, the absence of standardized methods to verify the contents of the vials before preparation, and reduced vigilance during administration. In all 22 cases reported during the 10-year review period, patients usually experienced dizziness, sweating, confusion, weakness, or loss of consciousness shortly after injection and reported blood glucose levels as low as 0–33 mg/dL in some of the cases. Although no deaths were reported, several patients needed to be hospitalized and thrown into an emergency situation.

The authors stated that a typical dose of insulin (0.5 mL) in the influenza vaccine would be approximately 50 U of U-100 insulin if insulin was improperly used, which would cause rapid and severe hypoglycemia. Systemic contributing factors were also mentioned in the review. Physical segregation was not performed to separate the insulin and influenza vaccine vials, which were stored in the same refrigerator. The primary cluster recorded reportedly checked refrigerator temperatures, which were not recorded, and the office of the nurse was not locked during the school day.

Additionally, the use of visual clues, as opposed to paying close attention to labeling, seemed to be a contributing factor. The authors addressed the possibility of confirmation bias, according to which the healthcare staff considers the appearance of the vials and does not read the entire label, thus risking error in the choice of products. Although few reported cases were compared to those of hundreds of millions of doses of influenza vaccines that were administered during the study period, the events were regarded as severe and avoidable. In this study, it was discovered that insulin–vaccine mix-ups are potentially severe never events that can be alleviated by adequate segregation in storage, standardization in preparation and administration protocols, compliance with advised vaccine handling procedures, and reinforcement of a culture that supports reporting and investigating mistakes (Clogston et al., 2016).

Tuberculin Confusion

Prior national surveillance has also demonstrated that there is a wide degree of confusion between vaccines and tuberculin-purified protein derivatives (PPDs). The 115 mix-up events, which involved more than 240 people, took place between 1969 and 2005, and the majority of them involved unintended administration of vaccines rather than PPD (Chang et al., 2008). Although local injection-site reactions were observed in most patients, some needed to be hospitalized, and others were wrongly initiated on tuberculosis prophylaxis because of misinterpretation of the vaccine reactions as positive skin tests. Both human and system factors contribute to LASA drugs, such as similar packaging, colocation in the refrigerator, use of confusing abbreviations (e.g., PPV vs. PPD), heavy workload in mass screening activities, and not reading labels right before administration.

Among these events, recurring underlying mechanisms are always involved. The most common indicators of vaccine–medication mix-ups include the sharing of space in the form of the costorage of vaccines and injectable drugs, similar vials or ampoules, poor organization of the workspace, the use of memory or visual identification, and a lack of barcode verification or second checking. Risk is further increased with high throughput and time pressure. Taken together, these instances prove that these mistakes are not a few instances of human lapses; instead, they indicate the existence of predictable weaknesses in the system that help the administration of high-alert medications to gain access to the processes of vaccination. System-level protection, such as physical separation of vaccines and medications, standardized storage maps, barcode scanning at the point of administration, and obligatory verification measures, is necessary to prevent such errors but not staff vigilance (Alj et al., 2024; Chang et al., 2008; Clogston et al., 2016).

Multicomponent Vaccine Errors

Reconstitution vaccines, or vaccines with multiple components, provide even more possibilities of severe administration mistakes when separate components are misinterpreted, separated, or omitted. Report analysis submitted to the ISMP VERP has indicated that component omission events, which are a category of vaccine error that occurs when a single manufacturer administers only the diluent or only a single component of a multicomponent vaccine, had the highest number of events in 2022–2023: approximately 15.9% of all vaccine error reports. The ISMP VERP data also revealed that meningococcal and combination pediatric vaccines were the most common products involved in such events, specifically, Menveo® (meningococcal groups A, C, Y, and W conjugate vaccine; MenACWY) and Pentacel® (diphtheria and tetanus toxoids and acellular pertussis adsorbed, inactivated poliovirus, and *Haemophilus influenzae* type b conjugate vaccine; DTaP-IPV/Hib).

Misunderstanding the vial that holds the active antigen, failure to mix the two parts before administration, and administration of the liquid part alone are the reported forms of failure. These mistakes are motivated by system vulnerabilities that can be anticipated, such as similar labeling between matching vials, poor visual distinction between antigen and diluent, poor reconstitution instructions, and storage procedures that permit physical separation of components. The risk is further increased by the high-throughput vaccination setting and staff's lack of familiarity with multivial products. These incidents highlight the inadequacy of relying on individual vigilance in cases when product design and workflow fail to make proper preparation evident (Shastay, 2016a). Notably, the ISMP highlights the point that such errors are not the fault of isolated human errors but of systems designed poorly. The mitigation measures that have been recommended include ensuring that paired components are kept in physical bundles, clearly labeling vials with the labels "Vial 1 of 2" and "Vial 2 of 2", dispensing multicomponent vaccines together, and ensuring the verification of the barcodes of both components before mixing and administration. The reduction in Menveo reconstitution errors also appears to persist after the implementation of improved labeling and barcode differentiation. Thus, upstream packaging and workflow redesign are more effective than education in the prevention of LASA-related component omission errors (Institute for Safe Medication Practices (ISMP), 2024; Shastay, 2016a).

The worst reconstitution-related vaccine errors occurred in 2014 in Syria, when atracurium, a neuromuscular blocking agent, was administered in place of sterile water during a measles immunization campaign that led to the death of at least 15 children in the aftermath. The WHO confirmed that ampoules of atracurium were inadvertently added to measles–rubella vaccination kits at a district distribution center in Idleb Governorate and subsequently supplied to four vaccination teams.

The neuromuscular blocking agent was then mistakenly used as a diluent during vaccine preparation. Subsequent analyses attributed the error to look-alike packaging and storage practices, as atracurium ampules closely resembled sterile water in size and appearance, facilitating wrong-product selection during reconstitution in a high-pressure campaign setting (Pakenham-Walsh & Ana, 2014; Roberts, 2014; World Health Organization, 2014). The mistake was termed an error that was waiting to occur, which indicated that there had been previous issues of unsafe packaging of high-alert drugs. In addition to the direct and immediate loss of life, the incident caused serious damage to the trust in the vaccination programs in an already vulnerable healthcare environment and triggered the demand to protect the vulnerable population at the system level by providing a clear distinction between hazardous drugs and nonharmful diluents and further controls in the vaccine production procedures.

Previous versions of Rotarix® had to be reconstituted with the help of a lyophilized vial with an oral dosing applicator, which presented extra preparatory procedures and increased the risk of dosing mistakes. A survey of reports by the Vaccine Adverse Event Reporting System (VAERS) and by the Centers for Disease Control and Prevention revealed 66 cases of rotavirus vaccine administration errors (39 cases were inadvertent injections (6 by RotaTeq® and 33 by Rotarix®). Some of the contributing factors were poor interpretation of the package insert instructions, interchangeability between the Rotarix oral applicator and injectable syringes, confusion between the Rotarix® vaccine vial and injectable vaccine vials, insufficient staff training, and not reading the package insert (Hibbs et al., 2014). As a follow-up to these risks, the current Rotarix® formulation is available in the form of a ready-to-use oral suspension in the liquid state, not requiring reconstitution or dilution, and in a prefilled oral-dosing applicator, eliminating any chances of preparation-related and route-of-administration errors (Park, 2022; Prescrire International, 2020; Shastay, 2016b), as shown in **Figure 2**.

Figure 2. The Rotarix® live oral rotavirus vaccine is currently formulated as an oral suspension in a prefilled oral dosage delivery device

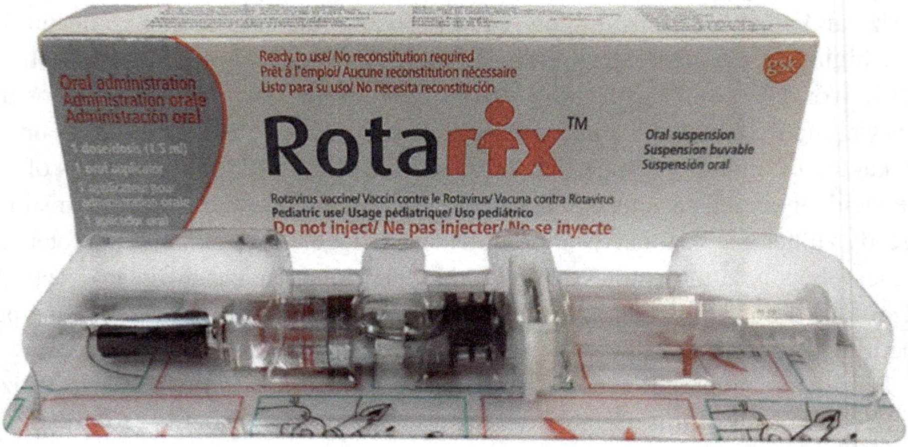

It has no reconstitution and no dilution and is strictly labeled as oral use only, indicating that the formulation and packaging modifications are of the manufacturer level intended to reduce the complexity of preparation and errors in wrong-route administration. The use of trade names and commercial sources is for identification purposes only and does not imply endorsement by the author

Formulation-Specific Errors

Additionally, mistakes can be caused by confusion among various formulations of the same vaccine, especially when products with different indications or age groups have similar names, packages, or storage sites. One of the worst incidences was reported in Pakistan, where 26 neonates accidentally received ONCO-BCG, a high-concentration intravesical preparation used to treat bladder cancer, rather than the routine neonatal BCG vaccine. The concentration of the ONCO-BCG preparation is approximately 80 times greater than that of the standard neonatal BCG. Clinical follow-up revealed that 16 babies (61.5%) had skin wounds at the injection site, three (11.5%) had coagulation abnormalities, and one (3.8%) had intracranial bleeding; however, no deaths or cases of disseminated tuberculosis among infants occurred after early multidisciplinary care and chemoprophylaxis were received (Jamil et al., 2025; Qureshi et al., 2019). This was ascribed to the fact that look-alike packaging depicts the situation, and the pharmacy dispensing and verifying services failed, which highlights the fact that formulation confusion may lead to severe yet avoidable damage in neonatal groups.

Preventable errors related to age-specific vaccine formulations represent one of the most common and avoidable categories of immunization errors. Numerous vaccines are sold in separate pediatric and adult formulations, which contain different antigen levels and doses but have similar names and packaging, posing a high LASA risk. An example of this issue is the use of influenza vaccines, where various age-restricted products are on the market, and the use of an age-dependent formulation that is administered beyond the approved age range has been reported as the most frequent error related to influenza. These incidences have often been linked visually to similar labeling and incomplete checking during preparation and administration. Taken together, these results indicate that the lack of differentiation of age-specific products, coupled with workflow stress and age-range mislabeling on storage containers, and the physical separation of pediatric and adult formulations are the main safety considerations that allow the formation of anticipatable wrong-age vaccinations (Condon & Hayney, 2016).

As **Figure 3** illustrates, the errors in the LASA vaccines are caused by foreseeable weaknesses in the system and hence should be managed by upstream design, segregation, verification, and risk reduction measures specific to the product.

Figure 3. Key groups of LASA vaccine errors and systemic prevention measures. The figure shows the major LASA vaccine error trends, such as vaccine-to-medication errors, age-related formulation errors, and multicomponent or reconstitution errors, and upstream system redesign and product-level mitigation are the primary prevention approaches

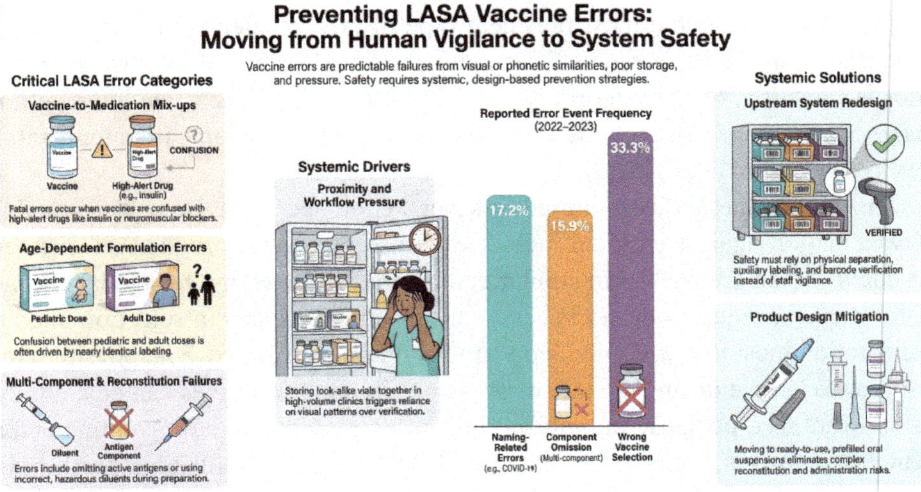

SPECIAL CONSIDERATIONS FOR VULNERABLE POPULATIONS

Neonates and Infants

Children—especially infants and preschool children—are the most vulnerable group in terms of immunization mistakes related to the prescription of drugs. A recent systematic review and meta-analysis revealed an overall prevalence of 0.044 vaccination errors for every 10,000 doses, although this prevalence was high among children under the age of five years and was found to be 0.334 per 10,000 doses. The most common clinical manifestations were fever, local pain, edema, and erythema, indicating both the direct physiological outcomes of such mistakes and the possible effects on the confidence of caregivers in vaccination programs (Tavares et al., 2024).

The imbalance in the number of children affected is also supported by national surveillance data. Most immunization errors were reported in children younger than five years, with almost one-third of these errors occurring in infants younger than one year. All these situations were most often linked to routine childhood vaccinations and were tied most often to improper vaccine indications, inappropriate dosage intervals, and administration technique errors. These results indicate the increased vulnerability of the early childhood immunization process, in which tight schedules, regular changes in formulation, and age- and weight-based dosage further impose cognitive and operational burdens on healthcare personnel (Barboza et al., 2020).

Similar tendencies can be found in large regional immunization systems. Infants under the age of one year contributed to approximately 39% of the reported immunization errors, and those under the age of four accounted for more than 50% of all pediatric cases. Immunization with a vaccine outside of the recommended age was found to be the most prevalent type of error, which is creating concern about the decrease in vaccine efficacy and posing a higher risk of adverse events after vaccination. Such pediatric errors were also linked to possible interruptions to the continuity of vaccinations and the low confidence of people in immunization services (Donnini et al., 2022).

This high vulnerability is caused by several child-specific factors. The schedule of vaccination against children includes the use of several products of different products, which are packed in similar containers with overlapping age labels and, in most cases, require booster vaccination, making mistakes in selection and administration most likely. Babies and young children can also have no physiological reserves to handle dosing deviations so that even minor mistakes can be a clinical issue. Moreover, pediatric immunization is often provided in large-volume outpatient environments, which puts the risk of LASA vaccine confusion at further risk because of workflow pressure, multitasking, and interruptions.

Taken together, these findings suggest that the risk of immunization errors in pediatrics is concentrated because of the interactions among developmental factors, complicated vaccination schedules, and risks at the system level. Young kids are still disproportionately affected, as they are the ones that are vaccinated the most in young stages of their lives and, in many cases, with similar formulations with different age-related dosing limits. These facts contribute to the necessity of pediatric-focused LASA prevention interventions, such as increased similarity screening of vaccine names, clear age-based labeling, standardized storage segregation, and the incorporation of clinical risk matrices, which rank high-risk pediatric situations. It is necessary to reinforce these safety measures to minimize avoidable damage and reduce confidence in childhood immunization programs.

Immunocompromised Patients

Patients with immunocompromised conditions are also vulnerable to nosocomial infections, especially when confined to an acute care hospital where conditions such as urinary tract infections, vagina-related problems, and LASA vaccine mistakes present specific risks to immunocompromised people. Live vaccines should not be used where contraindicated, as this can lead to an outbreak of the disease, whereas errors in administration or lack of active ingredients will leave them without sufficient protection against major diseases. Adverse events in this population are usually more severe and extended, and missed immunization opportunities have increased clinical implications. It has been repeatedly reiterated in the context of safety surveillance programs that immunocompromised patients are to be verified more, have their contraindications clearly documented, and have their products carefully chosen to alleviate the risks of LASA (Institute for Safe Medication Practices [ISMP], 2023).

Pregnant Women

Pregnant women are vulnerable to vaccine errors, which have health implications for the mother and the child. The administration of vaccines that were not advised during pregnancy was also noted as a common point of weakness of the vaccination system during pregnancy, as Brazilian surveillance data revealed it in approximately 10.8% of reported incorrect immunization injections (Donnini et al., 2022). In addition to possible biological hazards, e.g., exposing the fetus to transmitted ingredients in the vaccine, such inaccuracies often cause severe psychological trauma, anxiety, and mistrust toward the healthcare profession after the revelation. The following findings support the necessity of pregnancy-specific verification procedures, labeling, and decision-support systems in immunization processes.

As presented in **Figure 4**, immunization errors are disproportionately spread among vulnerable groups and must be explicitly addressed at the system level.

Figure 4. Populations at greater risk due to immunization errors and system-level protection. Key at-risk populations, including infants and young children, immunocompromised patients, and pregnant women, are highlighted, and safety actions, including LASA prevention, risk stratification, and increased verification procedures, are summarized

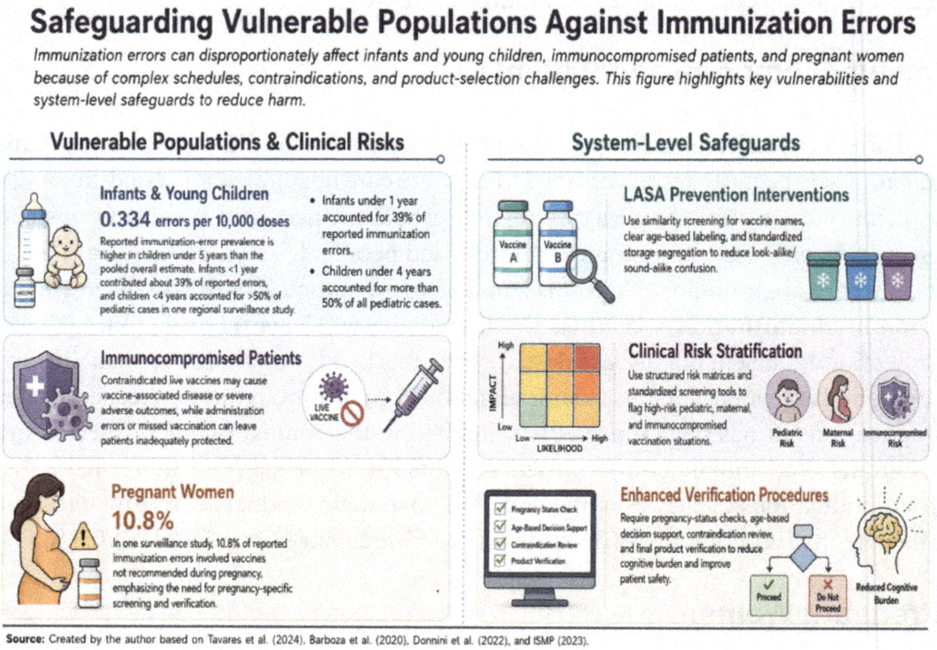

CASE STUDIES OF LASA VACCINE ERRORS

In-depth case studies help establish the necessary understanding of how LASA vulnerabilities spread within healthcare systems, particularly in cases of serious vaccine-related damage. There are two very educative neonatal events, one where a vaccine was confused with a high-alert medication and the other where different formulations of the same vaccine were mixed together, exemplifying the disastrous effect of LASA error when several latent failures in the system coincide. Six newborns in Morocco received the neuromuscular blocking agent rocuronium rather than the hepatitis B vaccine in a Moroccan maternity university hospital during routine vaccination against neonatal immunity. Every infant experienced acute clinical deterioration within minutes of injection, with some developing bradycardia, apnea, cyanosis, and seizures; emergency resuscitation and sugammadex use did not rescue one of them and gave the other a long-term sequela, whereas only four infants fully recovered (Alj et al., 2024).

The Moroccan Ministry of Health performed a root cause analysis that revealed that visual similarity in packaging was the major proximal cause and that the two products were packaged in the same white-and-blue package, with each having ten vials of 5 mL concentrated solution. These labels were exacerbated by unsafe storage conditions whereby vaccines and rocuronium were stored side-by-side in a darkly lit pharmacy cold room without warning labels or separation of high-alert drugs. Risk was also increased by organizational weaknesses, such as a lack of a full-time pharmacist, understanding on the day of the incident, and the fact that the hospital was still instituting neonatal hepatitis B vaccination without well-established immunization processes. Human factors also contributed significantly: the nurse who administered the drug misread the brand name of rocuronium as that of a vaccine and acted independently, without an independent check of their actions, while the pharmacy workers failed to verify the name twice before dispensing. This cluster shows that LASA errors associated with high-alert medications quickly lead to life-threatening consequences for neonates even when reversal agents are on hand, which explains why physical segregation, standardized labeling, processes of double checks, and staff education in vaccine safety systems are needed (Alj et al., 2024). A second major neonatal LASA error occurred in Karachi, a tertiary care hospital in Pakistan, where 26 (2–4-day-old) neonates (rather than the routine neonatal BCG vaccine) were accidentally injected with ONCO-BCG, a formulation used to treat intravesical bladder cancer, for more than two days. The dose of ONCO-BCG used was approximately 80 multiples of the recommended dose in neonates (Jamil et al., 2025; Qureshi et al., 2019).

The mistake that took place in the satellite pharmacy of the maternity ward started with a visual similarity of ONCO-BCG vials that the pharmacy provided to the satellite pharmacy and routine cross-checking errors that made the product reach the point of administration. All the affected infants were exposed to adverse drug reactions; 61.5% developed cutaneous lesions at the site of injection, 11.5% developed coagulation abnormalities, and one infant experienced intracranial hemorrhage (Qureshi et al., 2019). Spectacularly, there were no cases of tuberculosis spread or death. The prompt identification of the mistake led to a quick interdisciplinary intervention, open communication with families, and three months of orally administered chemoprophylaxis using isoniazid and rifampicin, combined with supportive and arranged follow-up for more than one year. All the infants eventually achieved clinical recovery. Researchers attributed the positive outcome to the timely detection of errors and coordinated control but noted that the event was a typical example of system failure, including similar packaging, poor product separation, staff turnover, and a lack of technological control (Jamil et al., 2025; Qureshi et al., 2019). This episode, as well as the earlier ones, underscores the very low probability (approximately 2.2 cases per million doses), although significantly underreported, that BCG is a threat to LASA in immunization efforts against newborn diseases (Qureshi et al., 2019).

The case studies are synthesized in **Table 2** by showing how risks caused by vaccine-specific LASA can be due to a small number of recurrent failures in the system rather than individual mistakes. There are also common contributing factors to wrong-product, wrong-route, and wrong-dose events; these factors include look-alike packaging, age-specific formulations, multicomponent products, proximity storage, and poor verification across vaccine types. As indicated in the table, high-impact prevention measures, such as physical segregation, high-profile labeling, double checks, barcode-enhanced workflows, and focused staff education, are cross-cutting controls that are used in immunization, regardless of the setting. The cases of neonatal outcomes above show that the lack of these controls can rapidly turn uncommon LASA vulnerabilities into life-threatening events; therefore, active, system-wide risk prioritization in vaccine safety programs is necessary.

Table 2. Vaccine-specific LASA risks, common error patterns, and key prevention strategies

Vaccine Type	Typical LASA Error Patterns	Key Contributing Factors	High-Impact Prevention Strategies	References
DTaP/Tdap/Td (pediatric combinations)	Wrong age formulation; confusion among DTaP, DT, Tdap, Td; mix-ups with combination products (DTaP-IPV, DTaP-IPV/Hib)	Case-sensitive abbreviations; similar packaging; complex schedules; multiple combination products	Verify DOB vs indication; include age ranges on labels; document generic + brand names; segregate formulations	Condon and Hayney (2016) Institute for Safe Medication Practices (ISMP) (2024)
Multicomponent pediatric vaccines (Pentacel®, ActHIB®, Menveo®)	Missing components; wrong diluent; administering only one vial	Look-alike components; generic diluent labels; unfamiliarity with 2-component products	Unit-dose kits; band components together; "vial 1 of 2/vial 2 of 2" labeling; barcode both components	Condon and Hayney (2016) Institute for Safe Medication Practices (ISMP) (2024) Shastay (2016a)
HPV vaccine	Storage errors; mix-ups with nearby vaccines	Temperature deviations; proximity storage; age-dependent schedules	Dedicated storage bins; temperature monitoring; staff education on schedules	Barboza et al. (2020) Condon and Hayney (2016)
Rotavirus (oral vaccines)	Wrong route (oral vs injection); component confusion	Oral applicator resembles syringe; route misunderstanding	Prominent "ORAL ONLY" labeling; route-specific devices; training	Institute for Safe Medication Practices (ISMP) (2024) Shastay (2016b)
COVID-19 vaccines	Wrong formulation (mono vs bivalent); wrong age; expired doses; documentation inconsistencies	Similar packaging/names/abbreviations; rapid rollout; workload pressure; knowledge gaps	Barcode scanning; age-specific EHR order sets; segregated storage by formulation; CDS alerts; targeted training	Institute for Safe Medication Practices (ISMP) (2024) Abdel-Qader et al. (2025)

continued on following page

Table 2. Continued

Vaccine Type	Typical LASA Error Patterns	Key Contributing Factors	High-Impact Prevention Strategies	References
BCG (neonatal vs ONCO-BCG)	Administration of ONCO-BCG to neonates; overdose	Similar appearance/labels; pharmacy dispensing errors; failed double-checks	Segregated storage; prominent warnings; mandatory independent verification; barcode scanning	Qureshi et al. (2019) Jamil et al. (2025)
Influenza vaccines	Wrong age formulation; confusion with insulin or heparin	Similar vials/cartridges; proximity storage; lack of standardized checks	Physical segregation; standardized verification; barcode administration	Clogston et al. (2016) Institute for Safe Medication Practices (ISMP) (2024)
Hepatitis A/B vaccines	Adult vs pediatric mix-ups; confusion with neuromuscular blockers (rocuronium/atracurium); insulin	Similar packaging; shared storage with medications; poor lighting; inadequate verification	Store away from medications; segregate by age; double checks; barcode scanning; clearer label age cues	Alj et al. (2024) Condon and Hayney (2016)
Meningococcal (Menveo)	Reconstitution errors; single-component administration	Similar labeling; identical barcodes (historical); small font	Manufacturer relabeling (unique barcodes, warnings); improved contrast	Institute for Safe Medication Practices (ISMP) (2024)

Abbreviations. DTaP = diphtheria and tetanus toxoids and acellular pertussis vaccine; Tdap = tetanus toxoid, reduced diphtheria toxoid, and acellular pertussis vaccine; Td = tetanus and diphtheria toxoids; IPV = inactivated poliovirus vaccine; Hib = *Haemophilus influenzae* type b vaccine; HPV = human papillomavirus vaccine; BCG = Bacillus Calmette–Guérin vaccine; ONCO-BCG = intravesical bacillus Calmette–Guérin formulation for bladder cancer; IIV4 = inactivated influenza vaccine, quadrivalent; HepA = hepatitis A vaccine; HepB = hepatitis B vaccine; RSV = respiratory syncytial virus; EHR = electronic health record; CDS = clinical decision support; DOB = date of birth; LASA = look-alike.

This evidence shows that LASA vaccine mistakes do not emerge because of the individual error of one person but rather because of the combination of weak points in product design, storage conditions, employee staffing, and clinical processes. They support the need to incorporate orthographic and visual similarity screening in the procurement decision-making process, physically separate vaccines and high-alert drugs, require independent double checks, and integrate risk-matrix frameworks that can be used to prioritize those situations with the potential to cause catastrophic harm, especially in neonatal settings where the physiological reserve is low and error margins are extremely narrow.

CLINICAL CONSEQUENCES AND SEVERITY SPECTRUM

The clinical outcomes of LASA vaccine errors contain a continuum of extremes, from no apparent effects to disastrous, life-threatening effects. Knowledge of this gradient of clinical effects is needed in risk stratification and prioritization of preventive measures in immunization systems.

No Harm or Minimal Clinical Impact

A significant percentage of LASA vaccine errors do not cause any clinical impact or only a slight clinical impact, especially when the error is the administration of a similar vaccine or a formulation that is age suited and used outside of recommended time periods. For example, combination vaccines that may be substituted include Pentacel® (DTaP-IPV/Hib) and Kinrix® (DTaP-IPV), which may result in an unnecessary extra dose of Hib but again are unlikely to cause clinically significant adverse effects. These mistakes are, however, operationally significant, as they must be documented, counseled, and frequently revaccinated, which adds to the burden of healthcare and causes anxiety to the caregiver (Institute for Safe Medication Practices (ISMP), 2024).

Inadequate Immunological Protection

Poorly preventable vaccine-preventable disease is among the most common downstream effects of LASA vaccine errors. This happens when only the diluent is used without the active component of the vaccine, when a single constituent of a two-component vaccine is used, or when a completely inappropriate vaccine is chosen. Mistakes in the area of omission of the active component or the wrongful reconstitution require a repeat vaccination, and it may postpone the process of achieving protection immunity and temporarily leave patients at risk of infection, as well as increase healthcare expenditures and workload (Shastay, 2016a, 2016b). Surveillance data from the ISMP and VAERS suggest that two-component vaccines are the most susceptible to such failures, with the most common products being Pentacel®, Menveo®, and ActHIB®, where errors in omissions occur because of the lack of familiarity with the preparation procedure and similarities in packaging (Institute for Safe Medication Practices (ISMP), 2024).

Adverse Events Following Immunization

There is also a range of adverse events following immunization (AEFI) that are linked to LASA vaccine errors. The most common types of reactions (mild to moderate) in surveillance studies of immunization errors are fever, local pain, edema, erythema, and flushing (Barboza et al., 2020; Tavares et al., 2024). Errors have also been reported to lead to more pronounced local reactions, such as in large inflammatory injection-site swellings. Systemic complications are less frequent, but they can occur, especially in cases of overdose or mistaken products. In terms of the incidence of ONCO-BCG in Pakistan, affected neonates develop cutaneous lesions (61.5%), coagulation abnormalities (11.5%), and lymphadenopathy, and in one case, intracranial hemorrhage, LASA errors may cause severe systemic morbidity without causing mortality (Qureshi et al., 2019).

Life-Threatening Complications

LASA errors associated with vaccines are devastating when the vaccines (or dilutions of vaccines) are mixed with high-alert drugs, especially neuromuscular blocking agents (NMBAs). Since NMBAs induce swift paralysis, when they are administered accidentally, acute respiratory failure that necessitates urgent resuscitation and ventilatory support may ensue. An example that was well documented was in Morocco, where seven newborns were injected with the wrong vaccine, rocuronium, rather than the hepatitis B (HepB) vaccine. All the affected infants experienced respiratory distress, and the look-alike packaging, as well as unsafe costorage of rocuronium with the vaccines and the absence of system gaps (e.g., a full-time pharmacist was not present on the unit, and the HepB vaccination was not implemented in the unit before), was defined as the significant factor. The administration of sugammadex and transfer to neonatal care led to the recovery of five new-borns, whereas one new-born died (Alj et al., 2024). Another significant pediatric tragedy associated with vaccine preparation was the mixing of a vaccine diluent and an NMBA.

In a 2014 campaign to immunize against measles in northern Syria, atracurium was inadvertently substituted with a solution to combine measles vaccines; up to 75 children are reported to have been exposed, and 15 of them died, with investigations indicating that similar packaging is a key factor (Griffiths, 2017). It is also an example mentioned by the CDC of serious injuries caused by improper reconstitution of a vaccine with atracurium rather than the recommended diluent (Shimabukuro, 2017). Taken together, these examples indicate that the most serious LASA vaccine incidents are usually system malfunctions as opposed to individual human error: the lack of a distinction (similarity hazard) between high-alert drugs and vaccines, the use of rapid visual identification, and inappropriate forcing functions (segregation, labeling differentiation, and pharmacist supervision) enable similarity hazards to transform into life-threatening outcomes (Alj et al., 2024; Griffiths, 2017; Hibbs et al., 2015; Shimabukuro, 2017).

PHARMACEUTICAL AND REGULATORY PERSPECTIVES

Vaccine Nomenclature and Naming Conventions

Vaccine nomenclature is a high-stakes upstream factor of LASA-based medication errors. In contrast to small-molecule medications, the name of the vaccine has to be informative at once; it is necessary to provide details regarding antigenic substances, routes of delivery, manufacture, and patient groups. This complexity has led to cognitive overload among healthcare professionals and the development of environments that favor selection errors and administration errors because of the increasing number of vaccines and the increase in the use of combination vaccines.

Initial regulatory and pharmacovigilance studies revealed significant deficiencies in nonproprietary systems for vaccine naming. Specifically, nonstandardized and inconsistent applications of descriptors such as "live," "inactivated," "adsorbed," "conjugate," and "recombinant" have been revealed to blur clinically significant product differences. Other confounding factors are the designation of the antigenic valency in a variable, microbe strain, production medium, and target age population in vaccine nomenclatures, particularly in regard to combination vaccines (Maurer, 2000). Such disparities make the labels of the vaccines less discriminable at the point of care and more dependent on the use of heuristics, including partial name recognition, first-letter correspondence, or abbreviations, all of which are known causes of LASA errors.

Real-world evidence of error reporting systems underpins the contribution of the complexity of nomenclature in vaccine errors. An examination of reports made to the ISMP National Vaccine Errors Reporting Program (VERP) from 2022–2023 revealed that confusion over the name of the selected product was most prevalent during the preparation and product selection phases of product selection, where name-based confusion was the leading cause (Institute for Safe Medication Practices (ISMP), 2024). Such findings can be compared to those of prior observational research performed in the United Kingdom, which revealed that similarity in vaccine names was a common contributing factor to medication errors reported to dedicated vaccine advisory clinics (Lang et al., 2014).

Although abbreviated vaccine nomenclature was developed to ease documentation and communication, this has been well documented as a source of look-alike/sound-alike (LASA) vulnerability. Misunderstanding of naming codes and abbreviations has been found to be a significant cause of wrong-vaccine mistakes. Report analysis of reports submitted to the Institute for Safe Medication Practices National Vaccine Errors Reporting Program (VERP) for 2022–2023 revealed that a wrong-vaccine administration error was responsible for 25.2% of all reported vaccine errors. Some of these events included similar packaging, names, abbreviations, and storage conditions, which were the sources of 79.6% of the cases. Specific naming errors and abbreviations were the most common errors associated with COVID-19 vaccines (17.2) and vaccines containing diphtheria- and tetanus-containing vaccines (21.6) because of the high density of products with similar abbreviated names in the age-specific and formulation-specific categories (Institute for Safe Medication Practices (ISMP), 2024; Lang et al., 2014).

The similarity of vaccines such as DTaP, Tdap, DT, and dT and combination vaccines such as DTaP-IPV and DTaP-IPV/Hib highlights this danger. The abbreviations are highly similar in the way they are cased and the structure of letters, which emphasizes how abbreviated nomenclature can cause errors in selection during routine vaccination practice (**Figure 5**).

One such case involves diphtheria-, tetanus-, and pertussis-containing vaccines. The abbreviations approved by the Centers for Disease Control and Prevention distinguish between formulations by both casing and order; e.g., DTaP and DT can be used in children aged 6 months up to 6 years, whereas Tdap and Td are used in adolescents and adults (Td in those ≥7 years old). These are the small visual differences that are easily missed in handwritten orders, verbal communication, and electronic prescribing or inventory systems, particularly in high-throughput outpatient clinics and public health immunizations. Continuous misunderstandings about the vaccine against tetanus-containing vaccines even after decades of educational campaigns are yet another reminder of how vulnerable abbreviation-based nomenclature is to human factor-related errors (Hall et al., 2021).

Figure 5. Storage of vaccines showing several diphtheria-, tetanus-, and pertussis-containing vaccines with similar abbreviations (e.g., DTaP, Tdap, DT, dT, DTaP-IPV, and DTaP-IPV-Hib) indicates the possibility of LASA selection errors in the regular practice of vaccination.

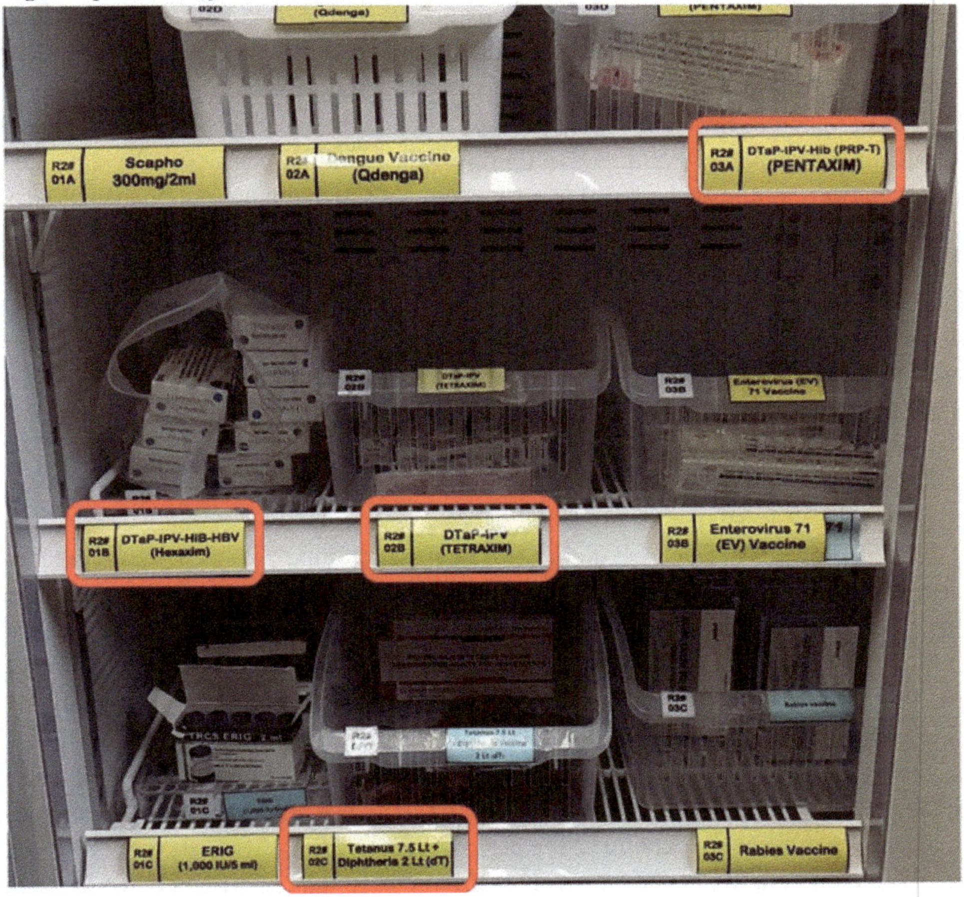

The use of trade names and commercial sources is for identification purposes only and does not imply endorsement by the author

In an in-depth study of 158 vaccine error reports submitted to an advice service on vaccines in the UK between 2009 and 2011, 33.3% of all reported vaccine error incidents involved administering the wrong vaccine, and a shared first letter of the vaccine name was reported in 13 wrong-vaccine incidents (Lang et al., 2014).

These findings support the conclusion that short or partially processed vaccine names increase LASA risk when interactions with time pressure, multitasking, and visual scanning behaviors are prevalent in immunization practice.

Brand Name vs. Nonproprietary Name Confusion

Confusion between brand names and nonproprietary names is another complexity that increases the problem of identifying vaccines. Several manufacturers can sell vaccines with the same antigenic constituents under varying proprietary brand names, whereas different valency or target populations can be referred to as similar or umbrella brand names. Maurer (2000) reported that long and cumbersome scientific names of vaccines are not often applied to final container labels because of space constraints that force healthcare workers to use brand names or locally accepted abbreviations, both of which differ across countries and languages (Maurer, 2000).

This inconsistency compromises the pharmacovigilance, documentation, and real-time checks at the time of administration. ISMP has consequently suggested regulatory strategies that focus on more evident discrepancies of vaccine products in marking, including more pronounced displays of distinguishing factors and less use of abbreviations with no inbuilt significance (Institute for Safe Medication Practices (ISMP), 2024).

Standardization Processes and Phases of Regulations

The European Official Medicines Control Laboratories (OMCL) Vaccine Nomenclature Drafting Group reported that the current nomenclature systems have shortcomings and proposed a three-letter code system that was intended to be used as a concise standardized name assigned to each vaccine antigen (Maurer, 2000).

In this system, an antigenic constituent corresponds to a fixed three-letter code (ex.: DIP: diphtheria, TET: tetanus, HIB: *Haemophilus influenzae* type b), and a combination vaccination would be represented as a hyphenated combination of these codes. That system was clearly meant to complement—not replace—brand names and serve as a final checkpoint at the point of care.

The main benefits of the suggested solution were that small labels would have better readability and that cross-language consistency would be enhanced with fewer disputes in documentation and pharmacovigilance reporting. Nevertheless, it lacks mass adoption, although it is technically feasible and conceptually clear. The obstacles are the necessity of regulatory harmonization internationally, the unwillingness to change existing naming systems, and the fact that encapsulating all the clinically relevant attributes of vaccines into a small set of names is intrinsically difficult.

Modern vaccine safety measures have therefore focused on an incremental nomenclature standardization approach together with complementary measures that include barcode scanning, standardized storage protocols, and, specifically, education about high-risk vaccine name pairs. Nomenclature reform is also a fundamental, but not sufficient, intervention from a medication safety standpoint, which needs to be incorporated into more comprehensive system-wide risk-reduction measures.

Packaging and Labeling Design

The design of packaging and labeling is a critical level of the manufacturer's determinants of look-alike/sound-alike (LASA) vaccine errors. In contrast to downstream clinical failures, vulnerabilities related to packaging are introduced at the stage of product design and spread throughout the entire process of medication usage, affecting storage, selection, preparation, and administration. Hundreds of cases of catastrophic vaccine-related mistakes have been shown to be a recurring proximal cause because of the visual similarity of primary and secondary packaging, especially when vaccines are stored alongside other injectable drugs or high-end drugs (Alj et al., 2024; Cohen, 2007).

Studies of human factors have revealed that in cases of time pressure, poor lighting, and heavy workload, the recognition of visual patterns is highly important to healthcare professionals. In situations where the packaging aspects (color schemes, vial size, typography, and carton structure) are alike, the chances of confirmation bias and automaticity are much higher, and errors are not blocked by various relationships of safety (Cohen, 2007).

Look-Alike Packaging Issues

Several well-documented vaccine-related incidents show how look-alike packaging may directly cause severe harm to a patient. The most common example is the *Morocco rocuronium*-hepatitis B vaccine incident, where six newborns were accidentally given rocuronium in place of the hepatitis B vaccine, and one of them experienced respiratory distress and died. In-depth root cause analysis revealed that the two products had almost the same packaging features (white-and-blue color scheme, the same number of vials per package (10 vials), and the same concentration and volume labeling (10 mg/mL in 5 mL vials). Colocation in the same cold room and poor lighting were noted as the main issues of the proximal cause of the error (Alj et al., 2024).

The second high-impact case involved a case in Pakistan where ONCO-BCG, a preparation that was to be used in intravesical therapy for bladder cancer in adults, was mistakenly used to treat the baby as a routine vaccination of BCG instead. In this case, 26 newborns were given ONCO-BCG within the span of two days. The investigations revealed that the ONCO-BCG and neonatal BCG products were similar in terms of vials and labeling. Thus, the pharmacy and nursing practitioners mistakenly identified the product during dispensing and administration. The dose administered was approximately 80 times the recommended dose at the neonatal level, leading to a high incidence of adverse effects, such as cutaneous lesions and adverse hematological events, that were avoidable (Jamil et al., 2025; Qureshi et al., 2019).

In addition to case-specific vaccine-related situations, the more general literature on medication safety supports the extent of the risk posed by packaging. According to Schnoor et al. (2015), similar packaging and labeling are the causes of approximately 30% of medication errors, and LASA mechanisms contribute to 7–20% of all reported medication errors in the healthcare environment. Their research indicated that even economically driven products, including the replacement of more expensive products by generic ones, may inadvertently increase the error rates in cases when the packaging similarity is not properly evaluated, although the costs are saved (Schnoor et al., 2015).

Problems of Multicomponent Vaccine Labeling

Multicomponent vaccines add extra labeling levels that may hinder proper preparation and administration procedures. A good example described in the literature is Menveo® (meningococcal conjugate vaccine), which comes in two separate parts that must be reconstituted before administration. The early labeling designs applied the same barcodes or similar colors and fonts to both components, but the fonts were small, and the color applied was similar, which created a risk of the vaccine being viewed as a single-component product. This design defect led to mistakes in which a single component was used, which undermined the efficacy of the vaccine (Institute for Safe Medication Practices (ISMP), 2024).

A highly dangerous category of labeling problems is represented by diluents. They are usually generic in nature, and they do not necessarily have a direct association with the particular product of the vaccine they are used in. This leaves room for wrong-diluent errors, particularly in places where vaccines and injectable drugs are kept together. The resulting case of fatalities in Syria involving a neuromuscular blocking agent as a dilution agent of the measles vaccine highlights the disastrous effects of poor diluent labeling and differentiation (Alj et al., 2024). These results are in line with those of previous human-factor studies on how critical warnings or differing information when pushed into secondary packaging or tiny text are unlikely to be noticed during clinical practice (Cohen, 2007).

Evidence Regarding Improvement and Risk Reduction of Labels

Notably, LASA risks associated with packaging can be changed, and a number of examples prove that specific label redesign may lead to the achievement of quantifiable safety benefits. After the errors associated with Menveo became actively publicized, the manufacturer made numerous design revisions, which included special barcoding of individual components, the addition of color contrast, and clear warnings, such as "NOT TO BE USED ALONE" printed prominently. ISMP revealed that there was a steady decrease in the number of reported Menveo preparation errors, which provides real-world evidence that manufacturer-level interventions may be effective at reducing error rates (Institute for Safe Medication Practices (ISMP), 2024).

Wider redesign efforts on packaging, as outlined by Cohen (2007), also affirm this conclusion. The implementation of changes, including larger fonts on drug names, improved hierarchy of information, refusal to use similar color palettes, and explicit identification of high-risk products, has been linked to a persistent decrease in reported medication errors in a variety of drug classes (Cohen, 2007). In the case of vaccines, especially in neonatal and mass immunization efforts, look-alike packaging errors at both the manufacturing and regulatory stages can lead to significant adverse effects that may cause acute harm on a large scale that downstream safety checks may not be able to handle.

Vaccine Packaging, Labeling, and LASA Risk Regulatory Frameworks

The intended areas of regulatory scrutiny of vaccine packaging and labeling are to identify the product, traceability, and safe usage; nevertheless, the experience of the past years shows that strict adherence to the existing regulatory standards is not enough to prevent LASA vaccine errors in the real setting. In the United States, the Food and Drug Administration (FDA) regulates the labeling of vaccines as a biologic and prescription drug under labeling requirements, including the use of proprietary and nonproprietary names, strength, route of administration, storing conditions, and lot name on immediate containers and external packaging (U.S. Food and Drug Administration, 2013). Although they present the minimum safety standard, they do not prescribe systematic premarket assessments of LASA risk or formal human factor tests based on immunization processes. Therefore, the vaccines can be used in clinical practice with packaging and labeling provisions that are legally acceptable but are not distinguished effectively in circumstances of time constraints, multitasking, and high patient flow.

The European Medicines Agency (EMA) in the European Union has been more explicit with respect to the issue of packaging-related medication safety. The regulation of pack design and labeling by EMA focuses on avoiding visual similarity between medicinal products, such as differentiating them by color, typography, and layout, to minimize the likelihood of selection error (European Medicines Agency (EMA), 2009, 2011). Regardless of these instructions, investigations of severe vaccine-related cases indicate that a breakdown in packaging differentiation still occurs and can directly cause patient injury. On the international front, the World Health Organization (WHO) has been dealing with concerns of vaccine safety using systems-based methods as opposed to prescriptive label design. The WHO safety in immunization guidance always suggests physical separation of vaccines with other injectable medicines, especially high-alert drugs, as a preventive approach to avoid errors in vaccine selection and administration (World Health Organization, 2016). Root cause analyses of disastrous vaccine-related errors follow this recommendation and regularly show that the mixing of the vaccines and neuromuscular blocking agents is a decisive factor (Alj et al., 2024). All these regulatory methods demonstrate one common weakness: although they recognize the importance of safe labeling and storage, they are mostly reactive and do not always involve proactive LASA risk eradication during product development and lifecycle management.

Medication safety bodies have been trying to fill these regulatory loopholes by converting surveillance data into action guidelines. Relying on reports to the National Vaccine Errors Reporting Program (VERP), the Institute for Safe Medication Practices (ISMP) has reported steadily occurring patterns of incorrect selection of vaccines, errors in preparation, and partial administration of multicomponent vaccines that can be defined by flaws in labeling and packaging (Institute for Safe Medication Practices (ISMP), 2024). On this basis, the ISMP has many times stressed that the effective labeling of vaccines should facilitate quick visual discrimination and reduce the use of memory- or abbreviation-based shortcuts. These postulates are consistent with the fundamental research on human factors, which has shown that clinicians who experience cognitive load tend to exhibit confirmation bias and errors in pattern recognition in the case of similar visual characteristics between products (Cohen, 2007).

In addition to labeling, the actual process of packaging design has been found to be a strong predictor of the risk of error. Traditional studies of medication errors have demonstrated that packaging characteristics such as vial size, shape, color scheme, and label surface area are significant factors in product selection and that these characteristics can both lessen and intensify LASA risk (Berman, 2004; Cohen, 2007). The literature concerning vaccine safety proves that these principles are directly applicable to the practice of immunization. As an illustration, two-component vaccines have a known failure mode in which one of the two vaccination components is given in an ineffective way, leading to poor immunization and the subsequent requirement for revaccination. Peer-reviewed studies on errors in vaccine administration, such as on meningococcal conjugate vaccination, have shown that the design of packaging and labeling that fail to clearly communicate the necessity of reconstitution contributes to this error trend (Bundy et al., 2009; Hibbs et al., 2015). Surveillance reports also show that these errors remain throughout time, and design-based forcing functions should be applied instead of depending on education (Institute for Safe Medication Practices (ISMP), 2024).

Even with the provision of regulatory guidance and recommendations from safety organizations, a number of systemic gaps still facilitate the occurrence of LASA vaccine errors. A major weakness is that there is no compulsory premarket LASA risk testing of vaccines compared with current products. Case reports and cluster studies have shown that potentially hazardously similar-looking vaccines and injectable drugs can be licensed and marketed without a systematic assessment of the risk of confusion worldwide (Alj et al., 2024; Schnoor et al., 2015). Moreover, voluntary reporting is central to postmarket surveillance systems such as the Vaccine Adverse Event Reporting System (VAERS) and the ISMP VERP, which also creates underascertainment and incomplete characterization of LASA mechanisms (Hibbs et al., 2015; Institute for Safe Medication Practices (ISMP), 2024). The difference in labeling and packaging standards around the world also makes it more challenging to train and recognize staff, especially when responding to a global outbreak and when acting during an emergency and when the enforcement system usually takes action only when it is too late (Cohen, 2007; World Health Organization, 2016).

In this regulatory environment, the major responsibility of avoiding LASA vaccine errors lies with the manufacturers. The literature on medication safety has repeatedly underscored the importance of preventing errors at an early design phase as opposed to in clinical practice, which happens lower down the line. It is therefore ethically and professionally the responsibility of manufacturers to take the LASA risk into account when they choose proprietary and nonproprietary names, design packaging and labeling, and test products under realistic conditions of use (Bundy et al., 2009; Cohen, 2007). Some of the key elements of this approach include usability testing with representative end users, the evaluation of storage and preparation settings, and the prediction of high-risk interfaces, including the storage of vaccines and medicines in the same place.

LASA risk management must also be spread through the product lifecycle. Timely redesign of packaging and labeling should be performed on the basis of postmarket surveillance data, and timely improvement should be made when confusion cues are observed. Vaccine error reporting shows that these kinds of redesigns can significantly reduce error rates, as reflected by decreases in the number of reported preparation mistakes after changes in the labeling and barcoding of multicomponent vaccines (Institute for Safe Medication Practices (ISMP), 2024). Notably, corrective action should not be reduced to the cases where the regulations require change; rather, a proactive approach must be taken with the principle of patient safety in mind.

Finally, it is imperative that the roles of manufacturers are not restricted to only designing physical products but also in communication and education. Clarity of the storage, preparation, and administration instructions; recognition of the risks accepted by LASA; and open dialog with healthcare institutions and regulators are essential for maintaining confidence in immunization programs. The cost effects of not being able to deal with LASA also intensify the significance of prevention. It was established that packaging-related medication errors neutralize cost savings gained because of procurement decisions and lead to high downstream costs related to adverse event management, revaccination, investigation, and liability (Hibbs et al., 2015; Schnoor et al., 2015). Even though the implementation of LASA prevention strategies involves some initial investment, the possible payoff (harm avoidance, system efficiency, and public confidence) is in favor of a preventive, design-centered strategy of vaccine safety. To avoid LASA vaccine errors, as illustrated in **Figure 6**, it is necessary to change the reactive compliance to the proactive human-based packaging design throughout the product lifecycle.

Figure 6. Future perspectives on the safety of vaccine packaging will help avoid LASA errors. The figure depicts the shortcomings of the existing regulatory standards and highlights design-based prevention designs, such as usability testing, design-based forcing functions, and lifecycle redesigning, to minimize errors in vaccine selection

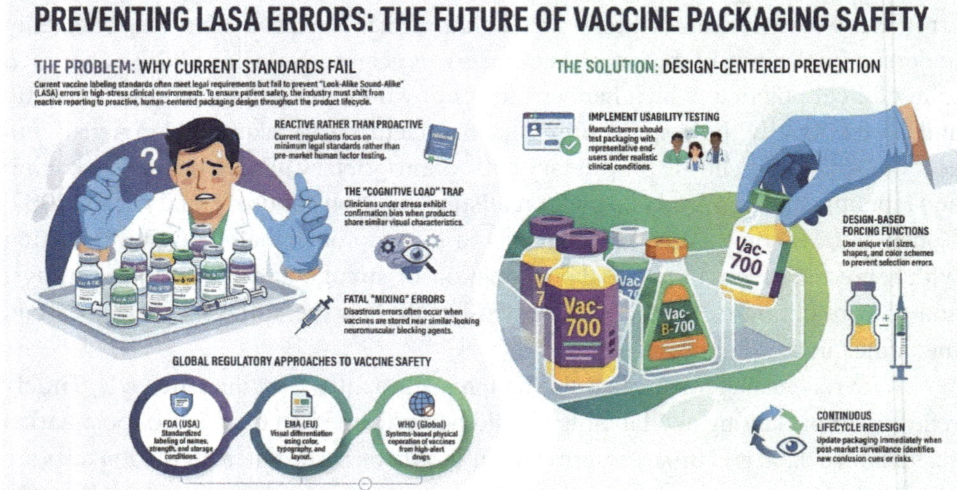

Healthcare System–Level Contributors to LASA Vaccine Errors

LASA vaccine errors are not caused by single individual errors. Rather, they are signs of the interaction between latent vulnerabilities in the system and the daily activities of immunization, such as product storage and retrieval practices, staffing and work pacing, verification design, information system support, and organizational reactions to near misses. According to the analysis of the ISMP National Vaccine Errors Reporting Program (VERP), wrong-vaccine selection incidents are always closely linked with work system circumstances comprising proximity storage, visual similarity amid products, and the absence of procedures that permit an inappropriate product to stay throughout the selection and preparation procedure to reach administration (Institute for Safe Medication Practices [ISMP], 2024). The most common antecedents of wrong-product selection mentioned in contributing-factor narratives include products placed adjacent to each other, similar appearances of containers and labels, and a lack of knowledge or communication between personnel (Institute for Safe Medication Practices (ISMP), 2024).

Upstream Risk Amplifiers of Storage and Organization

Storage design is among the core upstream factors that increase LASA vulnerability since vaccine selection is often performed under time pressure and is based largely on rapid visual scanning. Costoring vaccines—or vaccines and other injectable medicines—without physical separation of these two types of products increases the risk of selection error, usually among competent personnel. Proximate storage and look-alike labeling have been repeatedly found in analyses on ISMP as a frequent antecedent to wrong-vaccine selection events. This finding conforms to the recommendations of the U.S. Centers for Disease Control and Prevention, which recommend the use of special and properly organized spaces to store vaccines and the separation of products to minimize selection errors and facilitate the safe management of cold chains (Institute for Safe Medication Practices (ISMP), 2024; U.S. Centers For Disease Control and Prevention (CDC), 2024).

Manpower, Workload, and Peak-Hour Pressure

Staffing situations and workload are system-level factors contributing to errors in immunization, including LASA mechanisms, because they create interruptions and lessen compliance with verification processes. A review of vaccine error reports reported to a nationwide online reporting program revealed that errors were common in environments with a high demand for service, e.g., outpatient clinics and mass immunization endeavors (Barboza et al., 2020). Brazilian surveillance data also show that mistakes in immunization are highly concentrated in high-throughput healthcare facilities and overrepresented in infants and young children, who are in routine immunization programs during hectic clinical practice (Donnini et al., 2022). Although these studies do not prove the existence of shortages in staffing as a direct cause factor, they do indicate that times of workload stress and operational pressure are predictable situations where LASA risks are likely to be exaggerated.

Technology Infrastructure, Workflow Design, and Verification

The mechanism of preventing LASA should always be integrated into daily routine working processes and should not be dependent on personal alertness. Reports on vaccine errors and preventive measures published by the ISMP also highlight the significance of standardized preparation procedures, an independent second check on high-risk vaccines, and barcode-assisted verification and should be coupled with immunization information systems to curtail product selection and documentation errors (Barboza et al., 2020; Institute for Safe Medication Practices (ISMP), 2024). Additional practice-based reviews mention that simplification of the workflow and physical separation of similar vaccine products are also viable measures in terms of minimizing the amount of selection error in clinical practice (Condon & Hayney, 2016). Simultaneously, regulatory directions issued by the U.S. Food and Drug Administration and the European Medicines Agency emphasize that time-pressured and visually scanning behavior and storage density in terms of minimizing look-alike selection errors in relation to packaging and presentation should be considered in the design of labels and cartons (European Medicines Agency (EMA), 2009, 2011; U.S. Food and Drug Administration, 2013).

Safety Culture, Error Reporting, and Organizational Learning

In addition to technical controls, the organizational response to errors is also an important factor in LASA risk management. Brazilian national surveillance studies revealed that the fear of punitive actions and a low level of awareness of the significance of reporting errors with no related adverse events were significant obstacles to reporting errors in immunization and added to underreporting and the maintenance of latent risks in the system (Donnini et al., 2022). Without the presence of psychologically safe reporting conditions, healthcare organizations cannot detect local LASA hazard factors, e.g., baffling storage arrangements, ambiguous abbreviations, and inappropriate selection procedures, until they cause harm to a patient. The same observation is aligned with the literature on patient safety, which argues that learning-driven reporting systems are needed to detect and prevent the vulnerability of the systems at an early stage.

Taken together, the evidence that is available helps us understand LASA vaccine errors as predictable results of amenable system states rather than as a single individual failure. Achieving effective prevention requires integrated system design, such as purposeful segregation of storage, staffing, and scheduling strategies sensitive to demand; uniform workflows with external confirmation of high-risk products; barcode-based verification coupled with immunization registries; and an organizational culture that is proactive in encouraging reporting and taking corrective action on time (Barboza et al., 2020; Condon & Hayney, 2016; Donnini et al., 2022; Institute for Safe Medication Practices (ISMP), 2024). LASA vaccine mistakes occur because of system-level vulnerability interactions, as depicted in **Figure 7**, and are most mitigated by a combination of physical, workflow, technological, and organizational barriers.

Figure 7. LASA vaccine error prevention, systems-based. The figure shows the role of storage design, workload pressure, workflow gaps, and punitive reporting cultures in LASA vaccine errors and the role of integrated preventive strategies, such as physical product segregation and multilayered verification and psychologically safe reporting systems

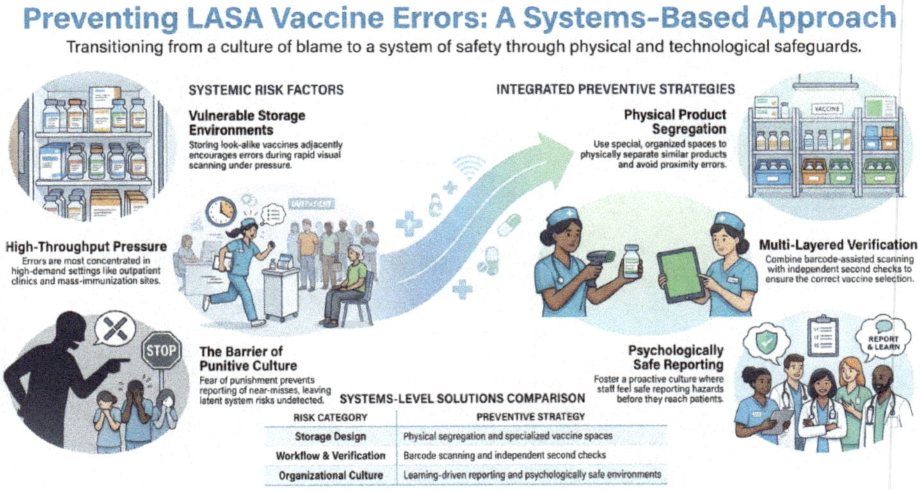

Table 3 describes the key system-level factors that contribute to LASA vaccine errors and system-level preventive strategies. The table illustrates that the occurrence of LASA events is fuelled by recurrent system states, such as those of storage and organizational configuration, workload pressure, workflow and verification holes, technology constraints, safety culture, and not single individual errors. The preventive strategies reviewed in Table 3 focus on preventive design of the system, i.e., physical product segregation, standardized workflow with independent checks, barcode-based verification, and enabling environments, and the summary of approaches that help

to minimize LASA risks in immunization practice is the primary application of integrated system-based methods.

Table 3. Healthcare system–level contributors to LASA vaccine errors and recommended system approaches

Domain	Key Contributing Factors	Examples	Implications for Practice	References
Storage & Organization	Proximity storage; inadequate segregation; suboptimal lighting; lack of structured layout	Proximity storage and visual similarity identified as contributors in severe wrong-product incidents; ISMP reports frequently cite environmental contributors to selection errors	Physically segregate LASA vaccines; separate vaccines from high-alert medications; improve lighting; use clearly labeled bins and standardized layouts	Alj et al. (2024); (Condon & Hayney, 2016; Institute for Safe Medication Practices (ISMP), 2024)
Staffing & Workload	High workload; peak-hour pressure; limited experience	Increased vaccination activity associated with higher frequency of administration errors; operational pressure described in outbreak and surveillance reports	Plan staffing to match demand; avoid excessive workload during campaigns; ensure supervision and appropriate skill mix	Abdel-Qader et al. (2025); (Barboza et al., 2020; Donnini et al., 2022)
Workflow & Process Design	Lack of standard operating procedures (SOPs); insufficient independent checks; interruptions	Case analyses show error progression when verification steps are absent; observational studies note interruptions as contributing factors	Implement SOPs; require independent double checks for high-risk vaccines; minimize interruptions; separate selection, preparation, and administration tasks	Institute for Safe Medication Practices (ISMP) (2024); Qureshi et al. (2019)
Technology & Information Systems	Absence of barcode scanning; weak Immunization Information System/ Electronic Health Record (IIS/EHR) integration; limited decision support	ISMP VERP reports describe information-system gaps contributing to wrong-vaccine events	Implement barcode-assisted administration; strengthen IIS–EHR integration; add age- and formulation-specific alerts	(Abdel-Qader et al., 2025); Institute for Safe Medication Practices (ISMP) (2024)
Safety Culture	Punitive responses; limited leadership engagement; poor communication	Underreporting of immunization errors associated with nonlearning environments	Promote nonpunitive reporting; visible leadership commitment; strengthen team communication	Donnini et al. (2022); Institute for Safe Medication Practices (ISMP) (2024)
Error Reporting & Learning	Limited access to reporting; weak feedback loops	ISMP VERP supports confidential reporting; postincident transparency enabled system learning	Maintain accessible reporting systems; analyze trends; provide structured feedback	Institute for Safe Medication Practices (ISMP) (2024); Qureshi et al. (2019)

continued on following page

Table 3. Continued

Domain	Key Contributing Factors	Examples	Implications for Practice	References
Training & Competency	Knowledge gaps; limited refreshers	Educational gaps identified in vaccine-error studies; training associated with improved practice	Provide vaccine-specific and LASA-focused training; conduct competency assessments	Alj et al. (2024); Institute for Safe Medication Practices (ISMP) (2024)
Multidisciplinary Coordination	Unclear role delineation; communication gaps	Error analyses describe coordination challenges during preparation and administration	Clarify responsibilities; support team-based workflows and training	Institute for Safe Medication Practices (ISMP) (2024)
Quality Improvement & Risk Management	Limited proactive risk assessment	Medication-safety literature recommends LASA lists and prospective risk analysis	Maintain LASA vaccine lists; conduct FMEA; perform environmental safety rounds	Institute for Safe Medication Practices (ISMP) (2024); Schnoor et al. (2015)
Process Standardization	Variable local practices	Standardized procedures associated with reduced variability in immunization delivery	Use standardized procedures and preparation checklists	Barboza et al. (2020); Institute for Safe Medication Practices (ISMP) (2024)
Infrastructure & Resources	Inadequate storage space; poor lighting; limited technology	Infrastructure constraints described in vaccine-error reports	Improve refrigeration capacity, lighting, workspace design, and monitoring	Condon and Hayney (2016); Institute for Safe Medication Practices (ISMP) (2024)

Abbreviations: LASA = look-alike/sound-alike; ISMP = Institute for Safe Medication Practices; VERP = Vaccine Errors Reporting Program; ISMP VERP = Institute for Safe Medication Practices National Vaccine Errors Reporting Program; SOPs = standard operating procedures; IIS = Immunization Information System; EHR = Electronic Health Record; FMEA = failure mode and effects analysis.

IMPACT OF PATIENTS AND PUBLIC HEALTH

LASA vaccine errors can produce cascading effects that extend beyond individual patients to public health systems and societal trust. At the clinical level, such errors may result in inadequate immunization, unnecessary risk, or adverse events ranging from mild local reactions to severe and life-threatening outcomes. Documented incidents include wrong-product administration, incorrect routes, and confusion with nonvaccine medications, which may necessitate revaccination, additional monitoring, or avoidable therapeutic interventions (Clogston et al., 2016; Shastay, 2016; Alj et al., 2024). High-profile events—such as the inadvertent administration of ONCO-BCG to neonates in Pakistan—also illustrate the psychological consequences for patients and families, including anxiety, loss of confidence in healthcare services, and persistent distress (Qureshi et al., 2019).

At the population level, immunization errors can undermine vaccination coverage and public confidence, thereby increasing the risk of outbreaks and threatening the sustainability of disease elimination and control programs. Surveillance and programmatic analyses suggest that errors affecting age-appropriate or schedule-appropriate vaccination may contribute to missed or delayed protection and reduced trust in immunization services (Donnini et al., 2022; Oliveira et al., 2022). These impacts are not evenly distributed: infants and young children, immunocompromised individuals, and socioeconomically disadvantaged people appear to be disproportionately affected, reflecting both higher exposure to routine vaccination encounters and lower tolerance for error (Barboza et al., 2020; Abdel-Qader et al., 2023). Although comprehensive economic evaluations remain limited, the available reports indicate meaningful direct and indirect costs related to clinical management, revaccination, investigation, and reputational harm. Importantly, several events have also prompted system-level improvements—such as barcode implementation and manufacturer-led label redesign (e.g., Menveo)—demonstrating how structured learning from errors can translate into safer immunization practices (Qureshi et al., 2019; Institute for Safe Medication Practices [ISMP], 2023).

Preventing LASA vaccine errors therefore requires layered, system-based controls spanning manufacturers, healthcare organizations, frontline clinicians, and patients, supported by effective learning systems. At the manufacturer level, evidence indicates that clear and standardized vaccine nomenclature, readable and differentiated labeling, component-specific barcoding, and human factor testing under realistic conditions of use can reduce confusion at the point of selection and preparation (ISMP, 2023; European Medicines Agency [EMA], 2011; U.S. Food and Drug Administration [FDA], 2013). At the healthcare organization level, high-impact approaches include physical segregation of LASA vaccines and separation from high-alert medications, clear bin labeling with age cues, reliable cold-chain and expiry controls, barcode verification at dispensing and administration, standardized operating procedures, and independent double checks for high-risk or multicomponent vaccines (Condon & Hayney, 2016; ISMP, 2023; Qureshi et al., 2019; Alj et al., 2024). At the clinician level, competency-based training, careful label reading, one-vaccine-at-a-time preparation, accurate documentation, and timely reporting of near misses strengthen defenses against wrong-product and wrong-route events (Condon & Hayney, 2016; ISMP, 2023). Finally, patient and family engagement—through Vaccine Information Statements (VIS) and encouragement of questions—adds an additional verification layer, while nonpunitive internal reporting and external surveillance systems (e.g., ISMP VERP, VAERS) enable root-cause analysis, shared learning, and continuous quality improvement (Donnini et al., 2022; ISMP, 2023).

Table 4 compiles prevention guidelines and system-wide optimal methods for decreasing LASA vaccine mistakes throughout the immunization-use continuum. The table shows that effective prevention is dependent on the layered controls adopted at various levels, which in this case starts with the manufacturer-controlled design measures, including the use of standardized nomenclature, readable labeling, differentiated packaging, barcoding, and human-factor validation, to minimize confusion within the point of product selection and preparation. Structural and process-based solutions, such as storage segregation, clear bin labeling, effective use of cold-chain solutions, barcode-enabled technology, standardized workflow, and independent verification steps, are vital safeguards against the spread of errors at the healthcare organization level. Frontline defenses can be further reinforced with clinician-focused practices, which can be facilitated by competency-based training and standardized preparation and administration behaviors, and with patient and family engagement, which offers further verification. Finally, in the absence of punitive reporting and learning systems, organizations cannot identify latent hazards, perform trend analysis, or implement corrective actions. Together, the measures listed in Table 4 highlight that both the integrated, system-based design and not individual vigilance alone can help achieve a sustainable reduction in LASA vaccine errors.

Table 4. Prevention protocols and system-level best practices for LASA vaccine errors

Level	System approach	Practical implementation examples
Manufacturer: Naming & nomenclature	Use clear, standardized vaccine names; avoid confusing similarities; consider multilingual contexts	Premarket name review; avoid near-homophones or similar abbreviations
Manufacturer: Label design	Improve readability; reduce clutter; emphasize critical cues (age, warnings); differentiate components	"Vial 1 of 2/Vial 2 of 2"; high-contrast warnings; larger fonts
Manufacturer: Barcoding	Unique barcode per component; scannable placement; encode lot and expiry	Distinct barcodes
Manufacturer: Packaging	Facilitate correct preparation; discourage partial use; differentiate from nonvaccine injectables	Integrated or connected components; distinct pack design
Manufacturer: Devices	Route-prompting or route-forcing devices	Oral applicators clearly distinct from syringes
Manufacturer: Human-factors & surveillance	Human-factors validation and postmarket redesign	Usability testing; monitoring error reports; proactive relabeling
Organization: Storage segregation	Separate LASA vaccines from each other and from high-alert medications; age-based segregation	Dedicated bins; separate refrigerator sections
Organization: Bin labeling & organization	Clear bin labels with age cues; limit products per bin	Age-band labels; structured layouts
Organization: Environment & cold chain	Adequate lighting and space; temperature and expiry controls	Twice-daily temperature checks; automated alerts
Organization: Technology	Barcode scanning; EHR order sets; clinical decision support; IIS integration	Age and interval alerts; verification of all components
Organization: SOPs & workflow	Standardized SOPs; minimize interruptions; manage peak-hour flow	Dedicated prep areas; surge staffing
Organization: Verification	Independent double checks at critical steps	Second-person verification for high-risk vaccines
Clinician: Competency	Initial and refresher training; LASA awareness	Training before new vaccine rollout; simulation
Clinician: Preadministration verification	Verify age, indication, history, lot, expiry	Compare DOB with VIS; confirm formulation
Clinician: Safe preparation/administration	One vaccine at a time; immediate syringe labeling; correct route	Avoid predrawing multiple syringes

continued on following page

Table 4. Continued

Level	System approach	Practical implementation examples
Patient/family engagement	Use VIS; encourage questions	Patient confirms vaccine name/ indication
Reporting & learning	Nonpunitive reporting; RCA; feedback loops; external reporting	Internal reporting plus ISMP VERP/VAERS submission

(Alj et al., 2024; Clogston et al., 2016; Condon & Hayney, 2016; Donnini et al., 2022; European Medicines Agency (EMA), 2011; Institute for Safe Medication Practices (ISMP), 2024; Maurer, 2000; Schnoor et al., 2015; Shastay, 2016a, 2016b, 2023)

Abbreviations: LASA = look-alike/sound-alike; ISMP = Institute for Safe Medication Practices; EMA = European Medicines Agency; FDA = U.S. Food and Drug Administration; SOPs = standard operating procedures; EHR = Electronic Health Record; IIS = Immunization Information System; VIS = Vaccine Information Statement; RCA = root cause analysis; VERP = Vaccine Errors Reporting Program; VAERS = Vaccine Adverse Event Reporting System.

CONCLUSION

LASA medication errors in vaccines are serious and mostly avoidable patient safety risks and threaten the health of the population. The analyzed evidence shows that these errors do not occur because of single individual errors but rather because of the interaction of human cognitive constraints and system-level vulnerabilities integrated in vaccine naming, labeling, packaging, storage, workflow design, and organizational culture. An analysis of surveillance data and cases regularly revealed that these groups of people are at disproportionate risk—neonates, infants, and young children—and that high-throughput settings such as mass immunization and the response to pandemics are also stress factors in LASA that impose time pressures, multitasking, and dependence on visual cues.

Clinical outcomes of LASA vaccine errors lie in the wide spectrum of severity, with no apparent harm and insufficient immunological coverage or severe morbidity and death in the case of vaccines perplexing with high-alert drugs or the wrong formula. In addition to causing harm to individual patients, these types of errors negatively affect societal trust in immunization initiatives, vaccine hesitancy, and disease response and can create clinical and financial overheads for medical institutions. These extended effects indicate that LASA vaccine error is not only a medication safety problem but also a health care issue.

The results underscore the idea that sustainable prevention requires system-oriented design but not personal attention. Interventions at the manufacturer level, such as the use of standard nomenclature, human-factor-based labeling and packaging, and component barcoding, are important upstream controls. Physical separation of vaccines and high-alert drugs, standardized operations, verification with barcodes, and an additional check of high-risk resources are effective protections at the healthcare-organization level. These defenses are further enhanced by frontline clinician practices that are supported by competency-based training and definite preparation standards. Just as crucial is a nonpunitive safety culture that supports reporting, allows learning about near misses, and helps to improve continuously with the help of internal and external surveillance systems.

LASA vaccine errors are considered predictable malfunctions of complicated immunization systems instead of occasional exceptions. To minimize these risks, the coordinated activity of manufacturers, regulators, healthcare organizations, and practitioners on the basis of human-factor principles and with the help of efficient learning systems is appropriate. Healthcare systems can advance the idea of focusing on integrated system-level interventions to defend vulnerable populations and maintain societal confidence in vaccination as a pillar of societal health.

REFERENCES

Abdel-Qader, D. H., Abdel-Qader, H., Silverthorne, J., Kongkaew, C., Al Nimrawi, M., Al Meslamani, A. Z., & Arabi, S. Z. (2025). Investigating the point prevalence, types, severity, causes and predictors of vaccines administration errors during COVID-19 pandemic in Jordan. *PLoS One*, *20*(1), e0312050. DOI: 10.1371/journal.pone.0312050 PMID: 39752371

Alj, L., Tebaa, A., Talibi, I., Moubarik, S., Benazzouz, M., & Soulaymani Bencheikh, R. (2024). Lessons learned from a cluster of immunization errors in newborns. *Therapeutic Advances in Vaccines and Immunotherapy*, *12*, 25151355231221009. DOI: 10.1177/25151355231221009 PMID: 38178960

Barboza, T. C., Guimarães, R. A., Gimenes, F. R. E., & Silva, A. (2020). Retrospective study of immunization errors reported in an online Information System. *Revista Latino-Americana de Enfermagem*, *28*, e3303. DOI: 10.1590/1518-8345.3343.3303 PMID: 32578753

Berman, A. (2004). Reducing medication errors through naming, labeling, and packaging. *Journal of Medical Systems*, *28*(1), 9–29. DOI: 10.1023/B:JOMS.0000021518.60670.10 PMID: 15171066

Bryan, R., Aronson, J. K., Williams, A., & Jordan, S. (2021). The problem of look-alike, sound-alike name errors: Drivers and solutions. *British Journal of Clinical Pharmacology*, *87*(2), 386–394. DOI: 10.1111/bcp.14285 PMID: 32198938

Bundy, D. G., Shore, A. D., Morlock, L. L., & Miller, M. R. (2009). Pediatric vaccination errors: Application of the "5 rights" framework to a national error reporting database. *Vaccine*, *27*(29), 3890–3896. DOI: 10.1016/j.vaccine.2009.04.005 PMID: 19442422

Centers for Disease Control and Prevention. (2021). E*pidemiology and prevention of vaccine-preventable diseases*. 14th ed. Washington, DC: Public Health Foundation. https://stacks.cdc.gov/view/cdc/252997

Chang, S., Pool, V., O'Connell, K., Polder, J. A., Iskander, J., Sweeney, C., Ball, R., & Braun, M. M. (2008). Preventable mix-ups of tuberculin and vaccines: Reports to the US Vaccine and Drug Safety Reporting Systems. *Drug Safety*, *31*(11), 1027–1033. DOI: 10.2165/00002018-200831110-00007 PMID: 18840022

Clogston, J., Hudanick, L., Suragh, T. A., Jankosky, C., Lewis, P., Martin, D., Schembri, C., Zinderman, C., Maslov, Y., Mistry, M., Pippins, J. R., Vee, S., Wyeth, J., Shimabukuro, T. T., & Leighton, J. (2016). Unintentional administration of insulin instead of influenza vaccine: A case study and review of reports to US vaccine and drug safety monitoring systems. *Drugs & Therapy Perspectives*, *32*(10), 439–446. DOI: 10.1007/s40267-016-0333-2

Cohen, M. R. (2007). The role of drug packaging and labeling in medication errors. In Cohen, M. R. (Ed.), *Medication Errors* (2nd ed., pp. 111–152). The American Pharmacists Association. https://doi.org/doi:10.21019/9781582120928.ch7

Condon, A. J., & Hayney, M. S. (2016). Strategies to minimize vaccine errors. *Journal of the American Pharmacists Association*, *56*(3), 339–341. DOI: 10.1016/j.japh.2016.03.016 PMID: 27156943

Donnini, D. A., Silva, C. M. B., Gusmão, J. D., Matozinhos, F. P., Silva, R. B., Amaral, G. G., & Oliveira, V. C. (2022). Incidence of immunization errors in the state of Minas Gerais, Brazil: A cross-sectional study, 2015-2019. *Epidemiologia e Serviços de Saúde: Revista do Sistema Unico de Saúde do Brasil*, *31*, e2022055. DOI: 10.1590/s2237-96222022000300008 PMID: 36351058

Emmerton, L. M., & Rizk, M. F. (2012). Look-alike and sound-alike medicines: Risks and 'solutions'. *International Journal of Clinical Pharmacy*, *34*(1), 4–8. DOI: 10.1007/s11096-011-9595-x PMID: 22193703

European Medicines Agency (EMA). (2009). *Guideline on the readability of the label and package leaflet of medicinal products for human use*. Retrieved 11 June from https://health.ec.europa.eu/system/files/2016-11/2009_01_12_readability_guideline_final_en_0.pdf

European Medicines Agency (EMA). (2011). *QRD recommendations on pack design and labeling for centrally authorized non-prescription human medicinal products*. Retrieved 10 Feb from https://www.ema.europa.eu/en/documents/regulatory-procedural-guideline/draft-quality-review-documents-recommendations-pack-design-and-labelling-centrally-authorised-non-prescription-human-medicinal-products_en.pdf

Griffiths, M. (2017). Beware of 'lookalikes'. *Nursing Standard*, *31*(25), 28. DOI: 10.7748/ns.31.25.28.s26 PMID: 28198315

Hibbs, B. F., Miller, E. R., & Shimabukuro, T. (2014). Notes from the field: Rotavirus vaccine administration errors—United States, 2006-2013. *MMWR. Morbidity and Mortality Weekly Report*, *63*(4), 81. PMID: 24476980

Hibbs, B. F., Moro, P. L., Lewis, P., Miller, E. R., & Shimabukuro, T. T. (2015). Vaccination errors reported to the Vaccine Adverse Event Reporting System, (VAERS) United States, 2000–2013. *Vaccine*, *33*(28), 3171–3178. DOI: 10.1016/j.vaccine.2015.05.006 PMID: 25980429

Institute for Safe Medication Practices (ISMP). (2024). ISMP National Vaccine Errors Reporting Program 2022-2023 analysis: New vaccines, new errors. ISMP Medication Safety Alert! *Acute Care*, *29*(21), 1–6.

Jamil, H., Sama, G., Nohri, A. R., & Malik, N. A. (2025). Medical Error in Pediatric Vaccination: Case Report of Accidental ONCO-BCG Administration in Neonates. *Journal of Health, Wellness, and Community Research*, e190-e190.

Lang, S., Ford, K. J., John, T., Pollard, A. J., & McCarthy, N. D. (2014). Immunization errors reported to a vaccine advice service: Intelligence to improve practice. *Quality in Primary Care*, *22*(3), 139–146. PMID: 24865341

Maurer, W. (2000). Vaccine nomenclature: The three-letter code. OMCL Vaccine Nomenclature Drafting Group. *Vaccine*, *18*(15), 1539–1542. DOI: 10.1016/S0264-410X(99)00435-1 PMID: 10618552

Pakenham-Walsh, N., & Ana, J. (2014). Confusing drug packaging contributes to death of 15 children. *The Lancet. Global Health*, *2*(11), e634. DOI: 10.1016/S2214-109X(14)70328-6 PMID: 25442687

Park, B. (2022). *New Formulation of Rotarix Removes the Need for Reconstitution.* Retrieved 10 Feb from https://www.empr.com/home/news/new-formulation-of-rotarix-removes-the-need-for-reconstitution/

Prescrire International. (2020). *Rotarix° oral vaccine: wrong-route errors.* Retrieved 10 Feb from https://english.prescrire.org/en/81/168/58487/0/NewsDetails.aspx

Qureshi, S., Ahmad, K., Fatima, P., Hassan, R. M., Sherali, F., Lalani, N., Jehan, F., Ali, S. A., & Qamar, F. N. (2019). Outcome of inadvertent high dose BCG administration in newborns at a tertiary care hospital, Karachi- Case series. *PLoS One*, *14*(7), e0219324. DOI: 10.1371/journal.pone.0219324 PMID: 31291329

Roberts, L. (2014). At least 15 children in Syria die in measles immunization campaign. *Science*. Retrieved February 10, 2026, from https://www.science.org/content/article/least-15-children-syria-die-measles-immunization-campaign

Samad, F., Burton, S. J., Kwan, D., Porter, N., Smetzer, J., Cohen, M. R., Tuttle, J., Baker, D., & Doherty, D. E. (2021). Strategies to reduce errors associated with 2-component vaccines. *Pharmaceutical Medicine*, *35*(1), 1–9. DOI: 10.1007/s40290-020-00362-9 PMID: 33151497

Schnoor, J., Rogalski, C., Frontini, R., Engelmann, N., & Heyde, C. E. (2015). Case report of a medication error by look-alike packaging: A classic surrogate marker of an unsafe system. *Patient Safety in Surgery*, *9*(1), 12. DOI: 10.1186/s13037-014-0047-0 PMID: 25767564

Shastay, A. (2016a). Administering Just the Diluent or One of Two Vaccine Components Leaves Patients Unprotected. *Home Healthcare Now*, *34*(4), 218–220. DOI: 10.1097/NHH.0000000000000371 PMID: 27023298

Shastay, A. (2016b). Liquid Oral Vaccine Mistakenly Given by Injection; Topical Anesthetics for Teething Infants. *Home Healthcare Now*, *34*(1), 43–44. DOI: 10.1097/NHH.0000000000000318 PMID: 26645844

Shastay, A. (2023). Look-alike Packaging. *Home Healthcare Now*, *41*(3), 168–169. DOI: 10.1097/NHH.0000000000001170 PMID: 37144934

Shimabukuro, T. (2017). *Vaccination Errors: Advisory Committee on Immunization Practices*. Retrieved 09 Feb from https://stacks.cdc.gov/view/cdc/58808

Supapaan, T. S., Napaporn, J., Ruthirakanok, R., Srichathum, S., Songmuang, A., & Pitchayajittipong, C. (2024). Look-alike sound-alike (LASA) medication errors in Thai hospitals. *Pharmacy Practice*, *22*(1), 2886.

Talbird, S. E., Carrico, J., La, E. M., Carias, C., Marshall, G. S., Roberts, C. S., Chen, Y.-T., & Nyaku, M. K. (2022). Impact of Routine Childhood Immunization in Reducing Vaccine-Preventable Diseases in the United States. *Pediatrics*, *150*(3), e2021056013. DOI: 10.1542/peds.2021-056013 PMID: 35821599

Tavares, L. O. M., Silva, M. A., Oliveira, B. R., Amaral, G. G., Guimarães, E. A. A., Couto, R. O., & Oliveira, V. C. (2024). Prevalence of errors causing events allegedly attributable to vaccination/immunization: Systematic review and meta-analysis. *Revista Gaúcha de Enfermagem*, *45*, e20230097. DOI: 10.1590/1983-1447.2024.20230097.pt PMID: 38477748

U.S. Centers For Disease Control and Prevention (CDC). (2024). *Vaccine Storage and Handling Toolkit*. Retrieved 10 Feb from https://www.cdc.gov/vaccines/hcp/downloads/storage-handling-toolkit.pdf

U.S. Food and Drug Administration. (2013). *Guidance for Industry: Labeling for Human Prescription Drug and Biological Products –Implementing the PLR Content andFormat Requirements*. Retrieved 10 Feb from https://www.fda.gov/media/71836/download

Whitney, C. G., Zhou, F., Singleton, J., & Schuchat, A. (2014). Benefits from immunization during the vaccines for children program era - United States, 1994-2013. *MMWR. Morbidity and Mortality Weekly Report, 63*(16), 352–355. PMID: 24759657

World Health Organization. (2014). *Statement regarding interim findings of WHO assessment of deaths of children in Idleb Governorate, Syria*. Retrieved 08 Feb from https://www.who.int/news/item/27-09-2014-statement-regarding-interim-findings-of-who-assessment-of-deaths-of-children-in-idleb-governorate-syria#:~:text=A%20WHO%20assessment%20of%20the,diluent%20for%20Measles%2FRubella%20vaccine

World Health Organization. (2016). *Global manual on surveillance of adverse events following immunization*. Retrieved 10 Feb from https://iris.who.int/server/api/core/bitstreams/12fbc390-517d-4c27-8c4c-8377eac4575d/content

ABBREVIATIONS

AEFI: Adverse Events Following Immunization
BCG: Bacillus Calmette–Guérin
CDC: Centers for Disease Control and Prevention
CDS: Clinical Decision Support
CoV-mRNA: mRNA coronavirus disease 2019
CRM197: Cross-Reactive Material 197 (nontoxic mutant diphtheria toxin used as a carrier protein)
DTaP: Diphtheria and tetanus toxoids and acellular pertussis vaccine
DTaP-HepB-IPV: Diphtheria and tetanus toxoids and acellular pertussis vaccine, hepatitis B vaccine, inactivated poliovirus vaccine
DTaP-IPV: Diphtheria and Tetanus Toxoids and Acellular Pertussis Vaccine, Inactivated Poliovirus Vaccine
DTaP-IPV/Hib: Diphtheria and Tetanus Toxoids and Acellular Pertussis Vaccine, Inactivated Poliovirus Vaccine, *Haemophilus influenzae* type B Vaccine
EHR: Electronic Health Record
EMA: European Medicines Agency
FDA: U.S. Food and Drug Administration
FMEA: Failure Mode and Effects Analysis
HepA: Hepatitis A Vaccine
HepB: Hepatitis B vaccine
Hib: *Haemophilus influenzae* type B
IIS: Immunization Information System
IIV4: Inactivated Influenza Vaccine, Quadrivalent

ISMP: Institute for Safe Medication Practices

ISMP VERP: Institute for Safe Medication Practices National Vaccine Errors Reporting Program

LASA: Look-Alike, Sound-Alike

MenACWY-CRM: Meningococcal (Serogroups A, C, W, and Y) Conjugate Vaccine (CRM197 carrier protein)

MMR: Measles, Mumps, and Rubella Vaccine

MMRV: Measles, Mumps, Rubella, and Varicella Vaccine

mRNA: Messenger ribonucleic acid

NMBA: Neuromuscular Blocking Agent

OMCL: Official Medicines Control Laboratories

ONCO-BCG: Intravesical Bacillus Calmette–Guérin for bladder cancer

PPD: Purified Protein Derivative

PPSV23: Pneumococcal polysaccharide vaccine, 23-Valent

RCA: Root Cause Analysis

RSV: respiratory syncytial virus

RZV: Recombinant Zoster Vaccine (Shingrix®)

SOPs: Standard Operating Procedures

Td: Tetanus and Diphtheria Toxoids

Tdap: Tetanus Toxoid, Reduced Diphtheria Toxoid, and Acellular Pertussis Vaccine

VAERS: Vaccine Adverse Event Reporting System

VIS: Vaccine Information Statement

WHO: World Health Organization

Chapter 12
Look-Alike, Sound-Alike Medication Errors in Injectable Drugs

ABSTRACT

Injectable drugs are among the most dangerous groups of medications in terms of medication safety due to the rapid systemic reactions and low safety margin. Look-Alike, Sound-Alike (LASA) errors in injectable medications are usually caused by the similarity in the name, similarity in packaging, limitations on label design, differences in concentration, and closeness in storage. Neuromuscular blockers, insulin, vasopressors, opioids, and concentrated electrolytes are often involved, and severely harming patients may be likely. The chapter reviews the common drug pairs, contributory factors, and regulatory measures associated with injectable LASA errors, with a focus on systemic prevention and human-factors-based safety measures.

INTRODUCTION

Injectable medications represent one of the highest-risk categories in contemporary medication safety practice. Compared with oral dosage forms, oral drugs that are administered intravenously are instantly absorbed into the system bloodstream and have fast pharmacological actions with minimal or no chance of being detected before the drug is absorbed into the system. The cost of medication error and the extent of damage are more devastating with intravenous administration than with other administration routes (Kuitunen et al., 2021; Westbrook et al., 2024). This is because of the unique susceptibility of injectable medications to catastrophic effects. Errors should be committed because of a combination of high bioavailability, narrow therapeutic indices, and the frequent use of high-alert medications, such as

DOI: 10.4018/979-8-3373-5478-1.ch012

vasoactive agents, neuromuscular blockers, concentrated electrolytes, insulin, and opioids (Institute for Safe Medication Practices (ISMP), 2022; Valentin et al., 2009).

This vulnerability is manifested in the perioperative and critical care setting. Clinicians tend to take on the role of the complete process of medication use, which can include prescribing, preparation, labeling, administration, documentation, and monitoring in circumstances of time constraints, environmental distractions, heavy cognitive load, etc. The literature on incident monitoring has repeatedly shown that syringe swaps, wrong-ampule choice, and labeling errors are frequent factors in anesthetic medication errors (Abeysekera et al., 2005; Currie et al., 1993). Notably, the Australian Incident Monitoring Study database analysis revealed that syringe or drug-preparation errors were thought to be the cause of most reported anesthetic drug errors, which included substitution errors (wrong drugs), which constituted a significant percentage (Abeysekera et al., 2005). These results highlight the fact that injectable medication errors are rarely stand-alone incidents but are symptomatic of weaknesses in the system that are engraved in workflow design.

Cases of medication errors during both anesthesia and critical care are thoroughly documented as contributors to preventable iatrogenic harm, including transient physiological instability to irreversible neurological damage and death (Nanji et al., 2016; Thomas & Mollon, 2018). In particular, intravenous administration error is linked to disproportionate severity because reversal options can be distributed once a drug has been administered (Kuitunen et al., 2021). A systematic review of in-hospital intravenous medication errors revealed that administration, prescription, and preparation were the stages of the medication-use process where errors are most likely to occur, and confusion between look-alike/sound-alike (LASA) medications consistently turned out to be a systemic factor at the different stages (Kuitunen et al., 2021).

Look-Alike Sound-Alike (LASA) medication errors are the types of patient safety threats that are here to stay on the global level. LASA errors occur when drugs that have orthographic (visual) or phonetic (auditory) resemblances are mixed during prescription, dispensing, preparation, and administration. This confusion can be based on brand-brand, brand-generic, and generic-generic names; similar packaging; labeling; vial size; or ampule shape (Institute for Safe Medication Practices (ISMP), 2022). Clinicians often use rapid visual recognition, as opposed to the intentional reading of labels, in high-acuity environments, especially in the presence of interruptions or other distracting activities, which predisposes them to LASA substitution errors (Cohen, 2007b; Nanji et al., 2016).

Injections of LASA are particularly high risk since most of them are high-vigilance drugs and cannot go through physiological protective measures that involve slower absorption pathways. In their systemic review, Kuitunen et al. (2021) reported confusion between LASA medications as one of the most frequent systemic causes of intravenous errors during the prescribing, preparation, and administration stages (Kuitunen et al., 2021). Additionally, mixing similar ampules, syringes, and infusion bags, especially when the products are removed from the outer cartons and kept in resistance proximity, has been repeatedly reported to be involved in substitution incidence (Cohen, 2007b). Similar and poor labeling practices have been attributed to errors associated with neuromuscular blocking agents, opioids, benzodiazepines, vasopressors and local anesthetics in practice (Abeysekera et al., 2005).

System LASA errors can hardly be traced to individual negligence. Research on human factors has shown that clinicians experience an attitudinal shift in recognition strategies that are heuristic in nature under conditions of heavy workload, fatigue, and time pressure, increasing their susceptibility to perceptual similarity traps (Abeysekera et al., 2005; Reason, 2000). Medication systems, including injectable systems that rely on manual double checks and handwritten labels on syringes or use memory to discriminate one kind of product against another, are fragile in nature. The literature highlights that latent factors that enable substitution errors to reach patients include a lack of standardization in labeling, inadequate segregation of high-alert drugs, deficiencies in the use of double-checking systems, and insufficient technological barriers (e.g., barcode verification and smart infusion pumps) (Institute for Safe Medication Practices (ISMP), 2018, 2022; Kuitunen et al., 2021).

Medication errors are among the most common causes of harm that are preventable across the globe. Medication safety is among the key patient safety priorities determined by the World Health Organization, which estimates that medication-related harm and its costs are billions every year and lead to significant morbidity and mortality (World Health Organization [WHO], 2017). Injectable LASA errors form an example of a high-impact, avoidable category of system failures in this broader context. According to the reports of studies of hospital incident reporting systems, LASA incidents are common in terms of injectable formulations and are often underreported regardless of their lethality (Michelet-Huot et al., 2017).

The concept of injectable LASA errors necessitates a multidimensional approach that involves human factors, system engineering, regulation design, packaging standards, environmental factors, and organizational safety culture. The combination of high-vigilance pharmacology, similar perceptions, and time-sensitive clinical decision-making leads to an anticipable risk environment, as opposed to a sequence of random disasters. The prevention methods should also be wider than personal awareness of systemic redesign—the use of standardized labels, tall man lettering, physical separation of potentially harmful drugs, barcode medication administration units, smart libraries of infusion pumps, and organized double checks based on the principles of reliability science (Institute for Safe Medication Practices (ISMP), 2018, 2022; Kuitunen et al., 2021).

Objectives of the Chapter

The aims of this chapter are as follows:

(1) To explain LASA issues, establish significant terms, and provide a cursory overview of the history of medication errors.
(2) To explore the frequency of injectable LASA errors and determine the clinical settings most prone to errors.
(3) To classify types of similarities that result in injectable medication errors, such as confusion in names, packaging, and appearance, and reasons behind their occurrence.
(4) To identify frequent LASA drug combinations among injectable drugs related to reported harm.
(5) To examine the contributory and risk factors for injectable LASA errors.
(6) To describe processes, prevention measures, and regulatory policies regarding the minimization of injectable LASA medication errors.

Organization of the Chapter

Chapter 12 begins with a brief overview of LASA concerns and the historical background of medication errors, emphasizing injectable medications as one of the highest-risk categories in medication safety. Unlike oral drugs, injectable medications, particularly intravenous agents, produce immediate systemic effects, with little opportunity to intercept errors after administration. The chapter then defines key terminology and reviews the prevalence of injectable LASA errors and the clinical settings most affected. It categorizes similarity mechanisms, names, packaging, and appearance confusion and presents common injectable LASA drug pairs associated with harm. The final sections analyze contributing and risk factors and outline prevention strategies, procedural safeguards, and relevant regulatory and labeling standards to reduce injectable LASA medication errors.

INJECTABLE LASA ERRORS PREVALENCE

One of the most clinically significant types of injectable medication errors in perioperative and critical care practice is incorrect drug administration. Since intravenous drugs obtain immediate systemic bioavailability and often require high-vigilance pharmacologic agents, substitution errors can result in acute physiologic degradation and little to no chance to intervene before the drug is taken. The evidence provided by epidemiologists supports the idea that wrong-drug errors are measured and are clinically reliable enough to occur at quantifiable rates. In another 24-hour multinational prospective study, which was carried out in 113 intensive care units (ICUs) in 27 countries, 861 parenteral medication errors were reported, representing 74.5 errors per 100 patient-days (95% CI 69.5–79.4) (Valentin et al., 2009). These mistakes were divided into five major categories: wrong time of administration (n = 386), missed medication (n = 259), wrong dose (n = 118), wrong drug (n = 61), and wrong route (n = 37). Wrong drug errors thus represented approximately 7% of all reported parenteral errors and had a rate of 5.3 events/100 patient-days. Notably, 0.9% of patients who experienced parenteral medication errors experienced irreversible damage or died. Vasopressors and catecholamines, insulin, coagulation-related agents, electrolytes, antimicrobials, and sedatives or analgesic drugs were included with drug classes associated with serious harm, with many of them being high-alert injectable drugs.

Similar results have been reported in perioperative practice. Nanji et al. (2016) conducted a prospective observational study of 3671 perioperative medication administrations and reported that in the case of 3,671, a minimum of 5% of the medication administrations were medication errors or adverse drug events—just 1 in 20 medication events. There were nine cases of incorrect medication errors (5.9% of the identified medication errors) (Nanji et al., 2016). Among the 896 anesthetic drug error reports examined in the Australian Incident Monitoring Study, 452 cases (50%) were syringe- or drug preparation mechanism-related (Abeysekera et al., 2005). Concentrating on real mistakes (not on preerrors), 155 cases (34%) were syringe swaps, 125 cases (28%) were ampule labeling errors, and 49 cases (11%) were preparation errors; the other reasons included 41 cases (9%). These results suggest that injectable wrong-drug errors occur most commonly during manual preparation and administration and not during prescription and that the similarity at the point of drug handling is a major weakness.

Together, these studies prove that injectable wrong-drug errors are not rare or isolated phenomena. Rather, they are patterned risks that are recurrent and systemically patterned risks that are highly concentrated in high-acuity settings, especially during the preparation and administration of high-alert injectable drugs.

Over a period of more than 20 years, the evidence has been reported and comprises incident monitoring databases, prospective observational studies, regulatory studies, national surveillance systems, systematic reviews, and international safety guidelines (summarized in **Table 1**). Together, the studies indicate that there are recurring tendencies in syringe swaps, similarity of ampules and vials, confusion in naming/packaging, and system susceptibility that mostly arise in pharmaceutical preparation and administration. The alignment of results between case reports, observational studies, national surveillance systems, and international guidance is indicative of the fact that injectable LASA error is neither a one-time event nor a unique structural threat to medication-use systems.

Epidemiologic data from anesthesiology and perioperative practice provide some of the most accurate incidence estimates. A large Norwegian prospective study revealed 0.11% medication errors (63 of 55,426 anesthetics, or 1 in 880 operations). However, 45 (0.08%) drug errors were incorrect, accounting for most of the recorded incidents. Syringe swaps caused 28 of 63 drug mistakes (44%), with muscle relaxants being the most common (Fasting & Gisvold, 2000). Similarly, an Australian study with 896 reports of anesthetic drug errors revealed that almost half of the errors involved syringe or preparation stage errors, with 34 and 28% syringe swaps and ampule labeling errors, respectively (Abeysekera et al., 2005). The preparation stage is always among the key points of weakness. Another example of the underreporting of passive surveillance systems is the approximately 5% rate of perioperative medication errors or adverse drug events in direct observational data from a U.S. academic hospital, which is significantly higher than the rates identified with voluntary reporting (Nanji et al., 2016).

Table 1. Injectable wrong-drug and LASA evidence base across case reports, observational studies, surveillance systems, narrative review, systematic reviews, international guidelines

Setting	Design	Sample/ Scope	Wrong-Drug Findings	LASA Mechanism Identified	High-Alert Drugs Involved	Key Contribution	Study (Year)
Australian anesthesia practice	Incident monitoring analysis	896 anesthetic drug error reports	~50% involved syringe/ preparation errors; 34% syringe swaps; 28% ampule labeling error	Syringe swaps, ampule labeling error	Neuromuscular blockers, vasopressors	Preparation-stage vulnerability	Abeysekera et al. (2005)
479 Thai public hospitals (national survey)	Descriptive national survey with interview validation	7,964 LASA pairs reported; 3,205 unique pairs identified	590 look-alike injectable ampule/ vial pairs (same manufacturer) and 417 injectable ampule/vial pairs (different manufacturers); (12.64% of all reported LASA pairs)	Look-alike ampule/vial labeling; similar font, size, color; strength differentiation failure; same-manufacturer packaging similarity	Injectable cardiovascular agents, sedatives, and other high-alert injectables implicated through packaging similarity	Provides national-level quantification showing injectable ampule/vial similarity accounts for >12% of LASA burden; highlights packaging-driven risk in parenteral medications	Chumchit et al. (2015)
Tertiary hospital (India)	Retrospective (36 months)	1,311 errors; 35 LASA (2.67%)	64.71% of LASA involved injectables; majority near-miss (74.28%)	68.57% phonetic similarity; 22.85% drug container or packaging similarity	Dopamine–Dobutamine; $MgSO_4$–Ondansetron; Inj.Doxorubicin vial – Inj. Cisplatin vial	Resource-limited injectable LASA vulnerability	Dhande et al. (2021)

continued on following page

Table 1. Continued

Setting	Design	Sample/ Scope	Wrong-Drug Findings	LASA Mechanism Identified	High-Alert Drugs Involved	Key Contribution	Study (Year)
Tertiary anesthesia practice (India)	Observational correspondence/ case examples	Reported multiple look-alike ampule and vial combinations	Numerous injectable look-alike pairs identified (e.g., ranitidine–chlorpheniramine; midazolam–heparin; atracurium–noradrenaline; potassium chloride–sodium bicarbonate)	Look-alike ampule/vial packaging; color and font similarity; procurement-driven packaging similarity	Vasopressors; muscle relaxants; electrolytes; sedatives	Highlights real-world packaging-driven injectable LASA hazards in resource-limited systems; emphasizes high-alert injectable risk	Dsouza and Kulkarni (2017)
Simulated operating room crisis (US)	Randomized controlled simulation study	89 anesthesia trainees	40% incorrect medication selection with standard labels vs 63% correct with redesigned labels; lidocaine–hetastarch look-alike IV bag confusion replicated	Label design deficiencies; visual similarity; stocking error; failure to detect incorrect IV bag	Lidocaine (500 mL IV) vs Hetastarch (500 mL IV)	Provides experimental evidence that improved label design significantly reduces wrong-drug selection in high-stress settings	Estock et al. (2018)

continued on following page

Table 1. Continued

Setting	Design	Sample/ Scope	Wrong-Drug Findings	LASA Mechanism Identified	High-Alert Drugs Involved	Key Contribution	Study (Year)
University hospital anesthesia department (Norway)	Prospective 36-month observational study (18 months before and after color-coded syringe labels)	55,426 procedures	63 drug errors (0.11%; 1:880); 45 were wrong-drug errors (0.08%; 1:1230). 28 syringe swaps (44%), 9 ampule swaps (14%), 8 other wrong-drug (13%). Muscle relaxants most frequently involved.	Syringe swaps between equal-size syringes; ampule similarity (e.g., glycopyrrolate vs glycopyrrolate/ neostigmine); visual similarity; reliance on pattern recognition	Neuromuscular blockers (succinylcholine, nondepolarizing agents), glycopyrrolate/ neostigmine, opioids	Provides prospective incidence data; demonstrates limited effect of color-coded syringe labels; confirms muscle relaxants as highest-risk injectable class	Fasting and Gisvold (2000)
FDA medication error analysis (US)	Regulatory review of 265 medication error reports	265 FDA error reports (2001 analysis)	20% attributed to labeling issues; 3% packaging/ design; 13% name confusion	Label readability, packaging similarity, proprietary name confusion	Not drug specific; applies broadly including high-alert injectables	Quantifies labeling- and name-related contributions to medication errors	Fontaine (2004)

continued on following page

Table 1. Continued

Setting	Design	Sample/ Scope	Wrong-Drug Findings	LASA Mechanism Identified	High-Alert Drugs Involved	Key Contribution	Study (Year)
Spinal anesthesia (orthopedic surgery)	Case report (Letter)	1 patient (76 M)	Intrathecal injection of dopamine (~80 mg) instead of intended 0.5% bupivacaine for spinal anesthesia; no long-term neurologic sequelae reported	Look-alike ampules (dopamine and bupivacaine similar in size, color, and shape); failure to verify prior to neuraxial injection	Dopamine (vasoactive agent; high-risk if administered via wrong route)	Demonstrates classic ampule-level LASA substitution in neuraxial anesthesia with catastrophic potential; underscores need for ampule differentiation and independent verification	Hong et al. (2014)

continued on following page

Table 1. Continued

Setting	Design	Sample/ Scope	Wrong-Drug Findings	LASA Mechanism Identified	High-Alert Drugs Involved	Key Contribution	Study (Year)
Perioperative anesthesia (thoracic surgery with thoracic epidural catheter)	Case report	1 patient (69F)	Wrong-route administration: IV-prepared sugammadex 200 mg + ramosetron 0.3 mg administered epidurally instead of intended epidural analgesic mixture	Wrong-syringe selection during delegation/ handoff; coexisting syringes prepared for different routes; inadequate verification prior to neuraxial injection	Sugammadex (neuromuscular blockade reversal agent; perioperative critical med) + ramosetron (antiemetic)	Illustrates high-severity risk of neuraxial wrong-route error driven by syringe similarity and workflow breakdown; supports route-specific safeguards and independent double-checks	Kim et al. (2026)

continued on following page

Table 1. Continued

Setting	Design	Sample/ Scope	Wrong-Drug Findings	LASA Mechanism Identified	High-Alert Drugs Involved	Key Contribution	Study (Year)
22 Thai hospitals (perioperative anesthesia)	Prospective multicenter observational incident-report study	85 medication errors from 2,206 anesthesia incident reports (4.25%)	Wrong-drug administration accounted for 19 cases (22.4%), including syringe swaps and wrong ampule selection; 18.8% of events caused temporary harm (NCC MERP E–F)	Syringe swaps; wrong ampule selection; labeling problems (17.6%); haste (62.4%); miscommunication; look-alike manufacturer packaging	Opioids, neuromuscular blockers, vasoactive agents (e.g., ephedrine–morphine substitution; fentanyl–pancuronium)	Provides national Thai epidemiologic data demonstrating high proportion of perioperative wrong-drug errors driven by labeling and look-alike ampule issues; confirms pediatric vulnerability and preventability	Lerdsirisopon et al. (2018)
University hospital	Retrospective 36-month analysis	28 LASA incidents (6.4% of total medication errors)	60.7% involved injectable forms; 57% LASA drug occurred during drug administration	Confusion between similar drug names and same ATC-class drugs (71.4%)	Opioids (28.6%), antibiotics (14.3%)	Demonstrates high proportion of injectable LASA events and severity risk during administration stage	Michelet-Huot et al. (2017)

continued on following page

Table 1. Continued

Setting	Design	Sample/ Scope	Wrong-Drug Findings	LASA Mechanism Identified	High-Alert Drugs Involved	Key Contribution	Study (Year)
Perioperative (US academic hospital)	Direct observation + chart review	3,671 perioperative medication administrations	~5% medication error/ADE rate; substitution a meaningful subset	Selection and labeling errors	Opioids, anesthetics, vasoactive agents	Demonstrates higher error detection with active surveillance	Nanji et al. (2016)
Tertiary hospital anesthesia practice (Nigeria)	Case reports + literature review	2 near-fatal perioperative cases	Case 1: Pancuronium administered instead of suxamethonium (substitution error); Case 2: Thiopentone overdose due to vial strength confusion (1 g mistaken for 500 mg)	Look-alike ampules; vial strength similarity; human error; failure to verify before administration	Neuromuscular blockers; induction agents (thiopentone)	Illustrates classic substitution and strength-confusion errors in anesthesia; reinforces role of look-alike packaging and need for standardized color coding and vigilance	Ogboli-Nwasor (2013)

continued on following page

Table 1. Continued

Setting	Design	Sample/ Scope	Wrong-Drug Findings	LASA Mechanism Identified	High-Alert Drugs Involved	Key Contribution	Study (Year)
Pharmacy and perioperative settings (Anesthetics Department, PACU) in a regional Australian tertiary hospital	Retrospective incident-report analysis with concurrent MedSCIM safety culture assessment.	246 medication incidents over 5 years (46 LASA-related; 18.7%)	LASA errors accounted for 18.7% of medication incidents; "incorrect medication" and "incorrect dose" common; majority involved packaging-related confusion; high-risk medications frequently implicated in perioperative area	Naming similarity (34.8%); packaging similarity (41.3%); naming + packaging (15.2%); syringe swaps (8.7%); medication selection based on packaging familiarity or storage location	High-risk medications per ISMP/ Australian Classification of a high-risk medication definitions; perioperative classes frequently involved: adrenergic agents, anesthetics, opioids, benzodiazepines, anticoagulants	Quantifies burden of LASA incidents in perioperative environment; demonstrates packaging-driven risk predominance (65.2%); links LASA errors to reactive safety culture, supporting system-level mitigation strategies	Ryan et al. (2025)
128 Thai hospitals	Cross-sectional survey	2,510 LASA pairs	427 injection pairs (17.01% of LASA); injections frequently Category B errors; harmful injectable pairs reported	63.14% name similarity; 29.10% injection packaging similarity	Ceftriaxone–Ceftazidime; insulin mixtures	National-level quantification of injectable LASA burden	Supapaan et al. (2024)

continued on following page

Table 1. Continued

Setting	Design	Sample/ Scope	Wrong-Drug Findings	LASA Mechanism Identified	High-Alert Drugs Involved	Key Contribution	Study (Year)
113 ICUs, 27 countries	Prospective 24-hr observational study	861 parenteral administration errors	5.3 wrong-drug errors per 100 patient-days; 0.9% permanent harm/ death	Drug confusion during administration	Vasopressors, sedatives, electrolytes	Provides population-level incidence of injectable wrong-drug errors	Valentin et al. (2009)
Large tertiary hospital, China (10 Operating room)	Prospective randomized open-label clinical trial	10,812 anesthesia medication administrations (1,066 cases)	Total error rate: 11.9% (manual carts) vs 7.3% (automated carts); substitution errors 1.1%	Manual drawer selection; substitution errors; documentation errors; reliance on human memory; cart layout vulnerability	Not stratified by specific drug class (perioperative injectable medications overall)	Demonstrates that automation reduces documentation errors but does not eliminate substitution (wrong-drug) errors, confirming persistent human-factor vulnerability in injectable selection	Wang et al. (2017)

continued on following page

Table 1. Continued

Setting	Design	Sample/ Scope	Wrong-Drug Findings	LASA Mechanism Identified	High-Alert Drugs Involved	Key Contribution	Study (Year)
Statewide healthcare facilities (127 facilities; acute care, ICU, ED, surgical units, etc.)	Retrospective surveillance analysis of mandatory reporting database (the Pennsylvania Patient Safety Reporting System (PA-PSRS)	450 wrong-drug events (WDEs) that reached patients in 2023	Wrong-drug events represented clinically significant medication errors; 12 classified as serious events; insulin most frequently involved; omission, unintended administration, and route errors reported	Orthographic/phonetic name similarity (shared stems), same-class confusion (e.g., insulin–insulin, epinephrine–norepinephrine), packaging similarity, ADC selection errors, storage and selection proximity	High-alert medications prominent: insulin (29.8% of high-alert meds), opioids, IV adrenergic agonists, neuromuscular blockers, magnesium sulfate, oxytocin, antithrombotics	Provides large-scale real-world evidence that wrong-drug events—including LASA mechanisms—contribute to serious harm; quantifies high-alert injectable involvement and highlights same-class naming vulnerability	Ro and Jones (2025)

continued on following page

Table 1. Continued

Setting	Design	Sample/ Scope	Wrong-Drug Findings	LASA Mechanism Identified	High-Alert Drugs Involved	Key Contribution	Study (Year)
International acute care & perioperative settings	Evidence-based practice guidelines/ consensus recommendations	Focus on high-alert IV and perioperative medications across healthcare systems	Wrong-drug and wrong-route errors frequently occur during manual IV preparation, syringe swaps, and perioperative medication handling; neuraxial and reversal-agent mix-ups highlighted as high-severity risks	Inadequate syringe labeling, look-alike packaging, storage proximity, failure of barcode scanning, ADC overrides, manual compounding outside pharmacy control	Insulin, IV vasopressors, opioids, neuromuscular blockers, reversal agents, concentrated electrolytes	Establishes system-level prevention standards for high-alert IV use; defines engineering controls (barcode verification, standardized labeling, segregation, pharmacy-prepared syringes) as core safeguards	Institute for Safe Medication Practices (ISMP) (2022)

continued on following page

Table 1. Continued

Setting	Design	Sample/ Scope	Wrong-Drug Findings	LASA Mechanism Identified	High-Alert Drugs Involved	Key Contribution	Study (Year)
Asia and Australia (multicountry healthcare settings)	Systematic review (PRISMA-guided; JBI quality appraisal)	39 eligible studies (2017–2022) from 7,799 screened records	Wrong-drug errors frequently reported within dispensing and prescribing categories; 14 studies identified wrong-drug incidents; wrong-dose also highly prevalent; injectable-related errors reported in hospital settings	Contributing factors: high workload, human factors, system failures, environmental issues, look-alike/sound-alike drug names reported in multiple studies	Not drug-specific in pooled analysis; hospital-based errors frequently involved high-alert classes (e.g., opioids, anticoagulants, insulin, pediatric dosing)	Provides regional epidemiologic synthesis demonstrating persistent burden of wrong-drug and wrong-dose errors in Asia–Australia; identifies workload and system weaknesses as dominant drivers, supporting need for structural safeguards	Annisa et al. (2023)

continued on following page

Table 1. Continued

Setting	Design	Sample/ Scope	Wrong-Drug Findings	LASA Mechanism Identified	High-Alert Drugs Involved	Key Contribution	Study (Year)
Perioperative setting (US)	Narrative review	Literature synthesis including observational and closed-claims data	Drug administration error rate ~0.75% in anesthesia; accidental substitution 30%; incorrect dose 20%; 63% IV bolus-related; ~1 in every 250 drug errors potentially fatal	Syringe substitution; similar vial appearance	Neuromuscular blockers, vasopressors, opioids, induction agents	Defines the abbreviated OR medication workflow; frames syringe swaps and injectable substitution as systemic perioperative vulnerability	Hanna and Levine (2011)
In-hospital IV medication systems (six countries)	Systematic review (11 observational studies)	11 studies examining systemic causes of IV medication errors	LASA confusion identified as a recurrent systemic cause across prescribing, preparation, dispensing, and administration stages	Name and packaging similarity; confusion between similar drug names and packages	Catecholamines, insulin, electrolytes, opioids (highlighted as high-alert IV drugs in ICU settings)	Establishes LASA as a cross-stage systemic risk factor in IV medication processes	Kuitunen et al. (2021)
Operating room medication safety	Narrative review	Literature synthesis	Wrong-drug and substitution errors common in OR; manual preparation and high-acuity environment amplify risk	Syringe swaps; similar packaging; lack of standardized preparation; environmental stressors	Neuromuscular blockers; vasopressors; opioids	Synthesizes perioperative injectable error mechanisms; supports system redesign and standardization	Wahr et al. (2017)

Analysis of the state of the United States revealed 450 wrong-drug events to reach patients in one year, with 12 severe events; regularly involved were insulin and other high-risk injectable drugs (Ro & Jones, 2025). Thailand registered 427 injectable LASA pairs, which is 17.01% of the reported LASA pairs, which confirmed that the injections were a significant type of burden (Supapaan et al., 2024). In a national survey of 479 public hospitals in Thailand, 1,007 of 7,964 reported LASA pairs (12.6) were associated with load-like injectable ampule and vial products: packaging-based injectable confusion is an important factor in national medication safety risk (Chumchit et al., 2015). One of the most commonly reported injectable LASA pairs is diazepam (10 mg/2 mL) and furosemide (20 mg/2 mL), which are manufactured by the Government Pharmaceutical Organization (GPO). These products were identified as look-alike ampules because of their highly similar packaging appearance (Bueng Kan Hospital, 2021; Chumchit et al., 2015) (**Figure 1**).

Figure 1. Diazepam (10 mg/2 mL) and furosemide (20 mg/2 mL) injections resulted in a similar ampule appearance

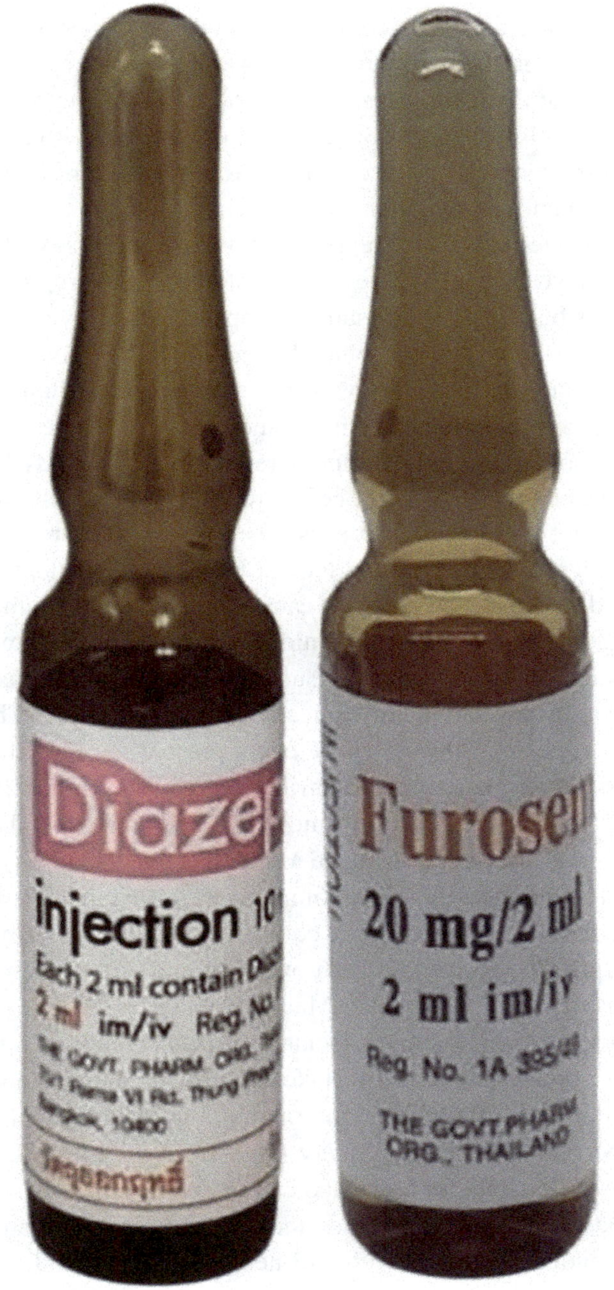

The pharmaceutical products shown are presented solely for academic and educational purposes. Their inclusion does not imply the endorsement, promotion, or advertising of any specific manufacturer, distributor, or brand.

Asian, Australian, and multicountry hospital-based systematic reviews also supported the idea that LASA confusion represents a systematic contributor that occurs repeatedly at different stages of prescription, preparation, dispensing, and administration (Annisa et al., 2023; Kuitunen et al., 2021). Taken together, these results support the idea that incorrect drug errors that occur in an injectable form are neither infrequent nor geographically isolated.

In the same manner, a statewide review of wrong drug events (WDEs) in healthcare facilities in Pennsylvania in 2023 revealed that the wrong-drug error was an issue with medications belonging to the same therapeutic category or with medications that were phonetically or orthographically similar (Ro & Jones, 2025). The most affected class was insulin products, which are often mixed with other insulins that have the same stems (e.g., lispro, regular, and glargine). There was also a general interchange of vasopressors (epinephrine-norepinephrine), opioids (hydromorphone-morphine), and antibiotics (cefazolin-ceftriaxone). These results confirm that LASA mechanisms are not one-time occurrences but are recurrent sources of incorrect drug occurrences. According to further reports of the Pennsylvania Patient Safety Authority, wrong-drug and wrong-dose events are caused by medication name confusion and unsafe abbreviation practices. As an example, mix-ups of MSO4 (morphine sulfate) and MgSO4 (magnesium sulfate) and insulin dosing mistakes in cases where U was used to denote units have all led to clinically significant events (The Pennsylvania Patient Safety Advisory, 2005a). These cases present the idea that orthographic similarity and unsafe notation can contribute directly to medication substitution errors. The systemic vulnerability of injectable medications is also facilitated by magnitude-of-error analyses. Cavell and Mandaliya conducted a seven-year search of the literature covering the incidence of incorrect dosing in hospitals and reported that errors in doses two and tenfold were common across the prescribing, dispensing, and administering phases and that both overdose and underdose were reported in adult and pediatric practice (Cavell & Mandaliya, 2021). Mistakes associated with such a scale were most commonly associated with calculations, an incorrect choice of units (mg vs. micrograms), and mistakes in infusion programming.

Owing to this body of evidence, international guidelines, including the ISMP IV and Perioperative Medication Safety Guidelines, highlight system-level prevention measures (Institute for Safe Medication Practices (ISMP), 2022). Some of the recommended protective measures include pharmacy-prepared standardized syringes, independent double-checking of neuraxial and high-alert drugs, barcode verification before administration, physical separation of like drugs, reducing automated dispensing cabinet overrides, and using engineering controls instead of the vigilance mode. The evolution of evidence, which progresses from individual case reports to national surveillance studies and finally to systematic international guidelines, logically demonstrates that the system's structure needs to be redesigned rather than placing blame on individuals. Overall, wrong-drug and LASA errors are cross-national patient safety risks that continue to persist because of the similarity of syringes, ampule packaging similarity, confusion of names and high-at-risk drugs, and workflow failure. Prevention has multilayered needs that involve engineering controls, standardized labeling, optimal storage, sound verification procedures, and a proactive safety culture (Fasting & Gisvold, 2000).

LASA Mechanisms Underlying Injectable Wrong-Drug Errors

LASA mechanisms are often the cause of incorrect injectable drug errors. In-hospital intravenous medication errors identified in the systematic review were found to be caused by similar drug names and drug packaging as common systemic factors at all stages of prescription, preparation, and administration (Kuitunen et al., 2021). Such weaknesses are enforced in settings that involve time pressure, interruptions, and a dependence on the quick speed of visual recognition.

The influence of physical similarity is especially strong for injectables. The ampules and vials frequently include withdrawals of outer cartons and are placed in close proximity within the anesthesia carts or automated dispensing cabinets. In these circumstances, clinicians can use pattern recognition rather than deliberate label verification. Syringe swaps are often related to the use of syringes of a similar size, which highlights the role played by physical design attributes in determining substitution risk.

Vulnerability is further exacerbated by labeling and packaging features. Perioperative safety studies have reported that approximately 20% of medication errors are a result of labeling flaws, 3% are a result of packaging similarity, and 13% are a result of name confusion (Al-Nasser, 2005; Fontaine, 2004). Although these percentages represent more general categories of medication errors, they represent the quantifiable role played by perceptual similarity in causing wrong drug events.

Injectable substitution errors are disproportionate with regard to high-alert medications. Intravenous catecholamines, insulin, opioids, and concentrated electrolytes are often linked to severe injury. The most frequent drug classes that were related to administration errors in multinational ICU data were sedatives and analgesics (9%), antimicrobials (9%), vasopressors (8%), and electrolytes (6%) (Valentin et al., 2009). When LASA mechanisms interact with high-alert drugs, the probability of irreversible or severe damage is significant.

Methodological Considerations and Underreporting

The incorrect drug incidence associated with injected drugs should be interpreted with consideration of the error-detection methodology. Compared with voluntary reporting systems, potential structured surveillance always has high error rates. The latter article by Valentin et al. (2009) on multinational ICUs revealed that a specific 24-hour observational system revealed 861 parenteral medication errors in one day, with 61 incorrect drug events. This proactive surveillance method is in contrast to passive reporting systems, which rely on the recognition of clinicians, perceived severity, and the desire to report—elements that are also known to play a role in systematic underestimation (Valentin et al., 2009).

Evidence from systematic reviews also presents a problem in terms of methodological limitations. Kuitunen et al. (2021) reviewed systematic factors of in-hospital intravenous medication errors and reported that the included studies included observational studies, and many often used voluntary or retrospective reporting. The authors highlighted that the stages of the process that were most susceptible to systemic error were administration, prescription, and preparation and that LASA confusion is a common cross-stage factor (Kuitunen et al., 2021).

Mechanistically, incident monitoring systems are useful in the sense that they can provide valuable insights, but they cannot give us rates on a population level. A study by Australian Incident Monitoring reported that approximately 50% of anesthetic drug errors occurred through syringe or preparation mechanisms (Abeysekera et al., 2005). LASA surveillance at the hospital also revealed that most of the reported cases of LASA were related to injectable preparations and that a significant percentage of the cases were categorized as potentially lethal (Michelet-Huot et al., 2017). Since the analyses are based on the reported incidents, there is probably a higher incidence than is indicated by the documented statistics.

The evidence of a systematic review proves that medication confusion, of similar names and packaging, is a frequent systemic factor in intravenous medication procedures (Kuitunen et al., 2021). Hospital LASA analyses go on to show that injectable forms are often involved and mostly portray high severity potential.

Three convergent trends are identified: errors related to injectable wrong drugs have quantifiable rates; the preparation and administration phases are the most susceptible locations; and high-risk medications such as vasopressors, neuromuscular blockers, insulin, opioids, and concentrated electrolytes are the most prone to causing serious harm. Since injectable drugs have systemic effects immediately and are often eliminated by secondary verification as soon as they are ready, the severity potential of substitution is increased.

Pediatric and Neonatal Injectable Wrong-Drug Intention.

Children and newborns are two especially vulnerable groups in terms of injectable drug delivery systems. The effects of substitution errors are increased by weight-based dosing, a small physiologic reserve, a small therapeutic index, and a dependence on intravenous therapy.

The multinational ICU cohort consisted of pediatric and neonatal units, but the rates of incorrect drug use were not stratified by age and were not reported separately (Valentin et al., 2009). Evidence from a systematic review (studies of neonatal intensive care) revealed LASA confusion as a common systemic factor in the occurrence of intravenous medication errors (Kuitunen et al., 2021). Serious outcomes were disproportionately related to high-alert agents, e.g., catecholamines, insulin, opioids, and concentrated electrolytes.

Neonatal injectable systems further add structural weaknesses, such as bedside dilution, manual syringe preparation, small quantities of administration, and the cognitive load of weight-based prescriptions. At least there are not enough pediatric-specific incidence numbers, but the existing statistics show increased susceptibility to serious injuries in the case of injectable substitution. In this respect, pediatric and neonatal injectable practices should be considered among the priority domains in which structured LASA mitigation strategies are implemented.

TYPES OF SIMILARITIES LEADING TO INJECTABLE MEDICATION ERRORS

LASA errors associated with injectable medications constitute one of the high-risk groups for medication safety incidents. In contrast to oral preparations, injectable drugs, particularly those in anesthetic or emergency practice and critical care, usually exhibit instantaneous physiological action, small therapeutic indices, and a scant possibility of error correction after the medicine is given.

The presence of injectable LASA errors is proven by available published case studies and institutional studies, which indicate that most errors are the result of five interrelated similarity mechanisms that include visual similarity between ampules and vials, similarity in packaging of the products by manufacturers, variability of concentration in the same injectable drug, constraint of label layout and typing techniques, and storage set-ups and workflow.

Visual Similarity

Local Anesthetic vs. Diluent: Levobupivacaine and Saline

One near-miss event was recorded with 10 mL of 0.75 mL of levobupivacaine, which is a high-concentration local anesthetic very closely resembling 10 mL of 0.9% sodium chloride after the redesign of the packaging. Its redesign made the ampules look physically similar in size, color, and general appearance. The authors stressed the idea that a potentially cardiotoxic anesthetic agent must not resemble a nontoxic diluent, and the situation was defined as a dangerous incident with latent risk (Astin et al., 2015).

Neuromuscular Blocking Agent vs. Sedative: Cisatracurium and Midazolam

One of the severe medication errors was the accidental delivery of cisatracurium rather than midazolam as a result of look-alike ampules (Graudins et al., 2016). Before proper anesthesia was achieved, the patient was in paralysis while she was awake. Similar labeling, leftover ampules on the anesthetic cart, and no independent double-checking were the factors that were identified in the root cause analysis (Graudins et al., 2016). The corrective actions included auxiliary red labeling, separation of neuromuscular blocking agents, and reinforcement of verification procedures.

Other Look-Alike Injectable Pairs

Correspondence records indicated that there were numerous visually similar injectable pairs, such as atracurium versus noradrenaline, midazolam versus heparin, sodium bicarbonate versus potassium chloride, and ranitidine versus chlorpheniramine. According to the authors, approximately one-third of confusing cases of medication are associated with analogous packaging and labeling (Dsouza & Kulkarni, 2017).

Manufacturer Packaging Similarity in Infusion Products

One of the hospitals reported an error of 500 mg of metronidazole in 100 mL of intravenous infusion (IV) and 0.9% sodium chloride in 100 mL of intravenous infusion (IV) provided by the same manufacturer but with different packaging arrangements. The resemblance was discovered when the products were introduced following changes in the procurement process. The mitigation measures included product separation and manufacturer replacement (Ramaswamy & Naik, 2014).

Concentration Variability Within the Same Injectable Drug

Alfentanil Concentration of 500 mcg/mL versus 5 mg/mL

One of the documented near misses was caused by the confusion of the two injectable concentrations of alfentanil, 500 mcg/mL and 5 mg/mL. Ampules with higher concentrations were drawn up twice, which led to a syringe holding 10 mg of ampules, as opposed to the originally planned 1 mg. The authors demonstrated that the similarity of the appearance of ampules of different strengths contributes greatly to the risk of overdose (Pandey & Philip, 2011).

Label Layout and Typography

The design constraints of labels were directly involved in the epidemic of cisatracurium-midazolam (Graudins et al., 2016). Equally, Astin et al. (2015) reported that regulatory advice contributing to prudent application of color might be wanting when human factor considerations are not implemented in the latter (Astin et al., 2015).

Storage Configuration and Workflow Factors

The case of cisatracurium involves the presence of discarded ampules from a previous operation on the anesthetic cart when the next urgent case was being considered, which also contributed to the missed opportunity (Graudins et al., 2016). There was also an incident of dispensing near misses, as injectable fosphenytoin was sent back into the incorrect storage place and almost dispensed rather than paricalcitol because of visual similarity (Cohen, 2008). The transmission of incorrect information to patients was avoided.

These confirmable cases reveal that injectable LASA mechanisms are recurrently reported in anesthesia and in the inpatient hospital environment. To prevent this event, it is necessary to segregate high-alert injectables, label auxiliary items, perform a double-check, conduct a proactive packaging review, and carry out a human-factor-informed design assessment (Astin et al., 2015; Graudins et al., 2016).

COMMON LASA DRUG PAIRS INJECTABLE MEDICATIONS

Neuromuscular Blocking Agents (NMBAs)

Neuromuscular blocking agents (NMBAs) are always reported to be high-risk injectable agents in perioperative medication error reports, especially in wrong-drug substitution incidents. A retrospective study of 896 Australian Incident Monitoring Study (AIMS) drug error reports revealed a 50.4% rate of syringe and drug preparation errors, with the most commonly involved drugs being neuromuscular blocking agents (Abeysekera et al., 2005). In these reports, errors in the choice of the wrong ampule and the replacement of the syringe were the most noticeable mechanisms, which may have occurred in the circumstances of inattention, haste, labeling confusion, and fatigue.

An in-depth analysis of quality improvements at Johns Hopkins Hospital revealed six cases where vecuronium was accidentally used in place of cefazolin because of the similarity in the appearance of the vials and the boat-like neighbors to be stored on automated dispensing systems (Herzer et al., 2013). Neuromuscular blocking agents can induce an awake-paralyzed state in which patients are awake but unable to breathe upon the use of these drugs as a single agent. Factors such as similar packaging, the nature of labels, and storage closeness were contributing factors. This incident resulted in institutional corrective measures and a nationwide recall of the product in question (Herzer et al., 2013). The Institute of Safe Medication Practices (ISMP) has reported several incidences of accidental introduction of neuromuscular blocking drugs because of package and labeling look-alikes. The incidents reported are confusion over pancuronium and vaccine diluents, influenza vaccines, and heparin flush solutions, which in some cases have resulted in respiratory arrest (Smetzer & Cohen, 2006). These reports indicate that the comparability of the vial size, label color emphasis, and storage proximity are common contributing variables.

A recent scoping review of look-alike drugs during the perioperative situation also supported the idea that incorrect drug errors were the most common look-alike incident, and neuromuscular blocking drugs were consistently mentioned among the high-risk injectable drugs (Ryan et al., 2024). The review revealed that the strategies for reducing risks often included the standardization of storage, look-alike product separation, labeling, and system-level protection as opposed to the use of technology alone. These results confirm the important fact that neuromuscular blocking agents constitute an urgent group of injectable LASA drugs for use in the perioperative room.

Mistakes are usually a result of ampule selection errors, the switching of syringes, and confusion during storage. Since these agents cause skeletal muscle paralysis, unintended administration is life-threatening to patients, especially in cases of unforeseen ventilation. Visual similarity during high-intensity perioperative selection is also more prone to increased orthographic patterns observed in neuromuscular blocking agents, such as the suffixes -curium and -ethonium. Although cisatracurium and suxamethonium are not pharmacologically similar, their similarity in terms of their naming structure, as well as being presented in the same way, reflects how similar orthographic patterns can be used to create look-alike risk. An example of an NMBA is shown in **Figure 2**.

Figure 2. Representative examples of neuromuscular blocking agents (suxamethonium and cisatracurium) illustrating naming structure and orthographic similarity

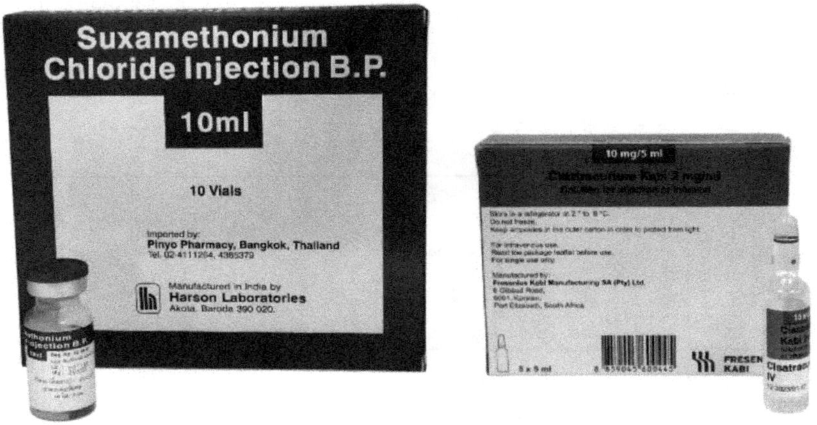

This figure does not depict a documented medication error involving this drug pair or their respective brands.

The pharmaceutical products shown are presented solely for academic and educational purposes. Their inclusion does not imply the endorsement, promotion, or advertising of any specific manufacturer, distributor, or brand.

Table 2 presents evidence that NMBA substitution errors take place in various clinical nodes, comprising pharmacy preparation and dispensing, automated dispensing cabinet (ADC) stockings, operating room administration and ICU infusion management, emergency department vaccination environments, and pediatric wards. The scope of the settings indicates the extensive spread of injectable drugs in hospitals and the systemic risk of LASA. The data in Table 2 also demonstrate that NMBA-related LASA events are multifactorial and involve human factors, packaging design, vulnerabilities in the electronic system, and storage practices. These similar mechanisms, which are repeated in various institutions, indicate that prevention should be instituted through structural protection and not just through the keenness of individuals.

Table 2. Documented LASA substitution pairs involving neuromuscular blocking agents (NMBAs), summarizing the drug classes involved, primary error mechanisms, clinical context, reported consequences, contributing system factors, recommended prevention strategies, and supporting references

LASA Pair	Drug Classes Involved	Primary LASA Mechanism	Clinical Context/Node of Error	Reported Clinical Consequence	System-Level Contributing Factors	Key Prevention Strategies Identified	Reference
Atracurium – Hepatitis B Vaccine	NMBA vs. Vaccine	Look-alike packaging; unsafe storage; atracurium injected instead of hepatitis B vaccine	Nursery refrigerator; pediatric setting	Respiratory distress; permanent injury; death reported	Inappropriate anesthesia drug floor stock; visual similarity	Restrict NMBA access; segregate refrigeration; limit availability to ventilated areas	Smetzer and Cohen (2006)
Atracurium – Sterile water	NMBA vs. Diluent	Similar vial color accents; atracurium nearly used instead of sterile water (near miss)	Respiratory box in the refrigerator	Near miss (intercepted)	Inadvertent return to storage box	Segregated storage; labeling safeguards	Smetzer and Cohen (2006)
Atracurium – Protamine	NMBA vs. Antidote (heparin reversal agent)	Incorrect cart storage; atracurium administered instead of protamine	Operating room (postvascular surgery)	Respiratory compromise; no reported awareness; patient recovered	Atracurium stored in incorrect cart; missing red warning label; failure to double-check	Cart standardization; ongoing storage audits; reinforcement of labeling policy; double-check compliance	Graudins et al. (2016)
Atracurium – Vecuronium	NMBA vs. NMBA	Name similarity; preparation error; vecuronium prepared instead of atracurium infusion	Pharmacy infusion preparation	Wrong NMBA administered	Similar naming within NMBA class	Segregated storage; verification prior to dispensing	Santell (2006)

continued on following page

Table 2. Continued

LASA Pair	Drug Classes Involved	Primary LASA Mechanism	Clinical Context/Node of Error	Reported Clinical Consequence	System-Level Contributing Factors	Key Prevention Strategies Identified	Reference
Cisatracurium – Antibiotic Infusion (Unintended IV bag)	NMBA vs. Antibiotic	Similar IV bag labeling; interruption during verification; cisatracurium infused instead of prescribed antibiotic	ICU/medical unit; infusion preparation	Respiratory arrest requiring ventilation	Similar label color; interruption; stacked infusions	Read-back verification; avoid stacked IV bags; double check before administration	Smetzer and Cohen (2006)
Cisatracurium – Cisplatin	NMBA vs. Antineoplastic	Electronic mnemonic autocomplete; orthographic similarity; cisatracurium prepared and dispensed instead of cisplatin	Pharmacy computer order entry and dispensing	Potential catastrophic substitution (high-alert NMBA dispensed instead of chemotherapy)	Mnemonic autofill rule; insufficient verification of generated label	Review mnemonic rules; computerized cross-check alerts; independent double verification	Santell (2006)
Cisatracurium – Midazolam	NMBA vs. Benzodiazepine	Selection error; midazolam administered instead of intended cisatracurium	Emergency Department (intubated patient)	Extra dose of midazolam; no permanent harm reported	Look-alike ampules; incomplete implementation of safeguards	In-house NMBA warning labels; mandatory double check; storage audit; red-barrel syringes	Graudins et al. (2016)
Cisatracurium – Midazolam	NMBA vs. Benzodiazepine	Selection error; cisatracurium administered instead of intended midazolam	Radiology (intubated patient during imaging)	Unintended paralysis; mechanical ventilation increased; no permanent harm	Look-alike ampules; labeling similarity; workflow interruption	Auxiliary red warning labels; segregation; mandatory double check; guideline implementation	Graudins et al. (2016)

continued on following page

Table 2. Continued

LASA Pair	Drug Classes Involved	Primary LASA Mechanism	Clinical Context/Node of Error	Reported Clinical Consequence	System-Level Contributing Factors	Key Prevention Strategies Identified	Reference
Doxazosin – Doxacurium	Cardiovascular agent vs. NMBA	Orthographic similarity; computer entry error; doxacurium entered instead of doxazosin	Pharmacy computer entry	High-risk wrong-drug substitution potential	Similar drug names; data entry error	Careful review of entered orders; system alerts	Santell (2006)
Mivacurium – Metronidazole	NMBA vs. Antibiotic	Foil overwrap similarity; labeling error; mivacurium dispensed instead of metronidazole	Pharmacy stocking and dispensing	Respiratory arrest; death; serious injury	Trial stock; mislabeling; look-alike packaging	Sequester NMBA stock; enhanced pharmacy verification	Smetzer and Cohen (2006)
Norcuron® (vecuronium) – Narcan® (naloxone)	NMBA vs. Opioid antagonist	Brand–generic name confusion; verbal clarification error; vecuronium administered instead of naloxone	ICU automated dispensing cabinet	Respiratory arrest (recovered)	Generic name unfamiliarity; verbal confusion	Education; brand–generic cross-reference alerts	Smetzer and Cohen (2006) Santell (2006)
Pancuronium – Sodium Chloride (Vaccine Diluent)	NMBA vs. Diluent	Look-alike vial; pancuronium used instead of sodium chloride diluent for measles/BCG vaccines	Vaccine preparation; ward/nursery setting	Respiratory arrest; infant death	Identical vial size; similar label color; inappropriate floor stock	Physical segregation; fluorescent warning labels	Smetzer and Cohen (2006)
Pancuronium – Influenza vaccine	NMBA vs. Vaccine	Look-alike vial and label; pancuronium administered instead of influenza vaccine	Emergency department (ED) vaccination setting	Dyspnea; respiratory depression	Adjacent refrigerator storage; similar labeling	Physical separation; auxiliary warnings	Smetzer and Cohen (2006)

continued on following page

Table 2. Continued

LASA Pair	Drug Classes Involved	Primary LASA Mechanism	Clinical Context/Node of Error	Reported Clinical Consequence	System-Level Contributing Factors	Key Prevention Strategies Identified	Reference
Pancuronium – Heparin flush solution	NMBA vs. Flush solution	Look-alike vial; bin mix-up; pancuronium flushed instead of heparin solution	ICU central line flush	Cardiac arrest (recovered)	Misplaced vial in storage bin	Sequestered storage; warning labels	Smetzer and Cohen (2006)
Pavulon® (Pancuronium) – Papaverine	NMBA vs. Vasodilator	Sound-alike drug names; preparation error; papaverine prepared instead of pancuronium infusion	Pharmacy infusion preparation	Wrong-drug administration risk	Similar pronunciation; preparation error	Independent double check; clear labeling	Santell (2006)
Rocuronium – Pancuronium	NMBA vs. NMBA	Look-alike/sound-alike drug names; stocking error; pancuronium dispensed instead of rocuronium	Pharmacy dispensing; ADC stocking	Wrong drug administration risk	Similar vial appearance; improper stocking; performance deficit; Similar naming ("-curonium" stem)	Segregated storage; avoid similar strengths in same drawer; barcode verification	Santell (2006)
Vecuronium – Cefazolin	NMBA vs. Antibiotic	Look-alike vial presentation and adjacent storage; vecuronium administered instead of cefazolin.	Automated dispensing cabinet (ADC); perioperative setting	Unintended paralysis requiring ventilatory support	Similar packaging; noncompliant warning labeling; adjacent storage in ADC	Removal from stock; mandatory "Paralyzing Agent" labeling; segregation; national recall	Herzer et al. (2013)
Vecuronium – Vancomycin	NMBA vs. Antibiotic	Orthographic similarity (ve**cur**onium vs. van**comy**cin); transcription misreading; vecuronium dispensed instead of vancomycin	Pharmacy order entry; dispensing	Intercepted prior to harm (near miss); risk of respiratory arrest	Handwritten order misinterpretation; insufficient auxiliary differentiation	Prominent warning labels; independent double check; improved order clarity	Smetzer and Cohen (2006)

continued on following page

Table 2. Continued

LASA Pair	Drug Classes Involved	Primary LASA Mechanism	Clinical Context/Node of Error	Reported Clinical Consequence	System-Level Contributing Factors	Key Prevention Strategies Identified	Reference
Vecuronium – Vancomycin	NMBA vs. Antibiotic	Look-alike vial stocking in ADC; vecuronium stocked with vancomycin 1 g vials	Operating room automated dispensing cabinet	High-risk wrong-drug potential	Similar vial appearance; costorage	Avoid costocking; segregate high-alert NMBAs	Santell (2006)
Vecuronium – Potassium chloride infusion	NMBA vs. Electrolyte infusion	Postdiscontinuation infusion mix-up; vecuronium infused instead of potassium chloride	ICU after extubation	Cardiac arrest; reintubation; ventilation ~6 h	Discontinued NMBA left in room; failure to remove/sequester	Prompt removal of discontinued NMBAs; sequestered bin for pickup; warnings	Smetzer and Cohen (2006)
Vecuronium – Saline flush (unlabeled syringe)	NMBA vs. Flush solution	Unlabeled syringe; vecuronium flushed instead of saline	ED pediatric setting	Respiratory paralysis; intubation required	Batch-prepared unlabeled syringes	Mandatory labeling; eliminate syringe batching	Smetzer and Cohen (2006)

Insulin Products

Insulin is a High-Alert LASA Medication

Insulin is among the drugs most commonly involved in LASA errors and wrong-drug events (WDEs) in healthcare systems worldwide. It is a high-alert drug of the universal category in that minor changes in dose can cause rapid onset of severe hypoglycemia, seizures, coma, irreversible neurological damage, or even death (Health and Disability Commissioner, 2017; Institute for Safe Medication Practices (ISMP), 2018; Ro & Jones, 2025). In contrast to several other LASA drugs, where substitution can only lead to therapeutic failure, insulin errors can have life-threatening physiologic effects.

Modern evidence from surveillance proves the existence of the systemic risk that is inherent in insulin treatment. The Pennsylvania Patient Safety Reporting System (PA-PSRS) was used, where 10.3% of all medications implicated in wrong drug events and 29.8% of all high-alert medications were reported as insulin as the most frequently reported medication class in wrong drug events (Ro & Jones, 2025). Earlier statewide precautionary messages also indicated an imbalance of insulin-related injuries, where almost 16% of severe medication incidents involved insulin treatment, and 12.8% of these were directly classified as wrong-drug errors (The Pennsylvania Patient Safety Advisory, 2005a, 2010). These values have been clinically important even after insulin pen devices, barcode medication administration devices, and electronic prescribing platforms have been improved, highlighting the inherent nature of insulin administration complexity.

The risk profile of insulin as a LASA drug is based on various confounding factors, such as increased formulations, product name similarity, unit-based dosing, packaging similarity, color differentiation, distance to other injectable drugs, and human cognition risks such as confirmation bias. **Table 3** shows a summary of representative insulin-related LASA incidents and safety advisories. It shows the pattern of orthographic similarity and packaging resemblance.

Table 3. Selected studies and incident reports describing insulin-related LASA errors involving name similarity, packaging similarity, or combined mechanisms

Country/Setting	LASA Pair(s)	Error Mechanism*	Reported Outcome/Harm	Study
Pennsylvania healthcare facilities	-Humalog®/ HumulinR®; -Humalog®75/25/ Humulin®70/30; -NovoLog®/ NovoLin R®	Shared brand stems ("Hum-", "Novo-") combined with look-alike vial and pen labeling; selection errors during prescribing, transcription, and dispensing	2,685 insulin-related events reported; 374 (13.9%) classified as wrong-drug events; 49 reached the patient and resulted in patient harm.	Pennsylvania Patient Safety Advisory review, 2008–2009 The Pennsylvania Patient Safety Advisory (2010) The Pennsylvania Patient Safety Advisory (2004)
Inpatient hospital	-Lantus®/Lente®; -dose misinterpretation using "U"	Sound-alike drug names; Unsafe abbreviation "U" for units misread as "0" or "4"; e.g., "4U" misread as 44 units; omission of mix ratio (e.g., 70/30 vs 75/25)	Tenfold overdoses; severe hypoglycemia; emergency treatment needed; documented transcription-related wrong-drug events; Tenfold overdoses; severe hypoglycemia; emergency dextrose treatment; some intercepted through patient verification ("I take 4 units, not 44").	Pennsylvania Patient Safety Advisory – Insulin Abbreviations & Complexity The Pennsylvania Patient Safety Advisory (2005a, 2005b)
Community pharmacy, Ontario	-Novolin® ge 30/70 and NovoRapid® cartriges	Look-alike cartridge and carton design; shared "Novo-" prefix; incomplete barcode scanning	Patient administered ultrarapid insulin instead of premix; symptomatic hypoglycemia; blood glucose approximately 2.5 mmol/L	ISMP Canada Safety Bulletin The Institute for Safe Medication Practices Canada (ISMP Canada) (2007)
Outpatient self-administration, USA	Lantus® (insulin glargine) and Humalog® (insulin lispro)	Patient-level selection error when both insulins were used concurrently; confusion due to similar visual appearance of the insulin preparations; patient inadvertently withdrew lispro instead of glargine despite distinct labeling	Two adults developed significant hypoglycemia after injecting lispro in place of scheduled glargine; one required IV glucose; blood glucose dropped to 57 mg/dL in one case	Adlersberg et al. (2002)

continued on following page

Table 3. Continued

Country/Setting	LASA Pair(s)	Error Mechanism*	Reported Outcome/Harm	Study
Hospital inpatient (TPN preparation)	Insulin versus Heparin (vial mix-ups)	Similar 10 mL vial presentation; both measured in "units"; storage adjacency under IV hood; transcription errors (e.g., insulin 10 units misread as heparin 10 units; 500 units heparin entered as insulin 500 units)	Severe hypoglycemia; neonatal case with blood glucose 17 mg/dL; fatalities reported in TPN admixture errors (insulin added instead of heparin, e.g., 200–1,000 units)	Cohen (2007a); Grissinger (2011)
Hospital inpatient	Insulin pens shared between patients	Device similarity; workflow failure; needle change but pen reused; lack of awareness of contamination risk	Risk of biological cross-contamination (hemoglobin detected in cartridges in published studies); institutional safety alert issued; policy revision required	Cohen (2008)

Sources of LASA Risk in Insulin Therapy

Currently used forms of insulin therapy include rapid-acting analogs (e.g., insulin lispro and insulin aspart), short-acting regular insulin, intermediate-acting neutral protamine Hagedorn (NPH), long-acting basal analogs (e.g., insulin glargine and insulin detemir), and a variety of premixed mixtures. Although such therapeutic diversification has significantly enhanced personalized glycemic control in individuals, it has also enhanced the structural susceptibility to LASA error. Wrong drug events have been attributed to the proliferation of insulin products, which have orthographic and phonetic similarities, especially those that belong to brand families such as Humalog®, Humulin®, NovoLog®, NovoLIN®, Lantus®, and Lente® (The Pennsylvania Patient Safety Advisory, 2005a). Pennsylvania surveillance data revealed confusion between Humalog® and Humulin R®, Humulin R® and Humulin 70/30®, Humalog 75/25® and Humulin 70/30®, Lente® and Lantus®, and NovoLog® and NovoLIN®; 12.8% of all insulin-related errors were incorrect drug occurrences (The Pennsylvania Patient Safety Advisory, 2005a). Recent studies support the view that insulin is the most commonly reported high-alert medication implicated in wrong-drug events; in a systematic review of 2023 data statewide, insulin was the most commonly involved medication, and 29.8% (93 of 312) of high-alert medications were implicated in wrong-drug events (Ro & Jones, 2025).

Insulin LASA is not an accident but is actually part of the organization of names and product differentiation. Ready-to-use formulations cause even more complexity. Humalog Mix 75/25®, NovoLog Mix 70/30®, Novolin 70/30®, and Humulin 70/30® are different products depending on the brand history as well as the pharmacokinetic ratio. Cases of errors, which include the omission of the strength of the mixtures by the clinician, errors in transcribing the ratio, and the adjacent premixed product having been selected in case of time rush, have been reported (The Pennsylvania Patient Safety Advisory, 2005a). These replacements are clinically consequential in the sense that the types of insulin vary significantly in their onset, peak, and duration of action. Substitution between long-acting and rapid-acting insulin might lead to the development of sustained hyperglycemia and insufficient glycemic regulation, and substitution between basal and rapid-acting insulin may cause severe hypoglycemia. In this way, insulin LASA mistakes often are pharmacokinetic errors and not mere duplication of treatment.

There is also a unit-based dosing convention concerning insulin, which contributes to the danger. Insulin is not administered in milligrams like most drugs; it is measured in units, and the historical "U" abbreviation has been implicated in ghastly 10-fold dosing errors many times over. Cases, as reported to the Pennsylvania Patient Safety Reporting System, of mistakenly reading "8 U" as 80, "5 U" as 54, and "10 U" as 100, resulting in severe hypoglycemia that necessitated emergent care, were reported (The Pennsylvania Patient Safety Advisory, 2005a). Confusion of the letter U with 0 or 4 has been specifically noted as a common cause of insulin overdoses, and a formal guideline has been given to spell out the word "units" in any prescribing paperwork (The Pennsylvania Patient Safety Advisory, 2005a). These examples demonstrate that prescribing-level orthographic ambiguity can be directly converted into the harm of high severity in patients.

Similar appearances occur because the majority of the insulin products are clear, colorless solutions provided in similar-sized vials; hence, differentiation through visual appearance is not reliable. This can result in the use of basal insulin in a bolus formulation or the opposite, and it adds to the notching of hypoglycemia at night or inadequate glycemic regulation. The issue of similarity in packaging has also been involved with international reports, such as confusion between Novolin® GE 30/70 Penfill® and NovoRapid® Penfill® cartridges that are similar in terms of their labeling color scheme and cartridge design, leading to the possibility of increasing selection error and subsequent severe symptomatic hypoglycemia (The Institute for Safe Medication Practices Canada (ISMP Canada), 2007). To synthesize the recurring patterns identified in these reports, **Table 4** maps insulin LASA errors across the three core mechanisms and their corresponding clinical consequences. As illustrated in **Figure 3**, visually similar vial sizes, labeling layouts, and color schemes may create perceptual overlap between insulin products, increasing the likelihood of selection errors under time pressure.

Collectively, these processes demonstrate the manner in which insulin LASA risk is evident in language, visual, and structural areas. Another less widely appreciated risk factor for insulin-related LASA is the role played by color differentiation. Manufacturers often use unique color patterns on the vial covers, pen bodies, labels, and packaging strips as a way of identifying rapid-action, basal, and premixed insulin products. In medical cases, color can be used as a quick visual aid when dispensing and administering medication. Color distinction could aid in distinguishing between basal therapy and bolus therapy in patients who are self-administering various types of insulin. There are, however, limitations to the dependence on color. No universal regulatory standard exists to regulate the insulin color coding among manufacturers, and biosimilar or reformulated medications can change the existing color associations. Furthermore, relying on color more than checking labels may encourage confirmation bias, in which clinicians make decisions regarding the identity of a product by its anticipated appearance without reading the label. Similar white labels with red resonance in the study of errors in insulin-influenza vaccine substitution led to misunderstandings in cases where the contents of the vials were not correctly checked (Clogston et al., 2016). Therefore, the differentiation of color must be a facilitating tool and not a key form of identification.

Table 4. Conceptual mapping of insulin-related LASA errors across the three core mechanisms: name similarity, appearance similarity, and packaging similarity

LASA Mechanism	How It Manifests in Insulin Products (Documented Cases)	Typical Clinical Consequences	References
Name similarity			
Name similarity – same brand stem	Confusion among "Hum-" products (e.g., Humalog, Humalog 75/25, Humulin R, Humulin 70/30, Humulin N); "Novo-" products (e.g., Novolog, Novolin R, Novolog 70/30, Novolin 70/30). Example: Humalog ordered instead of Humulin 70/30; Novolog 70/30 confused with Novolin 70/30.	Rapid-acting insulin administered instead of premix or regular insulin; inappropriate pharmacokinetic profile resulting in acute hypoglycemia or sustained hyperglycemia.	The Pennsylvania Patient Safety Advisory (2004, 2005a)
Name similarity – basal vs rapid analogs	Insulin glargine interchanged with insulin lispro; insulin lispro interchanged with insulin regular (most frequently reported insulin WDE pairs).	Basal insulin omitted or replaced with bolus insulin; severe hypoglycemia requiring intervention; unstable glycemic control.	Ro and Jones (2025)
Name similarity – Lente vs Lantus	Confusion between Lente (insulin zinc suspension) and Lantus (insulin glargine) due to orthographic similarity.	Long-acting insulin substitution errors; altered onset and duration increasing the risk of nocturnal hypoglycemia or hyperglycemia.	The Pennsylvania Patient Safety Advisory (2005b)
Abbreviation-related name/ dose confusion	Use of "U" for units misread as "0" or "4" (e.g., 5U read as 50 units; 4U misread as 44 units).	Tenfold overdose; severe hypoglycemia; emergency intervention needed.	The Pennsylvania Patient Safety Advisory (2005b)
Appearance similarity			
Appearance similarity – solution clarity & vial size	Clear, colorless solutions in similar 10 mL vials or pen cartridges; insufficient differentiation between lispro, regular, glargine, NPH.	Basal insulin administered as bolus or vice versa; repeated dosing errors; inpatient hypoglycemia events.	Ro and Jones (2025); The Pennsylvania Patient Safety Advisory (2005b)
Packaging similarity			

continued on following page

Table 4. Continued

LASA Mechanism	How It Manifests in Insulin Products (Documented Cases)	Typical Clinical Consequences	References
Packaging similarity – pen cartridges & labeling	Look-alike labeling between Novolog Mix 70/30 and Humulin 70/30; adjacent storage in refrigerators; insufficient tall man differentiation.	Rapid-acting insulin administered instead of premix; symptomatic hypoglycemia; delayed recognition of error.	The Pennsylvania Patient Safety Advisory (2004, 2005a)
Others			
Concurrent dual insulin therapy due to failure to discontinue	Patient received both Humalog and regular insulin, or Lantus plus NPH due to switching error and failure to stop prior insulin.	Additive hypoglycemic effect; hospitalization due to insulin stacking.	The Pennsylvania Patient Safety Advisory (2004, 2005a)
High-alert wrong drug events involving insulin	Insulin comprised 10.3% of all reported WDE medications and 29.8% of high-alert WDEs; multiple serious events involved unintended insulin administration.	Severe hypoglycemia requiring IV dextrose or emergency management; classified as serious events in PA-PSRS.	Ro and Jones (2025)
Strength omission in premixed products	Failure to specify mix ratio (e.g., 70/30 vs 75/25 vs 50/50); transcription errors in strength component.	Incorrect proportion of rapid vs intermediate insulin resulting in unpredictable glucose excursions.	The Pennsylvania Patient Safety Advisory (2005b)

Figure 3. Examples of visually similar insulin products demonstrating look-alike vial size, labeling layout, and color scheme

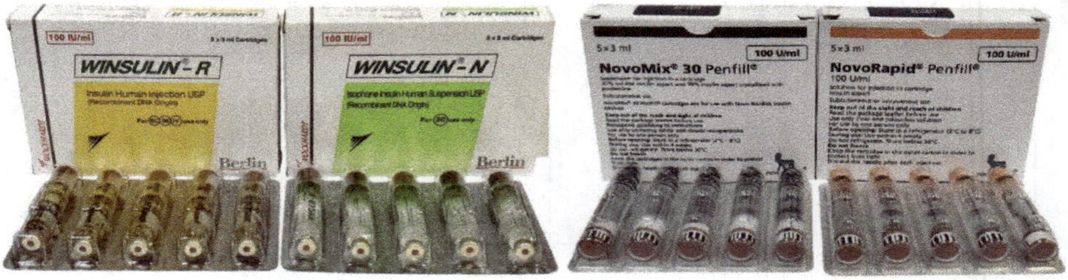

The pharmaceutical products shown are presented solely for academic and educational purposes. Their inclusion does not imply the endorsement, promotion, or advertising of any specific manufacturer, distributor, or brand.

Insulin Vaccine Mix-Ups

Another, but clinically important, LASA mechanism is the error of insulin-vaccine substitution, especially in influenza vaccination campaigns. A review of the reports published in the Vaccine Adverse Event Reporting System (VAERS) and the FDA Adverse Event Reporting System (FAERS) over ten years revealed 22 cases in which insulin was mistakenly used instead of an influenza vaccine (Clogston et al., 2016). In a cluster outbreak case, five adults had acute hypoglycemia after receiving an insulin that was thought to be an influenza vaccine; two patients had a minimum blood glucose level of 23 mg/dl and were taken to emergency care. Some of the contributing factors were the costorage of insulin and vaccine vials in the same refrigerator, failure to physically separate them, similarity in the size of the vials and their labeling appearance, and the lack of checking the labels prior to preparation (Clogston et al., 2016). In contrast to phonetically similarity-driven classical LASA errors, the events are container- and workflow-based substitution errors that are based on similarity on a visual basis and failure in environmental design.

Clinical Consequences of Insulin LASA Errors

In the same manner, a statewide review of wrong drug events (WDEs) in healthcare facilities in Pennsylvania in 2023 revealed that the wrong-drug error was an issue with medications belonging to the same therapeutic category or with medications that were phonetically or orthographically similar (Ro & Jones, 2025). The most affected class was insulin products, which are often mixed with other insulins that have the same stems (e.g., lispro, regular, and glargine).

There was also a general interchange of vasopressors (epinephrine-norepinephrine), opioids (hydromorphone-morphine), and antibiotics (cefazolin-ceftriaxone). These results confirm that LASA mechanisms are not one-time occurrences but are recurrent sources of incorrect drug occurrences. According to further reports of the Pennsylvania Patient Safety Authority, wrong-drug and wrong-dose events are caused by medication name confusion and unsafe abbreviation practices. As an example, mix-ups of MSO_4 (morphine sulfate) and $MgSO_4$ (magnesium sulfate) and insulin dosing mistakes in cases where U was used to denote units have all led to clinically significant events (The Pennsylvania Patient Safety Advisory, 2005a). These cases present the idea that orthographic similarity and unsafe notation can contribute directly to medication substitution errors.

Magnitude-of-error analyses also facilitate the systemic vulnerability of injectable medications. Cavell and Mandaliya conducted a seven-year search of the literature covering the incidence of incorrect dosing in hospitals and reported that errors in doses two and tenfold were common across the prescribing, dispensing, and administering phases and that both overdose and underdose were reported in adult and pediatric practice (Cavell & Mandaliya, 2021). Mistakes associated with such a scale were most commonly associated with calculations, an incorrect choice of units (mg vs. micrograms), and mistakes in infusion programming.

Prevention Strategies at the System Level

Eliminating insulin LASA errors would require a multilayer approach to the system. Environmental controls that need to be implemented include physical separation of insulin and vaccines and heparin, the use of distinctly marked storage containers, and not keeping look-alike products in close contact with each other (Clogston et al., 2016; The Pennsylvania Patient Safety Advisory, 2005a). The measures used to protect prescribing safety include spelling out of words, removing abbreviations that cause errors, and reducing verbal insulin orders. Tall man typing (e.g., NovoLOG® versus NovoLIN®) can help minimize orthographic confusion. Risk-reducing measures are important, and they include independent double checks prior to dispensing and administration, barcode scanning during pharmacy compounding and bedside checking, and structured protocols of TPN preparation (Grissinger, 2011). Continuous training on insulin pharmacokinetics, onset, and formulation variations strengthens cognitive protection. Additionally, pen-type insulins should not be shared among patients, as they can be contaminated (Cohen, 2008). Color differentiation is useful, but it should be integrated into this overall safety framework and, instead of entirely replacing label checks and standard storage procedures, strengthen them.

Insulin is a high-risk LASA drug whose risk history is due to various types of product, orthographic and phonetic similarity, unit-based dosing conventions, packaging similarity, inconsistent differentiation of colors, proximity of stored medications to insulin, and human cognitive bias. According to current surveillance data, insulin is always the most commonly reported high-alert medication implicated in adverse drug events (Ro & Jones, 2025). Because the effects of substitution or administering a wrong dosage may be disastrous, prevention is no longer an issue of naming safeguards but of an environmental design, use of technology to verify drug administration, systematic checks and balances, standardized labeling routines, and safety-oriented organizational culture. The persistence of insulin as the culprit in wrong-drug events highlights the importance of taking a proactive approach to risk evaluation and redesign of the system in both hospital and ambulatory care facilities. An example of structured insulin refrigerator storage with clearly segregated and labeled bins to reduce selection errors is shown in **Figure 4**.

Figure 4. Organized refrigerator bins for insulin

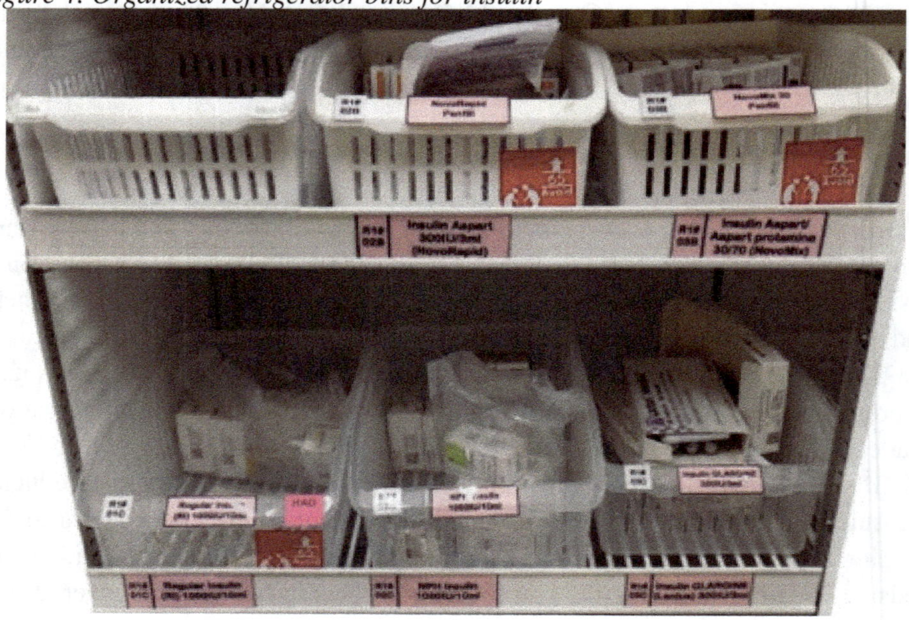

Each plastic bin is clearly labeled with the insulin subtype, strength, and rack location.

The pharmaceutical products shown are presented solely for academic and educational purposes. Their inclusion does not imply the endorsement, promotion, or advertising of any specific manufacturer, distributor, or brand.

Antibiotics

One of the most commonly implicated LASA injection-related medication errors in hospitals is antibiotics. Antibiotics are repeatedly found as the common source of wrong-drug incidents by hospital-based surveillance systems, as well as by national surveys, mostly because of the similarity of stems in terms of names, similarity in orthography, and similar vial display (Supapaan et al., 2024). LASA errors are caused by the similarity of names (orthographic and phonetic resemblance) and packages, and the probability of mistakes is higher in cases where agents have common prefixes or long character sequences (Basco et al., 2016; Bryan et al., 2015; Bryan et al., 2021a).

Cephalosporins

The most common subgroup of LASA antibiotics reported is cephalosporins. There are many orthographic overlaps among many other agents that share the root "cef." Both experimental and real-world studies prove that this type of similarity heightens the risk of selecting a wrong drug, especially in high-pressure clinical settings (Bryan et al., 2021a).

According to the MEDMARX Data Report (Hicks et al., 2008), there are many cephalosporin–cephalosporin LASA pairs, such as cefazolin, cefotaxime, ceftriaxone, cefepime, cefotetan, cefoxitin, and ceftazidime, with incidents ranging between Category A (possibility of error) and Category E-H (error leading to harm). Such statistics suggest that although many mistakes are detected even prior to reaching the patient, some of them cause clinically significant injury.

In addition to intraclass substitution, cases of cross-class confusion have been documented. An example that is described in detail is cefazolin and vecuronium, where the appearance of the vials and the proximity during storage caused a neuromuscular blocking agent to be given instead of prophylactic antibiotic therapy, which led to respiratory compromise (Herzer et al., 2013). The case at hand serves as an example in which mistakes in the use of LASA antibiotics can vary between changes in antimicrobial coverage and immediate life-threatening effects. Clinically, substitution between cephalosporins can change the antimicrobial spectrum, pharmacokinetics, and dosing schedules, but substitution between classes (e.g., cefazolin-vecuronium) can result in acute respiratory failure.

Penicillins

Antibiotics belonging to the penicillin class are also very vulnerable to LASA. Confusion may occur between single-agent and combination-agent products, e.g., ampicillin vs. ampicillin/sulbactam, and generic-generic names, e.g., penicillin and penicillamine. According to Ryan et al. (2024), one of the documented perioperative LASA pairs is ampicillin/ampicillin-sulbactam. Since ampicillin/sulbactam has a beta-lactamase inhibitor, which expands the antimicrobial spectrum, the unintentional use of ampicillin in place of the combination product may result in treatment failure in infections caused by beta-lactamase-producing organisms (Ryan et al., 2024; Ryan et al., 2025). Data from MEDMARX also record the misinterpretation between penicillin and penicillamine, and it shows that LASA risk is not just a brand name but also a threat to internationally standardized generic names (Hicks et al., 2008). Even though most of the documented cases were classified as either Category A or B, the cases that persisted reveal system weaknesses in the name-based system.

Orthographic similarity (similar spelling), phonetic similarity (similar sound), and packaging resemblance are identified worldwide as the causes of LASA medication errors, which have been linked to a large number of patients on the patient safety list (Bryan et al., 2021a; Bryan et al., 2021b; World Health Organization, 2023). In response, regulatory and safety organizations have adopted measures such as confusing drug name lists, lettering by tall man, and assisting with medication verification through barcodes. Regardless of such interventions, surveillance data still reveal the incidence of LASA in patients with various levels of severity, including one reported case of patient injury (Hicks et al., 2008).

As Table 5 demonstrates, the antibiotic-related LASA errors reported in the MEDMARX Data Report represent both intraclass (antibiotic–antibiotic) and cross-class (antibiotic–other drug class) substitutions. These are predominantly cephalosporins, with the most common combinations being cefazolin with ceftriaxone, cefotaxime, cefepime, cefotetan, cefoxitin, and ceftazidime because of the common prefix "cef-" and the high level of orthographic similarity. Notably, such cases do not qualify exclusively as near-miss cases, with MEDMARX severity scales spanning between the potential error of Category A to the error leading to harm of Category E-H, which means that there were some instances of antibiotic LASA use that produced clinically significant damage.

Table 5 also illustrates that penicillin-class agents cause both intraclass and generic-generic confusion, even between penicillin and penicillamine. Moreover, the example of cross-class substitution, e.g., cefazolin-vecuronium, explains how the malpractices of the antibiotic LASA can be expanded beyond therapeutic mis-selection to life-threatening administration of a drug with which the antibiotic is pharmacologically unrelated.

Table 5. Example of a documented LASA Injection drug in antibiotic pairs

Drug 1	Drug 2	NCC MERP Category*	Source
A. Antibacterial Agents			
Ampicillin	Amoxicillin	A, B, C–D	(Hicks et al., 2008)
Ampicillin	Ampicillin/Sulbactam (Unasyn®)	A, B, C–D, E-H	(Hicks et al., 2008)
Ampicillin 125 mg	Ampicillin 250 mg	A, B	(Supapaan et al., 2024)
Ampicillin	Cloxacillin	B	(Supapaan et al., 2024)
Ampicillin	Nafcillin	B, C-D	(Hicks et al., 2008)
Ampicillin	Oxacillin	C-D	(Hicks et al., 2008)
Ampicillin	Penicillin G Sodium	C-D	(Hicks et al., 2008)
Ampicillin	Piperacillin	C-D	(Hicks et al., 2008)
Azithromycin	Azathioprine	A, B, C–D	(Hicks et al., 2008)
Azithromycin	Aztreonam	B, C–D	(Hicks et al., 2008)
Cefazolin	Ampicillin	B, C–D	(Hicks et al., 2008)
Cefazolin	Ceftriaxone	A, B, C–D	(Hicks et al., 2008; Supapaan et al., 2024)
Cefazolin	Cefotaxime	A, B, C–D	(Hicks et al., 2008; Supapaan et al., 2024)
Cefazolin	Cefotetan	A, B, C–D, E–H	(Hicks et al., 2008)
Cefazolin	Cefepime	A, B, C–D	(Hicks et al., 2008)
Cefazolin	Cefoxitin	A, B	(Hicks et al., 2008)
Cefazolin	Ceftazidime	A, B, C–D	(Hicks et al., 2008; Supapaan et al., 2024)
Cefazolin	Cefuroxime	B, C–D	(Hicks et al., 2008)
Cefazolin	Oxacillin	C–D	(Hicks et al., 2008)
Cefazolin	Piperacillin/Tazobactam (Zosyn®)	B, C–D	(Hicks et al., 2008)
Cefdinir	Cefprozil	C–D	(Hicks et al., 2008)
Cefuroxime	Ceftriaxone	A, B, C–D	(Hicks et al., 2008)
Cefuroxime	Cefadroxil	B	(Hicks et al., 2008)
Cefepime	Ceftriaxone	A, B, C–D	(Hicks et al., 2008)

continued on following page

Table 5. Continued

Drug 1	Drug 2	NCC MERP Category*	Source
Ceftriaxone	Ceftazidime	A, B, C–D, E–H	(Hicks et al., 2008; Supapaan et al., 2024)
Ceftriaxone	Cefotaxime	B	(Supapaan et al., 2024)
Clindamycin	Gentamicin	A	(Supapaan et al., 2024)
Clarithromycin	Clindamycin	C–D	(Hicks et al., 2008)
Ertapenem	Imipenem/Cilastatin	C–D	(Hicks et al., 2008)
Ertapenem	Meropenem	C–D	(Hicks et al., 2008)
Penicillin	Penicillin G Benzathine	A, B	(Hicks et al., 2008)
Penicillin G Sodium	Ampicillin	A	(Hicks et al., 2008)
Penicillin	Penicillamine (Antirheumatic agent)	A, B	(Hicks et al., 2008)
Piperacillin/Tazobactam	Imipenem/Cilastatin	A	(Supapaan et al., 2024)
Cefazolin	Vecuronium (Neuromuscular blocker)	N/A	(Herzer et al., 2013)
Ceftriaxone	Omeprazole (Proton pump inhibitor)	B	(Supapaan et al., 2024)
Ciprofloxacin	Levofloxacin	C–D	(Hicks et al., 2008)
Ciprofloxacin	Moxifloxacin	B, C–D	(Hicks et al., 2008)
Meropenem	Metronidazole	C–D	(Hicks et al., 2008)
Meropenem	Midazolam (Benzodiazepine)	B	(Hicks et al., 2008)
Vancomycin	Clindamycin	A, B	(Hicks et al., 2008)
Vancomycin	Gentamicin	A	(Hicks et al., 2008)
Vancomycin	Tobramycin	A	(Hicks et al., 2008)
Vancomycin	Vibramycin® (Doxycycline; Tetracycline antibiotic)	B, C–D	(Hicks et al., 2008)
Vancomycin	Valacyclovir (Antiviral agent)	B, C–D	(Hicks et al., 2008)
Vancomycin	Vecuronium (Neuromuscular blocker)	B, C–D, E–H	(Hicks et al., 2008)
B. Antifungal Agents			
Abelcet® (Amphotericin B lipid complex)	AmBisome® (Liposomal amphotericin B)	A, B, C–D, E–H	(Hicks et al., 2008)
Amphotericin B Lipid Complex	Amphotericin B Desoxycholate	C–D	(Hicks et al., 2008)

continued on following page

Table 5. Continued

Drug 1	Drug 2	NCC MERP Category*	Source
Amphotericin B Liposome	Amphotericin B (conventional formulation)	A, B, C–D, E–H	(Hicks et al., 2008)
Amphotericin B	Streptokinase	B	(Supapaan et al., 2024)
Vfend® (Voriconazole)	Venofer® (Iron sucrose; Parenteral iron preparation)	A, B	(Hicks et al., 2008)
C. Antiviral Agents			(Hicks et al., 2008)
Viracept® (Nelfinavir)	Viramune® (Nevirapine)	A, B, C–D	(Hicks et al., 2008)
Viread® (Tenofovir)	Venofer® (Iron sucrose; Parenteral iron preparation)	B	(Hicks et al., 2008)
Ganciclovir	Acyclovir	B, C–D, E–H	(Hicks et al., 2008)

(Hicks et al., 2008; Supapaan et al., 2024)

*NCC MERP Category = National Coordinating Council for Medication Error Reporting and Prevention (NCC MERP) Index for Categorizing Medication Errors

Opioid Analgesics

Opioid analgesics have been consistently listed as high-alert injectable drugs that are often involved in harmful medication errors, especially LASA name confusion and dosing. National reporting systems have repeatedly shown that opioids are the cause of a disproportionate number of serious medication events. In Canada, an examination of voluntarily reported harmful medication events revealed that the use of morphine and hydromorphone, two of the highest-ranked drugs most frequently reported to cause patient harm, occurred between 2001 and 2005 (Institute for Safe Medication Practices (ISMP) Canada, 2006). The findings highlight clinical susceptibility to the use of injectable opioids, particularly in the institutional setting.

Reported Incidents Involving Injectable Opioid LASA Pairs

Injectable opioid analgesics, especially hydromorphone and morphine, are regularly listed in safety surveillance systems as high-risk drugs and are commonly involved in the occurrence of adverse medication errors. Hydromorphone is a semisynthetic opioid agonist that is synthetic and a derivative of morphine and is approximately five to seven times more powerful than morphine is (Lowe et al., 2017). In patients who are unable to tolerate morphine or who have to be opioid-rotated, it is typically chosen as an alternative. Although the latter is stronger in terms of its effects, it has not been proven to have a clinical advantage over morphine when moderate to severe pain is managed. Hydromorphone can be introduced through various routes, such as intravenous, subcutaneous, and oral routes (Lowe et al., 2017).

Morphine (n = 43) and hydromorphone (n = 32) were among the top 10 drugs reported to cause harm as a result of medication error between 2001 and 2005 (Institute for Safe Medication Practices (ISMP) Canada, 2006). The replacement of hydromorphone with morphine is among the most reported LASA opioid mistakes.

Analysis of wrong-drug medication errors involving HYDR omorphone revealed that 70% of the errors were attributable to mix-ups with morphine (Pennsylvania Patient Safety, 2010). The difference in potency between the two agents is quite high and enhances the clinical risk of this LASA pair. When administered intravenously, hydromorphone is approximately 7.5 times stronger than intravenous morphine is, and the reported equianalgesic ratios are between 4:1 and 8:1 (Pennsylvania Patient Safety, 2010). This difference has not been taken into consideration, and severe cases of overdosing, especially in conversion or substitution, have been reported.

An Ontario case series was able to identify eight accidental fatal opioid overdoses, including hydromorphone and morphine, among hospital inpatients and long-term care residents in 2007–2012. The range of the decedents was between 19 and 91 years. A structured medication use process framework that included five stages (prescribing, order processing (including transcription), dispensing, administration, and monitoring) was used in every case. Two or more possible intervention points were identified in seven out of eight instances, meaning that the deadly consequences were due to several system failures as opposed to single, stage failures. The size of the dosing discrepancies was large. There were 4 instances of approximately fivefold overdoses of opioids, two instances of tenfold overdoses of opioids, and one instance of an estimated 2.5 overdose of opioids because of morphine and hydromorphine coadministration. Failure to monitor was eminent; 6 out of the eight fatalities were deemed avoidable with better clinical monitoring. These results prove that fatal injectable hydromorphone-morphine incidents are typified by dose miscalculations, which are quantifiable, vulnerabilities in multiple stages of the processes, and avoidable monitoring shortfalls in institutional care environments (Lowe et al., 2017).

Clinical Consequences

Injection of opioid LASA errors has serious clinical effects, including respiratory depression, overdose, and death. In the Ontario case series, the patients were given excessive doses, in most cases, five- to tenfold, which caused lethal opioid toxicity (Lowe et al., 2017). Pennsylvania adverse drug reaction (ADR) statistics continue to reveal that 47.9% of all reports on hydromorphone-related adverse drug reactions involve the central nervous system and/or respiratory depression (Pennsylvania Patient Safety, 2010). Interestingly, 65 percent of such incidents seemed to be preventable, often in cases of inappropriate doses or combinations of additive sedatives. The ability of hydromorphone to bind with μ-opioid receptors in medullary respiratory centers explains why a foreseeable risk of clinically significant respiratory depression can be expected when the drug is overused (Dahan et al., 2010; Pattinson, 2008). Substitution errors of look-alike injectable drugs, including opioids, were also frequently reported in the first 4,000 anesthetic incident report categories in the Web-based Anesthetic Incident Reporting System (webAIRS) (Meyer TA & McAllister RK, 2023), which confirms that look-alike injectable medications, including opioids, do not have a unique impact on ward settings but are still reported in perioperative settings.

Management and Risk-Reduction Strategies

Evidence from reported incidents supports the implementation of system-level safeguards targeting injectable opioid LASA risks.

1. Dose Standardization and Conservative Initiation

Given the high potency of IV hydromorphone relative to morphine (approximately 7.5:1) (Pennsylvania Patient Safety, 2010), initial IV dosing for opioid-naïve patients should follow conservative dosing guidance (e.g., 0.2–0.6 mg IV every 2–3 hours as needed) rather than higher legacy starting doses.

2. Independent Double Checks for Intravenous (IV) Opioids

Pennsylvania analyses recommend independent double checks prior to IV hydromorphone administration as a harm-reduction strategy (Pennsylvania Patient Safety, 2010), particularly given the frequency of administration-node errors (78.9%).

3. Patient-Controlled Analgesia (PCA) Safeguards and Programming Controls

Wrong-dose errors frequently involve infusion device programming errors and PCA therapy (Pennsylvania Patient Safety, 2010). Standardized PCA order sets, restrictions on basal infusions in opioid-naïve patients, and concentration standardization are recommended risk-reduction approaches.

4. Storage and Physical Separation

Hydromorphone and morphine are in close proximity, contributing to selection errors (Pennsylvania Patient Safety, 2010). Physical separation in narcotic drawers and differentiated labeling reduce selection risk.

5. Tall man Lettering and Electronic Alerts

Anesthesia safety literature emphasizes the use of tall man lettering and enhanced labeling for high-alert LASA medications (Meyer TA & McAllister RK, 2023) to visually differentiate similar names (e.g., HYDROmorphone versus morphine).

6. Enhanced Monitoring

In the Ontario fatal case series, additional monitoring could have prevented several deaths (Lowe et al., 2017). Continuous respiratory monitoring and early recognition of oversedation are essential when administering injectable opioids.

Additional Injectable Opioid LASA Pairs Beyond Hydromorphone–Morphine

Although hydromorphone–morphine represents the most frequently documented and clinically consequential injectable opioid LASA pair, surveillance data confirm that additional opioid–opioid substitution errors occur in hospital practice. These errors similarly involve high-alert injectable narcotics and arise from orthographic similarity, shared storage environments, and vulnerabilities at the administration stage.

Morphine–Meperidine

The Pennsylvania Patient Safety Authority identified name confusion between morphine and meperidine among reported opiate narcotic errors. These events were classified into high-alert medication categories because of the serious risk associated with opioid substitution. Opioid narcotics were explicitly noted among the most serious name confusion errors reported to Pennsylvania surveillance systems (The Pennsylvania Patient Safety Advisory, 2004). In injectable contexts, such substitution may result in central nervous system depression, respiratory compromise, or inadequate analgesia depending on the direction of the error.

Hydromorphone–Meperidine

Wrong drug reports involving hydromorphone also identified meperidine as a substituted medication

(Pennsylvania Patient Safety, 2010). In the hydromorphone-related medication error analyses (January 2008–October 2009), wrong-drug errors accounted for 10.9% of the reported events (n = 185). Hydromorphone-meperidine was the most common medication pair (6 cases; 3.2%) and led to incorrect drug hydromorphone errors. The clinical outcomes of such replacements can be observed through case narratives. In one of the reports, an adult patient who presented with abdominal pain was prescribed 25 mg of IV meperidine, after which 2 mg of IV hydromorphone was repeated several hours later. The patient was also discovered to have shallow breaths and loss of responsiveness and had to be administered naloxone; subsequently, the dose of hydromorphone was reduced.

These reports highlight the risk of central nervous system depression and respiratory compromise posed by injectable opioid exposure. Notably, incorrect drug hydromorphone incidence analysis revealed that 78.9% of the errors were at the administration node, which indicates weakness in drug access and administration operations (Pennsylvania Patient Safety, 2010).

Hydromorphone-Lorazepam

Substitutions between hydromorphone and lorazepam were also found in the same dataset (6 cases; 3.2% of wrong-drug hydromorphone events) (Pennsylvania Patient Safety, 2010). An instance was reported of an older postoperative patient who was given 0.5 mg of lorazepam IV, after which he was given doses of hydromorphone 2 mg IV repeatedly. The patient then developed a low level of consciousness and had to be administered naloxone. Even though lorazepam is not an opioid, this combination is a high-risk injectable LASA scenario, as the central nervous system suppressants are additive.

Hydromorphone-Oxycodone

There were also incorrect drug reports of oxycodone-hydromorphone substitutions (5 cases; 2.7% of wrong-drug hydrocodone incidences) (Pennsylvania Patient Safety, 2010). These incidents indicate that several injectable opioid pairs are involved in the failure of selection and administration-stage errors in hospital practice.

Clinical Implications

Taken together, the Pennsylvania surveillance data validate the assumption that in addition to the most common hydromorphone–morphine pair, other injectable LASA replacements, such as hydromorphone–meperidine, hydromorphone–lorazepam, and oxycodone–hydromorphone, do take place in clinical practice, mostly at the administration stage. While hydromorphone–morphine remains the most frequently reported and fatal injectable opioid LASA pair, surveillance evidence confirms that additional opioid combinations, particularly morphine–meperidine and hydromorphone–meperidine, also pose significant safety risks. These errors consistently involve the following:

- High-alert injectable narcotics
- Administration-stage vulnerabilities
- Concentration variability
- Inadequate monitoring following administration

Given that 65% of adverse central nervous system and respiratory reactions involving hydromorphone are preventable (Pennsylvania Patient Safety, 2010), the extension of prevention strategies beyond a single opioid pair is warranted. Injectable opioid LASA risk should therefore be conceptualized as a class-level safety vulnerability rather than a single drug-pair phenomenon (Pennsylvania Patient Safety, 2010).

Vasopressors and Cardiovascular Agents

Vasopressors and cardiovascular agents that are injectable are especially susceptible to LASA errors since they are high-alert medications with a high incidence of intravenous use in acute care and are frequently under time pressure. Large surveillance systems affirm that wrong-drug mistakes take place during the administration phase and are commonly linked to parenteral drugs. In intensive care units, parenteral medication errors are categorized into defined numbers, which can lead to permanent injury or even mortality due to incorrect drug administration (Valentin et al., 2009).

LASA risk is further increased in perioperative and critical care settings because of the similarity of the ampule and vial's visual appearance, limited space on labels, and on-packaging similarity depending on the manufacturer, as well as proximity to storage (Ryan et al., 2024). Look-alike labeling and packaging, especially when small-volume injectable products are involved, is a phenomenon listed repeatedly as the cause of medication incidents (Bryan et al., 2021a; Cohen, 2007b). According to the WHO (2023) framework, the most frequent instances of LASA errors are observed during dispensing and administration if the products are stored close to each other or when the differences in strength are not clearly distinguished (World Health Organization, 2023).

In accordance with the MedMARX data, cardiovascular agents and catecholamines are represented in the list of wrong-drug pairs that were documented, and the errors were classified in the high-alert category of medications (Hicks et al., 2008). Despite the varying accounts of cases, the mechanisms reported always contain orthographic similarity, packaging similarity, and storage structure.

Since the therapeutic index of vasopressors is narrow and their effect is rapid in terms of hemodynamic changes, unintended substitution can lead to acute hypertension, hypotension, arrhythmias, or cardiovascular collapse. As highlighted in the international guidance, mitigation efforts should focus on lettering, segregation, and independent double-checking, as well as system-level safeguards against high-risk injectable medicines (Bryan et al., 2021a; World Health Organization, 2023).

LASA errors related to vasopressors and cardiovascular agents have always been recorded in anesthetic and critical care settings because drugs are ordered in an emergency and are applied intravenously. One of the most common and clinically important LASA pairs that are most often reported is confusion between ephedrine and epinephrine. Syringe label confusion was initially reported as a correlation between anesthesia and a change from adrenaline to epinephrine, resulting in the accidental replacement of ephedrine (James, 1998). The author noted that clinicians tend to read by word form as opposed to individual letters, which predisposes them to orthographic similarity. Although there was no harm in the cases mentioned, the incident demonstrated inherent LASA risk when anesthetic drugs were prepared.

Ephedrine–Epinephrine

ISMP Canada reported the case of a severe case in which epinephrine (1 mg/mL) was given instead of ephedrine (5 mg IV) for epidural-induced hypotension. The patient had acquired severe hypertension, tachycardia, vomiting, and probable subendocardial myocardial infarction (Institute for Safe Medication Practices (ISMP) Canada, 2007). The bulletin also referred to the data reported by the Closed Claims Project of the American Society of Anesthesiologists, according to which, in the majority of reported cases, there were errors related to epinephrine, and those cases were connected with either death or significant morbidity. Orthographic similarity, proximity of stored alphabets, and presentation of ampules of similar types were the LASA mechanisms attributed to other ISMP Medication Safety Alerts, such as near misses and actual substitutions of ephedrine and epinephrine, and some of the mistakes made during the preparation of ephedrine in cases of emergent hypotension (Institute for Safe Medication Practices (ISMP) Canada, 2007).

The Institute of Safe Medication Practices (ISMP) in the United States has been relentless in its recommendation of the ephedrine–epinephrine combination in its tall man lettering. The use of ePHEDrine-EPINEPHrine is specifically encouraged to avoid visual confusion in drug and pharmacy systems, automated dispensing cabinets, and labeling (Grissinger, 2012). This information proves that the LASA risk remains high even with increased awareness efforts and is increased in high-acuity settings.

All of the evidence points to the fact that LASA errors involving vasopressors, specifically ephedrine and epinephrine, are not hypothetical threats, but documented instances of medication errors causing severe cardiovascular damage are frequent. The similarity of name, high-alert category, IV administration, and similar packaging of the pair (see **Figure 5**) render it a sentinel warning of injectable LASA risk in perioperative and critical care practice.

Most recently, according to Majeed et al. (2025), there was a life-threatening dispensing error during living-donor liver transplantation in which a norepinephrine infusion bag provided by the pharmacy contained epinephrine instead of norepinephrine. This mistake became evident when progressive tachycardia, lactic acidosis, hyperglycemia, hypokalemia, and graft congestion worsened with increasing doses of what was believed to be "norepinephrine." Replacement with a newly prepared norepinephrine infusion resulted in rapid normalization of physiologic parameters. Toxicologic examination confirmed that the labeled bag contained epinephrine. Root cause analysis revealed LASA name similarity, similar appearance of multidose vials, label switching during the preparation phase, workflow design flaws, and staff overwork and fatigue as contributing factors. This case illustrates how serious LASA dispensing errors can be when high-alert vasopressors are involved and highlights the importance of physical separation, independent double-checking, and handling only one high-risk medication at a time (Majeed et al., 2025).

Figure 5. Norepinephrine, epinephrine, and ephedrine injections result in similar drug names and ampule appearances

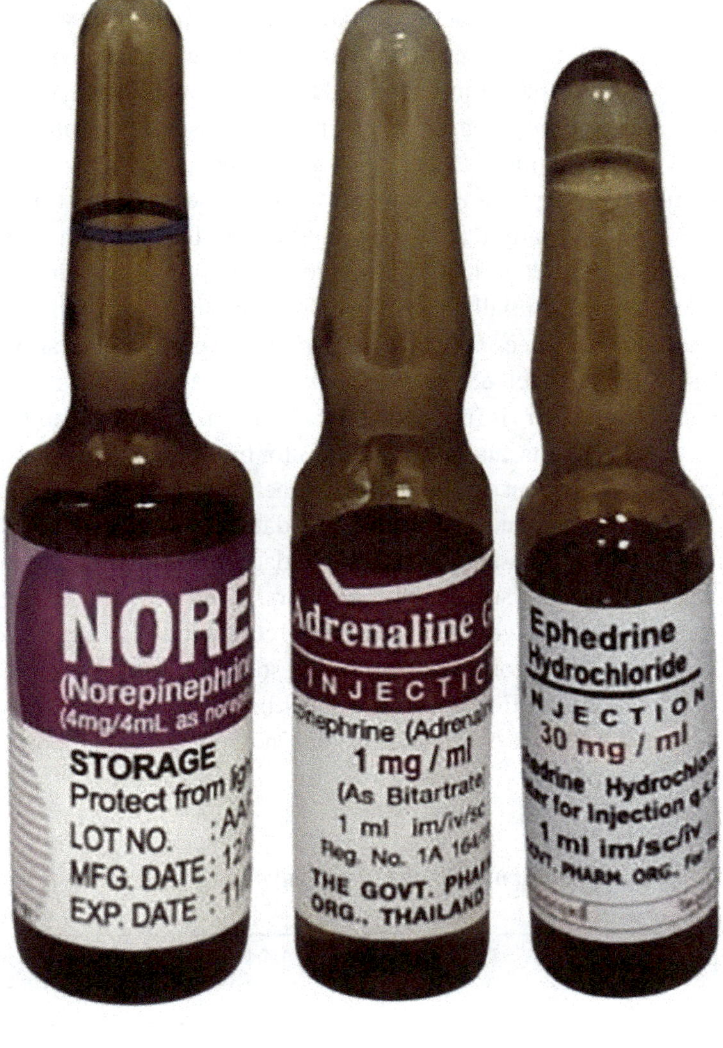

The pharmaceutical products shown are presented solely for academic and educational purposes. Their inclusion does not imply the endorsement, promotion, or advertising of any specific manufacturer, distributor, or brand

Errors with Epinephrine Intravenous Administration

In addition to confusion by name, formulation and route mistakes increase the risk of using epinephrine. In one of the pediatric cases, epinephrine was accidentally given intravenously at a concentration of 1:100,000, which is supposed to be administered intramuscularly. The authors reported that the most common concentrations of epinephrine are 1:1,000 (1 mg/mL), which is to be used as an intramuscular injection, and 1:10,000 (0.1 mg/mL), which is to be used as an intravenous injection. The old system of labeling based on ratios is also a cause of calculational error and clinical confusion, especially during emergent cases. In one of the retrospective reviews mentioned in the report, 2.4% of patients with improper administration of epinephrine developed potentially life-threatening complications, such as cardiogenic shock, coronary artery dissection, pulmonary edema, ventricular dysrhythmia, and myocardial ischemia (Garlich & Nelson, 2010). These results show that LASA risk associated with vasopressors is frequently associated with the availability of various concentrations, route effects, and dose variables for high-alert medication and under acute clinical stress, where an error is likely to reach the patient before it is detected.

LASA pairs were found in the MEDMARX database, but the route of administration was not stated (Hicks et al., 2008). The data in **Table 6** indicate that high-alert cardiovascular agents, such as vasopressors, inotropes, and other injectable therapies, were associated with reported name confusion mistakes. Most events did not harm patients (Category A, B, C-D), but some of them experienced greater levels of severity (Category E-H). These results highlight the clinical risk of LASA mistakes associated with critical cardiovascular injectables and support the idea of considerable safety control.

Table 6. Example of documented LASA pairs involving vasopressors and cardiovascular injectable agents

Drug 1	Drug 2	Pharmacologic Category	NCC MERP Category*	Potential Clinical Consequence
Dopamine	Dobutamine	Inotropes/Vasopressors	A, B, C–D, E-H	Inappropriate inotropy vs vasoconstriction; arrhythmia or shock worsening
Ephedrine	Adrenalin (Epinephrine)	Sympathomimetic vasopressors	A, B, C–D	Excess adrenergic stimulation; tachyarrhythmia
Epinephrine	Norepinephrine	Catecholamine vasopressors	B, C–D	Hemodynamic instability from wrong vasopressor selection
Epinephrine	Phenylephrine	Catecholamine/Alpha-agonist	B, C–D	Excess vasoconstriction or reflex bradycardia

continued on following page

Table 6. Continued

Drug 1	Drug 2	Pharmacologic Category	NCC MERP Category*	Potential Clinical Consequence
Pitocin (Oxytocin)	Pitressin (Vasopressin)	Uterotonic/Vasopressin analog	B, C–D	Hypertension or unintended vasopressin exposure
Propranolol	Propofol	Beta-blocker/Sedative	A	Bradycardia vs unintended deep sedation
Protamine Sulfate	Protirelin	Anticoagulation antidote/ Endocrine diagnostic agent	B	Failure to undo the effect of heparin results in persistent anticoagulation and bleeding; incorrect administration of protamine can result in hypotension, pulmonary hypertension, or anaphylaxis.

(Hicks et al., 2008)

*NCC MERP Category = National Coordinating Council for Medication Error Reporting and Prevention (NCC MERP) Index for Categorizing Medication Errors

Benzodiazepines, Sedatives, and High-Alert Parenteral Substitution

According to national reporting systems, injectable benzodiazepines, such as diazepam, midazolam, lorazepam, and clonazepam (where parenteral formulations exist), have been found to be recurring LASA pairs because of orthographic similarity, overlapping indications (e.g., seizure control and procedural sedation), and emergent administration situations (Hicks et al., 2008).

Diazepam, a benzodiazepine used for acute seizure control and procedural sedation, has been reported to be confused with other benzodiazepines, such as clonazepam, lorazepam, midazolam, temazepam, alprazolam, and oxazepam, most commonly distributed across NCC MERP Categories A–H, indicating intercepted events, no-harm errors, or temporary harm requiring intervention. Additional orthographic confusion extends beyond the benzodiazepine class, including diazepam–diltiazem, diazepam–DiaBeta® (glyburide), diazepam–Ditropan® (oxybutynin), and diazepam–doxepin. Among these, diazepam–diltiazem pairs have reached harm categories (category E-H), reflecting the potential for clinically significant consequences when a cardiovascular agent is substituted for a sedative. Overall, the distribution of MEDMARX shows that diazepam-related LASA events predominantly cluster within Categories A–D, with rare progression to fatal outcomes (Hicks et al., 2008).

Clonazepam is a long-acting benzodiazepine mainly used as an agent to treat seizures and panic disorders. It has a pharmacologic resemblance to other benzodiazepines, which is a risk factor for class-based confusion. The use of the

MEDMARX drug name index shows the extent and severity of distribution of the clonazepam-induced LASA events. The paired confusion involving clonazepam-alprazolam and clonazepam-clonidine both belong to categories A–H, meaning that the occurrences were between circumstances of the ability to induce an error and those where the treatments were life-sustaining. Other combinations, such as clonazepam-Ativan (lorazepam), clonazepam-diazepam, clonazepam-lorazepam, and clonazepam-clozapine, were distributed mainly into Categories A–D on the basis of errors of intercepted and no-harm and temporary harm to be dealt with. Overall, despite the events associated with clonazepam that span both ends of the NCC MERP spectrum to Category E–H, most of these events occur within Categories A–D, resulting in reversible clinical outcomes without causing permanent injury or death (Hicks et al., 2008).

This severity pattern is supported by the results of the Australian Incident Monitoring Study (AIMS). Among 896 drug errors as a result of anesthesia, half were comparative errors in syringe or drug preparation; benzodiazepines were the drugs involved (Abeysekera et al., 2005). The patterns that were documented and included as intended were as follows: midazolam intended but neuromuscular blocker administered (n = 16), neuromuscular blocker intended but midazolam administered (n = 5), and midazolam-rocuronium ampule labeling errors (n = 14). Although the total amount of data involved significant morbidity (4.7%) and fatality (0.3%), the syringe swaps related to sedation were more adjusted to reversible events (Abeysekera et al., 2005).

Depot hormonal injections exhibit a similar severity profile. MEDMARX finds that there is confusion between Depo-Medrol, Depo-Provera, and Lupron Depot (Hicks et al., 2008). Although these replacements can lead to accidental exposure to corticosteroids, endocrine deregulation, or unintended contraception, endocrine deregulation and accidental corticosteroid exposure usually require follow-up management or monitoring rather than life preservation, once again concentrating mostly on categories B–H.

In contrast, LASA substitutions with high-alert parenteral agents are significantly more severe. Mistaking magnesium sulfate and morphine sulfate, e.g., can lead to respiratory depression, arrhythmia, or cardiovascular collapse, which often go into categories A–D (Hicks et al., 2008). The other end of the spectrum is oncology agents. Vinca alkaloids, injectable vincristine, vinblastine, vinorelbine, and vindesine are also referred to as having catastrophic effects, which may cause serious consequences, including death, as a result of their misuse (Schulmeister, 2006).

IV-Fluid Look-ALike (LASA) Problems during Perioperative and Procedural Settings

LASA incidents related to intravenous (IV) fluids in the perioperative unit are strongly influenced by the similarity of containers and confusion of route rather than similarity of names. The preparation of irrigation solutions and IV infusion fluids is often performed in flexible bags of the same kind and processed in the same area of an operating room. Grissinger (2019) reported documented cases in which a 1,000 mL bag of the Lactated Ringer solution with 50,000 units of heparin to be used for intraoperative irrigation was mistakenly injected intravenously because of the similarity of labels and bags (Grissinger, 2019). Other main contributing factors that have been identified in the report are mix-ups between irrigation and parenteral solution bags, similar packaging and compatible access ports, unlabeled or poorly labeled additives, cluttered workspaces, and depending on the expected location of the bag as opposed to actual label verification. These are all the attributes of a defining appearance-based IV-fluid LASA substitution error. The accidental insertion of heparinized irrigation solution is a risk factor for high doses of anticoagulation for patients with a high risk of bleeding. The patients, as in the reported cases, needed protamine to be administered immediately to reverse the anticoagulant effect of heparin. Potential clinical consequences might be postoperative bleeding, hematoma formation, prolonged clotting times (elevated aPTT), and hemodynamic instability in severe cases. Although the reported patients have fully recovered because of early detection and reversal, the potential for high morbidity remains (Grissinger, 2019).

Cohen and Smetzer (2011) reported a similar wrong-route occurrence, but in this case, the solution ordered to be used (topical wound irrigation) was diluted sodium hypochlorite, which was given by mistake as an intravenous solution. In the case under report, a patient with severe burns was introduced to an IV catheter later, and the part of the catheter that was not covered by dressing was placed around the wound. The nurse made an incorrect assumption that the capped IV catheter was actually an irrigation catheter and then injected Dakin solution into it. When the patient complained of a burning sensation, the administration was terminated, with approximately 15 mL and less administered (Cohen & Smetzer, 2011). Although the patient did not develop any permanent sequelae, the solution proposed by Dakin includes sodium hypochlorite, which is a chemically irritating and cytotoxic substance. Larger volumes or delayed recognition might cause vascular injury, tissue damage, or systemic toxicity. Grissinger (2019) also reported that unintentional IV delivery of irrigation solution, such as hypotonic solution or irrigation solution that has additives, such as Dakin solution, can cause patient injury. Taken together, these findings support the notion that IV-fluid LASA incidents in perioperative units are mostly appearance-based, route-confusion events that can involve severe clinical outcomes (Cohen & Smetzer, 2011; Grissinger, 2019).

The ISMP perioperative protocols also warn against keeping 1,000 mL of sterile injectable or irrigating water and inhalation air bags of sterile water stock in patient care units since accidental IV injection is fatal. To prepare dantrolene as an emergency in malignant hyperthermia, the guidelines advise the use of sterile vials of water or 2–3-liter bags and placing them in different locations in the malignant hyperthermia cart to minimize look-alike risk (Institute for Safe Medication Practices (ISMP), 2022). The rationale is that the size of 1,000 mL sterile water bags is similar to that of standard IV fluids in terms of size, shape, and hanging geometry; thus, they have higher chances of inadvertent selection and connection to IV tubing (see Figure 6). Containers or vials with greater volume offer added visual distinction and contextual discontinuity with infusion fluids. IV-fluid LASA incidents in operating rooms are mostly superficial errors related to substitution, such as the design of bags that are similar, have compatible connectors and are located in conjunction with irrigation and infusion products. In the event that there are additives such as heparin, the clinical effects entail inadvertent systemic anticoagulation and bleeding, which is reversible with therapeutic intervention. This strategy is thus based on clear labels, the segregation of storage, the use of route-specific connectors, and environmental controls, all of which reduce misidentification because of the similarity of containers (Cohen & Smetzer, 2011; Institute for Safe Medication Practices (ISMP), 2022).

Figure 6. Images of intravenous fluid containers of the same size and shape may lead to look-alike selection errors in the perioperative environment

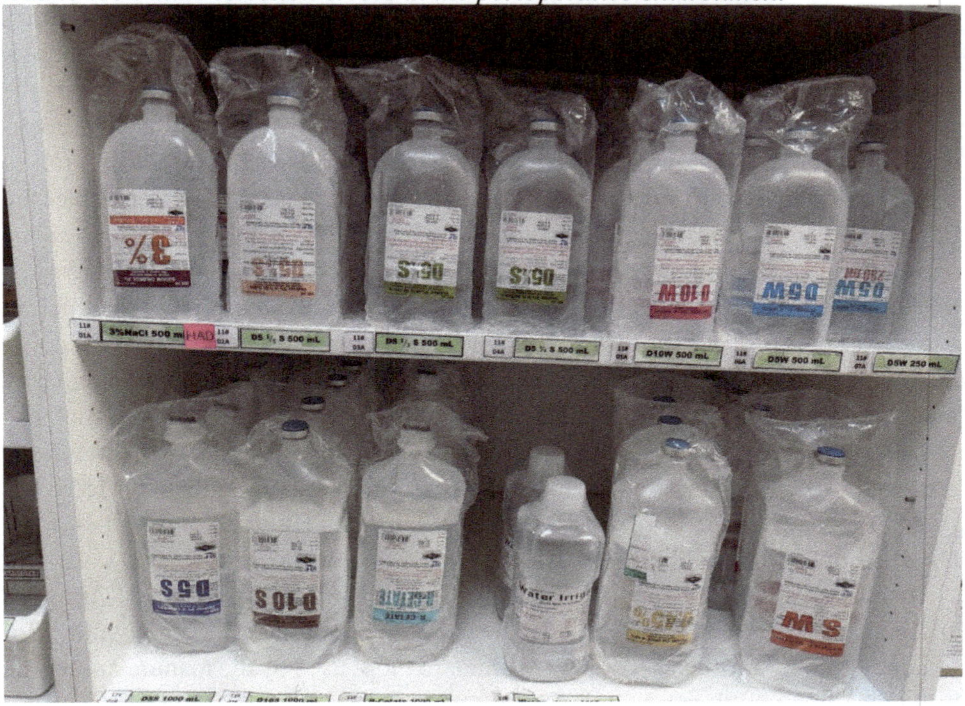

The pharmaceutical products shown are presented solely for academic and educational purposes. Their inclusion does not imply the endorsement, promotion, or advertising of any specific manufacturer, distributor, or brand.

CONTRIBUTING FACTORS AND RISK FACTORS OF INJECTABLE LASA ERRORS

LASA error with injectable drugs is a particularly risky type of medication safety event and is often used in critically ill clinical units. Reviews of perioperative safety and analyses of national wrong-drug events have continuously shown that injectable drugs (in particular, high-alert drugs) are disproportionately related to clinically significant harm in cases of confusion (Ro & Jones, 2025; Ryan et al., 2024).

In contrast to oral medications, injectable drugs do not undergo the first-pass metabolic process, whose effects are felt immediately and systemically; thus, substitutions in terms of the wrong drug can lead to immediate respiratory depression, paralysis, arrhythmia, severe hypoglycemia, or cardiovascular collapse before corrective measures can be taken.

The role of human factors in LASA injection events is important. Clinicians working in perioperative and emergency environments are frequently forced to choose, prepare, label, and administer IV drugs in a time-pressured environment when it is necessary to be near unstable patients at the same time. Haste, multitasking, interruptions, fatigue, and high cognitive load were identified as recurring contributors to look-alike incidents involving ampules and vials (Ryan et al., 2024). Injectables are often placed in anesthesia carts or an emergency tray where several high-alert drugs, such as benzodiazepines, opioids, neuromuscular blocking agents, vasopressors, and electrolyte concentrates, are closely stacked. In these circumstances, clinicians can trust the use of visual pattern recognition as opposed to consciously reading the entire label, which predisposes them to the effects of orthographic similarity and packaging similarity. Regulatory reviews also emphasize that the resemblance of packaging and a lack of eminence of important data, especially the name of the drug and its strength and route, can promote selection errors (European Medicines Agency (EMA), 2011; U.S. Department of Health and Human Services Food and Drug Administration, 2022).

This risk is increased by the physical nature of injectable products. Ampules and vials are small and restrict the label space, and the font size, layout, and color schemes used by various products are similar to those used by the manufacturer. The difference in strength can be minor (e.g., mg and mcg per mL), and concentrated preparations can appear similar to standard preparations. Moreover, more vulnerability is introduced by preparation-stage processes. Drawing up multiple syringes simultaneously, delayed labeling, or delegation without independent verification removes key safety barriers. Syringe swaps after the selection of a visually similar ampule have been reported as a frequent error etiology in the practice of anesthesia (Ryan et al., 2024).

The clinical importance of these vulnerabilities is supported by national surveillance data. High-alert drugs, such as insulin, electrolyte solutions, opioids, and neuromuscular blocking agents, were often represented in the Pennsylvania Patient Safety Reporting System analysis of 2023 wrong-drug events that reached patients (Ro & Jones, 2025; The Pennsylvania Patient Safety Advisory, 2005a, 2005b, 2010).

Owing to the immediate action with a low therapeutic index of injectable agents, incorrect drug errors with injectable agents have a greater likelihood of worsening into severe harm than false errors with lower-risk oral medications do. The administration stage therefore represents the final and most critical point in the injectable medication-use process.

Injectable LASA risk is further increased by environmental and organizational factors. Poor lighting, emergency conditions, frequent interruptions, and fragmented communication during handoffs reduce attention and increase cognitive strain. Disorganized storage, the presence of look-alike vials in the same place, and automated dispensing cabinet misfills are latent system failures that transform human slips into harm to the patient. Regulatory guidance emphasizes that important information should be well represented in the same field of view and that the similarity in the packaging should be minimized to avoid confusion (Bryan et al., 2021a; Bryan et al., 2021b; The Pennsylvania Patient Safety Advisory, 2005a).

The combination of evidence proves that injectable LASA error is caused by the combination of human cognitive impairments, high-alert drugs, packaging structure, storage system, and process complexity. The rapid onset of action of injectable agents, which can be severe in nature, leads to a unique harm profile, which requires a correspondingly higher level of safeguarding. Multilayered prevention methods such as physical segregation of high-alert injectables, the standard arrangement of anesthesia carts, independent second checks, labeling of syringes immediately after preparation, barcode checking at the point of care, and regulatory optimization of label design are needed to prevent these. LASA risk is not only a naming or packaging similarity issue in injectable medication systems but also a vulnerability at the systems level, which is exacerbated by the pharmacologic potency and immediacy of the effect.

CLINICAL SETTINGS MOST AFFECTED

LASA errors involving injectable medications disproportionately occur in high-acuity clinical environments where rapid pharmacologic intervention, cognitive load, and system complexity converge. Evidence from perioperative safety research, intensive care investigations, and emergency medicine literature consistently demonstrates that operating rooms, intensive care units (ICUs), emergency departments (EDs), and postanesthesia care units (PACUs) are the most vulnerable to clinically significant injectable LASA errors (Abeysekera et al., 2005; Nanji et al., 2016; Ryan et al., 2024).

Operating Rooms and Perioperative Settings

The operating room is widely recognized as one of the highest-risk environments for injectable medication errors. In anesthesia practice, a single clinician frequently assumes responsibility for medication selection, preparation, labeling, administration, and physiologic monitoring. This consolidation of the medication use process reduces redundancy and increases reliance on individual cognitive performance.

In a landmark analysis of 896 anesthesia-related drug error reports from the Australian Incident Monitoring Study (AIMS), syringe and drug preparation errors accounted for approximately 50% of reported events, with substitution and ampule confusion representing recurrent mechanisms (Abeysekera et al., 2005). The perioperative environment is characterized by urgent intravenous administration, multiple similar ampules stored in anesthesia carts, and frequent use of high-alert medications such as neuromuscular blockers, opioids, vasopressors, and sedatives.

To further support this vulnerability, in a prospective observational study, Nanji et al. (2016) reported that medication errors and adverse drug events occurred in approximately 1 in 20 perioperative medication administrations, with labeling, syringe swaps, and incorrect drug selection among the identified causes. The rapid onset of injectable agents amplifies the clinical impact of incorrect drug substitutions in this setting (Nanji et al., 2016).

Intensive Care Units

ICUs share many risk factors with operating rooms, including the frequent administration of high-alert injectable medications, continuous infusions, and complex titration regimens. ICU patients typically receive multiple simultaneous intravenous infusions, which require concentration calculations, dose adjustments, and pump programming.

High-alert medications—such as insulin, potassium chloride, magnesium sulfate, sedatives, and vasopressors—are regularly administered intravenously in this setting. The Institute for Safe Medication Practices (ISMP) and related national surveillance systems have repeatedly identified these classes as disproportionately represented in harmful wrong-drug events (Hicks et al., 2008).

The ICU environment also introduces infusion line complexity. Multiple pumps, visually similar tubing, and shared access ports increase the risk of line mix-ups and misidentification. Interruptions and alarm fatigue further decrease attention and increase error susceptibility. Research on human factors consistently shows that such high-cognitive-demand environments are associated with increased medication error risk (Nanji et al., 2016).

Emergency Departments

Emergency departments (EDs) present distinct LASA vulnerabilities because of unpredictability, time-critical decision-making, and reliance on verbal communication. Clinicians must rapidly initiate treatment for undifferentiated patients, often under noisy and chaotic conditions. The need for immediate intravenous medication administration can shorten verification steps and increase susceptibility to sound-alike confusion.

Errors related to injectables due to concentration in the perioperative and emergency care setting have also been reported where a range of similar agents of various strengths are stored in ampules or vials that look visually similar (Abeysekera et al., 2005; Nanji et al., 2016).

Additionally, EDs often stock a wide range of medications to address diverse clinical scenarios, increasing the number of potential LASA pairs within a single medication storage area. High ambient noise levels and frequent verbal order further contribute to the risk of phonetic misinterpretation.

Post-Anesthesia Care Units (PACUs)

PACUs represent a high-risk transition environment where patients are handed off from anesthesia providers to nursing staff. Handoffs are recognized as critical vulnerability points in medication safety. Errors during this stage may arise from syringe similarity, inadequate communication regarding prepared medications, or task delegation without independent verification (Ryan et al., 2024).

Patients in PACUs often require rapid administration of analgesics, antiemetics, vasopressors, or sedatives but are still physiologically unstable. The combination of fluctuating consciousness levels, multiple medication needs, and concurrent management of several patients creates workload pressures that may compromise verification practices.

Occurs Across Settings but is Most Severe in Critical Areas

Although injectable LASA errors have been documented across medical-surgical units, procedural suites, and outpatient infusion centers, the severity profile is concentrated in high-acuity areas. Statewide analyses of wrong-drug events demonstrate that serious outcomes disproportionately involve high-alert injectable medications (Figure 7) (Hicks et al., 2008).

Collectively, perioperative, ICU, ED, and PACU settings exhibit a convergence of risk-enhancing features:

- Rapid intravenous drug administration
- High-alert pharmacotherapy
- Visually similar ampules and vials
- Concentrated responsibility for medication preparation
- Frequent interruptions and cognitive overload

- Urgent clinical decision-making

Literature consistently demonstrates that these environmental and process characteristics amplify the consequences of LASA vulnerabilities when injectable medications are involved. Accordingly, targeted interventions—including standardized anesthesia cart organization, barcode-assisted medication verification, independent double checks for high-alert injectables, human factors–informed labeling, and structured handoff protocols—are essential in these high-risk settings.

Figure 7. Examples of High-Alert Injectable Drugs (HADs)

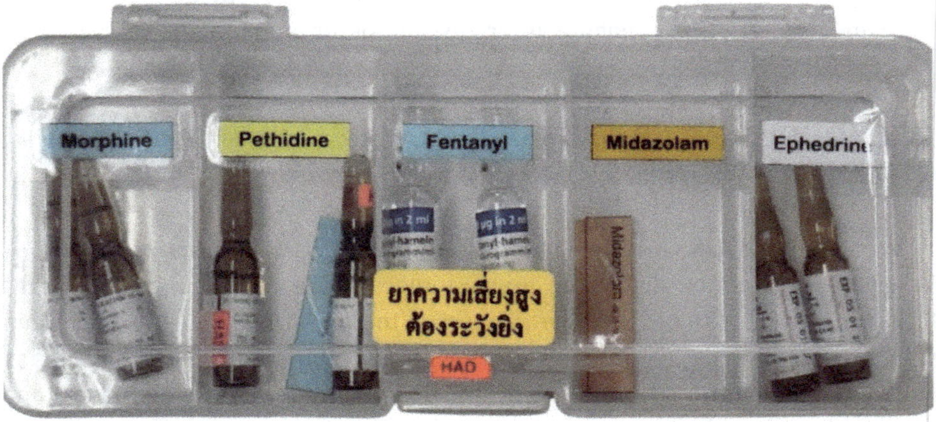

(A) Compartmentalized storage box filled with high-alert injectable drugs with an orange sticker of the letters HAD on it. The orange label of HAD signifies High-Alert Drugs, which is a medication with an increased risk of causing a serious harm to the patient in case of an error and should be subjected to better storage conditions, labeling, and handling.

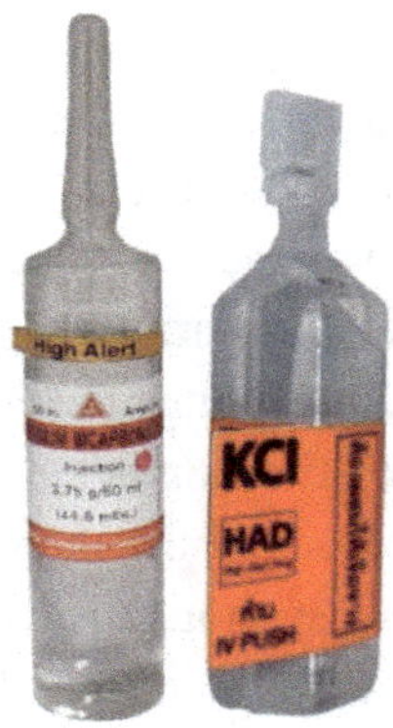

(B) To minimize selection errors, individual injectable high-alert ampules (e.g., sodium bicarbonate and potassium chloride [KCl]) should be labeled with large orange high-alert labels so that they can be distinguished among other injectable drugs.

Storage boxes or individual ampules have an orange sticker marked with the abbreviation HAD (High-Alert Drug) to clearly indicate that they are high-risk medications. The label HAD indicates that more precautions are needed during the storage, labeling, and handling of these drugs since they may cause severe harm to patients when they are used inappropriately.

The pharmaceutical products shown are presented solely for academic and educational purposes. Their inclusion does not imply the endorsement, promotion, or advertising of any specific manufacturer, distributor, or brand.

PROCEDURES TO REDUCE INJECTABLE LASA MEDICATION ERRORS

The concept of LASA errors with injectable medications implies the use of multilayered reductions that touch upon storage design and labeling standards, integration of technologies, standardization of the workflow, and organizational culture. The rapid absorption of injectable agents and their narrow therapeutic index require preventive efforts to function at the drug-use system level, not only at the individual level but also throughout the drug-use system.

Storage and Physical Segregation

Among the most evidence-based and basic methods for preventing wrong-drug and wrong-route errors, physical separation of high-alert injectable drugs must be mentioned. Ampule similarity and the proximity of storage have been consistently found among the factors associated with LASA events in perioperative and critical care settings (Abeysekera et al., 2005). Neuromuscular blocking agents (NMBAs) are especially dangerous since when they are administered accidentally without sedation, they can leave one awake and paralyzed or cause respiratory arrest. The safety literature in the area of ISMP and anesthesia focuses on segregation and sequestration as well as on the clear distinction between NMBAs and other injectable drugs in any place where they are stored (Abeysekera et al., 2005; Merry et al., 2011).

Colocation of intrathecal and intravenous drugs should be removed in stores to avoid incorrect route errors. Analyses of oncological safety indicate that the physical division of intrathecal and intravenous chemotherapy agents is highly important, especially in the case of vinca alkaloids, for which wrong-route administration has led to fatal consequences (Schulmeister, 2006). The same holds true for injectable LASA risk management: physical barriers make it less dependent on memory and visual pattern recognition.

Simplifying inventory is another way of minimizing risk. A reduction in similar ampules in anesthesia carts and ICU medication stations will reduce mental load and complexity of choice (Nanji et al., 2016). A regular examination of stock presentation is needed since modifications in the supplier packaging might result in LASA gaps.

Improper storage configurations and visual similarity of injectable drugs can increase the likelihood of LASA mistakes. Costorage can be unintentional and can readily take place when a drug is brought back into hospital wards and stored again in the wrong bins or compartments without proper verification. As shown in Figure 8(A), chlorpromazine and hydroxyprogesterone ampules have similar amber glasses and sizes, as well as similar label designs, which can be a source of visual confusion during quick choices. Similarly, as shown in Figure 8(B), magnesium sulfate and fentanyl can be costored in the same storage trays. Pharmacologically different but similar ampule sizes, label designs, and locations of storage could increase the potential for incorrect drug choice if entire label verification is not carried out. Previous studies have reported that storage proximity in automated dispensing cabinets and other packaging-related features are important environmental factors contributing to LASA errors (Bryan et al., 2021a; Lizano-Díez et al., 2020; Ruutiainen et al., 2021; Tseng et al., 2018).

Figure 8. Illustrations on the similarity of packaging and proximity of storage as possible causes of injectable LASA errors

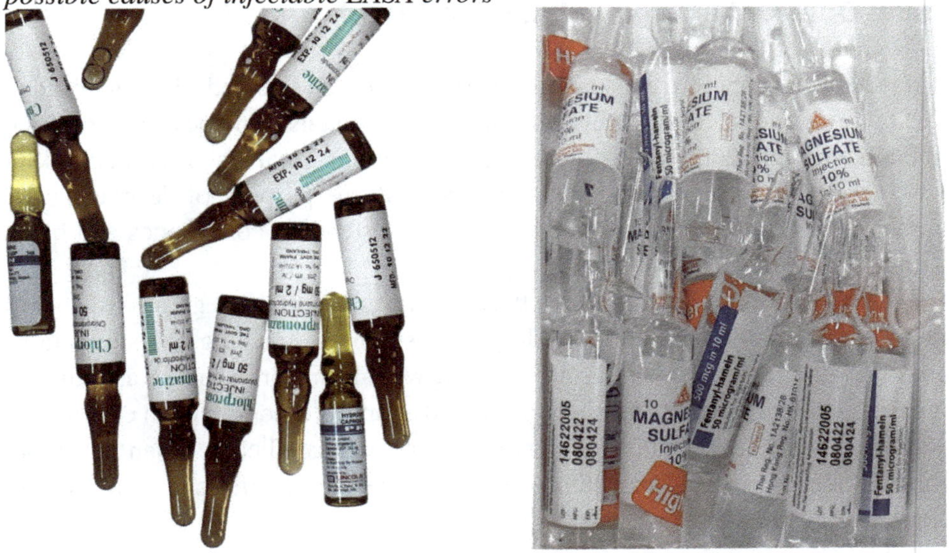

(A) Ampules of chlorpromazine and hydroxyprogesterone share similar amber glass presentation, size, and labeling layout, which may contribute to visual confusion during rapid selection.

(B) Co-storage of fentanyl (opioid analgesic) and magnesium sulfate (electrolyte/anticonvulsant) in the same storage tray, which demonstrates the similarity of packaging with its proximity as a potential risk factor.

According to the principle of similar appearance:

(A) Ampules include chlorpromazine (an antipsychotic agent) and hydroxyprogesterone (a progesterone hormone), which are similar and have similar amber glass looks and labels, which can lead to confusion in visual perception.
(B) Costorage of fentanyl (opioid analgesic) and magnesium sulfate (electrolyte/anticonvulsant) in the same storage tray, which demonstrates the similarity of packaging with its proximity as a potential risk factor. Wards may make inappropriate selections in terms of improperly storing or mixing the medications during ward medication returns.

These photos are shown as illustrative figures and do not show recorded medication error occurrences or particular incidents in the hospital.

The pharmaceutical products shown are presented solely for academic and educational purposes. Their inclusion does not imply the endorsement, promotion, or advertising of any specific manufacturer, distributor, or brand.

Visual Differentiation and Labeling Standards

Injectable medication safety depends on clear and standardized labeling. Syringe labeling errors are a common drug substitution mechanism in anesthesia practice (Abeysekera et al., 2005). Specific standards of international labeling, such as ISO 26825 (anesthetic drug labels), were created with the purpose of decreasing the number of cases of syringe swap errors by using standard color codes and high-contrast typography.

There is evidence that tall man lettering is an effective strategy for enhancing the visual differentiation of similar drug names. An eye-tracking and simulation-controlled study revealed that tall man lettering was much more effective at minimizing errors in identification and changing visual attention among critical care nurses (Lohmeyer et al., 2023). This intervention is especially applicable when injectable high-alert drugs such as morphine versus HYDROmorphone and vinCRIStine versus vinBLAStine are used.

Nonetheless, color coding is not enough. Merry and Webster note that the use of color without a label can lead to an illusion of security. A good label design must have high contrast, a standardized format, and a prominent drug name and concentration. Labeling should be readable even under low-light conditions in the operating room, and handwritten labels, which are related to the variability of legibility, should be avoided as much as possible (Merry et al., 2011).

Interventions Based on Technology

Barcode medication administration (BCMA) implemented with electronic medication administration records (e-MARs) effectively reduced medication administration and transcription errors in the inpatient environment. Poon et al. (2010) examined 14,041 medication administrations in a large tertiary-care hospital in a prospective before-and-after study and reported that nontiming medication administration errors decreased by 41.4% relative to the baseline (11.5 to 6.8) with the implementation of bar-code e-MAR ($p < 0.001$). Notably, the potential adverse drug events related to these errors decreased to 1.6% compared with 3.1%, which is a relative reduction of 50.8% ($p < 0.001$). In addition, transcription errors, which previously existed in 6.1% of the medication orders, were removed after the bar-code e-MAR system was implemented (Poon et al., 2010).

The use of technology-based interventions is instrumental in eliminating LASA errors associated with injectable medications. Nanji et al. (2016) reported that systems using barcodes at the point of care, tools that help with specific drug decisions, and electronic alerts are key technological safeguards. Barcode-assisted systems can minimize labeling and wrong-drug errors, particularly when they scan syringe labels immediately before administration. Wrong-dose and wrong-medication selection can be prevented with the help of drug-specific decision support tools (e.g., dose calculators and maximum dose checks). Strategically graded electronic notifications installed on anesthesia information systems were approximated to avoid more than half of medication errors and most of the related adverse drug events (Nanji et al., 2016). In the case of LASA injectable drugs, these technologies offer stratified electronic checks at the points of preparation, documentation, and administration, which minimize the probability of swapping syringes and selecting incorrect vials in high-intensity perioperative settings.

Independent Double Checks and Verification

Dual verification is also an essential safety measure for superior-alert injectable drugs. When addressed appropriately—meaning that each checker individually identifies errors related to the drug, concentration, dose, and patient—the double checks can detect mistakes before administration (Merry et al., 2011). To be effective, the process should truly be independent rather than confirmatory.

Immediate verification of the final read-back and label before injection is essential in time-sensitive situations. Perioperative medication error studies have shown that the lack of this last verification step is a widespread contributing factor (Nanji et al., 2016).

Physical, technological, workflow, and human-factor controls are needed to prevent injectable LASA errors in the future, as illustrated in Figure 9, not just by individual vigilance.

Figure 9. A layered system for preventing injectable LASA errors. The figure depicts combined precautions for injectable medication safety, such as physical separation of high-risk drugs, tall man typography and standardized syringe labeling, barcoded-based medication administration, autonomous duplicate checks, and supportive regulatory and safety-culture action

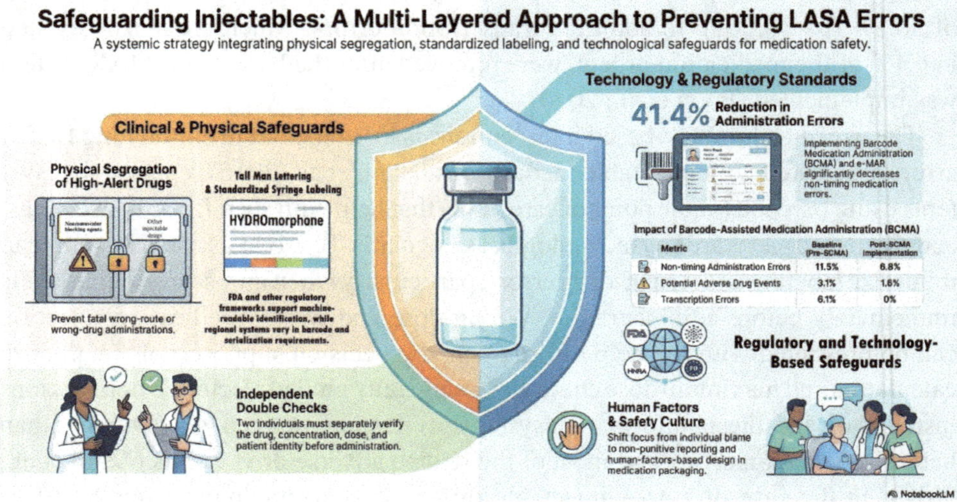

Organizational and Cultural Strategies

A reduction in injectable LASA errors should be performed sustainably, which means that quality improvement methods should be at the system level. Multidisciplinary safety review processes, nonpunitive reporting mechanisms, and organized hazard analysis have been found to enhance medical safety culture (Herzer et al., 2013). Resilience is enhanced by organizational commitment to uniform storage, procurement audits in light of LASA risk, and routine observation of near-miss incidents.

Education needs to be more than procedural training; it should also incorporate human factor awareness, identification of cognitive bias, and practice in high-risk scenarios by using simulation. Learning is supported by the publication and discussion of near-miss cases and normalization of the reporting of errors (Cohen et al., 2007).

REGULATORY FRAMEWORKS AND LABELING STANDARDS

The management of LASA risk in injectable drugs is not determined by an individual statute or technical standard but rather by an integrated ecosystem of regulatory requirements, international standards, national safety guidance, and supply chain harmonization processes and instruments. Injectable products, especially intravenous, intrathecal, epidural, and perioperative agents, present an unequal risk of catastrophic medication harm because of their immediate bioavailability, and once they have been given, there is no opportunity to stop the catastrophic harm. This leads to labeling and packaging controls of injectables being conceptualized in terms of regulatory authorities, rather than aesthetic conventions, as regulated risk-control measures based on incident data and human-factors science.

The ISO 26825:2008 standard defines the conditions of user-applied labels on syringes containing anesthetic drugs, including the color, size, design, overall features, and typographical features of the drug name. The standard only applies to user-affixed labels and not to syringe labels that are placed by the manufacturer. Test strips should be self-adhesive stickers that do not lift, curl, or move when subjected to tests that include a 50% solution of isopropanol. The length and width of each label ranged from 25–40 mm and 10–15 mm, respectively. The name of a drug to be used should be printed in a plain (sans serif) font, at least 2.5 mm high, with either regular capitalization or tall man font; there can be no all-capital font. Notably, the standard states that color should not be used as a substitute for the need to read and check the name of the drugs before administration but rather as a way of identification (International Organization for Standardization, 2008).

This limitation is supported by postmarket surveillance. Multincident analysis conducted by the ISMP Canada involving a study on high-alert medications provided in vials and ampules revealed common vulnerabilities associated with similar colors, similar label designs and layouts, and similar medication names (Institute for Safe Medication Practices (ISMP) Canada, 2023). The bulletin also observes structural limitations of injectable packages, the limited space on labels, the small size of containers, and the visual indistinguishability of clear solutions, which diminishes the discriminative strength of color or layout alone. The analysis revealed substitution errors involving high-alert injectables despite the presence of warning elements (e.g., neuromuscular blocking agent caps), underscoring the necessity of layered safeguards beyond appearance-based differentiation.

In the United States, most prescription drug products must include a linear bar code, which includes at least the National Drug Code (NDC) under 21 CFR §201.25 (The Code of Federal Regulations (CFR), 2004). The bar code should be displayed on the drug label, which includes the immediate container, to ensure the electronic identification of products and minimize medication errors with the help of barcode verification systems. In conjunction with that necessity, the FDA instructions on safety factors in product design focus on preventing medication errors actively by designing proprietary names, labeling containers, and structuring packaging, which is intended to make manufacturers apply human factor principles to their product development (Center for Drug Evaluation and Research (CDER), 2016).

Similar regulatory frameworks exist internationally, with direct relevance to injectable medicines that are commonly supplied in small containers (e.g., vials and ampules) where the label space is constrained and selection often occurs under time pressure. In the United Kingdom, the Human Medicines Regulations 2012 set legal requirements for packaging information, including particulars such as the medicinal product name and strength on outer and immediate packaging, and these requirements are supported by the Medicines and Healthcare products Regulatory Agency (MHRA) best-practice guidance, which is intended to be read alongside the Part 13 legislative framework for labeling and packaging (Medicines and Healthcare products Regulatory Agency, 2012; Medicines and Healthcare products Regulatory Agency (MHRA), 2020; UK Government, 2012).

In Canada, the Food and Drug Regulations (C.R.C., c. 870) provide binding labeling requirements, whereas Health Canada's *Good Label and Package Practices Guide for Prescription Drugs* offers design-oriented recommendations for inner and outer labels and packages across prescription pharmaceuticals, biologics/radiopharmaceuticals, and certain healthcare-directed products, including examples such as injectable epinephrine (Health Canada, 2019, 2025).

At the European Union level, Directive 2011/62/EU (the Falsified Medicines Directive) amended Directive 2001/83/EC to require harmonized safety features on certain medicinal products to prevent falsified medicines from entering the legal supply chain. The directive mandates that prescription medicines (subject to defined exemptions) bear a unique identifier enabling verification of authenticity and identification of individual packs, together with "a device allowing verification of whether the outer packaging has been tampered with" (European Parliament and Council, 2011) (**Table 7**).

Table 7. Global regulatory and standards-based governance of injectable LASA risk

	Regulatory/ Standards Body	Formal Instrument/ Legal Framework	Authority Type	Scope Relevant to Injectables	Core Standardization Elements	LASA Risk-Control Mechanism	References
United States	U.S. Food and Drug Administration	21 CFR §201.25 (Bar Code Final Rule, 2004)	Federal regulation (binding law)	Prescription drugs & biologics (including injectables)	Mandatory linear barcode (NDC)	Enables electronic verification prior to administration	The Code of Federal Regulations (CFR) (2004).
United States	U.S. Food and Drug Administration	Safety Considerations for Product Design to Minimize Medication Errors (2020)	Regulatory guidance	Labeling, container design, proprietary naming	Premarket error-risk evaluation	Design-level LASA differentiation	Center for Drug Evaluation and Research (CDER) (2016).
United Kingdom	Medicines and Healthcare products Regulatory Agency	Human Medicines Regulations 2012	Statutory regulation	Labeling and packaging requirements	Legal labeling content standards; name review oversight	Reduces labeling/ naming confusion	Medicines and Healthcare products Regulatory Agency (2012)
United Kingdom	Medicines and Healthcare products Regulatory Agency	Best Practice Guidance on the Labeling and Packaging of Medicines (2022)	National regulatory guidance	Label differentiation	Strength prominence; layout clarity	Mitigates visual similarity risk	Medicines and Healthcare products Regulatory Agency (MHRA) (2020)
Canada	Health Canada	Food and Drug Regulations (C.R.C., c. 870)	Federal regulation	Drug labeling & packaging	Label clarity and required content	Legal framework for differentiation	Health Canada (2025)
Canada	Institute for Safe Medication Practices Canada	Safety Bulletin: High-Alert Medication Label Analysis (2023)	National safety authority guidance	High-alert injectable vials & ampules	Incident-based differentiation recommendations	Packaging improvement based on error reports	Institute for Safe Medication Practices (ISMP) Canada (2023)

continued on following page

Table 7. Continued

	Regulatory/ Standards Body	Formal Instrument/ Legal Framework	Authority Type	Scope Relevant to Injectables	Core Standardization Elements	LASA Risk-Control Mechanism	References
European Union	European Medicines Agency	Directive 2001/83/ EC; Directive 2011/62/ EU (Falsified Medicines Directive)	EU regulation	Prescription medicine labeling	Mandatory 2D barcode (unique identifier); anti-tampering device	Machine-verification and traceability	European Parliament and Council (2011).
Australia	Therapeutic Goods Administration	Therapeutic Goods Act 1989	National regulation	Labeling, naming approval	Proprietary name risk review; labeling oversight	Prevents look-alike name approval	Therapeutic Goods Adminitration (TGA) (1990)
Australia	Australian Commission on Safety and Quality in Health Care	NSQHS Standards	National safety standards	High-risk injectable management	Standardized infusion concentration initiatives	Reduces preparation variability	Australian Commission on Safety and Quality in Health Care (ACSQHC) (2021)
Singapore	Health Sciences Authority	Health Products Act	National regulation	Labeling & packaging requirements	Label content control; name review	Reduces packaging similarity	Health Sciences Authority (HSA) (2026)
International	International Organization for Standardization	ISO 26825:2008	International consensus standard	Syringe labeling in anesthesia	Standardized color coding; typography standards	Reduces syringe swaps	International Organization for Standardization (2008)
International	GS1	GS1 Global Standards (GTIN; DataMatrix)	International supply-chain standard	Global medication identification	Unique product identifiers; machine-readable barcodes	Supports interoperable electronic verification	General Specifications Association Internationale Sans But Lucratif (GS1 AISBL) (2024)

CONCLUSION

The combination of high pharmacological potency, perceptual similarity, and complicated healthcare systems results in injectable drugs. Unlike oral therapies, injectable drugs enter the bloodstream immediately and are instant; thus, little time is left to determine or correct a mistake once the drugs are administered. The evidence reviewed in this chapter reveals that incorrect drug and LASA errors associated with injectable medications are not unique or rare. They are system failures that are recurrent and are reported across countries and clinical environments such as operating rooms, intensive care units, emergency departments, and, in general, hospital practice.

Epidemiologic studies always point to the preparation and administration phases as the most susceptible to the injectable medication-use procedure. They may include syringe swaps, look-alike ampules and vials, unclear or poorly developed labels, the storage of look-alike products near each other, and misunderstandings arising because of similarities in the names of drugs. High-alert injectable drugs such as neuromuscular blocking drugs, insulin, opioids, vasopressors, concentrated electrolytes, and some antibiotics are overrepresented in adverse events. In the case of LASA mechanisms with these high-risk drugs, the consequences are likely to rapidly develop into respiratory arrest, cardiovascular collapse, severe hypoglycemia, or permanent neurologic damage or even death.

As shown in the examples presented in this chapter, the risk associated with injectable LASA is multifactorial and crosscuts across different classes of drugs. Compared with sedatives or antibiotics, the substitution of neuromuscular blockers can be catastrophic in cases of paralysis. Insulin demonstrates the structural vulnerability of similarity of product variety, similarity of brand prefixes, unit-based dosing, and product packaging. Substitutes of opioids, especially hydromorphone-morphine, amplify differences in potency and harm. The similarity in names in the emergency context is a risk, as is evident in vasopressor confusion, e.g., ephedrine-epinephrine. Substitution with antibiotics and antifungals can result in treatment failure or acute physiologic instability, whereas name confusion is not inevitable since container similarity and route confusion can also cause a severe wrong-route event in the absence of name confusion.

Research on human factors clarifies that human error is not the main reason these errors occur. Perceptual traps are predictable because of high workload, fatigue, interruptions, time pressure, and the use of visual pattern recognition. When a system relies on memory to a great extent, handwritten labels, or even double checks, which are informal, it is by definition fragile. Under these conditions, even experienced clinicians may be deceived by the similarity of orthography or similar packaging.

The control of the injectable LASA errors is hence not possible within the framework of isolated education but within the framework of structural redesign. Multilayered risk controls, such as physical separation of high-alert drugs, standardized labeling and tall man lettering, adherence to syringe-labeling standards, including ISO 26825, barcode checks on the point-of-care, smart infusion pumps with dose-range limitations, high-risk and neuraxial drug-specific attention, simplified inventory choices, prudent procurement scrutiny of packaging similarity, robust postadministration observations, and a nonpunitive safety culture that favors near-miss reporting and analysis, are effective at reducing risks.

Regulatory frameworks and international supply chain standards endorse such efforts by mandating barcodes, anti-tampering, and organized labeling. Nonetheless, the similarity in perception cannot be eradicated through regulation. The active practice of local hazard evaluation, prevention of packaging, and cross-disciplinary quality enhancement are part of a secure injectable drug system.

Finally, LASA injection mistakes are predictable because of the susceptible system design and the use of powerful drugs. These events are structural hazards and not accidental ones, as the same patterns can be traced in terms of settings and decades of safety data. Owing to the grave effects of injectable drugs, which may result in instant and severe damage, their application requires an extremely high degree of reliability in the system. The prevention of injectable LASA errors is not merely a naming or packaging problem; it is a systems engineering problem that can be solved only by incorporating human factors, regulatory and technological protective measures, workflow redesign, and organizational dedication to patient safety.

REFERENCES

Abeysekera, A., Bergman, I. J., Kluger, M. T., & Short, T. G. (2005). Drug error in anaesthetic practice: A review of 896 reports from the Australian Incident Monitoring Study database. *Anaesthesia*, *60*(3), 220–227. DOI: 10.1111/j.1365-2044.2005.04123.x PMID: 15710005

Adlersberg, M. A., Fernando, S., Spollett, G. R., & Inzucchi, S. E. (2002). Glargine and Lispro: Two cases of mistaken identity. *Diabetes Care*, *25*(2), 404–405. DOI: 10.2337/diacare.25.2.404 PMID: 11815523

Al-Nasser, B. (2005). Labeling as a tool to reduce drug error in anesthesia practice. *Regional Anesthesia and Pain Medicine*, *30*(3), 311. DOI: 10.1097/00115550-200505000-00020 PMID: 15898042

Annisa, A. T., Yasin, N. M., & Kristina, S. A. (2023). Medication errors analysis in Asia and Australia: A systematic review. *Pharmaceutical Sciences Asia*, 50(2).

Astin, J., Steynberg, S., & Cook, T. (2015). Time for mandatory color coding of drug ampoules and packaging – yet again. *Anesthesia*, 70(4), 502-502. https://doi .org/https://doi.org/10.1111/anae.13055

Australian Commission on Safety and Quality in Health Care (ACSQHC). (2021). *The National Safety and Quality Health Service (NSQHS) Standards*. Retrieved 25 Feb from https://www.sydneyprivate.com.au/wp-content/uploads/2024/04/national_safety_and_quality_health_service_nsqhs_standards_second_edition_-_updated_may_2021-compressed.pdf

Basco, W. T.Jr, Garner, S. S., Ebeling, M., Freeland, K. D., Hulsey, T. C., & Simpson, K. (2016). Evaluating the potential severity of look-alike, sound-alike drug substitution errors in children. *Academic Pediatrics*, *16*(2), 183–191. DOI: 10.1016/j.acap.2015.06.014 PMID: 26946271

Bryan, R., Aronson, J. K., ten Hacken, P., Williams, A., & Jordan, S. (2015). Patient safety in medication nomenclature: Orthographic and semantic properties of International Nonproprietary Names. *PLoS One*, *10*(12), e0145431. DOI: 10.1371/journal.pone.0145431 PMID: 26701761

Bryan, R., Aronson, J. K., Williams, A., & Jordan, S. (2021a). The problem of look-alike, sound-alike name errors: Drivers and solutions. *British Journal of Clinical Pharmacology*, *87*(2), 386–394. DOI: 10.1111/bcp.14285 PMID: 32198938

Bryan, R., Aronson, J. K., Williams, A. J., & Jordan, S. (2021b). A systematic literature review of LASA error interventions. *British Journal of Clinical Pharmacology*, *87*(2), 336–351. DOI: 10.1111/bcp.14644 PMID: 33197079

Bueng Kan Hospital. (2021). *Look Alike Sound Alike Drug*. Retrieved 17 Jan from https://bkh.moph.go.th/bkhweb/uploads/media/202303310725123_4.LASA_update -_2566.pdf#page=6.00

Cavell, G. F., & Mandaliya, D. (2021). Magnitude of error: A review of wrong dose medication incidents reported to a UK hospital voluntary incident reporting system. *European Journal of Hospital Pharmacy : Science and Practice*, *28*(5), 260–265. DOI: 10.1136/ejhpharm-2019-001987 PMID: 34426478

Center for Drug Evaluation and Research (CDER). (2016). *Safety Considerations for Product Design to Minimize Medication Errors: Guidance for Industry*. Retrieved 25 Feb from https://www.fda.gov/media/84903/download

Chumchit, C., Amrumpai, Y., & Treesak, C. (2015). Recognition on medication safety and look-alike/sound-alike medication problems in Thai public hospitals. *Silpakorn U Science & Tech J*, *9*(2), 40–51.

Clogston, J., Hudanick, L., Suragh, T. A., Jankosky, C., Lewis, P., Martin, D., Schembri, C., Zinderman, C., Maslov, Y., Mistry, M., Pippins, J. R., Vee, S., Wyeth, J., Shimabukuro, T. T., & Leighton, J. (2016). Unintentional administration of insulin instead of influenza vaccine: A case study and review of reports to US vaccine and drug safety monitoring systems. *Drugs & Therapy Perspectives*, *32*(10), 439–446. DOI: 10.1007/s40267-016-0333-2

Cohen, M. R. (2007a). Action needed to prevent dangerous heparin-insulin confusion; sorting things out; staff unaware of fentanyl patch starting doses. *Hospital Pharmacy*, *42*(8), 675–679. DOI: 10.1310/hpj4208-675

Cohen, M. R. (2007b). The role of drug packaging and labeling in medication errors. In Cohen, M. R. (Ed.), *Medication Errors* (2nd ed., pp. 111–152). The American Pharmacists Association. https://doi.org/doi:10.21019/9781582120928.ch7

Cohen, M. R. (2008). Cross Contamination with Insulin Pens; Look-Alike Vials; Kids and Medication Patches; New Look-Alike Name Pair; Preventing Dosing Errors with Methotrexate Injection. *Hospital Pharmacy*, *43*(6), 445–447. DOI: 10.1310/hpj4306-445

Cohen, M. R., & Smetzer, J. L. (2011). ISMP Medication Error Report Analysis-Dakin's Solution Accidentally Given Intravenously; Perilous Infection Control Practices With Needles, Syringes, and Vials Suggest Stepped-up Monitoring Is Needed; Taxotere Concentration and Preparation; Update on Metal in Drug Patches. *Hospital Pharmacy*, *46*(2), 82–86. DOI: 10.1310/hpj4602-82

Cohen, M. R., Smetzer, J. L., Tuohy, N. R., & Kilo, C. M. (2007). High-alert medications: safeguarding against errors. In Cohen, M. R. (Ed.), *Medication Errors* (2nd ed., pp. 317–412). The American Pharmacists Association. DOI: 10.21019/9781582120928.ch14

Currie, M., Mackay, P., Morgan, C., Runciman, W. B., Russell, W. J., Sellen, A., & Williamson, J. A. (1993). The Australian Incident Monitoring Study. The "wrong drug" problem in anesthesia: An analysis of 2000 incident reports. *Anaesthesia and Intensive Care*, *21*(5), 596–601. DOI: 10.1177/0310057X9302100517 PMID: 8273881

Dahan, A., Aarts, L., & Smith, T. W. (2010). Incidence, Reversal, and Prevention of Opioid-induced Respiratory Depression. *Anesthesiology*, *112*(1), 226–238. DOI: 10.1097/ALN.0b013e3181c38c25 PMID: 20010421

Dhande, P. P., Mule, A. V., & Chaudhari, A. P. (2021). Retrospective analysis of look-alike and sound-alike drug incidents in a tertiary care hospital. *Indian Journal of Pharmacy Practice*, *14*(2), 115. DOI: 10.5530/ijopp.14.2.21

Dsouza, S., & Kulkarni, A. (2017). The hazards of look alike packaging in anesthesia practice. *Asian Journal of Anesthesiology*, *55*(4), 91–92. DOI: 10.1016/j.aja.2017.10.003 PMID: 29239830

Estock, J. L., Murray, A. W., Mizah, M. T., Mangione, M. P., Goode, J. S.Jr, & Eibling, D. E. (2018). Label Design Affects Medication Safety in an Operating Room Crisis: A Controlled Simulation Study. *Journal of Patient Safety*, *14*(2), 101–106. DOI: 10.1097/PTS.0000000000000176 PMID: 25760652

European Medicines Agency (EMA). (2011). *QRD recommendations on pack design and labeling for centrally authorized nonprescription human medicinal products*. Retrieved 10 Feb from https://www.ema.europa.eu/en/documents/regulatory-procedural-guideline/draft-quality-review-documents-recommendations-pack-design-and-labelling-centrally-authorised-non-prescription-human-medicinal-products_en.pdf

European Parliament and Council. (2011). *Directive* 2011/62/*EU of the European Parliament and of the Council of* 8 *June* 2011 *amending Directive* 2001/83/*EC on the Community code relating to medicinal products for human use, as regards the prevention of the entry into the legal supply chain of falsified medicinal products. Official Journal of the European Union, L* 174, 74–87. Retrieved 25 Feb from https://health.ec.europa.eu/document/download/7bd5d800-08de-47a3-be9f-d5832682c262_en?

Fasting, S., & Gisvold, S. E. (2000). Adverse drug errors in anesthesia, and the impact of colored syringe labels. *Canadian Journal of Anaesthesia*, *47*(11), 1060–1067. DOI: 10.1007/BF03027956 PMID: 11097534

Fontaine, A. L. (2004). Current requirements and emerging trends for labeling as a tool for communicating pharmacovigilance findings. *Drug Safety*, *27*(8), 579–589. DOI: 10.2165/00002018-200427080-00009 PMID: 15154829

Garlich, F. M., & Nelson, L. S. (2010). Inadvertent IV administration of IM epinephrine. *Emerg Med*, *42*, 24–27.

General Specifications Association Internationale Sans But Lucratif (GS1 AISBL). (2024). *GS*1 *General Specifications Standard*. Retrieved 15 Aug from https://ref.gs1.org/standards/genspecs/

Graudins, L. V., Downey, G., Bui, T., & Dooley, M. J. (2016). Recommendations and Low-Technology Safety Solutions Following Neuromuscular Blocking Agent Incidents. *Joint Commission Journal on Quality and Patient Safety*, *42*(2), 86–91. DOI: 10.1016/S1553-7250(16)42010-6 PMID: 26803037

Grissinger, M. (2011). Action is neeeded to prevent heparin-insulin mixups. *P&T : a Peer-Reviewed Journal for Formulary Management*, *36*(4), 177–202. PMID: 21572772

Grissinger, M. (2012). Tall man letters are gaining wide acceptance. *P&T : a Peer-Reviewed Journal for Formulary Management*, *37*(3), 132–148. PMID: 22605902

Grissinger, M. (2019). Accidental IV Infusion of Heparinized Irrigation in the Operating Room. *P&T : a Peer-Reviewed Journal for Formulary Management*, *44*(7), 389–390. PMID: 31258307

Hanna, G. M., & Levine, W. C. (2011). Medication safety in the perioperative setting. *Anesthesiology Clinics*, *29*(1), 135–144. DOI: 10.1016/j.anclin.2010.11.009 PMID: 21295758

Health and Disability Commissioner. (2017). *Incorrect dispensing of insulin (Case* 16*HDC*01665). Retrieved 9 July from https://www.hdc.org.nz/decisions/search-decisions/2017/16hdc01665/

Health Canada. (2019). *Good label and package practices guide for prescription drugs*. Retrieved 15 March from https://www.canada.ca/en/health-canada/services/drugs-health-products/reports-publications/medeffect-canada/good-label-package-practices-guide-prescription-drugs-profile/guidance-document.html

Health Canada. (2025). *Food and Drug Regulations (C.R.C., c.* 870). Retrieved 25 Feb from https://laws-lois.justice.gc.ca/eng/regulations/c.r.c.%2C_c._870/page-62.html?

Health Sciences Authority (HSA). (2026). *Therapeutic Products Guidance on Therapeutic Product Registration in Singapore*. Retrieved 25 Feb from https://www.hsa.gov.sg/docs/default-source/hprg-tpb/guidances/guidance-on-therapeutic-product-registration-in-singapore.pdf?sfvrsn=cd174383_62

Herzer, K. R., Lim, C., Li, M., Xie, Y., Doyle, P. A., Cover, R., & Mark, L. J. (2013). Q-tip: From local quality improvement to national drug recall. *American Journal of Medical Quality : The Official Journal of the American College of Medical Quality*, *28*(3), 265. DOI: 10.1177/1062860613478730 PMID: 23508529

Hicks, R., Becker, S., & Cousins, D. (2008). *MEDMARX data report. A report on the relationship of drug names and medication errors in response to the institute of Medicine's call for action*. Center for the Advancement of Patient Safey, US Pharmacopeia.

Hong, J.-M., Cho, A.-R., & Choi, S.-A. (2014). Accidental intrathecal injection of dopamine hydrochloride resulting in analgesic effects. *Korean Journal of Anesthesiology*, *67*(Suppl), S49–S50. DOI: 10.4097/kjae.2014.67.S.S49 PMID: 25598904

Institute for Safe Medication Practices (ISMP). (2018). *ISMP guidelines for optimizing safe implementation and use of basal insulin*. Retrieved 9 July from https://www.ismp.org/sites/default/files/attachments/2018-09/ISMP138D-Insulin%20Guideline-090718.pdf

Institute for Safe Medication Practices (ISMP). (2022). *ISMP Guidelines for Safe Medication Use in Perioperative and Procedural Settings*. Retrieved 28 Jan from https://www.ismp.org/system/files/resources/2022-08/ISMP198-Periop-Guidelines-FINAL.pdf

Institute for Safe Medication Practices (ISMP) Canada. (2006). Top 10 Drugs Reported as Causing Harm through Medication Error. *ISMP Canada Safety Bulletin*, *6*(1), 1–2.

Institute for Safe Medication Practices (ISMP) Canada. (2007). Risk of Mix-ups between Ephedrine and Epinephrine. *ISMP Canada Safety Bulletin*, *7*(2), 1–3.

Institute for Safe Medication Practices (ISMP) Canada. (2023). *Reported Concerns with Labeling and Packaging of High-Alert Medications in Vials and Ampoules: A Multi-Incident Analysis*. Retrieved 25 Feb from https://ismpcanada.ca/wp-content/uploads/ISMPCSB2023-i2-Label-Package-High-Alert-Meds.pdf

International Organization for Standardization. (2008). *ISO* 26825:2008*(E). Anesthetic and respiratory equipment —User-applied labels for syringes containing drugs used during anesthesia — Colors, design and performance*. Retrieved 25 Feb from https://cdn.standards.iteh.ai/samples/43811/3572a136579d4e3691196a4df1c4b1f5/ISO-26825-2008.pdf

James, R. H. (1998). Ephedrine/Epinephrine drug label confusion. *Anaesthesia, 53*(5), 511. DOI: 10.1046/j.1365-2044.1998.04771.x PMID: 9659030

Kim, J. W., Ko, T. Y., & Kang, D. (2026). Accidental epidural administration of sugammadex and ramosetron - A case report. *Anesthesia and Pain Medicine*, *21*(1), 67–71. DOI: 10.17085/apm.25330 PMID: 41667250

Kuitunen, S., Niittynen, I., Airaksinen, M., & Holmström, A.-R. (2021). Systemic Causes of In-Hospital Intravenous Medication Errors: A Systematic Review. *Journal of Patient Safety*, *17*(8), e1660–e1668. DOI: 10.1097/PTS.0000000000000632 PMID: 32011427

Lerdsirisopon, S., Angkasuvan, W., Viengteerawat, S., Limapichat, R., Prapongsena, P., Ariyanuchitkul, T., & Chongarunngamsang, W. (2018). Medication Errors and Adverse Drug Events: Analysis from Perioperative Anesthetic Adverse Events in Thailand (PAAd Thai Study). *Journal of the Medical Association of Thailand*, *101*(6).

Lizano-Díez, I., Figueiredo-Escribá, C., Piñero-López, M., Lastra, C. F., Mariño, E. L., & Modamio, P. (2020). Prevention strategies to identify LASA errors: Building and sustaining a culture of patient safety. *BMC Health Services Research*, *20*(1), 63. DOI: 10.1186/s12913-020-4922-3 PMID: 31996197

Lohmeyer, Q., Schiess, C., Wendel Garcia, P. D., Petry, H., Strauch, E., Dietsche, A., Schuepbach, R. A., Buehler, P. K., & Hofmaenner, D. A. (2023). Effects of tall man lettering on the visual behavior of critical care nurses while identifying syringe drug labels: A randomized in situ simulation. *BMJ Quality & Safety*, *32*(1), 26–33. DOI: 10.1136/bmjqs-2021-014438 PMID: 35260415

Lowe, A., Hamilton, M., Greenall, B. M. J., Ma, J., Dhalla, I., & Persaud, N. (2017). Fatal overdoses involving hydromorphone and morphine among inpatients: A case series. *CMAJ Open*, *5*(1), E184–e189. DOI: 10.9778/cmajo.20160013 PMID: 28401133

Majeed, A., Chaiah, Y., Hammad, A., Alkhani, S., Amer, M. A., & Broering, D. C. (2025). Adrenaline rush: Unsuspicious dispensing error causing life threatening wrong drug infusion during living donor liver transplantation. *Saudi Journal of Anaesthesia, 19*(3), 416–418. DOI: 10.4103/sja.sja_602_24 PMID: 40642627

Medicines and Healthcare products Regulatory Agency. (2012). *The Human Medicines Regulations* 2012. Retrieved 25 Feb from https://www.legislation.gov.uk/uksi/2012/1916/contents/made

Medicines and Healthcare products Regulatory Agency (MHRA). (2020). *Best practice guidance on the labeling and packaging of medicines. Medicines and Healthcare products Regulatory Agency.* Retrieved 13 July from https://assets.publishing.service.gov.uk/media/5fe09fa48fa8f51489f14374/Best_practice_guidance_labelling_and_packaging_of_medicines.pdf

Merry, A. F., Shipp, D. H., & Lowinger, J. S. (2011). The contribution of labeling to safe medication administration in anesthetic practice. *Best Practice & Research. Clinical Anaesthesiology, 25*(2), 145–159. DOI: 10.1016/j.bpa.2011.02.009 PMID: 21550540

Meyer, T. A., & McAllister, R. K. (2023). Medication errors related to look-alike, sound-alike drugs—How big is the problem and what progress is being made? *APSF Newsletter, 38*(2), 47–49.

Michelet-Huot, E., Bacouillard, J. B., Quillet, P., Bonnet, M., Mongaret, C., & Hettler, D. (2017). PS-106 Look-alike and sound-alike drug incidents in a hospital: A retrospective analysis. *European Journal of Hospital Pharmacy : Science and Practice, 24*(Suppl 1), A274. DOI: 10.1136/ejhpharm-2017-000640.612

Nanji, K. C., Patel, A., Shaikh, S., Seger, D. L., & Bates, D. W. (2016). Evaluation of Perioperative Medication Errors and Adverse Drug Events. *Anesthesiology, 124*(1), 25–34. DOI: 10.1097/ALN.0000000000000904 PMID: 26501385

Ogboli-Nwasor, E. (2013). Medication errors in anesthetic practice: A report of two cases and review of the literature. *African Health Sciences, 13*(3), 845–849. DOI: 10.4314/ahs.v13i3.46 PMID: 24250330

Pandey, R., & Philip, A. (2011). Concentrate on the Concentration! Double Checkin g Avoids Another Potential Disaster. *Journal of Anesthesia & Clinical Research, 2*(7), 148. DOI: 10.4172/2155-6148.1000148

Pattinson, K. T. S. (2008). Opioids and the control of respiration. *British Journal of Anaesthesia, 100*(6), 747–758. DOI: 10.1093/bja/aen094 PMID: 18456641

Poon, E. G., Keohane, C. A., Yoon, C. S., Ditmore, M., Bane, A., Levtzion-Korach, O., Moniz, T., Rothschild, J. M., Kachalia, A. B., Hayes, J., Churchill, W. W., Lipsitz, S., Whittemore, A. D., Bates, D. W., & Gandhi, T. K. (2010). Effect of Bar-Code Technology on the Safety of Medication Administration. *The New England Journal of Medicine*, *362*(18), 1698–1707. DOI: 10.1056/NEJMsa0907115 PMID: 20445181

Ramaswamy, G., & Naik, R. (2014). Saline and metronidazole. *British Journal of Anaesthesia*, *112*(6), 1123. DOI: 10.1093/bja/aeu177 PMID: 24829428

Reason, J. (2000). Human error: Models and management. *BMJ (Clinical Research Ed.)*, *320*(7237), 768–770. DOI: 10.1136/bmj.320.7237.768 PMID: 10720363

Ro, M., & Jones, R. (2025). Wrong Drug Events Across Pennsylvania Healthcare Facilities: A Systematic Analysis of Medication Pairs, Class Patterns, and Clinical Safety Implications. *Patient Safety*, *7*(2). Advance online publication. DOI: 10.33940/001c.134046

Ruutiainen, H. K., Kallio, M. M., & Kuitunen, S. K. (2021). Identification and safe storage of look-alike, sound-alike medicines in automated dispensing cabinets. *European Journal of Hospital Pharmacy : Science and Practice*, *28*(e1, Suppl 2), e151–e156. DOI: 10.1136/ejhpharm-2020-002531 PMID: 33452109

Ryan, A. N., Robertson, K. L., & Glass, B. D. (2024). Look-alike medications in the perioperative setting: Scoping review of medication incidents and risk reduction interventions. *International Journal of Clinical Pharmacy*, *46*(1), 26–39. DOI: 10.1007/s11096-023-01629-2 PMID: 37688737

Ryan, A. N., Robertson, K. L., & Glass, B. D. (2025). Look-alike, sound-alike medication perioperative incidents in a regional Australian hospital: Assessment using a novel medication safety culture assessment tool. *International Journal for Quality in Health Care*, *37*(1), mzaf018. DOI: 10.1093/intqhc/mzaf018 PMID: 40037610

Safety, P. P. (2010). Adverse drug events with HYDROmorphone: How preventable are they. *Pennsylvania Patient Safety Advisory*, *7*(3), 69–75.

Santell, J. P. (2006). Medication errors involving neuromuscular blocking agents. *Jt Comm J Qual Patient Saf*, 32(8), 470-475, 417. DOI: 10.1016/S1553-7250(06)32062-4

Schulmeister, L. (2006). Look-alike, sound-alike oncology medications. *Clinical Journal of Oncology Nursing*, *10*(1), 35–41. DOI: 10.1188/06.CJON.35-41 PMID: 16482726

Smetzer, J. L., & Cohen, M. R. (2006). Preventing errors with neuromuscular blocking agents. *Joint Commission Journal on Quality and Patient Safety*, *32*(1), 56–59. DOI: 10.1016/S1553-7250(06)32008-9 PMID: 16514940

Supapaan, T. S., Napaporn, J., Ruthirakanok, R., Srichathum, S., Songmuang, A., & Pitchayajittipong, C. (2024). Look-alike sound-alike (LASA) medication errors in Thai hospitals. *Pharmacy Practice*, *22*(1), 2886.

The Code of Federal Regulations (CFR). (2004). *§* 201.25 *Bar code label requirements*. Retrieved 25 Feb from https://www.ecfr.gov/current/title-21/chapter-I/subchapter-C/part-201/subpart-A/section-201.25

The Institute for Safe Medication Practices Canada (ISMP Canada). (2007). Patient Report of Insulin Mix-Up Shared. *ISMP Canada Safety Bulletin*, *7*(6), 1–2.

The Pennsylvania Patient Safety Advisory. (2004). Medication errors linked to drug name confusion. *PA PSRS Patient Saf Advis*, *1*(4), 7–8.

The Pennsylvania Patient Safety Advisory. (2005a). Abbreviations: A shortcut to medication errors. *PA PSRS Patient Saf Advis*, *2*(1), 19–21.

The Pennsylvania Patient Safety Advisory. (2005b). Complexity of insulin therapy. *PA PSRS Patient Saf Advis*, *2*(2), 30–31.

The Pennsylvania Patient Safety Advisory. (2010). Medication Errors with the Dosing of Insulin: Problems across the Continuum. *PA PSRS Patient Saf Advis*, *7*(1), 9–17.

Therapeutic Goods Adminitration (TGA). A. G. (1990). *Therapeutic Goods Act* 1989. Retrieved 25 Feb from https://www.tga.gov.au/resources/legislation/therapeutic-goods-act-1989

Thomas, P. B. M., & Mollon, J. D. (2018). Syringe labels seen through the eyes of the color-deficient clinician. *British Journal of Anaesthesia*, *121*(6), 1370–1373. DOI: 10.1016/j.bja.2018.07.023 PMID: 30442268

Tseng, H. Y., Wen, C. F., Lee, Y. L., Jeng, K. C., & Chen, P. L. (2018). Dispensing errors from look-alike drug trade names. *European Journal of Hospital Pharmacy : Science and Practice*, *25*(2), 96–99. DOI: 10.1136/ejhpharm-2016-001019 PMID: 31156995

UK Government. (2012). *The Human Medicines Regulations* 2012 (*SI* 2012/1916). Retrieved 25 Feb from https://www.legislation.gov.uk/uksi/2012/1916/pdfs/uksi_20121916_en.pdf?

U.S. Department of Health and Human Services Food and Drug Administration. (2022). *Safety considerations for container labels and carton labeling design to minimize medication errors guidance for industry*. Retrieved 11 July from https://www.fda.gov/media/158522/download

Valentin, A., Capuzzo, M., Guidet, B., Moreno, R., Metnitz, B., Bauer, P., & Metnitz, P. (2009). Errors in administration of parenteral drugs in intensive care units: Multinational prospective study. *BMJ (Clinical Research Ed.)*, *338*(mar12 1), b814. DOI: 10.1136/bmj.b814 PMID: 19282436

Wahr, J. A., Abernathy, J. H.III, Lazarra, E. H., Keebler, J. R., Wall, M. H., Lynch, I., Wolfe, R., & Cooper, R. L. (2017). Medication safety in the operating room: Literature and expert-based recommendations. *British Journal of Anaesthesia*, *118*(1), 32–43. DOI: 10.1093/bja/aew379 PMID: 28039240

Wang, Y., Du, Y., Zhao, Y., Ren, Y., & Zhang, W. (2017). Automated anesthesia carts reduce drug recording errors in medication administrations - A single center study in the largest tertiary referral hospital in China. *Journal of Clinical Anesthesia*, *40*, 11–15. DOI: 10.1016/j.jclinane.2017.03.051 PMID: 28625429

Westbrook, J. I., Li, L., Woods, A., Badgery-Parker, T., Mumford, V., Merchant, A., Fitzpatrick, E., & Raban, M. Z. (2024). Risk Factors Associated with Medication Administration Errors in Children: A Prospective Direct Observational Study of Pediatric Inpatients. *Drug Safety*, *47*(6), 545–556. DOI: 10.1007/s40264-024-01408-6 PMID: 38443625

World Health Organization. (2023). *Medication safety for look-alike, sound-alike medicines*. World Health Organization. Retrieved 3 June from https://iris.who.int/bitstream/handle/10665/373495/9789240058897-eng.pdf?sequence=1

ABBREVIATIONS

ADC: Automated Dispensing Cabinet
ADE: Adverse Drug Event
ADR: Adverse Drug Reaction
AIMS: Australian Incident Monitoring Study
BCMA: Barcode Medication Administration
ED: Emergency departments
eMAR: Electronic Medication Administration Record
HAD: High-Alert Injectable Drug
ICU: Intensive Care Unit

ISO: International Organization for Standardization
ISMP: Institute for Safe Medication Practices
IV: Intravenous
IU: International Unit
LASA: Look-Alike, Sound-Alike
MSO_4: Morphine sulfate
$MgSO_4$: Magnesium sulfate
NCC MERP: National Coordinating Council for Medication Error Reporting and Prevention
NCC MERP Category: NCC MERP Index for Categorizing Medication Errors
NMBA: Neuromuscular Blocking Agent
OR: Operating Room
PA-PSRS: Pennsylvania Patient Safety Reporting System
PCA: Patient-Controlled Analgesia
PPSA: Pennsylvania Patient Safety Authority
SC: Subcutaneous
U: Unit
U.S. FDA: United States Food and Drug Administration
webAIRS: Web-based Anesthetic Incident Reporting System
WHO: World Health Organization

Compilation of References

Abdel-Latif, M. M. (2016). Knowledge of healthcare professionals about medication errors in hospitals. *Journal of Basic and Clinical Pharmacy*, *7*(3), 87–92. DOI: 10.4103/0976-0105.183264 PMID: 27330261

Abdel-Qader, D. H., Abdel-Qader, H., Silverthorne, J., Kongkaew, C., Al Nimrawi, M., Al Meslamani, A. Z., & Arabi, S. Z. (2025). Investigating the point prevalence, types, severity, causes and predictors of vaccines administration errors during COVID-19 pandemic in Jordan. *PLoS One*, *20*(1), e0312050. DOI: 10.1371/journal.pone.0312050 PMID: 39752371

Abeysekera, A., Bergman, I. J., Kluger, M. T., & Short, T. G. (2005). Drug error in anaesthetic practice: A review of 896 reports from the Australian Incident Monitoring Study database. *Anaesthesia*, *60*(3), 220–227. DOI: 10.1111/j.1365-2044.2005.04123.x PMID: 15710005

Abrishami, R., Aghili, S. H., Farhang Ranjbar, M., & Lashgari, N.-A. (2024). Assessment of Transcription Errors and their Effects on Medical Approach, Hospitalization Duration, and Financial Costs of Traumatic Patients: How Can We Prevent Them? *Epidemiol Health System J*, *11*(3), 121–127. DOI: 10.34172/ehsj.26193

Academy of Managed Care Pharmacy (AMCP). (2023). *Medication errors*. Retrieved 16 Mar from https://www.amcp.org/about/managed-care-pharmacy-101/concepts-managed-care-pharmacy/medication-errors

Aceves-Gonzalez, C., Caro-Rojas, A., Rey-Galindo, J. A., Aristizabal-Ruiz, L., & Hernández-Cruz, K. (2024). Estimating the impact of label design on reducing the risk of medication errors by applying HEART in drug administration. *European Journal of Clinical Pharmacology*, *80*(4), 575–588. DOI: 10.1007/s00228-024-03619-3 PMID: 38282080

Adlersberg, M. A., Fernando, S., Spollett, G. R., & Inzucchi, S. E. (2002). Glargine and Lispro: Two cases of mistaken identity. *Diabetes Care*, *25*(2), 404–405. DOI: 10.2337/diacare.25.2.404 PMID: 11815523

Agency for Healthcare Research and Quality (AHRQ). (2017). *Guide to patient and family engagement in hospital quality and safety*. Retrieved 23 Jan from https://www.ahrq.gov/patient-safety/patients-families/engagingfamilies/guide.html

Agency for Healthcare Research and Quality (AHRQ)-Patient Safety Network (PS-NET). (2024). *Medication errors and adverse drug events*. Retrieved 22 Jan from https://psnet.ahrq.gov/primer/medication-errors-and-adverse-drug-events

Ahuja, A., & Ahuja, V. (2024). LASA (Look alike sound alike) medicament errors-What a dental personnel needs to know? *Journal of Dental Panaceal*, *6*(3), 113–114. DOI: 10.18231/j.jdp.2024.023

Alj, L., Tebaa, A., Talibi, I., Moubarik, S., Benazzouz, M., & Soulaymani Bencheikh, R. (2024). Lessons learned from a cluster of immunization errors in newborns. *Therapeutic Advances in Vaccines and Immunotherapy*, *12*, 25151355231221009. DOI: 10.1177/25151355231221009 PMID: 38178960

Allard, J., Carthey, J., Cope, J., Pitt, M., & Woodward, S. (2002). Medication errors: Causes, prevention and reduction. *British Journal of Haematology*, *116*(2), 255–265. DOI: 10.1046/j.1365-2141.2002.03272.x

Allie, J. (2022). *What different eye drop cap colors mean*. Retrieved 15 March from https://www.allaboutvision.com/treatments-and-surgery/drugs-medications/eye-drop-cap-color-meanings/

Almohammed, O. A., Alnogaidan, R. A., Ghannam, F. O., Alqahtani, R. S., Aloraini, S. K., & Abanmy, N. O. (2023). Public awareness of online pharmacies, consumers' motivating factors, experience and satisfaction with online pharmacy services, and current barriers and motivators for non-consumers: The case of Saudi Arabia. *Saudi Pharmaceutical Journal : SPJ : The Official Publication of the Saudi Pharmaceutical Society*, *31*(8), 101676. DOI: 10.1016/j.jsps.2023.06.009 PMID: 37576852

Al-Nasser, B. (2005). Labeling as a tool to reduce drug error in anesthesia practice. *Regional Anesthesia and Pain Medicine*, *30*(3), 311. DOI: 10.1097/00115550-200505000-00020 PMID: 15898042

Aluminium [Aluminum] Hydroxide, M. H., and Simeticone [Simethicone], (2025). *Lexi-Drugs Multinational. UpToDate Lexidrug. UpToDate Inc.* Retrieved 19 March from https://online.lexi.com

Ambroxol. (2025). *Lexi-Drugs Multinational. UpToDate Lexidrug. UpToDate Inc.* Retrieved 19 March from https://online.lexi.com

Amcon, T. E. S. C. (2025). *Know your ophthalmic eye drops by cap colors*. Retrieved 14 March from https://www.amconlabs.com/blog/why-ophthalmic-eye-drop-caps-colors/

American Society of Anesthesiologists. (2020). *Statement on Labeling of Pharmaceuticals for Use in Anesthesiology*. Retrieved 2024 from https://www.asahq.org/standards-and-practice-parameters/statement-on-labeling-of-pharmaceuticals-for-use-in-anesthesiology

American Society of Health-System Pharmacists (ASHP). (2018). *ASHP Guidelines on Preventing Medication Errors with Chemotherapy and Biotherapy*. Retrieved 14 Oct from https://www.ashp.org/-/media/assets/policy-guidelines/docs/guidelines/preventing-medication-errors-chemotherapy-biotherapy.pdf?utm

American Society of Health-System Pharmacists. (2009). ASHP statement on bar-code-enabled medication administration technology. *American Journal of Health-System Pharmacy*, *66*(6), 588–590. DOI: 10.2146/ajhp080414 PMID: 19265189

American Society of Health-System Pharmacists. (2011). ASHP statement on bar-code verification during inventory, preparation, and dispensing of medications. *American Journal of Health-System Pharmacy*, *68*(5), 442–445. DOI: 10.2146/sp100012 PMID: 21330687

Amoxicillin and Clavulanate. (2025). *Lexi-Drugs Multinational. UpToDate Lexidrug. UpToDate Inc.* Retrieved 19 March from https://online.lexi.com

Amoxicillin. (2025). *Lexi-Drugs Multinational. UpToDate Lexidrug. UpToDate Inc.* Retrieved 23 May from https://online.lexi.com

Anand, N., Prathibha, P., Purohit, P., Nalamitha, R., & Rajarao Padma, C. (2021). *Biometric enabled patient-centric automated medication dispenser using IoT*. Computer Networks and Inventive Communication Technologies. DOI: 10.1007/978-981-15-9647-6_43

Annisa, A. T., Yasin, N. M., & Kristina, S. A. (2023). Medication errors analysis in Asia and Australia: A systematic review. *Pharmaceutical Sciences Asia*, 50(2).

Archambault, G. F. (1983). USAN and the USP dictionary of drug names—Who needs it? *Drug Intelligence & Clinical Pharmacy*, *17*(7-8), 608. DOI: 10.1177/106002808301700741 PMID: 6347600

Arimura, J., Poole, R. L., Jeng, M., Rhine, W., & Sharek, P. (2008). Neonatal heparin overdose-a multidisciplinary team approach to medication error prevention. *The Journal of Pediatric Pharmacology and Therapeutics: The Official Journal of PPAG, 13*(2), 96–98. DOI: 10.5863/1551-6776-13.2.96 PMID: 23055872

Aronson, J. K. (2009). Medication errors: Definitions and classification. *British Journal of Clinical Pharmacology, 67*(6), 599–604. DOI: 10.1111/j.1365-2125.2009.03415.x PMID: 19594526

Ashcroft, D. M., Quinlan, P., & Blenkinsopp, A. (2005). Prospective study of the incidence, nature and causes of dispensing errors in community pharmacies. *Pharmacoepidemiology and Drug Safety, 14*(5), 327–332. DOI: 10.1002/pds.1012 PMID: 15386722

ASHP. *ASHP guidelines on preventing medication errors in hospitals*. Retrieved 12 May from https://www.ashp.org/-/media/assets/policy-guidelines/docs/guidelines/preventing-medication-errors-hospitals.ashx

Astin, J., Steynberg, S., & Cook, T. (2015). Time for mandatory color coding of drug ampoules and packaging – yet again. *Anesthesia*, 70(4), 502-502. https://doi.org/https://doi.org/10.1111/anae.13055

Australian Commission on Safety and Quality in Health Care (ACSQHC). (2012). *Consultation on labelling and packaging of medicines: Submission to the consultation on theTGA Medicine Labelling and Packaging Review* Retrieved 24 July from https://www.tga.gov.au/sites/default/files/consult-labelling-packaging-review-120524-submission-acsqhc.pdf?

Australian Commission on Safety and Quality in Health Care (ACSQHC). (2021). *The National Safety and Quality Health Service (NSQHS) Standards*. Retrieved 25 Feb from https://www.sydneyprivate.com.au/wp-content/uploads/2024/04/national_safety_and_quality_health_service_nsqhs_standards_second_edition_-_updated_may_2021-compressed.pdf

Australian Commission on Safety and Quality in Health Care (ACSQHC). (2024). *National mixed-case lettering list*. ACSQHC. Retrieved 18 March from https://www.safetyandquality.gov.au/sites/default/files/2024-04/national_mixed-case_lettering_list.pdf

Avigan, M. I., Mozersky, R. P., & Seeff, L. B. (2016). Scientific and Regulatory Perspectives in Herbal and Dietary Supplement Associated Hepatotoxicity in the United States. *International Journal of Molecular Sciences, 17*(3), 331. DOI: 10.3390/ijms17030331 PMID: 26950122

Bai, H. K., Ahearn, J. D., & Bartlett, M. G. (2021). Over-the-counter drugs: Regulatory analysis of warning letters between fiscal years 2015-2019. *Therapeutic Innovation & Regulatory Science*, *55*(2), 426–436. DOI: 10.1007/s43441-020-00231-2 PMID: 33095420

Bailey, R. L., Gahche, J. J., Miller, P. E., Thomas, P. R., & Dwyer, J. T. (2013). Why US adults use dietary supplements. *JAMA Internal Medicine*, *173*(5), 355–361. DOI: 10.1001/jamainternmed.2013.2299 PMID: 23381623

Barboza, T. C., Guimarães, R. A., Gimenes, F. R. E., & Silva, A. (2020). Retrospective study of immunization errors reported in an online Information System. *Revista Latino-Americana de Enfermagem*, *28*, e3303. DOI: 10.1590/1518-8345.3343.3303 PMID: 32578753

Barenie, R. E., Kesselheim, A. S., Gagne, J. J., Lu, Z., Campbell, E. G., Dutcher, S. K., & Sarpatwari, A. (2020). Preferences for and experiences with pill appearance changes: National surveys of patients and pharmacists. *The American Journal of Managed Care*, *26*(8), 340–347. DOI: 10.37765/ajmc.2020.44070 PMID: 32835461

Basco, W. T.Jr, Garner, S. S., Ebeling, M., Freeland, K. D., Hulsey, T. C., & Simpson, K. (2016). Evaluating the potential severity of look-alike, sound-alike drug substitution errors in children. *Academic Pediatrics*, *16*(2), 183–191. DOI: 10.1016/j.acap.2015.06.014 PMID: 26946271

Beckman, A., Bernsten, C., Parker, M. G., Thorslund, M., & Fastbom, J. (2005). The difficulty of opening medicine containers in old age: A population-based study. *Pharmacy World & Science*, *27*(5), 393–398. DOI: 10.1007/s11096-005-7903-z PMID: 16341746

Bekker, J. L., Flores, A., & Sinha, M. S. (2023). Re-regulating dietary supplements. *Journal of Food Law & Policy, 19*(2), 1–22. https://doi.org/10.54119/jflp.eqso5002

Bellis, J. R., Kirkham, J. J., Thiesen, S., Conroy, E. J., Bracken, L. E., Mannix, H. L., Bird, K. A., Duncan, J. C., Peak, M., Turner, M. A., Smyth, R. L., Nunn, A. J., & Pirmohamed, M. (2013). Adverse drug reactions and off-label and unlicensed medicines in children: A nested case–control study of inpatients in a pediatric hospital. *BMC Medicine*, *11*(1), 238. DOI: 10.1186/1741-7015-11-238

Bent, S., Tiedt, T. N., Odden, M. C., & Shlipak, M. G. (2003). The relative safety of ephedra compared with other herbal products. *Annals of Internal Medicine*, *138*(6), 468–471. DOI: 10.7326/0003-4819-138-6-200303180-00010 PMID: 12639079

Berman, A. (2004). Reducing medication errors through naming, labeling, and packaging. *Journal of Medical Systems*, *28*(1), 9–29. DOI: 10.1023/B:-JOMS.0000021518.60670.10 PMID: 15171066

Boaden, B. (2022). *Syringe labeling in anesthesia and critical care areas: review 2022*. Retrieved 15 March from https://anaesthetists.org/Home/Resources-publications/Guidelines/Syringe-labelling-in-anaesthesia-and-critical-care-areas-review-2022

Bone, R. G. (2015). Trademark Functionality Reexamined. *The Journal of Legal Analysis*, *7*(1), 183–246. DOI: 10.1093/jla/lav002

Bradley, S. H. (2022). *Know Your Drops by Color*. Retrieved 15 March from https://www.aao.org/young-ophthalmologists/yo-info/article/know-your-drops-by-color

Brand Institute, Inc. (2023). *Brand Institute's Vice President of Creative Nomenclature Explains the Pharmaceutical Brand Name Review Process Used by Japanese Regulators*. Retrieved 06 Sep from https://www.prnewswire.com/news-releases/brand-institutes-vice-president-of-creative-nomenclature-explains-the-pharmaceutical-brand-name-review-process-used-by-japanese-regulators-301734086.html

Brandt, J. D. (2015). Human Factors and Ophthalmic Drug Packaging: Time for a Global Standard. *Ophthalmology*, *122*(12), 2368–2370. DOI: 10.1016/j.ophtha.2015.08.035 PMID: 26592669

Brompheniramine and Phenylephrine. (2025). *Lexi-Drugs Multinational. UpToDate Lexidrug. UpToDate Inc.* Retrieved 19 March from https://online.lexi.com

Brown, S. G. A. (2004). Clinical features and severity grading of anaphylaxis. *The Journal of Allergy and Clinical Immunology*, *114*(2), 371–376. DOI: 10.1016/j.jaci.2004.04.029 PMID: 15316518

Bryan, R., Aronson, J. K., ten Hacken, P., Williams, A., & Jordan, S. (2015). Patient safety in medication nomenclature: Orthographic and semantic properties of International Nonproprietary Names. *PLoS One*, *10*(12), e0145431. DOI: 10.1371/journal.pone.0145431 PMID: 26701761

Bryan, R., Aronson, J. K., Williams, A. J., & Jordan, S. (2021b). A systematic literature review of LASA error interventions. *British Journal of Clinical Pharmacology*, *87*(2), 336–351. DOI: 10.1111/bcp.14644 PMID: 33197079

Bryan, R., Aronson, J. K., Williams, A., & Jordan, S. (2021a). The problem of look-alike, sound-alike name errors: Drivers and solutions. *British Journal of Clinical Pharmacology*, *87*(2), 386–394. DOI: 10.1111/bcp.14285 PMID: 32198938

Bueng Kan Hospital. (2021). *Look Alike Sound Alike Drug*. Retrieved 17 Jan from https://bkh.moph.go.th/bkhweb/uploads/media/20230331072512_4.LASA_update-_2566.pdf#page=6.00

Bundy, D. G., Shore, A. D., Morlock, L. L., & Miller, M. R. (2009). Pediatric vaccination errors: Application of the "5 rights" framework to a national error reporting database. *Vaccine, 27*(29), 3890–3896. DOI: 10.1016/j.vaccine.2009.04.005 PMID: 19442422

Campbell, J., & Sumner, W.II. (2005). OOPS: Test of a structure for recording patient safety events. *AMIA ... Annual Symposium Proceedings - AMIA Symposium. AMIA Symposium, 2005*, 910. PMID: 16779197

Carayon, P., Wetterneck, T. B., Rivera-Rodriguez, A. J., Hundt, A. S., Hoonakker, P., Holden, R., & Gurses, A. P. (2014). Human factors systems approach to healthcare quality and patient safety. *Applied Ergonomics, 45*(1), 14–25. DOI: 10.1016/j.apergo.2013.04.023 PMID: 23845724

Carayon, P., Wooldridge, A., Hoonakker, P., Hundt, A. S., & Kelly, M. M. (2020). SEIPS 3.0: Human-centered design of the patient journey for patient safety. *Applied Ergonomics, 84*, 103033. DOI: 10.1016/j.apergo.2019.103033 PMID: 31987516

Carter, D., & Sooknanan, D. (2024). *Long-acting oral opioids (MS Contin™, Oxycontin™)*. Retrieved 4 June from https://pain.ucsf.edu/opioid-analgesics/long-acting-oral-opioids-ms-contin%E2%84%A2-oxycontin%E2%84%A2

Castro-Gómez, A. (2023). Labeling of medications in anesthesia: Colors and letters that save lives. *Revista Colombiana de Anestesiología, 51*(2). Advance online publication. DOI: 10.5554/22562087.e1065

Catchpole, K., & McCulloch, P. (2010). Human factors in critical care: Toward standardized integrated human-centered systems of work. *Current Opinion in Critical Care, 16*(6), 618–622. DOI: 10.1097/MCC.0b013e32833e9b4b PMID: 20736826

Cavell, G. F., & Mandaliya, D. (2021). Magnitude of error: A review of wrong dose medication incidents reported to a UK hospital voluntary incident reporting system. *European Journal of Hospital Pharmacy : Science and Practice, 28*(5), 260–265. DOI: 10.1136/ejhpharm-2019-001987 PMID: 34426478

Cefaclor. (2025). *Lexi-Drugs Multinational. UpToDate Lexidrug. UpToDate Inc.* Retrieved 19 March from https://online.lexi.com

Cefixime. (2026). *Lexi-Drugs Multinational. UpToDate Lexidrug. UpToDate Inc.* Retrieved 25 Jan from https://online.lexi.com

Center for Drug Evaluation and Research (CDER). (2000). *Proprietary name review: Foradil aerolizer*. Retrieved 11 Jan from https://www.accessdata.fda.gov/drugsatfda_docs/nda/2001/20831_Foradil_admindocs_P1.pdf

Center for Drug Evaluation and Research (CDER). (2004). *Approval package for: Application number NDA* 21-615 *medical review (s)*. Retrieved 11 Jan from https://www.accessdata.fda.gov/drugsatfda_docs/nda/2004/021615s000_Razadyne_medr.pdf

Center for Drug Evaluation and Research (CDER). (2006). *Proprietary name review(s): Foradil certihaler*. https://www.accessdata.fda.gov/drugsatfda_docs/nda/2006/021592s000_NameR.pdf

Center for Drug Evaluation and Research (CDER). (2016). *Procedures for handling requests for proprietary name review*. Retrieved 15 June from https://www.fda.gov/files/about%20fda/published/Procedures-for-Handling-Requests-for-Proprietary-Name-Review.pdf

Center for Drug Evaluation and Research (CDER). (2016). *Safety Considerations for Product Design to Minimize Medication Errors: Guidance for Industry*. Retrieved 25 Feb from https://www.fda.gov/media/84903/download

Center for Food Safety and Applied Nutrition. U. S. F. a. D. A. (2018). *U4Life LLC dba Mitadone*. Retrieved 18 Jan from https://www.fda.gov/inspections-compliance-enforcement-and-criminal-investigations/warning-letters/u4life-llc-dba-mitadone-542731-01112018

Centers for Disease Control and Prevention. (2021). E*pidemiology and prevention of vaccine-preventable diseases*. 14th ed. Washington, DC: Public Health Foundation. https://stacks.cdc.gov/view/cdc/252997

Cetirizine (systemic). (2026). *Lexi-Drugs Multinational. UpToDate Lexidrug. UpToDate Inc.* Retrieved 25 Jan from https://online.lexi.com

Chanakit, T., Kumpalum, D., Kunwaradisai, N., Swatwongchai, Y., & Ragsawong, N. (2009).. . *Characteristics of Drug Information Service in Thailand Thai Pharmaceutical and Health Science Journal*, *4*(4), 490–499.

Chanakit, T., Napaporn, J., Chiempattanakajohn, T., Sangkhawan, S., & Wichakot, S. (2013). The survey of look alike/sound alike (LASA) drugs available in hospitals in Thailand. *African Journal of Pharmacy and Pharmacology*, *7*(6), 227–239. DOI: 10.5897/AJPP11.812

Chang, S., Pool, V., O'Connell, K., Polder, J. A., Iskander, J., Sweeney, C., Ball, R., & Braun, M. M. (2008). Preventable mix-ups of tuberculin and vaccines: Reports to the US Vaccine and Drug Safety Reporting Systems. *Drug Safety*, *31*(11), 1027–1033. DOI: 10.2165/00002018-200831110-00007 PMID: 18840022

Chen, F., Du, M., Blumberg, J. B., Ho Chui, K. K., Ruan, M., Rogers, G., & Zhang, F. F. (2019). Association Among Dietary Supplement Use, Nutrient Intake, and Mortality Among U.S. Adults: A Cohort Study. *Annals of Internal Medicine*, *170*(9), 604–613. DOI: 10.7326/M18-2478 PMID: 30959527

Cheung, R. Y., & Goodwin, S. H. (2013). What's in a drug name? *Canadian Pharmacists Journal/Revue des Pharmaciens du Canada*, 146(1), 8-9. DOI: 10.1177/1715163512472651

Chlorphenamine [Chlorpheniramine]. (2025). *Lexi-Drugs Multinational. UpToDate Lexidrug. UpToDate Inc.* Retrieved 19 March from https://online.lexi.com

Choi, Y. J., & Kim, H. (2019). Effect of pharmacy-led medication reconciliation in emergency departments: A systematic review and meta-analysis. *Journal of Clinical Pharmacy and Therapeutics*, *44*(6), 932–945. DOI: 10.1111/jcpt.13019 PMID: 31436877

Chotsampancharoen, T., Sripornsawan, P., & Wongchanchailert, M. (2016). Two Fatal Cases of Accidental Intrathecal Vincristine Administration: Learning from Death Events. *Chemotherapy*, *61*(2), 108–110. DOI: 10.1159/000441380 PMID: 26636546

Christie, I. W., & Hill, M. R. (2002). Standardized color coding for syringe drug labels: a National Survey. *Anesthesia, 57*(8), 778-817. https://doi.org/10.1046/j.1365-2044.2002.02698_3.x

Chu, G., Mantin, R., Shen, Y. M., Baskett, G., & Sussman, H. (1993). Massive cisplatin overdose by accidental substitution for carboplatin. Toxicity and management. Cancer, 72(12), 3707-3714. https://doi.org/10.1002/1097-0142

Chumchit, C., Amrumpai, Y., & Treesak, C. (2015). Recognition on medication safety and look-alike/sound-alike medication problems in Thai public hospitals. *Silpakorn U Science & Tech J*, *9*(2), 40–51.

Ciociano, N., & Bagnasco, L. (2014). Look alike/sound alike drugs: A literature review on causes and solutions. *International Journal of Clinical Pharmacy*, *36*(2), 233–242. DOI: 10.1007/s11096-013-9885-6 PMID: 24293334

Ciociano, N., Saullo, F., Pacillo, M., Romano, F., & Bagnasco, L. (2013). GRP-020 Analysis of Italian Hospital Pharmacist Activities to Prevent LASA Drug Errors in Treatment: First Results. *European Journal of Hospital Pharmacy: Science and Practice*, *20*(Suppl 1), A7–A8. DOI: 10.1136/ejhpharm-2013-000276.020

ClinicalTrials.gov. (2024). *A study to assess effect of Glucocil® on metabolic health in individuals with prediabetes and type 2 diabetes mellitus (ClinicalTrials.gov Identifier: NCT*06496893). *U.S. National Library of Medicine*. Retrieved 18 Jan from https://www.clinicaltrials.gov/study/NCT06496893#study-plan

Clogston, J., Hudanick, L., Suragh, T. A., Jankosky, C., Lewis, P., Martin, D., Schembri, C., Zinderman, C., Maslov, Y., Mistry, M., Pippins, J. R., Vee, S., Wyeth, J., Shimabukuro, T. T., & Leighton, J. (2016). Unintentional administration of insulin instead of influenza vaccine: A case study and review of reports to US vaccine and drug safety monitoring systems. *Drugs & Therapy Perspectives*, *32*(10), 439–446. DOI: 10.1007/s40267-016-0333-2

Cohen, M. R. (1991). Insulin overdoses that originated in the pharmacy IV admixture area. Hosp Pharm, 26, 998-999.

Cohen, M. R., Harris, D., Zanoletty, A., & Linvill-Neal, D. (2021). *The inside track on drug naming safety standards*. Retrieved 15 June from https://www.ismp.org/sites/default/files/attachments/2021-07/The%20Inside%20Track%20on%20Drug%20Naming%20Standards-%20Handouts.pdf

Cohen, A. (2014). Crazy for Ya Ba: Methamphetamine use among northern Thai youth. *The International Journal on Drug Policy*, *25*(4), 776–782. DOI: 10.1016/j.drugpo.2014.06.005 PMID: 25067795

Cohen, M. (1999). Celebrex, celexa, cerebyx. *Nursing*, *29*(7), 14. DOI: 10.1097/00152193-199907000-00006

Cohen, M. R. (2001). Another purpose for "purpose" look-alike unit-dose containers mixed up misinterpretation of sliding-scale insulin dose. *Hospital Pharmacy*, *36*(12), 1132–1133. DOI: 10.1177/001857870103601203

Cohen, M. R. (2006). Maalox brand name extension causes confusion near sight/sound dead hit! omacor–amicar look-alike tylenol packets. *Hospital Pharmacy*, *41*(1), 13–16. DOI: 10.1310/hpj4101-13

Cohen, M. R. (2007). Action needed to prevent dangerous heparin-insulin confusion; sorting things out; staff unaware of fentanyl patch starting doses. *Hospital Pharmacy*, *42*(8), 675–679. DOI: 10.1310/hpj4208-675

Cohen, M. R. (2007). The role of drug packaging and labeling in medication errors. In Cohen, M. R. (Ed.), *Medication Errors* (2nd ed., pp. 111–152). The American Pharmacists Association. https://doi.org/doi:10.21019/9781582120928.ch7

Cohen, M. R. (2008). Cross Contamination with Insulin Pens; Look-Alike Vials; Kids and Medication Patches; New Look-Alike Name Pair; Preventing Dosing Errors with Methotrexate Injection. *Hospital Pharmacy, 43*(6), 445–447. DOI: 10.1310/hpj4306-445

Cohen, M. R. (2020). Medication Errors. *Nursing, 50*(11), 72. https://doi.org/DOI-10.1097/01.NURSE.0000719696.41409.94. DOI: 10.1097/01.NURSE.0000719696.41409.94 PMID: 6907778

Cohen, M. R., & Davis, N. M. (1992). Dispensing the Wrong Medication. *American Pharmacy, 32*(5), 32. DOI: 10.1016/S0160-3450(15)31197-1

Cohen, M. R., & Davis, N. M. (1993a). Preventing errors: Errors caused by medical office personnel. *American Pharmacy, 33*(7), 18. DOI: 10.1016/S0160-3450(15)30726-1 PMID: 8342489

Cohen, M. R., & Davis, N. M. (1993b). Preventing errors: Mixups with Norvasc and Navane. *American Pharmacy, 33*(8), 26. DOI: 10.1016/S0160-3450(15)30717-0 PMID: 8213467

Cohen, M. R., & Davis, N. M. (1994a). Confusing name; tips for storing drugs. *American Pharmacy, 34*(2), 20–21. DOI: 10.1016/S0160-3450(15)30526-2 PMID: 8166041

Cohen, M. R., & Davis, N. M. (1994b). Preventing errors. *American Pharmacy, 34*(12), 18–74. DOI: 10.1016/S0160-3450(15)30239-7 PMID: 7856504

Cohen, M. R., & Smetzer, J. L. (2011). ISMP Medication Error Report Analysis-Dakin's Solution Accidentally Given Intravenously; Perilous Infection Control Practices With Needles, Syringes, and Vials Suggest Stepped-up Monitoring Is Needed; Taxotere Concentration and Preparation; Update on Metal in Drug Patches. *Hospital Pharmacy, 46*(2), 82–86. DOI: 10.1310/hpj4602-82

Cohen, M. R., & Smetzer, J. L. (2015). No unlabeled containers anywhere, ever! where did this come from? *Hospital Pharmacy, 50*(3), 185–188. DOI: 10.1310/hpj5003-185 PMID: 26405305

Cohen, M. R., & Smetzer, J. L. (2017). ISMP medication error report analysis. *Hospital Pharmacy, 52*(6), 390–393. DOI: 10.1177/0018578717715346 PMID: 29276260

Cohen, M. R., & Smetzer, J. L. (2018). Multifactorial Causes of Tacrolimus Errors: Confusion With Strength/Formulation, Look-Alike Names, Preparation Errors, and More Ensuring Safety of Recipes for Drug Compounding Please, no more teaspoon dosing. *Hospital Pharmacy*, *53*(3), 142–145. DOI: 10.1177/0018578718769757

Cohen, M. R., Smetzer, J. L., Westphal, J. E., Comden, S. C., & Horn, D. M. (2012). Risk models to improve safety of dispensing high-alert medications in community pharmacies. *Journal of the American Pharmacists Association*, *52*(5), 584–602. DOI: 10.1331/JAPhA.2012.10145 PMID: 23023839

Cohen, P. A. (2009). American Roulette — Contaminated Dietary Supplements. *The New England Journal of Medicine*, *361*(16), 1523–1525. DOI: 10.1056/NEJMp0904768 PMID: 19812394

Condon, A. J., & Hayney, M. S. (2016). Strategies to minimize vaccine errors. *Journal of the American Pharmacists Association*, *56*(3), 339–341. DOI: 10.1016/j.japh.2016.03.016 PMID: 27156943

Condren, M. E., & Desselle, S. P. (2015). The fate of pediatric prescriptions in community pharmacies. *Journal of Patient Safety*, *11*(2), 79–88. DOI: 10.1097/PTS.0b013e3182948a7d PMID: 25996644

Co-Trimoxazole [Sulfamethoxazole and Trimethoprim]. (2025). *Lexi-Drugs Multinational. UpToDate Lexidrug. UpToDate Inc*. Retrieved 19 March from https://online.lexi.com

Council of Europe. (2024). *European Directorate for the Quality of Medicines & Healthcare (EDQM)*. Retrieved 15 June from https://www.coe.int/en/web/civil-society/european-directorate-for-the-quality-of-medicines-healthcare-edqm-#:~:text=European%20Directorate%20for%20the%20Quality%20of%20Medicines%20%26%20Healthcare%20(EDQM),-Drugs%20and%20Addictions

Cunha, A., Adão, T., & Trigueiros, P. (2014). HelpmePills: A Mobile Pill Recognition Tool for Elderly Persons. *Procedia Technology*, *16*, 1523–1532. DOI: 10.1016/j.protcy.2014.10.174

Currie, M., Mackay, P., Morgan, C., Runciman, W. B., Russell, W. J., Sellen, A., & Williamson, J. A. (1993). The Australian Incident Monitoring Study. The "wrong drug" problem in anesthesia: An analysis of 2000 incident reports. *Anaesthesia and Intensive Care*, *21*(5), 596–601. DOI: 10.1177/0310057X9302100517 PMID: 8273881

da Silva, B. A., & Krishnamurthy, M. (2016). The alarming reality of medication error: A patient case and review of Pennsylvania and National data. *Journal of Community Hospital Internal Medicine Perspectives*, *6*(4), 31758. DOI: 10.3402/jchimp.v6.31758 PMID: 27609720

Dahan, A., Aarts, L., & Smith, T. W. (2010). Incidence, Reversal, and Prevention of Opioid-induced Respiratory Depression. *Anesthesiology*, *112*(1), 226–238. DOI: 10.1097/ALN.0b013e3181c38c25 PMID: 20010421

Davis, N. M., & Cohen, M. R. (1995). Preventing errors: Computer-generated prescription orders. *American Pharmacy*, *35*(9), 10. DOI: 10.1016/S0160-3450(15)30081-7 PMID: 7484808

Davis, T. C., Wolf, M. S., Bass, P. F.III, Middlebrooks, M., Kennen, E., Baker, D. W., Bennett, C. L., Durazo-Arvizu, R., Bocchini, A., Savory, S., & Parker, R. M. (2006). Low literacy impairs comprehension of prescription drug warning labels. *Journal of General Internal Medicine*, *21*(8), 847–851. DOI: 10.1111/j.1525-1497.2006.00529.x PMID: 16881945

de Almeida Lopes, D. M., Rabelo Néri, E. D., Santos Madeira, L., de Souza Neto, P. J., Araújo Lélis, A. R., de Souza, T. R., de Oliveira, A. B., Oliveira Costa, L., & de França Fonteles, M. M. (2012). Análise da rotulagem de medicamentos semelhantes: Potenciais erros de medicação. *Revista da Associação Médica Brasileira*, *58*(1), 95–103. DOI: 10.1590/S0104-42302012000100021 PMID: 22392323

Department of Pharmacy, Bueng Kan Hospital. (2023). *Look alike sound alike drug*. Retrieved 22 May from https://bkh.moph.go.th/bkhweb/uploads/media/20230331072512 3_4.LASA_update-_2566.pdf

Department of Pharmacy, Srinagarind Hospital. (2022a). *Medication error due to LASA mix-up on the shelf: levetiracetam vs hydrocortisone*. Retrieved 02 June from https://pharm.md.kku.ac.th/post/14

Department of Pharmacy, Srinagarind Hospital. (2022b). *Medication error due to LASA mix-up on the shelf: zinforo inj vs zavicefta inj*. Retrieved 02 June from https://pharm.md.kku.ac.th/post/13

Devine, E. B., Wilson-Norton, J. L., Lawless, N. M., Hazlet, T. K., Hansen, R., Kelly, K., . . . Wong, C. (2005). Preparing for ambulatory computerized prescriber order entry by evaluating preimplementation medication errors. Advances in Patient Safety: From Research to Implementation (Vol. 2). Concepts and Methodology.

Devine, E. B., Wilson-Norton, J. L., Lawless, N. M., Hazlet, T. K., Hansen, R., Kelly, K., . . . Wong, C. (2005). Preparing for ambulatory computerized prescriber order entry by evaluating preimplementation medication errors. In Henriksen K, Battles JB, Marks ES, et al. (eds.) Advances in Patient Safety: From Research to Implementation (Vol. 2: Concepts and Methodology). Rockville (MD): Agency for Healthcare Research and Quality (US); 2005 Feb. Available from: https://www.ncbi.nlm.nih.gov/books/NBK20508/

DeYoung, J. L., Vanderkooi, M. E., & Barletta, J. F. (2009). Effect of bar-code-assisted medication administration on medication error rates in an adult medical intensive care unit. *American Journal of Health-System Pharmacy*, *66*(12), 1110–1115. DOI: 10.2146/ajhp080355 PMID: 19498127

Dhande, P. P., Mule, A. V., & Chaudhari, A. P. (2021). Retrospective analysis of look-alike and sound-alike drug incidents in a tertiary care hospital. *Indian Journal of Pharmacy Practice*, *14*(2), 115. DOI: 10.5530/ijopp.14.2.21

Dicycloverine [Dicyclomine] and Simeticone [Simethicone]. (2025). *Lexi-Drugs Multinational. UpToDate Lexidrug. UpToDate Inc.* Retrieved 19 March from https://online.lexi.com

Dietlein, T. S., Jordan, J. F., Lüke, C., Schild, A., Dinslage, S., & Krieglstein, G. K. (2008). Self-application of single-use eyedrop containers in an elderly population: Comparisons with standard eyedrop bottle and with younger patients. *Acta Ophthalmologica*, *86*(8), 856–859. DOI: 10.1111/j.1755-3768.2007.01155.x PMID: 18494743

Dinwoodie, G. B., & Janis, M. D. (2008). *Trademark law and Theory: A handbook of contemporary research*. Edward Elgar Publishing. DOI: 10.4337/9781848441316

Diphenhydramine, A. C., and Sodium Citrate, (2025). *Lexi-Drugs Multinational. UpToDate Lexidrug. UpToDate Inc.* Retrieved 19 March from https://online.lexi.com

Domperidone. (2025). *Lexi-Drugs Multinational. UpToDate Lexidrug. UpToDate Inc.* Retrieved 19 March from https://online.lexi.com

Donaldson, M. S., Corrigan, J. M., & Kohn, L. T. (2000). To err is human: building a safer health system.

Donnini, D. A., Silva, C. M. B., Gusmão, J. D., Matozinhos, F. P., Silva, R. B., Amaral, G. G., & Oliveira, V. C. (2022). Incidence of immunization errors in the state of Minas Gerais, Brazil: A cross-sectional study, 2015-2019. *Epidemiologia e Serviços de Saúde: Revista do Sistema Unico de Saúde do Brasil*, *31*, e2022055. DOI: 10.1590/s2237-96222022000300008 PMID: 36351058

Dowse, R., & Ehlers, M. (2005). Medicine labels incorporating pictograms: Do they influence understanding and adherence? *Patient Education and Counseling*, *58*(1), 63–70. DOI: 10.1016/j.pec.2004.06.012 PMID: 15950838

Drug.com. (2025). *Pill Identifier*. Retrieved 30 July from https://www.drugs.com/pill_identification.html

DrugPatentWatch. (2025). *A Comprehensive Generic Drug Naming Resource: Decoding the Pharmaceutical Alphabet*. Retrieved 20 Oct from https://www.drugpatentwatch.com/blog/a-comprehensive-generic-drug-naming-resource/

Dsouza, S., & Kulkarni, A. (2017). The hazards of look alike packaging in anesthesia practice. *Asian Journal of Anesthesiology*, *55*(4), 91–92. DOI: 10.1016/j.aja.2017.10.003 PMID: 29239830

Dunne, S. S., & Dunne, C. P. (2015). What do people really think of generic medicines? A systematic review and critical appraisal of literature on stakeholder perceptions of generic drugs. *BMC Medicine*, *13*(1), 173. DOI: 10.1186/s12916-015-0415-3 PMID: 26224091

Dwyer, J. T., Coates, P. M., & Smith, M. J. (2018). Dietary Supplements: Regulatory Challenges and Research Resources. *Nutrients*, *10*(1), 41. Advance online publication. DOI: 10.3390/nu10010041 PMID: 29300341

Ehsani, S. R., Cheraghi, M. A., Nejati, A., Salari, A., Esmaeilpoor, A. H., & Nejad, E. M. (2013). Medication errors of nurses in the emergency department. *Journal of Medical Ethics and History of Medicine*, *6*(11). PMID: 24427488

Eiland, L. S., Benner, K., Gumpper, K. F., Heigham, M. K., Meyers, R., Pham, K., & Potts, A. L. (2018). ASHP-PPAG Guidelines for Providing Pediatric Pharmacy Services in Hospitals and Health Systems. *The Journal of Pediatric Pharmacology and Therapeutics*, *23*(3), 177–191. DOI: 10.5863/1551-6776-23.3.177 PMID: 29970974

Elmzughi, R. F., Abuhasina, A., & Abdulsalam, O. (2025). Impact of Illegible Handwritten Prescriptions on Dispensing Errors: A Focus on Look-Alike Sound-Alike Medications in Libyan Community Pharmacies. *Journal of Pharmacy and Pharmacology, 7*(3), 73–82. https://doi.org/10.36349/easjpp.2025.v07i03.004

Emmerton, L. M., & Rizk, M. F. (2012). Look-alike and sound-alike medicines: Risks and 'solutions'. *International Journal of Clinical Pharmacy*, *34*(1), 4–8. DOI: 10.1007/s11096-011-9595-x PMID: 22193703

Emmerton, L., Curtain, C., Swaminathan, G., & Dowling, H. (2020). Development and exploratory analysis of software to detect look-alike, sound-alike medicine names. *International Journal of Medical Informatics*, *137*, 104119. DOI: 10.1016/j.ijmedinf.2020.104119 PMID: 32172184

Endestad, T., Wortinger, L. A., Madsen, S., & Hortemo, S. (2016). Package design affects accuracy recognition for medications. *Human Factors*, *58*(8), 1206–1216. DOI: 10.1177/0018720816664824 PMID: 27591209

Estock, J. L., Murray, A. W., Mizah, M. T., Mangione, M. P., Goode, J. S.Jr, & Eibling, D. E. (2018). Label Design Affects Medication Safety in an Operating Room Crisis: A Controlled Simulation Study. *Journal of Patient Safety*, *14*(2), 101–106. DOI: 10.1097/PTS.0000000000000176 PMID: 25760652

European Commission. (2001). *Guidance concerning the Braille requirements for labeling and the package leaflet*. Retrieved 15 June from https://academy.gmp-compliance.org/guidemgr/files/BRAILLE_TEXT20050411.PDF

European Medicines Agency (EMA). (2009). *Guideline on the readability of the label and package leaflet of medicinal products for human use*. Retrieved 11 June from https://health.ec.europa.eu/system/files/2016-11/2009_01_12_readability_guideline_final_en_0.pdf

European Medicines Agency (EMA). (2011). *QRD recommendations on pack design and labeling for centrally authorized nonprescription human medicinal products*. Retrieved 10 Feb from https://www.ema.europa.eu/en/documents/regulatory-procedural-guideline/draft-quality-review-documents-recommendations-pack-design-and-labelling-centrally-authorised-non-prescription-human-medicinal-products_en.pdf

European Medicines Agency (EMA). (2011). *QRD recommendations on pack design and labeling for centrally authorized non-prescription human medicinal products*. Retrieved 10 Feb from https://www.ema.europa.eu/en/documents/regulatory-procedural-guideline/draft-quality-review-documents-recommendations-pack-design-and-labelling-centrally-authorised-non-prescription-human-medicinal-products_en.pdf

European Medicines Agency (EMA). (2021). *Recommendations on medication errors*. Retrieved 01 August from https://www.ema.europa.eu/en/human-regulatory/post-authorisation/pharmacovigilance/medication-errors/recommendations-medication-errors

European Medicines Agency (EMA). (2021a). *Pharmacovigilance Risk Assessment Committee (PRAC)*. Retrieved 16 Jan from https://www.ema.europa.eu/en/committees/pharmacovigilance-risk-assessment-committee-prac

European Medicines Agency (EMA). (2021b). *Signal management*. Retrieved 16 Jan from https://www.ema.europa.eu/en/human-regulatory-overview/post-authorisation/pharmacovigilance-post-authorisation/signal-management

European Medicines Agency (EMA). (2023). *Guideline on the acceptability of names for human medicinal products processed through the centralized procedure - Scientific guideline*. https://www.ema.europa.eu/en/documents/scientific-guideline/guideline-acceptability-names-human-medicinal-products-processed-through-centralised-procedure-revision-7_en.pdf

European Medicines Agency (EMA). (2023). *Guideline on the acceptability of names for human medicinal products processed through the centralized procedure - Scientific guideline*. Retrieved 11 June from https://www.ema.europa.eu/en/documents/scientific-guideline/guideline-acceptability-names-human-medicinal-products-processed-through-centralised-procedure-revision-7_en.pdf

European Medicines Agency (EMA). (2025). *Medicines*. Retrieved 31 July from https://www.ema.europa.eu/en/medicines

European Parliament and Council. (2011). *Directive* 2011/62/*EU of the European Parliament and of the Council of* 8 *June* 2011 *amending Directive* 2001/83/*EC on the Community code relating to medicinal products for human use, as regards the prevention of the entry into the legal supply chain of falsified medicinal products. Official Journal of the European Union, L* 174, 74–87. Retrieved 25 Feb from https://health.ec.europa.eu/document/download/7bd5d800-08de-47a3-be9f-d5832682c262_en?

Faculty of Pharmaceutical Sciences Ubon Ratchathani University. (2025). *Drug Identification Database, Ubon Ratchathani University*. Retrieved 31 July from https://drugiden2.ubu.ac.th/

Faculty of Pharmaceutical Sciences. U. R. U. (2022). *Drug identification database*. Retrieved 11 Oct from https://drugiden.ubu.ac.th/

Fadda, H. M., Weiler, H., Carvalho, M., Lee, Y. Z., Dassouki, H., AbuBlan, R., & Li, Z. (2024). Pediatric oral extemporaneous preparations and practices: International Pharmaceutical Federation (FIP) global study. *European Journal of Pharmaceutics and Biopharmaceutics : Official Journal of Arbeitsgemeinschaft für Pharmazeutische Verfahrenstechnik e.V*, *204*, 114483. DOI: 10.1016/j.ejpb.2024.114483

Fasting, S., & Gisvold, S. E. (2000). Adverse drug errors in anesthesia, and the impact of colored syringe labels. *Canadian Journal of Anaesthesia = Journal Canadien d'Anesthésie*, *47*(11), 1060–1067. DOI: 10.1007/BF03027956 PMID: 11097534

Ferrous Fumarate. (2025). *Lexi-Drugs Multinational. UpToDate Lexidrug. UpToDate Inc.* Retrieved 19 March from https://online.lexi.com

Filiatrault, P., & Hyland, S. (2009). Does color-coded labeling reduce the risk of medication errors? *The Canadian Journal of Hospital Pharmacy*, *62*(2), 154–156. DOI: 10.4212/cjhp.v62i2.446 PMID: 22478883

Filik, R., Purdy, K., Gale, A., & Gerrett, D. (2004). Drug name confusion: Evaluating the effectiveness of capital ("Tall Man") letters using eye movement data. *Social Science & Medicine*, *59*(12), 2597–2601. DOI: 10.1016/j.socscimed.2004.04.008 PMID: 15474212

Filik, R., Purdy, K., Gale, A., & Gerrett, D. (2006). Labeling of medicines and patient safety: Evaluating methods of reducing drug name confusion. *Human Factors*, *48*(1), 39–47. DOI: 10.1518/001872006776412199 PMID: 16696255

Fontaine, A. L. (2004). Current requirements and emerging trends for labeling as a tool for communicating pharmacovigilance findings. *Drug Safety*, *27*(8), 579–589. DOI: 10.2165/00002018-200427080-00009 PMID: 15154829

Food and Drug Administration. (2004). Bar code label requirement for human drug products and biological products. Final rule. *Federal Register*, *69*(38), 9119–9171. PMID: 14986679

Food and Drug Administration. (2020). *Best Practices in Developing Proprietary Names for Human Prescription Drug Products; Guidance for Industry*. Retrieved 15 Aug from https://www.fda.gov/regulatory-information/search-fda-guidance-documents/best-practices-developing-proprietary-names-human-prescription-drug-products-guidance-industry

Franklin, B. D., O'Grady, K., Donyai, P., Jacklin, A., & Barber, N. (2007). The impact of a closed-loop electronic prescribing and administration system on prescribing errors, administration errors and staff time: A before-and-after study. *Quality & Safety in Health Care*, *16*(4), 279–284. DOI: 10.1136/qshc.2006.019497 PMID: 17693676

Fyhr, A., & Akselsson, R. (2012). Characteristics of medication errors with parenteral cytotoxic drugs. *European Journal of Cancer Care*, *21*(5), 606–613. DOI: 10.1111/j.1365-2354.2012.01331.x PMID: 22335508

Gahche, J., Bailey, R., Burt, V., Hughes, J., Yetley, E., Dwyer, J., & Sempos, C. (2011). Dietary supplement use among U.S. adults has increased since NHANES III (1988-1994). *NCHS Data Brief*, (61), 1–8. PMID: 21592424

Galanter, W. L., Bryson, M. L., Falck, S., Rosenfield, R., Laragh, M., Shrestha, N., Schiff, G. D., & Lambert, B. L. (2014). Indication alerts intercept drug name confusion errors during computerized entry of medication orders. *PLoS One*, *9*(7), e101977. DOI: 10.1371/journal.pone.0101977 PMID: 25025346

Gallagher, T. H., Waterman, A. D., Ebers, A. G., Fraser, V. J., & Levinson, W. (2003). Patients' and physicians' attitudes regarding the disclosure of medical errors. *Journal of the American Medical Association*, *289*(8), 1001–1007. DOI: 10.1001/jama.289.8.1001 PMID: 12597752

Gandhi, T. K., Bartel, S. B., Shulman, L. N., Verrier, D., Burdick, E., Cleary, A., Rothschild, J. M., Leape, L. L., & Bates, D. W. (2005). Medication safety in the ambulatory chemotherapy setting. *Cancer*, *104*(11), 2477–2483. DOI: 10.1002/cncr.21442 PMID: 16245353

Gangakhedkar, G. R., Waghalkar, P. V., Shetty, A. N., & Dalvi, A. M. (2019). Look-Alike Drugs: Avoiding Potential Medical Errors. *International Journal of Preventive Medicine*, *10*(1), 9. DOI: 10.4103/ijpvm.IJPVM_331_18 PMID: 30774843

Gardiner, P., Sarma, D. N., Low Dog, T., Barrett, M. L., Chavez, M. L., Ko, R., & Giancaspro, G. I. (2008). The state of dietary supplement adverse event reporting in the United States. *Pharmacoepidemiology and Drug Safety*, *17*(10), 962–970. DOI: 10.1002/pds.1627 PMID: 18613260

Garfield, S., Furniss, D., Husson, F., Etkind, M., Williams, M., Norton, J., Ogunleye, D., Jubraj, B., Lakhdari, H., & Franklin, B. D. (2020). How can patient-held lists of medication enhance patient safety? A mixed-methods study with a focus on user experience. *BMJ Quality & Safety*, *29*(9), 764–773. DOI: 10.1136/bmjqs-2019-010194 PMID: 31949006

Garlich, F. M., & Nelson, L. S. (2010). Inadvertent IV administration of IM epinephrine. *Emerg Med*, *42*, 24–27.

Gaunt, M. (2007). Error Trifecta: Avandia, Coumadin, and Cardura. *Pharmacy Times*, *73*(11), 53.

Geller, A. I., Shehab, N., Weidle, N. J., Lovegrove, M. C., Wolpert, B. J., Timbo, B. B., Mozersky, R. P., & Budnitz, D. S. (2015). Emergency Department Visits for Adverse Events Related to Dietary Supplements. *The New England Journal of Medicine*, *373*(16), 1531–1540. DOI: 10.1056/NEJMsa1504267 PMID: 26465986

General Specifications Association Internationale Sans But Lucratif (GS1 AISBL). (2024). *GS1 General Specifications Standard*. Retrieved 15 Aug from https://ref.gs1.org/standards/genspecs/

Ghelardini, C., Di Cesare Mannelli, L., & Bianchi, E. (2015). The pharmacological basis of opioids. *Clinical Cases in Mineral and Bone Metabolism, 12*(3), 219–221. DOI: 10.11138/ccmbm/2015.12.3.219 PMID: 26811699

Gonzales, K. (2010). Medication Administration Errors and the Pediatric Population: A Systematic Search of the Literature. *Journal of Pediatric Nursing, 25*(6), 555–565. DOI: 10.1016/j.pedn.2010.04.002

Gopakumar, K. M., & Syam, N. (2007). A study on the use of International Nonproprietary Names in India. New Delhi: Centre for Trade & Development (Centad), in collaboration with the WHO India Country Office.

Government of Canada. (2014). *Guidance document for industry - review of drug brand names*. Retrieved 6 August from https://www.canada.ca/en/health-canada/services/drugs-health-products/reports-publications/medeffect-canada/guidance-document-industry-review-drug-brand-names.html

Grant, M., Remines, J., Nadpara, P., & Goode, J. K. R. (2020). Impact of live training on medication errors in a community-based pharmacy setting. *Innovations in Pharmacy, 11*(3), 11. Advance online publication. DOI: 10.24926/iip.v11i3.3291 PMID: 34007633

Graudins, L. V., Downey, G., Bui, T., & Dooley, M. J. (2016). Recommendations and Low-Technology Safety Solutions Following Neuromuscular Blocking Agent Incidents. *Joint Commission Journal on Quality and Patient Safety, 42*(2), 86–91. DOI: 10.1016/S1553-7250(16)42010-6 PMID: 26803037

Griffiths, M. (2017). Beware of 'lookalikes'. *Nursing Standard, 31*(25), 28. DOI: 10.7748/ns.31.25.28.s26 PMID: 28198315

Grissinger, M. (2008). Morphine and Hydromorphone: An Omnipresent Risk of Mix-ups. *P&T : a Peer-Reviewed Journal for Formulary Management, 33*(4), 194–247. PMID: 19750160

Grissinger, M. (2011). Action is neeeded to prevent heparin-insulin mixups. *P&T : a Peer-Reviewed Journal for Formulary Management, 36*(4), 177–202. PMID: 21572772

Grissinger, M. (2012). Color-coded syringes for anesthesia drugs-use with care. *P&T : a Peer-Reviewed Journal for Formulary Management, 37*(4), 199–201. PMID: 22593629

Grissinger, M. (2012). Tall man letters are gaining wide acceptance. *P&T : a Peer-Reviewed Journal for Formulary Management, 37*(3), 132–148. PMID: 22605902

Grissinger, M. (2013). Multiple brand names for the same generic drug can cause confusion. *P&T : a Peer-Reviewed Journal for Formulary Management*, *38*(6), 305. PMID: 23946623

Grissinger, M. (2016). Death and Neurological Devastation From Intrathecal Vinca Alkaloids. *P&T : a Peer-Reviewed Journal for Formulary Management*, *41*(8), 464–525. PMID: 27504060

Grissinger, M. (2019). Accidental IV Infusion of Heparinized Irrigation in the Operating Room. *P&T : a Peer-Reviewed Journal for Formulary Management*, *44*(7), 389–390. PMID: 31258307

GuaiFENesin. (2025). *Lexi-Drugs Multinational. UpToDate Lexidrug. UpToDate Inc.* Retrieved 19 March from https://online.lexi.com

Gulur, P., Koury, K., Arnstein, P., Lee, H., McCarthy, P., Coley, C., & Mort, E. (2015). Morphine versus Hydromorphone: Does Choice of Opioid Influence Outcomes? *Pain Research and Treatment*, *482081*, 1–6. Advance online publication. DOI: 10.1155/2015/482081 PMID: 26609431

Gupta, P. K., Ishihara, R., Zhao, Z., Owji, S., Anyama, E., Schmitz-Brown, M., Chacin, A. C., Iyer, B., Friedman, D., & Ladki, M. S. (2023). Novel tactile bottle neck adaptor facilitates eye drop adherence in visually impaired patients. *BMJ Open Ophthalmology*, *8*(1), e001462. Advance online publication. DOI: 10.1136/bmjophth-2023-001462 PMID: 38154911

Gutierrez, M. A., Todd, K., & Nagy, R. M. (1991). On the alert for clonazepam (Klonopin) versus clonidine. *Journal of Clinical Psychopharmacology*, *11*(4), 269–270. DOI: 10.1097/00004714-199108000-00018 PMID: 1918426

Hajibeglou, A., Zagheri Tafreshi, M., Kamrani, F., & Nasiri, M. (2018). The impact of training on medication error rate of the emergency department in hospitals affiliated to Golestan University of Medical Sciences. *Advances in Nursing & Midwifery*, *27*(4), 32–36.

Hanna, G. M., & Levine, W. C. (2011). Medication safety in the perioperative setting. *Anesthesiology Clinics*, *29*(1), 135–144. DOI: 10.1016/j.anclin.2010.11.009 PMID: 21295758

Hardy, L. (2015). *Name That Drop*. Retrieved 23 Nov from https://www.2020mag.com/article/name-that-drop

Hauben, M., & Aronson, J. K. (2009). Defining 'Signal' and its Subtypes in Pharmacovigilance Based on a Systematic Review of Previous Definitions. *Drug Safety*, *32*(2), 99–110. DOI: 10.2165/00002018-200932020-00003 PMID: 19236117

Health and Disability Commissioner. (2017). *Incorrect dispensing of insulin (Case 16HDC01665)*. Retrieved 9 July from https://www.hdc.org.nz/decisions/search-decisions/2017/16hdc01665/

Health Canada. (2004). *ARCHIVED - Issue analysis summary: Look-alike Sound-alike (LA/SA) health product names: the development of a comprehensive policy recommendation for Look-alike Sound-alike (LA/SA) health product names*. Retrieved 15 June from https://www.canada.ca/en/health-canada/services/drugs-health-products/biologics-radiopharmaceuticals-genetic-therapies/look-alike-sound-alike/issue-analysis-summary-look-alike-sound-alike-health-product-names-development-comprehensive-policy-recommendation-look-alike-sound-alike.html

Health Canada. (2014). *Guidance document: review of drug brand names* Government of Canada, Department of Health. Retrieved 04 Mar from https://www.canada.ca/content/dam/hc-sc/migration/hc-sc/dhp-mps/alt_formats/pdf/pubs/medeff/guide/2014-review-examen_drug-medicament_names-marques/2014-review-examen_drug-medicament_names-marques-eng.pdf

Health Canada. (2019). *Good label and package practices guide for prescription drugs*. Retrieved 15 March from https://www.canada.ca/en/health-canada/services/drugs-health-products/reports-publications/medeffect-canada/good-label-package-practices-guide-prescription-drugs-profile/guidance-document.html

Health Canada. (2025). *Drug Product Database (DPD)*. Retrieved 31 July from https://health-products.canada.ca/dpd-bdpp/index-eng.jsp

Health Canada. (2025). *Food and Drug Regulations (C.R.C., c.* 870). Retrieved 25 Feb from https://laws-lois.justice.gc.ca/eng/regulations/c.r.c.%2C_c._870/page-62.html?

Health Sciences Authority (HSA). (2026). *Therapeutic Products Guidance on Therapeutic Product Registration in Singapore*. Retrieved 25 Feb from https://www.hsa.gov.sg/docs/default-source/hprg-tpb/guidances/guidance-on-therapeutic-product-registration-in-singapore.pdf?sfvrsn=cd174383_62

Heck, J., Groh, A., Stichtenoth, D. O., Bleich, S., & Krause, O. (2020). Look-alikes, sound-alikes: Three cases of insidious medication errors. *Clinical Case Reports*, *8*(12), 3284–3287. DOI: 10.1002/ccr3.3409 PMID: 33363919

Heo, J., Kang, Y., Lee, S., Jeong, D. H., & Kim, K. M. (2023). An Accurate Deep Learning-Based System for Automatic Pill Identification: Model Development and Validation. *Journal of Medical Internet Research*, *25*, e41043. DOI: 10.2196/41043 PMID: 36637893

Herzer, K. R., Lim, C., Li, M., Xie, Y., Doyle, P. A., Cover, R., & Mark, L. J. (2013). Q-tip: From local quality improvement to national drug recall. *American Journal of Medical Quality : The Official Journal of the American College of Medical Quality, 28*(3), 265. DOI: 10.1177/1062860613478730 PMID: 23508529

Hibbs, B. F., Miller, E. R., & Shimabukuro, T. (2014). Notes from the field: Rotavirus vaccine administration errors—United States, 2006-2013. *MMWR. Morbidity and Mortality Weekly Report, 63*(4), 81. PMID: 24476980

Hibbs, B. F., Moro, P. L., Lewis, P., Miller, E. R., & Shimabukuro, T. T. (2015). Vaccination errors reported to the Vaccine Adverse Event Reporting System, (VAERS) United States, 2000–2013. *Vaccine, 33*(28), 3171–3178. DOI: 10.1016/j.vaccine.2015.05.006 PMID: 25980429

Hicks, R., Becker, S., & Cousins, D. (2008). MEDMARX data report. A report on the relationship of drug names and medication errors in response to the institute of Medicine's call for action. Center for the Advancement of Patient Safey, US Pharmacopeia.

Hicks, R. W., Becker, S. C., & Cousins, D. D. (2006). Harmful medication errors in children: A 5-year analysis of data from the USP's MEDMARX program. *Journal of Pediatric Nursing, 21*(4), 290–298. DOI: 10.1016/j.pedn.2006.02.002

Hicks, R., Becker, S., & Cousins, D. (2008). *MEDMARX data report. A report on the relationship of drug names and medication errors in response to the institute of Medicine's call for action*. Center for the Advancement of Patient Safey, US Pharmacopeia.

Hoffman, J. M., & Proulx, S. M. (2003). Medication errors caused by confusion of drug names. *Drug Safety, 26*(7), 445–452. DOI: 10.2165/00002018-200326070-00001 PMID: 12735783

Holbrook, A., Schulman, S., Witt, D. M., Vandvik, P. O., Fish, J., Kovacs, M. J., . . . Guyatt, G. H. (2012). Evidence-based management of anticoagulant therapy: Antithrombotic Therapy and Prevention of Thrombosis, 9th ed: American College of Chest Physicians Evidence-Based Clinical Practice Guidelines. *Chest*, 141(2 Suppl), e152S-e184S. DOI: 10.1378/chest.11-2295

Hong, J.-M., Cho, A.-R., & Choi, S.-A. (2014). Accidental intrathecal injection of dopamine hydrochloride resulting in analgesic effects. *Korean Journal of Anesthesiology, 67*(Suppl), S49–S50. DOI: 10.4097/kjae.2014.67.S.S49 PMID: 25598904

Huang, D., Luo, Z., Song, X., & Zou, K. (2024). Global research on sufentanil use in anesthesiology from 2003 to 2023: a bibliometric analysis [Systematic Review]. *Frontiers in Pharmacology, Volume* 15 - 2024. DOI: 10.3389/fphar.2024.1412726

Hughes, R. G., & Blegen, M. A. (2008). Medication administration safety. In Hughes, R. G. (Ed.), *Patient safety and quality: An evidence-based handbook for nurses*. Agency for Healthcare Research and Quality. https://www.ncbi.nlm.nih.gov/books/NBK2656/

HydrOXYzine. (2025). *Lexi-Drugs Multinational. UpToDate Lexidrug. UpToDate Inc.* Retrieved 19 March from https://online.lexi.com

Ibrahim, O. M., Ibrahim, R. M., Meslamani, A. Z. A., & Mazrouei, N. A. (2020). Dispensing errors in community pharmacies in the United Arab Emirates: Investigating incidence, types, severity, and causes. *Pharmacy Practice*, *18*(4), 2111. DOI: 10.18549/PharmPract.2020.4.2111 PMID: 33149793

Ibuprofen. (2025). *Lexi-Drugs Multinational. UpToDate Lexidrug. UpToDate Inc.* Retrieved 19 March from https://online.lexi.com

Iglesias Gomez, R., Font Noguera, I., Correa Ballester, M., Ruiz Caldes, M. J., & Poveda Andres, J. L. (2022). Tall man lettering application in medication information systems as a quality and safety strategy in hospital organization. *Journal of Clinical Pharmacy and Therapeutics*, *47*(10), 1570–1575. DOI: 10.1111/jcpt.13703 PMID: 35641241

Institute for Safe Medication Practices (ISMP) Canada. (2002). Confusion Between SEROQUEL® and SERZONE-5HT2® Reported in Canada. *ISMP Canada Safety Bulletin*, *2*(10), 1–2.

Institute for Safe Medication Practices (ISMP) Canada. (2006). Top 10 Drugs Reported as Causing Harm through Medication Error. *ISMP Canada Safety Bulletin*, *6*(1), 1–2.

Institute for Safe Medication Practices (ISMP) Canada. (2007). Risk of Mix-ups between Ephedrine and Epinephrine. *ISMP Canada Safety Bulletin*, *7*(2), 1–3.

Institute for Safe Medication Practices (ISMP) Canada. (2023). *Reported Concerns with Labeling and Packaging of High-Alert Medications in Vials and Ampoules: A Multi-Incident Analysis*. Retrieved 25 Feb from https://ismpcanada.ca/wp-content/uploads/ISMPCSB2023-i2-Label-Package-High-Alert-Meds.pdf

Institute for Safe Medication Practices (ISMP). (2015). *Community/ambulatory care IMSP Medication Safety Allert! Health alert! Avandia, not Coumadin*. Retrieved 16 Jan from https://www.ismp.org/sites/default/files/attachments/2018-03/community201512.pdf

Institute for Safe Medication Practices (ISMP). (2015). Open the bag to catch errors at the point-of-sale. *ISMP Medication Safety Alert! Community. Ambulatory Care, 14*(7), 1–2.

Institute for Safe Medication Practices (ISMP). (2016). *ISMP Medication Safety Alert! Do not let "Depo-" medications be a depot for mistakes*. Retrieved 11 Jan from https://www.ismp.org/sites/default/files/attachments/2018-03/20160324.pdf

Institute for Safe Medication Practices (ISMP). (2016). Prescribing and dispensing errors with oral solutions. *ISMP Medication Safety Alert! Community. Ambulatory Care, 15*(5), 1–6.

Institute for Safe Medication Practices (ISMP). (2018). *ISMP guidelines for optimizing safe implementation and use of basal insulin*. Retrieved 9 July from https://www.ismp.org/sites/default/files/attachments/2018-09/ISMP138D-Insulin%20Guideline-090718.pdf

Institute for Safe Medication Practices (ISMP). (2021). *ISMP targeted medication safety best practices for hospitals*. Retrieved 31 July from https://www.ismp.org/sites/default/files/attachments/2020-02/2020-2021%20TMSBP-%20FINAL_1.pdf

Institute for Safe Medication Practices (ISMP). (2022). *ISMP Guidelines for Safe Medication Use in Perioperative and Procedural Settings*. Retrieved 28 Jan from https://www.ismp.org/system/files/resources/2022-08/ISMP198-Periop-Guidelines-FINAL.pdf

Institute for Safe Medication Practices (ISMP). (2024). ISMP National Vaccine Errors Reporting Program 2022-2023 analysis: New vaccines, new errors. ISMP Medication Safety Alert! *Acute Care, 29*(21), 1–6.

Institute for Safe Medication Practices Canada. (2015). *TALLman lettering for look-alike/sound-alike drug names in Canada*. Retrieved 11 Sep from https://www.ismp-canada.org/download/TALLman/TALLman_lettering.pdf

Institute of Medicine Committee on Quality of Health Care in. A. (2000). To err is human: building a safer health system. In L. T. Kohn, J. M. Corrigan, & M. S. Donaldson (Eds.). National Academies Press (US). DOI: 10.17226/9728

International Organization for Standardization. (2008). *ISO* 26825:2008*(E). Anesthetic and respiratory equipment —User-applied labels for syringes containing drugs used during anesthesia — Colors, design and performance*. Retrieved 25 Feb from https://cdn.standards.iteh.ai/samples/43811/3572a136579d4e3691196a4df1c4b1f5/ISO-26825-2008.pdf

International Pharmaceutical Federation (FIP). (2020). *Pharmacists' Role in Medication Without Harm*. The Hague. International Pharmaceutical Federation.

International Union of Pure and Applied Chemistry. (2013). *Nomenclature of Organic Chemistry. IUPAC Recommendationsand Preferred Names* 2013. Retrieved 06 Sep from https://iupac.qmul.ac.uk/BlueBook/PDF/2013BlueBook.pdf

ISMP News/ECRI. (2020). *Due to ISMP Advocacy, VinCRIStine Labeling and Packaging Changed to Prevent Wrong Route Administration*. Retrieved 5 Sep from https://home.ecri.org/blogs/ismp-news/due-to-ismp-advocacy-vincristine-labeling-and-packaging-changed-to-prevent-wrong-route-administration?

ISMP. (2016). *FDA and ISMP lists of look-alike drug names with recommended tall man letters*. Retrieved 5 Sep from https://www.ismp.org/sites/default/files/attachments/2017-11/tallmanletters.pdf?

James, R. H. (1998). Ephedrine/Epinephrine drug label confusion. *Anaesthesia*, *53*(5), 511. DOI: 10.1046/j.1365-2044.1998.04771.x PMID: 9659030

Jamil, H., Sama, G., Nohri, A. R., & Malik, N. A. (2025). Medical Error in Pediatric Vaccination: Case Report of Accidental ONCO-BCG Administration in Neonates. *Journal of Health, Wellness, and Community Research*, e190-e190.

Jarernsiripornkul, N., Chaisrisawadsuk, S., Chaiyakum, A., & Krska, J. (2009). Patient self-reporting of potential adverse drug reactions to non-steroidal anti-inflammatory drugs in Thailand. *Pharmacy World & Science*, *31*(5), 559–564. DOI: 10.1007/s11096-009-9310-3 PMID: 19575308

Jeetu, G., & Anusha, G. (2010). Pharmacovigilance: A worldwide master key for drug safety monitoring. *Journal of Young Pharmacists : JYP*, *2*(3), 315–320. DOI: 10.4103/0975-1483.66802 PMID: 21042493

Jitanapakarn, P., Khunawaradisai, N., & Supapaan, T. (2023). Outcomes of medication reconciliation at patient ward in a community hospital in the Northeast. *Thai J Pharm Pract*, *15*(4), 1003–1014.

Jitruknatee, A., Martro, J., Tosanguan, K., Doangjai, Y., & Theantawee, W. (2020). National drug policies in Thailand: Evolution and lessons for the future. *J Health Sci*, *29*(Special Issue), S3–S14.

Joint Commission International. (2017). *Quick Safety Issue 37: Eliminating vincristine administration events*. Retrieved 5 Sep from https://www.jointcommission.org/en/knowledge-library/newsletters/quick-safety/issue-37?

Kalola, A. S., & Dean, R. (2019). The United States Food and Drug Administration and Prescription Drug Promotion. *The Journal of Innovations in Cardiac Rhythm Management*, *10*(3), 3588–3591. DOI: 10.19102/icrm.2019.100305 PMID: 32477722

Kapook. (2023). *Shampoo dispensed instead of cough syrup; 66-year-old patient spit it out after tasting*. Retrieved 23 Jan from https://hilight.kapook.com/view/233483

Karet, G. B. (2019). How do drugs get named? *AMA Journal of Ethics*, *21*(8), E686–E696. DOI: 10.1001/amajethics.2019.686 PMID: 31397664

Karet, G. B. (2023). Linguistic analysis of generic-generic drug name pairs prone to wrong-drug errors for which tall-man lettering is recommended. *Therapeutic Innovation & Regulatory Science*, *57*(4), 751–758. DOI: 10.1007/s43441-023-00526-0 PMID: 37171707

Kaushal, R., Bates, D. W., Landrigan, C., McKenna, K. J., Clapp, M. D., Federico, F., & Goldmann, D. A. (2001). Medication Errors and Adverse Drug Events in Pediatric Inpatients. *Journal of the American Medical Association*, *285*(16), 2114–2120. DOI: 10.1001/jama.285.16.2114 PMID: 11311101

Kelling, S. E. (2017). Look-alike/sound-alike dietary supplements. *Journal of the American Pharmacists Association*, *57*(3), 300–301. DOI: 10.1016/j.japh.2017.03.001 PMID: 28411012

Kemp, S. F., Lockey, R. F., & Simons, F. E. (2008). Epinephrine: The drug of choice for anaphylaxis. A statement of the World Allergy Organization. *Allergy*, *63*(8), 1061–1070. DOI: 10.1111/j.1398-9995.2008.01733.x PMID: 18691308

Kesselheim, A. S., Bykov, K., Avorn, J., Tong, A., Doherty, M., & Choudhry, N. K. (2014). Burden of changes in pill appearance for patients receiving generic cardiovascular medications after myocardial infarction: Cohort and nested case–control studies. *Annals of Internal Medicine*, *161*(2), 96–103. DOI: 10.7326/M13-2381 PMID: 25023248

Khaosod. (2023). *Hospital error: TCA acid dispensed instead of chloral hydrate in pediatric case*. Retrieved 23 Jan from https://www.khaosod.co.th/breaking-news/news_8000990

Khari, S., & Pazokian, M. (2022). Simulation of training solution for the prevention of medication errors in the emergency ward. *Pharmacy Education*, *22*(1), 492–497. DOI: 10.46542/pe.2022.221.492497

Khontum, A., & Chanthapasa, K. (2021). Perceptions of communities regarding Look-Twin Sound-Twin drugs: A case study of a sub-district in the Northeastern Region of Thailand. *Risk Management and Healthcare Policy*, *14*, 2345–2355. DOI: 10.2147/RMHP.S303899 PMID: 34113190

Khoo, Y. K., Lim, J., Tan-Koi, W., Kitikiti, N., & Sim-Devadas, A. (2023). Promoting collaboration of regulators and patients in improving drug safety and regulatory decision making. *Drug Safety*, *47*(3), 217–225. DOI: 10.1007/s40264-023-01385-2 PMID: 38082120

Khumsikiew, J., Sripa, S., Moolasarn, S., Toh, L. S., Anderson, C., & Supapaan, T. (2023). Facilitators and barriers of the rational drug use hospital program in Thailand. *Pharmacy Practice*, *21*(3), 1–11. DOI: 10.18549/PharmPract.2023.3.2815

Kierstan, B. (2019). *Eye medication mix-ups*. Retrieved 14 March from https://www.aao.org/eye-health/treatments/eye-medication-mix-ups

Kim, J. W., Ko, T. Y., & Kang, D. (2026). Accidental epidural administration of sugammadex and ramosetron - A case report. *Anesthesia and Pain Medicine*, *21*(1), 67–71. DOI: 10.17085/apm.25330 PMID: 41667250

Kimura, E., Kawakami, Y., Inoue, S., & Okajima, A. (2025). A dataset for mapping the Japanese drugs to RxNorm standard concepts. *Data in Brief*, *59*, 111418. DOI: 10.1016/j.dib.2025.111418 PMID: 40124300

Kloth, D. D. (2002). Prevention of Chemotherapy Medication Errors. *Journal of Pharmacy Practice*, *15*(1), 17–31. DOI: 10.1106/EXK5-5F5M-T5QV-45CW

Kondrak, G., & Dorr, B. (2006). Automatic identification of confusable drug names. *Artificial Intelligence in Medicine*, *36*(1), 29–42. DOI: 10.1016/j.artmed.2005.07.005 PMID: 16359851

Kopp, B. J., Erstad, B. L., Allen, M. E., Theodorou, A. A., & Priestley, G. (2006). Medication errors and adverse drug events in an intensive care unit: Direct observation approach for detection. *Critical Care Medicine*, *34*(2), 415–425. DOI: 10.1097/01.CCM.0000198106.54306.D7 PMID: 16424723

Kovacic, L., & Chambers, C. (2011). Look-alike, sound-alike drugs in oncology. *Journal of Oncology Pharmacy Practice*, *17*(2), 104–118. DOI: 10.1177/1078155209354135 PMID: 20118216

Kowing, D., & Kester, E. (2007). Keep an eye out for glaucoma. *The Nurse Practitioner*, *32*(7), 18–23. DOI: 10.1097/01.NPR.0000279566.70700.09 PMID: 17595584

Kuitunen, S., Niittynen, I., Airaksinen, M., & Holmström, A.-R. (2021). Systemic Causes of In-Hospital Intravenous Medication Errors: A Systematic Review. *Journal of Patient Safety*, *17*(8), e1660–e1668. DOI: 10.1097/PTS.0000000000000632 PMID: 32011427

Kutner, M., Greenberg, E., & Baer, J. (2006). *A First Look at the Literacy of America's Adults in the 21st Century. NCES 2006-470*. National Center for Education Statistics.

Kvarnström, K., Westerholm, A., Airaksinen, M., & Liira, H. (2021). Factors contributing to medication adherence in patients with a chronic condition: A scoping review of qualitative research. *Pharmaceutics*, *13*(7), 1100. Advance online publication. DOI: 10.3390/pharmaceutics13071100 PMID: 34371791

Lambert, B. L. (1997). Predicting look-alike and sound-alike medication errors. *American Journal of Health-System Pharmacy*, *54*(10), 1161–1171. DOI: 10.1093/ajhp/54.10.1161 PMID: 9161623

Lambert, B. L., Galanter, W., Liu, K. L., Falck, S., Schiff, G., Rash-Foanio, C., Schmidt, K., Shrestha, N., Vaida, A. J., & Gaunt, M. J. (2019). Automated detection of wrong-drug prescribing errors. *BMJ Quality & Safety*, *28*(11), 908–915. DOI: 10.1136/bmjqs-2019-009420 PMID: 31391313

Lambert, B. L., Lin, S. J., Chang, K. Y., & Gandhi, S. K. (1999). Similarity as a risk factor in drug-name confusion errors: The look-alike (orthographic) and sound-alike (phonetic) model. *Medical Care*, *37*(12), 1214–1225. DOI: 10.1097/00005650-199912000-00005 PMID: 10599603

Lambert, B. L., Lin, S.-J., & Tan, H. (2005). Designing Safe Drug Names. *Drug Safety*, *28*(6), 495–512. DOI: 10.2165/00002018-200528060-00003 PMID: 15924503

Lang, S., Ford, K. J., John, T., Pollard, A. J., & McCarthy, N. D. (2014). Immunization errors reported to a vaccine advice service: Intelligence to improve practice. *Quality in Primary Care*, *22*(3), 139–146. PMID: 24865341

Larmené-Beld, K. H. M., Alting, E. K., & Taxis, K. (2018). A systematic literature review on strategies to avoid look-alike errors of labels. *European Journal of Clinical Pharmacology*, *74*(8), 985–993. DOI: 10.1007/s00228-018-2471-z PMID: 29754215

Leape, L. L. (2007). Chapter 1. Systems Analysis and Redesign: The Foundation of Medical Error Prevention. In *Medication Errors, 2nd Edition*. The American Pharmacists Association. https://doi.org/doi:10.21019/9781582120928.ch1

Leape, L. L., Bates, D. W., Cullen, D. J., Cooper, J., Demonaco, H. J., Gallivan, T., & Edmondson, A. (1995). Systems Analysis of Adverse Drug Events. *Journal of the American Medical Association*, *274*(1), 35–43. DOI: 10.1001/jama.1995.03530010049034 PMID: 7791256

Lerdsirisopon, S., Angkasuvan, W., Viengteerawat, S., Limapichat, R., Prapongsena, P., Ariyanuchitkul, T., & Chongarunngamsang, W. (2018). Medication Errors and Adverse Drug Events: Analysis from Perioperative Anesthetic Adverse Events in Thailand (PAAd Thai Study). *Journal of the Medical Association of Thailand*, *101*(6).

Lexicomp. (2024). *Metformin: Drug information*. UpToDate. Retrieved 10 Fwb from https://www-uptodate-com

Lexi-Drugs. (2025). *UpToDate Lexidrug. UpToDate Inc.* Retrieved 19 March from https://online.lexi.com

Lizano-Díez, I., Figueiredo-Escribá, C., Piñero-López, M., Lastra, C. F., Mariño, E. L., & Modamio, P. (2020). Prevention strategies to identify LASA errors: Building and sustaining a culture of patient safety. *BMC Health Services Research*, *20*(1), 63. DOI: 10.1186/s12913-020-4922-3 PMID: 31996197

Lohmeyer, Q., Schiess, C., Wendel Garcia, P. D., Petry, H., Strauch, E., Dietsche, A., Schuepbach, R. A., Buehler, P. K., & Hofmaenner, D. A. (2023). Effects of tall man lettering on the visual behavior of critical care nurses while identifying syringe drug labels: A randomized in situ simulation. *BMJ Quality & Safety*, *32*(1), 26–33. DOI: 10.1136/bmjqs-2021-014438 PMID: 35260415

Lowe, A., Hamilton, M., Greenall, B. M. J., Ma, J., Dhalla, I., & Persaud, N. (2017). Fatal overdoses involving hydromorphone and morphine among inpatients: A case series. *CMAJ Open*, *5*(1), E184–e189. DOI: 10.9778/cmajo.20160013 PMID: 28401133

Lumbreras, B., Sanz-Valero, J., & López-Pintor, E. (2022). Impact of Variation in Pill/Package Appearance of Drugs on Patients' Behavior: A Systematic Review. *Journal of Patient Safety*, *18*(4), 310–317. DOI: 10.1097/PTS.0000000000000941 PMID: 35452203

Lustig, A. (2000). Medication error prevention by pharmacists-An Israeli solution. *Pharmacy World & Science*, *22*(1), 21–25. DOI: 10.1023/A:1008774206261 PMID: 10815296

Magnesium Hydroxide. (2025). *Lexi-Drugs Multinational. UpToDate Lexidrug. UpToDate Inc.* Retrieved 19 March from https://online.lexi.com

Mahidol University. (2025). *Medilet: Thailand drug database by Faculty of Pharmacy, Mahidol University*. Retrieved 31 July from https://pharmacy.mahidol.ac.th/medilet/

Majeed, A., Chaiah, Y., Hammad, A., Alkhani, S., Amer, M. A., & Broering, D. C. (2025). Adrenaline rush: Unsuspicious dispensing error causing life threatening wrong drug infusion during living donor liver transplantation. *Saudi Journal of Anaesthesia*, *19*(3), 416–418. DOI: 10.4103/sja.sja_602_24 PMID: 40642627

Manager Online. (2018). *Yaa Chud is dangerous! Thai FDA warns it can be fatal due to lack of control and regulation*. Retrieved 28 July from https://mgronline.com/onlinesection/detail/9680000053297

Manias, E., Rixon, S., Williams, A., Liew, D., & Braaf, S. (2015). Barriers and enablers affecting patient engagement in managing medications within specialty hospital settings. *Health Expectations : An International Journal of Public Participation in Health Care and Health Policy*, *18*(6), 2787–2798. DOI: 10.1111/hex.12255 PMID: 25186633

Marilyn Schwartz. (2007). *Look-Alike/Sound-Alike (LASA) drug names - review update -Health Canada's Perspective*. Retrieved 14 April from https://capra.ca/_uploads/archive/presentations/14-MarilynSchwartz-LA-SAGuidanceUpdate.pdf

Markert, A., Thierry, V., Kleber, M., Behrens, M., & Engelhardt, M. (2009). Chemotherapy safety and severe adverse events in cancer patients: Strategies to efficiently avoid chemotherapy errors in in- and outpatient treatment. *International Journal of Cancer*, *124*(3), 722–728. DOI: 10.1002/ijc.23991 PMID: 18989899

Marovino, E., Morgillo, A., Mancino, N., Di Feo, V., & Genito, E. (2022). Therapeutic error: Types and prevention strategies and focus about" Look Alike/Sound Alike" and" High Risk" drugs. *Journal of Pharmaceutical Research International*, *34*(48A), 9–16. DOI: 10.9734/jpri/2022/v34i48A36409

Mathew, P., Thomas, S. A., & Chandy, S. J. (2022). The role of Schedule H1 and Red Line campaign in improving antibiotic use in India. *Journal of Family Medicine and Primary Care*, *11*(6), 2656–2661. DOI: 10.4103/jfmpc.jfmpc_1811_21 PMID: 36119342

Maurer, W. (2000). Vaccine nomenclature: The three-letter code. OMCL Vaccine Nomenclature Drafting Group. *Vaccine*, *18*(15), 1539–1542. DOI: 10.1016/S0264-410X(99)00435-1 PMID: 10618552

Mazor, K. M., Simon, S. R., Yood, R. A., Martinson, B. C., Gunter, M. J., Reed, G. W., & Gurwitz, J. H. (2004). Health plan members' views about disclosure of medical errors. *Annals of Internal Medicine*, *140*(6), 409–418. DOI: 10.7326/0003-4819-140-6-200403160-00006 PMID: 15023706

Medicines and Healthcare products Regulatory Agency (MHRA). (2014). *Mercaptamine and mercaptopurine: confusion between drug names*. Retrieved 15 June from https://www.gov.uk/drug-safety-update/mercaptamine-and-mercaptopurine-confusion-between-drug-names

Medicines and Healthcare products Regulatory Agency (MHRA). (2014a). *Mercaptamine and mercaptopurine: confusion between drug names*. Retrieved 15 June from https://www.gov.uk/drug-safety-update/mercaptamine-and-mercaptopurine-confusion-between-drug-names

Medicines and Healthcare products Regulatory Agency (MHRA). (2014b). *Recent drug-name confusion*. Retrieved 11 July from https://www.gov.uk/drug-safety-update/recent-drug-name-confusion

Medicines and Healthcare products Regulatory Agency (MHRA). (2018). *Drug-name confusion: reminder to be vigilant for potential errors*. Retrieved 15 June from https://www.gov.uk/drug-safety-update/drug-name-confusion-reminder-to-be-vigilant-for-potential-errors

Medicines and Healthcare products Regulatory Agency (MHRA). (2019). *MHRA guideline for the naming of medicinal products and Braille requirements for nme on lbel*. Retrieved 15 June from https://assets.publishing.service.gov.uk/media/5d0cb4dd40f0b620109f090c/MHRA_Guideline_for_the_Naming_of_Medicinal_Products_and_Braille_Requirements_for_Name_on_Label.pdf

Medicines and Healthcare products Regulatory Agency (MHRA). (2020). *Best practice guidance on the labeling and packaging of medicines. Medicines and Healthcare products Regulatory Agency*. Retrieved 13 July from https://assets.publishing.service.gov.uk/media/5fe09fa48fa8f51489f14374/Best_practice_guidance_labelling_and_packaging_of_medicines.pdf

Medicines and Healthcare products Regulatory Agency. (2012). *The Human Medicines Regulations* 2012. Retrieved 25 Feb from https://www.legislation.gov.uk/uksi/2012/1916/contents/made

Medscape. (2000). *Prescribing alert sent to pharmacists about lamictal and lamisil*. Retrieved 22 May from https://www.medscape.com/viewarticle/411972?form=fpf

MedSnap. (2025). *MedSnap: Mobile drug verification using computer vision.* Retrieved 31 July from https://medsnap.com

Merative. (2025). *Micromedex: Clinical decision support.* Retrieved 31 July from https://www.merative.com/clinical-decision-support/micromedex

Meredith, P. A. (1996). Generic drugs: Therapeutic equivalence. *Drug Safety*, *15*(4), 233–242. DOI: 10.2165/00002018-199615040-00001 PMID: 8905248

Merry, A. F., Shipp, D. H., & Lowinger, J. S. (2011). The contribution of labeling to safe medication administration in anesthetic practice. *Best Practice & Research. Clinical Anaesthesiology*, *25*(2), 145–159. DOI: 10.1016/j.bpa.2011.02.009 PMID: 21550540

Meyer, T. A., & McAllister, R. K. (2023). Medication errors related to look-alike, sound-alike drugs—How big is the problem and what progress is being made? *APSF Newsletter*, *38*(2), 47–49.

Michelet-Huot, E., Bacouillard, J. B., Quillet, P., Bonnet, M., Mongaret, C., & Hettler, D. (2017). PS-106 Look-alike and sound-alike drug incidents in a hospital: A retrospective analysis. *European Journal of Hospital Pharmacy : Science and Practice*, *24*(Suppl 1), A274. DOI: 10.1136/ejhpharm-2017-000640.612

Miller, M. R., Robinson, K. A., Lubomski, L. H., Rinke, M. L., & Pronovost, P. J. (2007). Medication errors in pediatric care: A systematic review of epidemiology and an evaluation of evidence supporting reduction strategy recommendations. *Quality & Safety in Health Care*, *16*(2), 116–126. DOI: 10.1136/qshc.2006.019950

Ministry of Public Health Republic of Lebanon. (2024). *Look alike sound alike medicines.* Retrieved 15 June from https://www.moph.gov.lb/en/view/68527/look-alike-sound-alike-medicines

Mishra, D., Kaur, K., Gurnani, B., Heda, A., & Dwivedi, K. (2022). Clinical and diagnostic color-coding in ophthalmology - An indispensable educational tool for ophthalmologists. *Indian Journal of Ophthalmology*, *70*(9), 3191–3197. DOI: 10.4103/ijo.IJO_442_22 PMID: 36018086

Mitobe, J., & Higuchi, T. (2016). Does finger pointing toward drug names prevent confusion between similar names during rapid search? *Psychologia*, *59*(1), 38–49. DOI: 10.2117/psysoc.2016.38

Mohammed, A. (2022). *Instruments of local anesthesia.* Retrieved 17 March from https://uomus.edu.iq/img/lectures21/MUCLecture_2022_3111211.pdf

Momo, K., Shimano, M., Kanezaki, Y., Minagawa, A., Takagi, A., Seino, T., & Koinuma, M. (2019). Assessment of. *Die Pharmazie-An International Journal of Pharmaceutical Sciences, 74*(5), 310–312. PMID: 31109403

Momtahan, K., Burns, C. M., Jeon, J., Hyland, S., & Gabriele, S. (2008). Using human factors methods to evaluate the labeling of injectable drugs. *Healthc Q*, 11(3 Spec No.), 122-128. DOI: 10.12927/hcq.2013.19598

Monnier, A. A. C. S., Matin A, Kamath S, Sharmeen T, Khan WA, Bright HR, Mathew P, Wertheim HFL, (2024). What can be learned from Medicine Labeling Initiatives in Asia, with a focus on Antibiotics? *J Community Med Public Health, 8*(2), 432. https://doi.org/10.29011/2577-2228.100432

Monnier, A. A., Do, N. T. T., Asante, K. P., Afari-Asiedu, S., Khan, W. A., Munguambe, K., Sevene, E., Tran, T. K., Nguyen, C. T. K., Punpuing, S., Gómez-Olivé, F. X., van Doorn, H. R., Caillet, C., Newton, P. N., Ariana, P., Wertheim, H. F. L., Wertheim, H. F. L., Monnier, A. A., Newton, P. N., & van Doorn, H. R. (2023). Is this pill an antibiotic or a painkiller? Improving the identification of oral antibiotics for better use. *The Lancet. Global Health, 11*(8), e1308–e1313. DOI: 10.1016/S2214-109X(23)00258-9 PMID: 37474237

Monthly Index of Medical Specialties (MIMS) Thailand. (2025). *Pill identifier*. Retrieved 31 July from https://www.mims.com/thailand/image/advancedsearch

Mosa, A. S., Yoo, I., & Sheets, L. (2012). A systematic review of healthcare applications for smartphones. *BMC Medical Informatics and Decision Making, 12*(1), 67. DOI: 10.1186/1472-6947-12-67 PMID: 22781312

Muchu, P. (2024). Look Alike Sound Alike Drugs in Adults. *International Journal of Health Care and Biological Sciences, 5*(1), 18–23. DOI: 10.46795/ijhcbs.v5i1.609

Mulac, A., Mathiesen, L., Taxis, K., & Gerd Granås, A. (2021). Barcode medication administration technology use in hospital practice: A mixed-methods observational study of policy deviations. *BMJ Quality & Safety, 30*(12), 1021–1030. DOI: 10.1136/bmjqs-2021-013223 PMID: 34285114

Mumani, A. A. (2018). User-packaging interaction (UPI): A comprehensive research platform and techniques for improvement, evaluation, and design.

Munesh, G., & Bhavaraju, M. L. R. (2024). Regulatory framework for USFDA regulated drug product labeling update. *Pharmaceutical Sciences Asia*, 51(1), 10–18

Nagamotoo, Y., Lai, K., & Cavell, G. (2022). Measuring drug name similarity to prioritize the application of tall-man lettering in a computerized pharmacy dispensing system. *The International Journal of Pharmacy Practice*, *30*(S2), ii35–ii36. DOI: 10.1093/ijpp/riac089.041

Nanji, K. C., Patel, A., Shaikh, S., Seger, D. L., & Bates, D. W. (2016). Evaluation of Perioperative Medication Errors and Adverse Drug Events. *Anesthesiology*, *124*(1), 25–34. DOI: 10.1097/ALN.0000000000000904 PMID: 26501385

Napaporn, J., Buakaew, P., Suksakornthanawat, P., Sripa, S., Jinatongthai, P., & Supapaan, T. (2022). Analogous comparison of registered brand name drugs of tablets and capsules commercially available in Thailand: A retrospective study. *PLoS One*, *17*(10), e0276321. DOI: 10.1371/journal.pone.0276321 PMID: 36260612

Napaporn, J., Supapaan, J., Jinathongthai, P., Sripa, S., Kamnuek, J., Khakaew, C., & Pitchayajittipong, C. (2023). Analysis of similarity of physical appearances of pills in the forms of tablets and capsules commercially available in Thailand. *Thai J Pharm Pract*, *15*(4), 1060–1070.

Naseralallah, L., Stewart, D., Azfar Ali, R., & Paudyal, V. (2022). An umbrella review of systematic reviews on contributory factors to medication errors in health-care settings. *Expert Opinion on Drug Safety*, *21*(11), 1379–1399. DOI: 10.1080/14740338.2022.2147921 PMID: 36408597

National Center for Biotechnology Information. (2024a). *PubChem Compound Summary for CID* 1983, *Acetaminophen*. Retrieved 19 May from https://pubchem.ncbi.nlm.nih.gov/compound/Acetaminophen

National Center for Biotechnology Information. (2024b). *PubChem Compound Summary for CID* 2083, *Albuterol*. Retrieved 19 May from https://pubchem.ncbi.nlm.nih.gov/compound/Albuterol

National Center for Biotechnology Information. (2024c). *PubChem Compound Summary for CID* 3488, *Glyburide*. Retrieved 19 May from https://pubchem.ncbi.nlm.nih.gov/compound/Glyburide

National Center for Biotechnology Information. (2024d). *PubChem Compound Summary for CID* 4058, *Meperidine*. Retrieved 19 May from https://pubchem.ncbi.nlm.nih.gov/compound/Meperidine

National Center for Biotechnology Information. (2024e). *PubChem Compound Summary for CID* 27447, *Cephalexin*. Retrieved 19 May from https://pubchem.ncbi.nlm.nih.gov/compound/Cephalexin

National Center for Biotechnology Information. (2024f). *PubChem Compound Summary for CID* 41781, *Torsemide*. Retrieved 19 May from https://pubchem.ncbi.nlm.nih.gov/compound/Torsemide

National Center for Biotechnology Information. (2024g). *PubChem Compound Summary for CID* 135398735, *Rifampin*. Retrieved 19 May from https://pubchem.ncbi.nlm.nih.gov/compound/Rifampin

National Center for Biotechnology Information. (2024h). *ubChem Compound Summary for CID* 3715, *Indomethacin*. Retrieved 19 May from https://pubchem.ncbi.nlm.nih.gov/compound/Indomethacin

National Coordinating Council for Medication Error Reporting and Prevention (NCC MERP). (2022). *Types of Medication Errors*. Retrieved 11 Oct from https://www.nccmerp.org/types-medication-errors

National Institutes of Health. (2026a). *Dietary Supplement Label Database: Glucocil® product label*. Retrieved 18 Jan from https://dsld.od.nih.gov/label/301431

National Institutes of Health. (2026b). *Dietary Supplement Label Database: Luna Gentle Sleep Aid*. Retrieved 18 Jan from https://dsld.od.nih.gov/label/255959

National Library of Medicine. (2025). *The DailyMed database* Retrieved 17 Sep from https://dailymed.nlm.nih.gov/dailymed/index.cfm

National Patient Safety Agency. Patient Safety Division. (2008). *Design for patient safety: a guide to labeling and packaging of injectable medicines*. Retrieved 31 July from https://www.intmedsafe.net/wp-content/uploads/2014/01/0592_InjectablesBookV9_Web1.pdf

Naunton, M., Gardiner, H. R., & Kyle, G. (2015). Look-alike, sound-alike medication errors: A novel case concerning a Slow-Na, Slow-K prescribing error. *International Medical Case Reports Journal*, *8*, 51–53. DOI: 10.2147/IMCRJ.S78637 PMID: 25733932

Nchinech, N., Benhasna, O., Achour, S., Elkartouti, A., Bousliman, Y., Lamsaouri, J., & Tadlaoui, Y. (2023). Medication Errors Related to Look Alike and Sound Alike Medications: About a Moroccan City University Hospital and Community Pharmacies Experience. *Sch Acad J Pharm*, *12*(12), 271–277. DOI: 10.36347/sajp.2023.v12i12.003

NCPDP. (2021). NCPDP recommendations for standardizing dosing in metric units (mL) on prescription container labels of oral liquid medications, version 2.0. *American Journal of Health-System Pharmacy*, *78*(7), 578–605. DOI: 10.1093/ajhp/zxab023

Neelakantan, M., Sharma, P., & Kulkarni, A. (2024). Look-alike, sound-alike (LASA) drugs in India. *The Lancet Regional Health. Southeast Asia*, *26*, 100425. DOI: 10.1016/j.lansea.2024.100425 PMID: 38798984

Neuss, M. N., Gilmore, T. R., Belderson, K. M., Billett, A. L., Conti-Kalchik, T., Harvey, B. E., Hendricks, C., LeFebvre, K., Mangu, P., McNiff, K., Olsen, M. K., Schulmeister, L., Von Gehr, A., & Polovich, M. (2017). 2016 Updated American Society of Clinical Oncology/Oncology Nursing Society Chemotherapy Administration Safety Standards, Including Standards for Pediatric Oncology. *Oncology Nursing Forum*, *44*(1), 31–43. DOI: 10.1188/17.ONF.31-43 PMID: 28067033

News, N. B. C. (2005). *Zyprexa, Zyrtec similarities causing confusion*. Retrieved 15 Apr from https://www.nbcnews.com/health/health-news/zyprexa-zyrtec-similarities-causing-confusion-flna1c9439578

Newton, P. N., Hampton, C. Y., Alter-Hall, K., Teerwarakulpana, T., Prakongpan, S., Ruangveerayuth, R., White, N. J., Day, N. P. J., Tudino, M. B., Mancuso, N., & Fernández, F. M. (2008). Characterization of "Yaa Chud" Medicine on the Thailand-Myanmar border: Selecting for drug-resistant malaria and threatening public health. *The American Journal of Tropical Medicine and Hygiene*, *79*(5), 662–669. DOI: 10.4269/ajtmh.2008.79.662 PMID: 18981500

Nightingale, S. L. (1998). Guidance on industry-supported scientific and educational activities. *Journal of the American Medical Association*, *279*(5), 346–346. DOI: 10.1001/jama.279.5.346-JFD81013-2-1 PMID: 9459455

Noble, D. J., & Donaldson, L. J. (2010). The quest to eliminate intrathecal vincristine errors: A 40-year journey. *Quality & Safety in Health Care*, *19*(4), 323–326. DOI: 10.1136/qshc.2008.030874 PMID: 20211962

Nyström, M. E., Karltun, J., Keller, C., & Andersson Gäre, B. (2018). Collaborative and partnership research for improvement of health and social services: Researcher's experiences from 20 projects. *Health Research Policy and Systems*, *16*(1), 46. DOI: 10.1186/s12961-018-0322-0 PMID: 29843735

Ocvirk, J., Heeger, S., McCloud, P., & Hofheinz, R.-D. (2013). A review of the treatment options for skin rash induced by EGFR-targeted therapies: Evidence from randomized clinical trials and a metaanalysis. *Radiology and Oncology*, *47*(2), 166–175. DOI: 10.2478/raon-2013-0014 PMID: 23801914

Ogboli-Nwasor, E. (2013). Medication errors in anesthetic practice: A report of two cases and review of the literature. *African Health Sciences*, *13*(3), 845–849. DOI: 10.4314/ahs.v13i3.46 PMID: 24250330

Ostini, R., Roughead, E. E., Kirkpatrick, C. M., Monteith, G. R., & Tett, S. E. (2012). Quality use of medicines—Medication safety issues in naming; look-alike, sound-alike medicine names. *The International Journal of Pharmacy Practice*, *20*(6), 349–357. DOI: 10.1111/j.2042-7174.2012.00210.x PMID: 23134093

Otero López, M. J., Martín Muñoz, R., Sánchez Barba, M., Abad Sazatornil, R., Andreu Crespo, A., Arteta Jiménez, M.,…Cajaraville Ordoñana, G. (2011). Development of a List of Look-alike Drug Names With Recommended Tall Man Letters. *Farmacia Hospitalaria, 35*(5), 225-235. DOI: 10.1016/j.farmae.2011.06.001

Pakenham-Walsh, N., & Ana, J. (2014). Confusing drug packaging contributes to death of 15 children. *The Lancet. Global Health*, *2*(11), e634. DOI: 10.1016/S2214-109X(14)70328-6 PMID: 25442687

Palasuberniam, P., Chin, S., Thangiah, V., & Dsouza, U. J. A. (2018). Medication Errors: A Review of Classifications. *Borneo Journal of Medical Sciences*, *12*(3), 11–18. DOI: 10.51200/bjms.v12i3.1173

Pandey, R., & Philip, A. (2011). Concentrate on the Concentration! Double Checkin g Avoids Another Potential Disaster. *Journal of Anesthesia & Clinical Research*, *2*(7), 148. DOI: 10.4172/2155-6148.1000148

Pandolfini, C., & Bonati, M. (2005). A literature review on off-label drug use in children. *European Journal of Pediatrics*, *164*(9), 552–558. DOI: 10.1007/s00431-005-1698-8

Paracetamol [Acetaminophen]. (2025). *Lexi-Drugs Multinational. UpToDate Lexidrug. UpToDate Inc.* Retrieved 19 March from https://online.lexi.com

Park, B. (2022). *New Formulation of Rotarix Removes the Need for Reconstitution.* Retrieved 10 Feb from https://www.empr.com/home/news/new-formulation-of-rotarix-removes-the-need-for-reconstitution/

Patterson, E. S., Cook, R. I., & Render, M. L. (2002). Improving Patient Safety by Identifying Side Effects from Introducing Bar Coding in Medication Administration. *Journal of the American Medical Informatics Association*, *9*(5), 540–553. DOI: 10.1197/jamia.M1061 PMID: 12223506

Pattinson, K. T. S. (2008). Opioids and the control of respiration. *British Journal of Anaesthesia*, *100*(6), 747–758. DOI: 10.1093/bja/aen094 PMID: 18456641

Payne, C. H., Smith, C. R., Newkirk, L. E., & Hicks, R. W. (2007). Pediatric medication errors in the postanesthesia care unit: Analysis of MEDMARX data. *AORN Journal*, *85*(4), 731–740. DOI: 10.1016/S0001-2092(07)60147-1

Pelletier-Dattu, C. E. (2017). Pharmacologic Suffixes. In *Lange Smart Charts: Pharmacology, 2e*. McGraw-Hill Medical.

Perucca, P., & Gilliam, F. G. (2012). Adverse effects of antiepileptic drugs. *The Lancet. Neurology, 11*(9), 792–802. DOI: 10.1016/S1474-4422(12)70153-9 PMID: 22832500

Pervanas, H. C., Revell, N., & Alotaibi, A. F. (2016). Evaluation of medication errors in community pharmacy settings: A retrospective report. *The Journal of Pharmacy Technology : jPT : Official Publication of the Association of Pharmacy Technicians, 32*(2), 71–74. DOI: 10.1177/8755122515617199 PMID: 34861023

Pharmaceutical Braille. (2025). *Marburg medium Braille font standard*. Retrieved 11 July from https://www.pharmabraille.com/pharmaceutical-braille/marburg-medium-font-standard/

Pharmaceutical Services Division. M. o. H. M. (2012). *Guide on handling look alike, sound alike medications*. Retrieved 25 May from https://pharmacy.moh.gov.my/sites/default/files/document-upload/guide-handling-lasa.pdf

Pharmaceutical Services Division. Ministry of Health Malaysia. (2012). *Guide on handling look alike, sound alike medications*. Retrieved 25 May from https://pharmacy.moh.gov.my/sites/default/files/document-upload/guide-handling-lasa.pdf

Pharmaceuticals and Medical Devices Agency (PMDA). (2014). *Medication errors in prescription orders*. Retrieved 15 June from https://www.pmda.go.jp/files/000153905.pdf

Pharmaceuticals and Medical Devices Agency (PMDA). (2017). *Mix-up of drugs due to similarity of nonproprietary names* Retrieved 15 June from https://www.pmda.go.jp/files/000220148.pdf

Pharmaceuticals and Medical Devices Agency (PMDA). (2024). *Profile of services*. Retrieved 15 June from https://www.pmda.go.jp/files/000241469.pdf

Pharmaceuticals and Medical Devices Agency (PMDA). (2025). *PMDA English website*. Retrieved 31 July from https://www.pmda.go.jp/english/

Pharmacy Times. (2005). *Reminyl Is Now Razadyne*. Retrieved 11 Jan from https://www.pharmacytimes.com/view/2005-08-9769

Phatak, H. M., Cady, P. S., Heyneman, C. A., & Culbertson, V. L. (2005). Retrospective Detection of Potential Medication Errors Involving Drugs with Similar Names. *Journal of the American Pharmacists Association, 45*(5), 616–624. DOI: 10.1331/1544345055001247 PMID: 16295648

Pierrel, S. P. A. (2021). *The mechanics of the dental anesthetic cartridge*. Retrieved 17 March from https://www.orabloc.com/wp-content/uploads/Clinical-Tips-The-Mechanics-of-the-Dental-Anesthetic-Cartridge.pdf

Pitchayajittipong, C., Purachaka, S., Kruaysungnoen, A., Fangseekam, N., Noisri, A., Songmuang, T., & Prachuabaree, L. (2025). Extemporaneous compounding practices: Case study in Thai Hospitals. *Pharmacy Practice*, *23*(1), 1–16. DOI: 10.18549/PharmPract.2025.1.3134

Pitchayajittipong, C., Sriboon, S., Kulmee, S., Prachuabaree, L., Srisawai, K., Wattanawong, W., Sripa, S., Anderson, C., & Supapaan, T. (2021). An overview of pharmaceutical production in Thai hospitals. *Hospital Pharmacy*, *56*(4), 265–275. DOI: 10.1177/0018578719890090

Pollak, P. T., Pierce, S., & Cooke, C. (1998). Amrinone and amiodarone: Serious confusion in the intravenous line. *Archives of Internal Medicine*, *158*(2), 193–194. DOI: 10.1001/archinte.158.2.193 PMID: 9448563

Poon, E. G., Keohane, C. A., Yoon, C. S., Ditmore, M., Bane, A., Levtzion-Korach, O., Moniz, T., Rothschild, J. M., Kachalia, A. B., Hayes, J., Churchill, W. W., Lipsitz, S., Whittemore, A. D., Bates, D. W., & Gandhi, T. K. (2010). Effect of Bar-Code Technology on the Safety of Medication Administration. *The New England Journal of Medicine*, *362*(18), 1698–1707. DOI: 10.1056/NEJMsa0907115 PMID: 20445181

Pornwattanakavee, S., Petchsomrit, A., Methaneethorn, J., & Leelakanok, N. (2021). How to Know the Unknown Drugs: A Qualitative Study for Drug Identification Tools Used in Thai Community Pharmacies. *Teikyo Medical Journal*, *44*(3), 849–858.

Pottier, J., Chastang, R., Dumet, C., & Watier, H. (2017). Rethinking the INN system for therapeutic antibodies. *mAbs*, *9*(1), 5–11. DOI: 10.1080/19420862.2016.1255520 PMID: 27808597

Prescrire International. (2020). *Rotarix° oral vaccine: wrong-route errors*. Retrieved 10 Feb from https://english.prescrire.org/en/81/168/58487/0/NewsDetails.aspx

Prokop, D., Babigumira, J., & Lewis, A. (2020). Pill Identification using a Mobile Phone App for Assessing Medication Adherence and Post-Market Drug Surveillance. *arXiv preprint arXiv:*2004.11479.

Prompradith, V., & Chimvong, P. (2017). *Drug regulation in Thailand*. Retrieved 14 April from https://nsp.mohw.org.tw/dl-34-960f0775f3234877a9cde3b445548c62.html

Puttilerpong, C. (2006). System approach to resolve and prevent mediation error: experience of Prachuapkhirikhan hospital. In Chulavatnatol S, Montakantikul P, Chindavijak B, Suksomboon N, & S. T (Eds.), *Pharmacist and quality medication system* (pp. 38-61). The Association of Hospital Pharmacist (Thailand).

Qureshi, S., Ahmad, K., Fatima, P., Hassan, R. M., Sherali, F., Lalani, N., Jehan, F., Ali, S. A., & Qamar, F. N. (2019). Outcome of inadvertent high dose BCG administration in newborns at a tertiary care hospital, Karachi- Case series. *PLoS One*, *14*(7), e0219324. DOI: 10.1371/journal.pone.0219324 PMID: 31291329

Radimer, K., Bindewald, B., Hughes, J., Ervin, B., Swanson, C., & Picciano, M. F. (2004). Dietary Supplement Use by US Adults: Data from the National Health and Nutrition Examination Survey, 1999–2000. *American Journal of Epidemiology*, *160*(4), 339–349. DOI: 10.1093/aje/kwh207 PMID: 15286019

Rahman, Z., & Parvin, R. (2015). Medication errors associated with look-alike/sound-alike drugs: A brief review. *J Enam Med Col*, *5*(2), 110–117. DOI: 10.3329/jemc.v5i2.23385

Raj, N., Fernandes, S., Charyulu, N. R., & Dubey, A., G, S. R., & Hebbar, S. (. (2019). Postmarket surveillance: A review on key aspects and measures on the effective functioning in the context of the United Kingdom and Canada. *Therapeutic Advances in Drug Safety*, *10*, 2042098619865413. DOI: 10.1177/2042098619865413 PMID: 31384423

Ramaswamy, G., & Naik, R. (2014). Saline and metronidazole. *British Journal of Anaesthesia*, *112*(6), 1123. DOI: 10.1093/bja/aeu177 PMID: 24829428

Rameshkumar, T., Haputhanthrige, I. U., Misbahunnisa, M. Y., & Galappatthy, P. (2022). Patients' knowledge about medicines improves when provided with written compared to verbal information in their native language. *PLoS One*, *17*(10), e0274901. DOI: 10.1371/journal.pone.0274901 PMID: 36315507

Ranchon, F., Salles, G., Späth, H. M., Schwiertz, V., Vantard, N., Parat, S., Broussais, F., You, B., Tartas, S., Souquet, P. J., Dussart, C., Falandry, C., Henin, E., Freyer, G., & Rioufol, C. (2011). Chemotherapeutic errors in hospitalized cancer patients: Attributable damage and extra costs. *BMC Cancer*, *11*(1), 478. DOI: 10.1186/1471-2407-11-478 PMID: 22067636

Rastogi, S. (2012). Look alike sound alike drugs: From hospitals to homes. *Journal of Pediatric Intensive Care*, *1*(3), 125–126. DOI: 10.3233/PIC-2012-021 PMID: 31214397

Reallon, E., Yailian, A.-L., Marchand, C., Filali, S., Merienne, C., Pivot, C.,...Pirot, F. (2021). Medicine Identification New Database (MIND): A quick, simple and accurate tool for the identification of unlabeled medication in hospital pharmacies. *Spectroscopy Europe*, 33(6). https://doi.org/10.1255/sew.2021.a27

Reason, J. (2000). Human error: Models and management. *BMJ (Clinical Research Ed.)*, *320*(7237), 768–770. DOI: 10.1136/bmj.320.7237.768 PMID: 10720363

Reines, S. A. (2005). Look-alike, sound-alike drug errors with Reminyl and Amaryl. *American Journal of Health-System Pharmacy*, *62*(1), 35–36. DOI: 10.1093/ajhp/62.1.35 PMID: 15658069

Rider, B. B., Mehta, H., & Merchant, L. (2019). Special considerations for proprietary name review: Focus on products that may be prescribed "As Directed". *Therapeutic Innovation & Regulatory Science*, *53*(3), 381–386. DOI: 10.1177/2168479018782669 PMID: 29929377

Rinke, M. L., Shore, A. D., Morlock, L., Hicks, R. W., & Miller, M. R. (2007). Characteristics of pediatric chemotherapy medication errors in a national error reporting database. *Cancer*, *110*(1), 186–195. DOI: 10.1002/cncr.22742

Roberts, L. (2014). At least 15 children in Syria die in measles immunization campaign. *Science*. Retrieved February 10, 2026, from https://www.science.org/content/article/least-15-children-syria-die-measles-immunization-campaign

Rodziewicz, T. L., Houseman, B., & Hipskind, J. E. (2023). Medical error reduction and prevention. [Updated 2024 Feb 12]. StatPearls Publishing. Retrieved 22 May from https://www.ncbi.nlm.nih.gov/books/NBK499956/

Rodziewicz, T. L., Houseman, B., & Hipskind, J. E. (2023). Medical error reduction and prevention. StatPearls Publishing. https://www.ncbi.nlm.nih.gov/books/NBK499956

Rodziewicz, T. L., Houseman, B., & Hipskind, J. E. (2023). *Medical error reduction and prevention*. StatPearls Publishing.

Ro, M., & Jones, R. (2025). Wrong Drug Events Across Pennsylvania Healthcare Facilities: A Systematic Analysis of Medication Pairs, Class Patterns, and Clinical Safety Implications. *Patient Safety*, *7*(2). Advance online publication. DOI: 10.33940/001c.134046

Roy, P. K. (2001). To err is human, negligence is sin. *Medical Journal, Armed Forces India*, *57*(4), 326–328. DOI: 10.1016/S0377-1237(01)80015-0 PMID: 27365633

Ruutiainen, H. K., Kallio, M. M., & Kuitunen, S. K. (2021). Identification and safe storage of look-alike, sound-alike medicines in automated dispensing cabinets. *European Journal of Hospital Pharmacy : Science and Practice*, *28*(e1, Suppl 2), e151–e156. DOI: 10.1136/ejhpharm-2020-002531 PMID: 33452109

RxList. (2025). *RxList Pill Identification Tool*. Retrieved 30 July from https://www.rxlist.com/pill-identification-tool/article.htm

Ryan, A. N., Robertson, K. L., & Glass, B. D. (2024). Look-alike medications in the perioperative setting: Scoping review of medication incidents and risk reduction interventions. *International Journal of Clinical Pharmacy*, *46*(1), 26–39. DOI: 10.1007/s11096-023-01629-2 PMID: 37688737

Ryan, A. N., Robertson, K. L., & Glass, B. D. (2025). Look-alike, sound-alike medication perioperative incidents in a regional Australian hospital: Assessment using a novel medication safety culture assessment tool. *International Journal for Quality in Health Care*, *37*(1), mzaf018. DOI: 10.1093/intqhc/mzaf018 PMID: 40037610

Safety, P. P. (2010). Adverse drug events with HYDROmorphone: How preventable are they. *Pennsylvania Patient Safety Advisory*, *7*(3), 69–75.

Sakaeda, T., Tamon, A., Kadoyama, K., & Okuno, Y. (2013). Data Mining of the Public Version of the FDA Adverse Event Reporting System [Review]. *International Journal of Medical Sciences*, *10*(7), 796–803. DOI: 10.7150/ijms.6048 PMID: 23794943

Sakai, T., & Morimoto, Y. (2022). The history of infectious diseases and medicine. *Pathogens (Basel, Switzerland)*, *11*(10), 1147. Advance online publication. DOI: 10.3390/pathogens11101147 PMID: 36297204

Samad, F., Burton, S. J., Kwan, D., Porter, N., Smetzer, J., Cohen, M. R., Tuttle, J., Baker, D., & Doherty, D. E. (2021). Strategies to reduce errors associated with 2-component vaccines. *Pharmaceutical Medicine*, *35*(1), 1–9. DOI: 10.1007/s40290-020-00362-9 PMID: 33151497

Samaranayake, N. R., Cheung, D. S., Lam, M. P., Cheung, T. T., Chui, W. C., Wong, I. C., & Cheung, B. M. (2014). The effectiveness of a 'Do Not Use' list and perceptions of healthcare professionals on error-prone abbreviations. *International Journal of Clinical Pharmacy*, *36*(5), 1000–1006. DOI: 10.1007/s11096-014-9987-9 PMID: 25098946

Sangsuriyan, S., Duangkhan, S., Anekprasongkul, W., & Leelakanok, N. (2018). *Drug identification tools in pharmacies*. Faculty of Pharmaceutical Sciences, Burapha University.

Sanook. (2022). *Mother shocked: Infant fed lotion instead of cough syrup, admitted to ICU*. Retrieved 23 Jan from https://www.sanook.com/news/8700410/

Santell, J. P. (2006). Medication errors involving neuromuscular blocking agents. *Jt Comm J Qual Patient Saf*, 32(8), 470-475, 417. DOI: 10.1016/S1553-7250(06)32062-4

Santell, J. P., Hicks, R. W., McMeekin, J., & Cousins, D. D. (2003). Medication errors: Experience of the United States Pharmacopeia (USP) MEDMARX reporting system. *Journal of Clinical Pharmacology*, *43*(7), 760–767. DOI: 10.1177/0091270003254831

Sarpatwari, A., Gagne, J. J., Lu, Z., Campbell, E. G., Carman, W. J., Enger, C. L., Dutcher, S. K., Jiang, W., & Kesselheim, A. S. (2019). A Survey of Patients' Perceptions of Pill Appearance and Responses to Changes in Appearance for Four Chronic Disease Medications. *Journal of General Internal Medicine*, *34*(3), 420–428. DOI: 10.1007/s11606-018-4791-1 PMID: 30632102

Schnoor, J., Rogalski, C., Frontini, R., Engelmann, N., & Heyde, C. E. (2015). Case report of a medication error by look-alike packaging: A classic surrogate marker of an unsafe system. *Patient Safety in Surgery*, *9*(1), 12. DOI: 10.1186/s13037-014-0047-0 PMID: 25767564

Schroeder, S. R., Salomon, M. M., Galanter, W. L., Schiff, G. D., Vaida, A. J., Gaunt, M. J., Bryson, M. L., Rash, C., Falck, S., & Lambert, B. L. (2017). Cognitive tests predict real-world errors: The relationship between drug name confusion rates in laboratory-based memory and perception tests and corresponding error rates in large pharmacy chains. *BMJ Quality &amp. Safety (Basel, Switzerland)*, *26*(5), 395–407. DOI: 10.1136/bmjqs-2015-005099 PMID: 27193033

Schulmeister, L. (2006). Look-alike, sound-alike oncology medications. *Clinical Journal of Oncology Nursing*, *10*(1), 35–41. DOI: 10.1188/06.CJON.35-41 PMID: 16482726

Schwappach, D. L., & Wernli, M. (2010). Medication errors in chemotherapy: Incidence, types and involvement of patients in prevention. A review of the literature. *European Journal of Cancer Care*, *19*(3), 285–292. DOI: 10.1111/j.1365-2354.2009.01127.x PMID: 19708929

Scopolamine (hyoscine). (2026). *Lexi-Drugs Multinational. UpToDate Lexidrug. UpToDate Inc.* Retrieved 25 Jan from https://online.lexi.com

Scott, S. D., Hirschinger, L. E., Cox, K. R., McCoig, M., Brandt, J., & Hall, L. W. (2009). The natural history of recovery for the healthcare provider "second victim" after adverse patient events. *Quality & Safety in Health Care*, *18*(5), 325–330. DOI: 10.1136/qshc.2009.032870 PMID: 19812092

Senior Care Consultant Group (SCCG). (2006). *Appendix* 17: *sound alike/look alike medications*. Retrieved 22 May from http://mysccg.com/generalDocuments/Look%20and%20Sound%20Alike%20Meds.pdf

Serafini, M., Cargnin, S., Massarotti, A., Tron, G. C., Pirali, T., & Genazzani, A. A. (2021). What's in a Name? Drug Nomenclature and Medicinal Chemistry Trends using INN Publications. *Journal of Medicinal Chemistry*, *64*(8), 4410–4429. DOI: 10.1021/acs.jmedchem.1c00181 PMID: 33847110

Shah, M. B., Merchant, L., Chan, I. Z., & Taylor, K. (2017). Characteristics that may help in the identification of potentially confusing proprietary drug names. *Therapeutic Innovation & Regulatory Science*, *51*(2), 232–236. DOI: 10.1177/2168479016667161 PMID: 30231718

Shao, S. C., Lai, E. C., Owang, K. L., Chen, H. Y., & Chan, Y. Y. (2018). Look-Alike Medication Packages and Patient Safety. *Journal of Patient Safety*, *14*(3), e47–e48. DOI: 10.1097/PTS.0000000000000506 PMID: 29894438

Sharma, A. E., Rivadeneira, N. A., Barr-Walker, J., Stern, R. J., Johnson, A. K., & Sarkar, U. (2018). Patient engagement in health care safety: An overview of mixed-quality evidence. *Health Affairs (Project Hope)*, *37*(11), 1813–1820. DOI: 10.1377/hlthaff.2018.0716 PMID: 30395509

Shastay, A. (2016a). Administering Just the Diluent or One of Two Vaccine Components Leaves Patients Unprotected. *Home Healthcare Now*, *34*(4), 218–220. DOI: 10.1097/NHH.0000000000000371 PMID: 27023298

Shastay, A. (2016b). Liquid Oral Vaccine Mistakenly Given by Injection; Topical Anesthetics for Teething Infants. *Home Healthcare Now*, *34*(1), 43–44. DOI: 10.1097/NHH.0000000000000318 PMID: 26645844

Shastay, A. (2023). Look-alike Packaging. *Home Healthcare Now*, *41*(3), 168–169. DOI: 10.1097/NHH.0000000000001170 PMID: 37144934

Shaw, K. N., Lillis, K. A., Ruddy, R. M., Mahajan, P. V., Lichenstein, R., Olsen, C. S., & Network, P. E. C. A. R. (2013). Reported medication events in a pediatric emergency research network: Sharing to improve patient safety. *Emergency Medicine Journal : EMJ*, *30*(10), 815–819. DOI: 10.1136/emermed-2012-201642 PMID: 23117714

Shermock, S. B., Shermock, K. M., & Schepel, L. L. (2023). Closed-loop medication management with an electronic health record system in U.S. and Finnish hospitals. *International Journal of Environmental Research and Public Health*, *20*(17), 6680. DOI: 10.3390/ijerph20176680 PMID: 37681820

Shiffman, S., Gerlach, K. K., Sembower, M. A., & Rohay, J. M. (2011). Consumer understanding of prescription drug information: An illustration using an antidepressant medication. *The Annals of Pharmacotherapy*, *45*(4), 452–458. DOI: 10.1345/aph.1P477

Shimabukuro, T. (2017). *Vaccination Errors: Advisory Committee on Immunization Practices*. Retrieved 09 Feb from https://stacks.cdc.gov/view/cdc/58808

Shrank, W., Avorn, J., Rolon, C., & Shekelle, P. (2007). Effect of content and format of prescription drug labels on readability, understanding, and medication use: A systematic review. *The Annals of Pharmacotherapy*, *41*(5), 783–801. DOI: 10.1345/aph.1H582 PMID: 17426075

Siddiqui, D. E. (2020). Minimizing medication errors by triangle check of look-alike sound-alike medications from crash cart of gynecology and obstetrics in emergency. *Innovations in Pharmacy*, *11*(4), 18. Advance online publication. DOI: 10.24926/iip.v11i4.3480 PMID: 34007659

Siebert, J. N., Ehrler, F., Combescure, C., Lacroix, L., Haddad, K., Sanchez, O., Gervaix, A., Lovis, C., & Manzano, S. (2017). A mobile device App to reduce time to drug delivery and medication errors during simulated pediatric cardiopulmonary resuscitation: A randomized controlled trial. *Journal of Medical Internet Research*, *19*(2), e31. DOI: 10.2196/jmir.7005 PMID: 28148473

Simeticone [Simethicone]. (2025). *Lexi-Drugs Multinational. UpToDate Lexidrug. UpToDate Inc.* Retrieved 19 March from https://online.lexi.com

Sinha, H. K. (2014). Role of pharmacists in retailing of drugs. *Journal of Advanced Pharmaceutical Technology & Research*, *5*(3), 107. DOI: 10.4103/2231-4040.137383 PMID: 25126530

Smetzer, J. L., & Cohen, M. R. (2006). Preventing errors with neuromuscular blocking agents. *Joint Commission Journal on Quality and Patient Safety*, *32*(1), 56–59. DOI: 10.1016/S1553-7250(06)32008-9 PMID: 16514940

Smith, H. S., & Lesar, T. S. (2011). Analgesic prescribing errors and associated medication characteristics. *The Journal of Pain*, *12*(1), 29–40. DOI: 10.1016/j.jpain.2010.04.007 PMID: 21187270

Sobhani, P., Christopherson, J., Ambrose, P. J., & Corelli, R. L. (2008). Accuracy of Oral Liquid Measuring Devices: Comparison of Dosing Cup and Oral Dosing Syringe. *The Annals of Pharmacotherapy*, *42*(1), 46–52. DOI: 10.1345/aph.1K420

Sriboonruang, P., & Rattanamahattana, M. (2022). Barcode scanning technology to improve pre-dispensing errors. *Greater Mekong Subregion Medical J*, *3*(1), 7–12.

Srisuriyachanchai, W., Cox, A. R., Kampichit, S., & Jarernsiripornkul, N. (2023). Severity and management of adverse drug reactions reported by patients and healthcare professionals: A cross-sectional survey. *International Journal of Environmental Research and Public Health*, *20*(4), 3725. Advance online publication. DOI: 10.3390/ijerph20043725 PMID: 36834422

Studer, H., Imfeld-Isenegger, T. L., Beeler, P. E., Ceppi, M. G., Rosen, C., Bodmer, M., Boeni, F., Hersberger, K. E., & Lampert, M. L. (2023). The impact of pharmacist-led medication reconciliation and interprofessional ward rounds on drug-related problems at hospital discharge. *International Journal of Clinical Pharmacy*, *45*(1), 117–125. DOI: 10.1007/s11096-022-01496-3 PMID: 36327045

Sullivan, P. (2003, March 4). New US labeling to eliminate drug conFUSION. *Canadian Medical Association Journal*, *168*(5), 598. PMID: 12615765

Sunpuwan, M., Punpuing, S., Jaruruengpaisan, W., Kinsman, J., & Wertheim, H. (2019). What is in the drug packet?: Access and use of non-prescribed poly-pharmaceutical packs (Yaa Chud) in the community in Thailand. *BMC Public Health*, *19*(1), 971. DOI: 10.1186/s12889-019-7300-5 PMID: 31331304

Supapaan, T. S., Kamnuek, J., Khakaew, C., Jungsuwadee, T., Songmuang, A., Saksit, S., & Napaporn, J. (2024). Assessment of look-Alike, Sound-Alike similarities among brand names of tablets and capsules: A cross-sectional survey in Thailand. *Pharmacy Practice*, *22*(3), 2955. DOI: 10.18549/PharmPract.2024.3.2955

Supapaan, T. S., Low, B. Y., Anderson, C., Boonlue, T., Puripunyavanich, N., Khumsikiew, J., & Poonphol, P. (2023). Evaluation of the rational drug use (RDU) literacy among undergraduate students. *Pharmacy Practice*, *21*(4), 2867.

Supapaan, T. S., Napaporn, J., Ruthirakanok, R., Srichathum, S., Songmuang, A., & Pitchayajittipong, C. (2024). Look-alike sound-alike (LASA) medication errors in Thai hospitals. *Pharmacy Practice*, *22*(1), 2886.

Supapaan, T. S., Somsorn, S., Saensupha, N., Songmuang, T., Songmuang, A., Jaturapattarawong, A., & Napaporn, J. (2024). Development of drug information and drug images identification database for supporting the medical management system at Warinchamrab hospital. *Pharmacy Practice*, *22*(4). Advance online publication. DOI: 10.18549/PharmPract.2024.4.3057

Supapaan, T. S., Songmuang, A., Napaporn, J., Sangsukwow, P., Boonrod, P., Intarapongsakul, P., Jaturapattarawong, A., & Pitchayajittipong, C. (2024). Look-alike/sound-alike medication errors: An in-depth examination through a hospital case study. *Pharmacy Practice*, *22*(2), 2959. DOI: 10.18549/PharmPract.2024.2.2959

Supapaan, T., Jamlongpeng, C., Yangyuen, N., Srisawai, K., Prachuabaree, L., Wattanawong, W., & Pitchayajittipong, C. (2023). Enhancing extemporaneous preparations in Thai Hospitals: Exploring variation, common formulations, and challenges and needs related to extemporaneous preparations. *Pharmacy Practice*, *21*(4), 1–12. DOI: 10.18549/PharmPract.2023.4.2892

Supapaan, T., Pitchayajittipong, C., Sonrasawan, K., Chittawee, C., & Napaporn, J. (2024). Development of the database for look-alike, sound-alike drugs in Thailand. *Thai J Pharm Pract*, *16*(1), 112–125.

Svensk, J., & McIntyre, S. E. (2021). Using QR Code Technology to Reduce Self-Administered Medication Errors. *Journal of Pharmacy Practice*, *34*(4), 587–591. DOI: 10.1177/0897190019885245 PMID: 31835959

Talbird, S. E., Carrico, J., La, E. M., Carias, C., Marshall, G. S., Roberts, C. S., Chen, Y.-T., & Nyaku, M. K. (2022). Impact of Routine Childhood Immunization in Reducing Vaccine-Preventable Diseases in the United States. *Pediatrics*, *150*(3), e2021056013. DOI: 10.1542/peds.2021-056013 PMID: 35821599

Tansuwannarat, P., Vichiensanth, P., Sivarak, O., Tongpoo, A., Promrungsri, P., Sriapha, C., Wananukul, W., & Trakulsrichai, S. (2022). Characteristics and consequences of medication errors in pediatric patients reported to Ramathibodi Poison Center: A 10-year retrospective study. *Therapeutics and Clinical Risk Management*, *18*, 669–681. DOI: 10.2147/TCRM.S363638 PMID: 35795851

Tariq, R. A., Vashisht, R., Sinha, A., & Scherbak, Y. (2021). Medication dispensing errors and prevention. [Updated 2024 Feb 12]. StatPearls Publishing. Retrieved 22 May from https://www.ncbi.nlm.nih.gov/books/NBK519065/

Tariq, R. A., Vashisht, R., Sinha, A., & Scherbak, Y. (2021). Medication dispensing errors and prevention. In *StatPearls*. StatPearls Publishing.

Tavares, L. O. M., Silva, M. A., Oliveira, B. R., Amaral, G. G., Guimarães, E. A. A., Couto, R. O., & Oliveira, V. C. (2024). Prevalence of errors causing events allegedly attributable to vaccination/immunization: Systematic review and meta-analysis. *Revista Gaúcha de Enfermagem, 45*, e20230097. DOI: 10.1590/1983-1447.2024.20230097.pt PMID: 38477748

Thai Food and Drug Administration. (2025). *National Drug Information (NDI) database*. Retrieved 31 July from https://ndi.fda.moph.go.th/

Thailand Food and Drug Administration. (2025). Public pharmaceutical regulatory information: Details of medicinal product.

Thailand Food and Drug Administration. (2025). *Public pharmaceutical regulatory information: Details of medicinal product.* Retrieved 3 April from Thaipharmaitem. (2025). *Pill identifier*. Retrieved 31 July from https://thaipharmaitem.com/en/drug-identification-pill-identifier/

Thairath. (2018). *Hospital dispensed anti-itch lotion instead of cough syrup*. Retrieved 23 Jan from https://www.thairath.co.th/news/society/1206147

Thairath. (2023). *Hospital dispensed TCA (trichloroacetic acid) instead of chloral hydrate to* 1*-year-old; staff suspended*. Retrieved 23 Jan from https://www.thairath.co.th/news/society/2746607

Thakur, D. S., & Prashant, R. T. (2024). *India's problem — different drugs, identical brand names*. Retrieved 15 June from https://www.thehindu.com/opinion/op-ed/indias-problem-different-drugs-identical-brand-names/article67773569.ece

The 2023 American Geriatrics Society Beers Criteria® Update Expert Panel. (2023). American Geriatrics Society 2023 updated AGS Beers Criteria® for potentially inappropriate medication use in older adults. *Journal of the American Geriatrics Society*, *71*(7), 2052–2081. DOI: 10.1111/jgs.18372

The Academy of Managed Care Pharmacy (AMCP). (2019). *Medication errors*. Retrieved 16 Apr from https://www.amcp.org/about/managed-care-pharmacy-101/concepts-managed-care-pharmacy/medication-errors

The American Academy of Ophthalmology. (2015). *Color Codes for Topical Ocular Medications*. Retrieved 20 Nov from https://www.aao.org/about/policies/color-codes-topical-ocular-medications

The American Dental Association (ADA). (2023). *Anesthesia and Sedation: Color Coding of Local Anesthetic Cartridges*. Retrieved 23 Nov from https://www.ada.org/resources/ada-library/oral-health-topics/anesthesia-and-sedation

The American Society for Testing and Materials (ASTM). (2022). *Standard Specification for User Applied Drug Labels in Anesthesiology (Withdrawn 2022)*. Retrieved 21 Nov from https://www.astm.org/d4774-11r17.html

The Associated Press. (2005). *Zyprexa, Zyrtec similarities causing confusion*. Retrieved 8 Feb from https://www.nbcnews.com/health/health-news/zyprexa-zyrtec-similarities-causing-confusion-flna1c9439578

The Australian Commission on Safety and Quality in Health Care. (2020). *Principles for the safe selection and storage of medicines: guidance on the principles and survey tool*. Retrieved 22 June from https://www.safetyandquality.gov.au/sites/default/files/resources/attachments//survey_tool_-_principles_for_safe_selection_and_storage_of_medicines_-_final.pdf

The Code of Federal Regulations (CFR). (2004). *§ 201.25 Bar code label requirements*. Retrieved 25 Feb from https://www.ecfr.gov/current/title-21/chapter-I/subchapter-C/part-201/subpart-A/section-201.25

The Health and Disability Commissioner. (2003). *Antidepressant nefazodone (Serzone) dispensed instead of prescribed antipsychotic quetiapine (Seroquel)*. Retrieved 16 Jan from https://www.hdc.org.nz/media/exujf0qh/01hdc11914pharmacists.pdf

The Institute for Safe Medication Practices (ISMP) Canada. (2001). Multiple reports of confusion between lamotrigine (LAMICTAL®) and products with 'sound alike'/'look alike' name. *ISMP Canada Safety Bulletin*, 1(3).

The Institute for Safe Medication Practices (ISMP). (2011). *ISMP list of high-alert medications in community/ambulatory healthcare*. Retrieved 20 March from https://www.ismp.org/sites/default/files/attachments/2017-11/highAlert-community.pdf

The Institute for Safe Medication Practices (ISMP). (2015). *ISMP's list of confused drug names*. Retrieved 16 Apr from https://www.ismp.org/sites/default/files/attachments/2017-11/confuseddrugnames%2802.2015%29.pdf?

The Institute for Safe Medication Practices (ISMP). (2016). Hydralazine, hydroxyzine confused again. *America's Pharmacist*.

The Institute for Safe Medication Practices (ISMP). (2019). *ISMP list of confused drug names*. Retrieved 11 Oct from https://www.ismp.org/recommendations/confused-drug-names-list

The Institute for Safe Medication Practices (ISMP). (2022). *Adopt strategies to manage look-alike and/or sound-alike medication name mix-ups*. Retrieved 11 July from https://www.ismp.org/sites/default/files/newsletter-issues/20220602.pdf

The Institute for Safe Medication Practices (ISMP). (2023). *List of confused drug names*. Retrieved 16 Apr from https://www.ismp.org/recommendations/confused-drug-names-list

The Institute for Safe Medication Practices (ISMP). (2023a). *FDA and ISMP lists of look-alike drug names with recommended tall man (mixed case) letters*. Retrieved 16 Apr from https://www.ismp.org/system/files/resources/2023-01/ISMP_Tallman_Letters_012523_MS5087%20%282%29.pdf

The Institute for Safe Medication Practices (ISMP). (2023b). *List of confused drug names*. Retrieved 16 Apr from https://www.ismp.org/recommendations/confused-drug-names-list

The Institute for Safe Medication Practices (ISMP). (2023b). *List of confused drug names*. Retrieved 16 April from https://www.ismp.org/recommendations/confused-drug-names-list

The Institute for Safe Medication Practices (ISMP). (2023c). *Obstetrical patient receives ampule of digoxin instead of BUPivacaine for spinal anesthesia*. Retrieved 05 Sep from https://www.ismp.org/resources/obstetrical-patient-receives-ampule-digoxin-instead-bupivacaine-spinal-anesthesia

The Institute for Safe Medication Practices (ISMP). (2024). *ISMP List of Confused Drug Names*. Retrieved 07 Sep from https://online.ecri.org/hubfs/ISMP/Resources/ISMP_ConfusedDrugNames.pdf

The Institute for Safe Medication Practices (ISMP). (2024). *ISMP list of error-prone abbreviations, symbols, and dose designations*. Retrieved 12 April from https://www.ismp.org/recommendations/error-prone-abbreviations-list?check_logged_in=1

The Institute for Safe Medication Practices (ISMP). (2024a). *ISMP List of Confused Drug Names*. Retrieved 07 Sep from https://online.ecri.org/hubfs/ISMP/Resources/ISMP_ConfusedDrugNames.pdf

The Institute for Safe Medication Practices (ISMP). (2024b). *ISMP list of error-prone abbreviations, symbols, and dose designations*. Retrieved 12 April from https://www.ismp.org/recommendations/error-prone-abbreviations-list?check_logged_in=1

The Institute for Safe Medication Practices (ISMP). (2024c). ISMP list of high-alert medications in acute care settings. *ISMP An ECRI Affiliate*, *29*(1), 6.

The Institute for Safe Medication Practices Canada (ISMP Canada). (2007). Patient Report of Insulin Mix-Up Shared. *ISMP Canada Safety Bulletin*, *7*(6), 1–2.

The Institute for Safe Medication Practices Canada (ISMP Canada). (2016). *Drug labeling and the application of TALLman lettering project report*. Retrieved 15 June from https://www.ismp-canada.org/download/TALLman/TALLmanLettering-ProjectReport.pdf

The Joint Commission. (2016). *Managing Health Information: use of abbreviations, acronyms, symbols and dose designations - understanding the requirements*. Retrieved 19 May from https://www.jointcommission.org/standards/standard-faqs/hospital-and-hospital-clinics/information-management-im/000001457/

The Joint Commission. (2023). *Quick Safety Issue* 37: *Eliminating vincristine administration events*. Retrieved 07 Sep from https://www.jointcommission.org/en-us/knowledge-library/newsletters/quick-safety/issue-37

The Joint Commission. (2024). *Managing Health Information: use of abbreviations, acronyms, symbols and dose designations - understanding the requirements*. Retrieved 12 May from https://www.jointcommission.org/standards/standard-faqs/hospital-and-hospital-clinics/information-management-im/000001457/

The Pennsylvania Patient Safety Advisory. (2004). Medication errors linked to drug name confusion. *PA PSRS Patient Saf Advis*, *1*(4), 7–8.

The Pennsylvania Patient Safety Advisory. (2005). Abbreviations: A shortcut to medication errors. *PA PSRS Patient Saf Advis*, *2*(1), 19–21.

The Pennsylvania Patient Safety Advisory. (2005). Complexity of insulin therapy. *PA PSRS Patient Saf Advis*, *2*(2), 30–31.

The Pennsylvania Patient Safety Advisory. (2006). hydrOXYzine and hydrALAzine mix-ups. *PA PSRS Patient Saf Advis*, *3*(2), 21.

The Pennsylvania Patient Safety Advisory. (2007). Inadvertent mix-up of morphine and hydromorphone: A potent error. *PA PSRS Patient Saf Advis*, *4*(3), 86–88.

The Pennsylvania Patient Safety Advisory. (2010). Medication Errors with the Dosing of Insulin: Problems across the Continuum. *PA PSRS Patient Saf Advis*, *7*(1), 9–17.

Therapeutic Goods Administration. (2016). *Mercaptamine (cysteamine) and mercaptopurine*. Retrieved 13 Jan from https://www.tga.gov.au/safety/safety-monitoring-and-information/safety-alerts/mercaptamine-cysteamine-and-mercaptopurine

Therapeutic Goods Adminitration (TGA). A. G. (1990). *Therapeutic Goods Act* 1989. Retrieved 25 Feb from https://www.tga.gov.au/resources/legislation/therapeutic-goods-act-1989

Thomas, P. B. M., & Mollon, J. D. (2018). Syringe labels seen through the eyes of the color-deficient clinician. *British Journal of Anaesthesia, 121*(6), 1370–1373. DOI: 10.1016/j.bja.2018.07.023 PMID: 30442268

Timmers, T., Janssen, L., Kool, R. B., & Kremer, J. A. (2020). Educating patients by providing timely information using smartphone and tablet Apps: Systematic review. *Journal of Medical Internet Research, 22*(4), e17342. DOI: 10.2196/17342 PMID: 32281936

Tranchard, F., Gauthier, J., Hein, C., Lacombe, J., Brett, K., Villars, H., Sallerin, B., Montastruc, J.-L., & Despas, F. (2019). Drug identification by the patient: Perception of patients, physicians and pharmacists. *Thérapie, 74*(6), 591–598. DOI: 10.1016/j.therap.2019.03.003 PMID: 31014975

Travasso, C. (2016). India draws a red line under antibiotic misuse. *BMJ (Clinical Research Ed.), 352*, i1202. DOI: 10.1136/bmj.i1202 PMID: 26926703

Trbovich, P., & Hyland, S. (2017). Responding to the challenge of look-alike, sound-alike drug names. *BMJ Quality & Safety, 26*(5), 357-359. https://qualitysafety.bmj.com/content/26/5/357

Treejan, K., Jinatongthai, P., Moolasarn, S., Low, B. Y., Anderson, C., & Supapaan, T. (2022). Self-health care behaviors and knowledge of youth living with HIV. *J Am Pharm Assoc (*2003), 62(4), 1249-1259.e1247. DOI: 10.1016/j.japh.2022.02.006

Tseng, H. Y., Wen, C. F., Lee, Y. L., Jeng, K. C., & Chen, P. L. (2018). Dispensing errors from look-alike drug trade names. *European Journal of Hospital Pharmacy : Science and Practice, 25*(2), 96–99. DOI: 10.1136/ejhpharm-2016-001019 PMID: 31156995

Tu, C.-M., Taylor, K., & Chai, G. (2012). Use of proprietary names by prescribers for discontinued brand drug products with existing generic equivalents. *Drug Information Journal, 46*(6), 677–682. DOI: 10.1177/0092861512456282

U.S. Centers For Disease Control and Prevention (CDC). (2024). *Vaccine Storage and Handling Toolkit*. Retrieved 10 Feb from https://www.cdc.gov/vaccines/hcp/downloads/storage-handling-toolkit.pdf

U.S. Department of Health and Human Services Food and Drug Administration (FDA), Center for Drug Evaluation and Research (CDER). (2015). *Size, shape, and other physical attributes of generic tablets and capsules*. Retrieved 10 Jan from https://www.fda.gov/files/drugs/published/Size--Shape--and-Other-Physical-Attributes-of-Generic-Tablets-and-Capsules.pdf

U.S. Department of Health and Human Services Food and Drug Administration (FDA). (2005). Use of Color on Pharmaceutical Product Labels, Labeling and Packaging; Public Hearing. *Federal Register, 70*(22), 5687–5689.

U.S. Department of Health and Human Services Food and Drug Administration (FDA). (2014). *Nonproprietary naming of biological products guidance for industry*. Retrieved 15 June from https://www.fda.gov/files/drugs/published/Nonproprietary-Naming-of-Biological-Products-Guidance-for-Industry.pdf

U.S. Department of Health and Human Services Food and Drug Administration (FDA). (2019). *Procedures for handling requests for nonproprietary name suffix review for biological products newly licensed under section* 351*of the PHS Act*. Retrieved 15 June from https://www.fda.gov/media/123894/download

U.S. Department of Health and Human Services Food and Drug Administration (FDA). (2020). *FDA name differentiation project*. Retrieved 06 Aug from https://www.fda.gov/drugs/medication-errors-related-cder-regulated-drug-products/fda-name-differentiation-project

U.S. Department of Health and Human Services Food and Drug Administration (FDA). (2021). *Phonetic and Orthographic Computer Analysis (POCA) Program*. Retrieved 13 June from https://www.fda.gov/drugs/resources-drugs/phonetic-and-orthographic-computer-analysis-poca-program

U.S. Department of Health and Human Services Food and Drug Administration (FDA). (2022a). *Investigational New Drug (IND) Application*. Retrieved 15 June from https://www.fda.gov/drugs/types-applications/investigational-new-drug-ind-application

U.S. Department of Health and Human Services Food and Drug Administration (FDA). (2022b). *New Drug Application (NDA)*. Retrieved 15 June from https://www.fda.gov/drugs/types-applications/new-drug-application-nda

U.S. Department of Health and Human Services Food and Drug Administration (FDA). (2024). *Medication errors related to CDER-regulated drug products*. Retrieved 13 June from https://www.fda.gov/drugs/drug-safety-and-availability/medication-errors-related-cder-regulated-drug-products

U.S. Department of Health and Human Services Food and Drug Administration, Center for Drug Evaluation and Research (CDER). (2016). *Safety considerations for product design to minimize medication errors: guidance for industry*. Retrieved 8 June from https://www.fda.gov/files/drugs/published/Safety-Considerations-for-Product-Design-to-Minimize-Medication-Errors-Guidance-for-Industry.pdf

U.S. Department of Health and Human Services Food and Drug Administration. (1999). *Guidance for industry: container closure systems for packaging human drugs and biologics*. Retrieved 11 July from https://www.fda.gov/media/70788/download

U.S. Department of Health and Human Services Food and Drug Administration. (2015). *Galantamine hydrobromide (marketed as Razadyne, formerly Reminyl) Information*. Retrieved 11 Jan from https://www.fda.gov/drugs/postmarket-drug-safety-information-patients-and-providers/galantamine-hydrobromide-marketed-razadyne-formerly-reminyl-information

U.S. Department of Health and Human Services Food and Drug Administration. (2016). *October - December* 2016 *Report | Potential Signals of Serious Risks/New Safety Information Identified by the FDA Adverse Event Reporting System (FAERS)*. Retrieved 11 Jan from https://www.fda.gov/drugs/fdas-adverse-event-reporting-system-faers/october-december-2016-report-potential-signals-serious-risksnew-safety-information-identified-fda

U.S. Department of Health and Human Services Food and Drug Administration. (2022). *Safety considerations for container labels and carton labeling design to minimize medication errors guidance for industry*. Retrieved 11 July from https://www.fda.gov/media/158522/download

U.S. Department of Health and Human Services Food and Drug Administration. "Center for Drug Evaluation and Research (CDER). (2016). *Safety considerations for product design to minimize medication errors: guidance for industry*. Retrieved 8 June from https://www.fda.gov/files/drugs/published/Safety-Considerations-for-Product-Design-to-Minimize-Medication-Errors-Guidance-for-Industry.pdf

U.S. Department of Health and Human Services Food and Drug Administration. C. f. D. E. a. R. C. (2016). *Safety considerations for product design to minimize medication errors: guidance for industry*. Retrieved 8 June from https://www.fda.gov/files/drugs/published/Safety-Considerations-for-Product-Design-to-Minimize-Medication-Errors-Guidance-for-Industry.pdf

U.S. Food and Drug Administration. (2011). *Guidance for Industry: Substantiation for Dietary Supplement Claims Made Under Section* 403(*r*) (6) *of the Federal Food, Drug, and Cosmetic Act*. Retrieved 17 Jan from https://www.fda.gov/regulatory-information/search-fda-guidance-documents/guidance-industry-substantiation-dietary-supplement-claims-made-under-section-403r-6-federal-food

U.S. Food and Drug Administration. (2013). *Guidance for Industry: Labeling for Human Prescription Drug and Biological Products –Implementing the PLR Content andFormat Requirements*. Retrieved 10 Feb from https://www.fda.gov/media/71836/download

U.S. Food and Drug Administration. (2016). *Questions and Answers: FDA alerts companies to stop the illegal sale of products claiming to treat diabetes*. https://www.fda.gov/consumers/health-fraud-scams/questions-and-answers-fda-alerts-companies-stop-illegal-sale-products-claiming-treat-diabetes

U.S. Food and Drug Administration. (2018). *Illegally sold opioid cessation products*. Retrieved 18 Jan from https://www.fda.gov/consumers/health-fraud-scams/illegally-sold-opioid-cessation-products#:~:text=U4Life%2C%20LLC%20dba%20Mitadone%20%C2%B7%20Mitadone%20Anti%2DOpiate,Product%20name%20linked%20to%20Flickr%20image%20when

U.S. Food and Drug Administration. (2025). *National Drug Code Directory*. Retrieved 31 July from https://www.accessdata.fda.gov/scripts/cder/ndc/index.cfm

U.S. National Library of Medicine. (2025). *RxNorm overview*. https://www.nlm.nih.gov/research/umls/rxnorm/

UK Government. (2012). *The Human Medicines Regulations* 2012 (*SI* 2012/1916). Retrieved 25 Feb from https://www.legislation.gov.uk/uksi/2012/1916/pdfs/uksi_20121916_en.pdf?

United States Pharmacopeia (USP). (2020). *General Chapter <7> Labeling. USP–NF*. Retrieved 22 Aug from https://www.uspnf.com/sites/default/files/usp_pdf/EN/USPNF/revisions/gc-7-ira-20200731.pdf?

US Food and Drug Administration. (US FDA). (2015). *FDA Drug Safety Communication: FDA warns about prescribing and dispensing errors resulting from brand name confusion with antidepressant Brintellix (vortioxetine) and antiplatelet Brilinta (ticagrelor)*. Retrieved 10 Feb from https://www.fda.gov/drugs/drug-safety-and-availability/fda-drug-safety-communication-fda-warns-about-prescribing-and-dispensing-errors-resulting-brand-name

US Food and Drug Administration. (US FDA). (2024). *Utilizing Generic Drug Awareness to Improve Patient Outcomes with Dr. Sarah Ibrahim*. Retrieved 25 July from https://www.fda.gov/drugs/news-events-human-drugs/utilizing-generic-drug-awareness-improve-patient-outcomes-dr-sarah-ibrahim?

Vaismoradi, M., Jordan, S., Vizcaya-Moreno, F., Friedl, I., & Glarcher, M. (2020). PRN medicines optimization and nurse education. *Pharmacy (Basel, Switzerland), 8*(4), 201. Advance online publication. DOI: 10.3390/pharmacy8040201 PMID: 33114731

Valentin, A., Capuzzo, M., Guidet, B., Moreno, R., Metnitz, B., Bauer, P., & Metnitz, P. (2009). Errors in administration of parenteral drugs in intensive care units: Multinational prospective study. *BMJ (Clinical Research Ed.), 338*(mar12 1), b814. DOI: 10.1136/bmj.b814 PMID: 19282436

Veronin, M. (2011). Packaging and labeling of pharmaceutical products obtained from the internet. *Journal of Medical Internet Research, 13*(1), e22. DOI: 10.2196/jmir.1441 PMID: 21324833

Vlietinck, A., Pieters, L., & Apers, S. (2009). Legal requirements for the quality of herbal substances and herbal preparations for the manufacturing of herbal medicinal products in the European union. *Planta Medica, 75*(7), 683–688. DOI: 10.1055/s-0029-1185307 PMID: 19204891

Wahr, J. A., Abernathy, J. H.III, Lazarra, E. H., Keebler, J. R., Wall, M. H., Lynch, I., Wolfe, R., & Cooper, R. L. (2017). Medication safety in the operating room: Literature and expert-based recommendations. *British Journal of Anaesthesia, 118*(1), 32–43. DOI: 10.1093/bja/aew379 PMID: 28039240

Waknine, Y. (2005). *Zyprexa and Zyrtec substitution errors may lead to adverse events, relapse of schizophrenia or bipolar disorder*. Retrieved 14 Jan from https://www.medscape.com/viewarticle/499062?form=fpf

Wang, W., He, Q., Wang, M., Kang, Y., Ji, P., Zhu, S.,…Sun, X. (2022). Associations of Fentanyl, Sufentanil, and Remifentanil With Length of Stay and Mortality Among Mechanically Ventilated Patients: A Registry-Based Cohort Study [Original Research]. *Frontiers in Pharmacology, Volume* 13 - 2022. DOI: 10.3389/fphar.2022.858531

Wang, Y., Du, Y., Zhao, Y., Ren, Y., & Zhang, W. (2017). Automated anesthesia carts reduce drug recording errors in medication administrations - A single center study in the largest tertiary referral hospital in China. *Journal of Clinical Anesthesia, 40*, 11–15. DOI: 10.1016/j.jclinane.2017.03.051 PMID: 28625429

Waterman, A. D., Garbutt, J., Hazel, E., Dunagan, W. C., Levinson, W., Fraser, V. J., & Gallagher, T. H. (2007). The emotional impact of medical errors on practicing physicians in the United States and Canada. *Joint Commission Journal on Quality and Patient Safety, 33*(8), 467–476. DOI: 10.1016/S1553-7250(07)33050-X PMID: 17724943

Weingart, S. N., Toth, M., Sands, D. Z., Aronson, M. D., Davis, R. B., & Phillips, R. S. (2003). Physicians' decisions to override computerized drug alerts in primary care. *Archives of Internal Medicine*, *163*(21), 2625–2631. DOI: 10.1001/archinte.163.21.2625 PMID: 14638563

Weiss, B. D., Brega, A. G., LeBlanc, W. G., Mabachi, N. M., Barnard, J., Albright, K., Cifuentes, M., Brach, C., & West, D. R. (2016). Improving the Effectiveness of Medication Review: Guidance from the Health Literacy Universal Precautions Toolkit. *Journal of the American Board of Family Medicine : JABFM*, *29*(1), 18–23. DOI: 10.3122/jabfm.2016.01.150163 PMID: 26769873

West Virginia University School of Pharmacy. (2021). *Idecabtagene vicleucel (ABECMA®) drug monograph*. Retrieved 29 Dec from https://pharmacy.wvu.edu/media/3385/abecma-monograph.pdf

Westbrook, J. I., Li, L., Woods, A., Badgery-Parker, T., Mumford, V., Merchant, A., Fitzpatrick, E., & Raban, M. Z. (2024). Risk Factors Associated with Medication Administration Errors in Children: A Prospective Direct Observational Study of Pediatric Inpatients. *Drug Safety*, *47*(6), 545–556. DOI: 10.1007/s40264-024-01408-6

Wheeler, A. J., Scahill, S., Hopcroft, D., & Stapleton, H. (2018). Reducing medication errors at transitions of care is everyone's business. *Australian Prescriber*, *41*(3), 73–77. DOI: 10.18773/austprescr.2018.021 PMID: 29922001

Whitney, C. G., Zhou, F., Singleton, J., & Schuchat, A. (2014). Benefits from immunization during the vaccines for children program era - United States, 1994-2013. *MMWR. Morbidity and Mortality Weekly Report*, *63*(16), 352–355. PMID: 24759657

WHO Collaborating Centre for Patient Safety Solutions. (2007). *Look-alike, sound-alike medication names*. Retrieved 9 August from https://cdn.who.int/media/docs/default-source/patient-safety/patient-safety-solutions/ps-solution1-look-alike-sound-alike-medication-names.pdf?sfvrsn=d4fb860b_8

Winfield, A. J., Jessiman, D., Williams, A., & Esakowitz, L. (1990). A study of the causes of non-compliance by patients prescribed eyedrops. *The British Journal of Ophthalmology*, *74*(8), 477–480. DOI: 10.1136/bjo.74.8.477 PMID: 2390523

Wolters Kluwer. (2025). *Medi-Span: drug data for clinical and business decision support*. Retrieved 31 July from https://www.wolterskluwer.com/en/solutions/medi-span

Wongboonnak, P. (2017). Resolving the problems on look-alike sound-alike drugs at the system level. *Thai J Pharm Pract*, *9*(1), 251–258.

Wongboonnak, P. (2018). Look-alike sound-alike drugs situation in Thailand. *HCU Journal of Health Science, 22*, 205–216.

Woods, D., Dekker, S., Cook, R., Johannesen, L., & Sarter, N. (2017). *Behind human error*. CRC Press. DOI: 10.1201/9781315568935

World Health Organization. (1997). *Guidance on INN*. Retrieved 24 Dec from https://www.who.int/medicines/services/inn/innquidance/en/

World Health Organization. (2004). *WHO guidelines on safety monitoring of herbal medicines in pharmacovigilance systems*. Retrieved 18 Jan from https://www.who.int/publications/i/item/9241592214

World Health Organization. (2007). *The importance of pharmacovigilance: safety monitoring of medicinal products*. Retrieved 10 Sep from https://www.who.int/publications/i/item/10665-42493

World Health Organization. (2007). *WHO launches 'Nine patient safety solutions'*. Retrieved 12 Aug from https://www.who.int/news/item/02-05-2007-who-launches-nine-patient-safety-solutions

World Health Organization. (2014). *Reporting and learning systems for medication errors: the role of pharmacovigilance centers*. Retrieved 19 June from https://iris.who.int/bitstream/handle/10665/137036/9789241507943_eng.pdf?sequence=1

World Health Organization. (2014). *Statement regarding interim findings of WHO assessment of deaths of children in Idleb Governorate, Syria*. Retrieved 08 Feb from https://www.who.int/news/item/27-09-2014-statement-regarding-interim-findings-of-who-assessment-of-deaths-of-children-in-idleb-governorate-syria#:~:text=A%20WHO%20assessment%20of%20the,diluent%20for%20Measles%2FRubella%20vaccine

World Health Organization. (2016). *Global manual on surveillance of adverse events following immunization*. Retrieved 10 Feb from https://iris.who.int/server/api/core/bitstreams/12fbc390-517d-4c27-8c4c-8377eac4575d/content

World Health Organization. (2017). *Guidance on the use of International Nonproprietary Names (INNs) for pharmaceutical substances*. Retrieved 16 June from https://cdn.who.int/media/docs/default-source/international-nonproprietary-names-(inn)/who-pharm-s-nom-1570.pdf

World Health Organization. (2017). *Medication without harm*. Retrieved 10 Feb from https://www.who.int/initiatives/medication-without-harm

World Health Organization. (2017a). *Guidance on the use of International Non-proprietary Names (INNs) for pharmaceutical substances*. Retrieved 16 June from https://cdn.who.int/media/docs/default-source/international-nonproprietary-names-(inn)/who-pharm-s-nom-1570.pdf

World Health Organization. (2017b). *Medication without harm*. Retrieved 10 Feb from https://www.who.int/initiatives/medication-without-harm

World Health Organization. (2021). Global patient safety action plan 2021–2030: Towards eliminating avoidable harm in health care. Retrieved 10 Feb from https://iris.who.int/handle/10665/343477.

World Health Organization. (2021). Toward eliminating avoidable harm in health care. *Global patient safety action plan*, 2030.

World Health Organization. (2022). *WHO launches' Nine patient safety solutions'*. Retrieved 2 July from https://www.who.int/news/item/02-05-2007-who-launches-nine-patient-safety-solutions

World Health Organization. (2023). *Medication safety for look-alike, sound-alike medicines*. World Health Organization. Retrieved 3 June from https://iris.who.int/bitstream/handle/10665/373495/9789240058897-eng.pdf?sequence=1

World Health Organization. (2024). *Medication safety: WHO webinar on the Global Patient Safety Challenge Medication Without Harm*. Retrieved 24 July from https://cdn.who.int/media/docs/default-source/integrated-health-services-%28ihs%29/psf/medication-without-harm/medication-safety-who-webinar-7march2024.pdf

World Health Organization. (2024). *Promoting rational use of medicines*. Retrieved 6 Mar from https://www.who.int/activities/promoting-rational-use-of-medicines

World Health Organization. (2024). *Use of stems in the selection of International Nonproprietary Names (INN) for pharmaceutical substances*. World Health Organization. (Original work published 2024)

Wu, A. W. (2000). Medical error: the second victim. *The doctor who makes the mistake needs help too*, 320(7237), 726-727. DOI: 10.1136/bmj.320.7237.726

Yin, H. S., Dreyer, B. P., Moreira, H. A., van Schaick, L., Rodriguez, L., Boettger, S., & Mendelsohn, A. L. (2014). Liquid medication dosing errors in children: Role of provider counseling strategies. *Academic Pediatrics, 14*(3), 262–270. DOI: 10.1016/j.acap.2014.01.003

Yin, H. S., Mendelsohn, A. L., Wolf, M. S., Parker, R. M., Fierman, A., van Schaick, L., Bazan, I. S., Kline, M. D., & Dreyer, B. P. (2010). Parents' medication administration errors: Role of dosing instruments and health literacy. *Archives of Pediatrics & Adolescent Medicine*, *164*(2), 181–186. DOI: 10.1001/archpediatrics.2009.269 PMID: 20124148

Yuliani, S. H., Putri, D. C. A., Virginia, D. M., Gani, M. R., & Riswanto, F. D. O. (2023). Prevalence, risk, and challenges of extemporaneous preparation for pediatric patients in developing nations: A review. *Pharmaceutics*, *15*(3), 840. DOI: 10.3390/pharmaceutics15030840

Zafar, R., & Raza, M. L. (2020). Assessment of look-alike, sound-alike and read-alike (LASARA) medicine-errors in pharmacy. *Journal of the College of Physicians and Surgeons—Pakistan : JCPSP*, *30*(4), 425–428. DOI: 10.29271/jcpsp.2020.04.425 PMID: 32513366

About the Author

Teeraporn Sadira Supapaan received her PhD from the School of Pharmacy, University of Nottingham, United Kingdom, through a scholarship from the Royal Thai Government. She is currently an Associate Professor in the Division of Pharmacy Practice at the Faculty of Pharmaceutical Sciences, Ubon Ratchathani University, Thailand. Her academic experience spans more than two decades, with research interests in pharmacy practice, medication safety, pharmaceutical education, and rational drug use. She has authored several peer-reviewed publications in internationally recognized journals and has engaged in collaborative research at both national and international levels, particularly in the area of Look-Alike Sound-Alike (LASA) medication errors. She has also played a role in developing national drug identification databases to support patient safety initiatives in Thailand.

Index

A

B

C

D

E

I

L

M

N

O

P

R

S

T

U

V

www.ingramcontent.com/pod-product-compliance
Lightning Source LLC
LaVergne TN
LVHW062211200926
848484LV00006B/1369